Herbert J. Buchsbaum, M.D. Professor of Obstetrics and Gynecology
Director, Division of Gynecologic Oncology
University of Texas-Southwestern
Medical School
Dallas, Texas

Joseph D. Schmidt, M.D. Professor of Surgery/Urology
Head, Division of Urology
School of Medicine
University of California
San Diego, California

Second Edition

GYNECOLOGIC *and* OBSTETRIC UROLOGY

1982

W. B. Saunders Company
Philadelphia London Toronto Mexico City Rio de Janeiro Sydney Tokyo

W. B. Saunders Company: West Washington Square
Philadelphia, PA 19105

1 St. Anne's Road
Eastbourne, East Sussex BN21 3UN, England

1 Goldthorne Avenue
Toronto, Ontario M8Z 5T9, Canada

Apartado 26370—Cedro 512
Mexico 4, D.F., Mexico

Rua Coronel Cabrita, 8
Sao Cristovao Caixa Postal 21176
Rio de Janeiro, Brazil

9 Waltham Street
Artarmon, N.S.W. 2064, Australia

Ichibancho, Central Bldg., 22-1 Ichibancho
Chiyoda-Ku, Tokyo 102, Japan

Library of Congress Cataloging in Publication Data

Main entry under title:

Gynecologic and obstetric urology.

1. Urinary organs—Diseases. 2. Urinary organs—Surgery. 3.Generative organs, Female—Diseases. 4. Gynecology, Operative. 5. Pregnancy, Complications of. I. Buchsbaum, Herbert J. II. Schmidt, Joseph D. [DNLM: 1. Genital diseases, Female. 2. Obstetrics. 3. Urologic diseases WJ 190 G977]

RG484.G96 1982 616.6 81–40560
ISBN 0–7216–2173–2 AACR2

Gynecologic and Obstetric Urology ISBN 0-7216-2173-2

Last digit is the print number: 9 8 7 6 5 4 3 2 1

CONTRIBUTORS

MARGARET B. AYDELOTTE, Ph.D.
Assistant Professor of Biochemistry, Rush Medical College, Rush-Presbyterian-St. Luke's Medical Center, Chicago, Illinois
Developmental Anatomy

R. PETER BECK, M.D.C.M., F.R.C.O.G., F.A.C.O.G., F.R.C.S.(C)
Professor of Obstetrics and Gynaecology, University of Alberta and University Hospital, Edmonton, Alberta, Canada
The Sling Operation

ALVIN L. BREKKEN, M.D.
Associate Professor, University of Texas Health Science Center; Program Director, Obstetrics/Gynecology, St. Paul Hospital, Dallas, Texas
Age-Specific Urinary Problems: Adolescent/Sexually Active

WILLIAM A. BROCK, M.D., F.A.A.P.
Associate Clinical Professor of Surgery/Urology, School of Medicine, University of California, San Diego; Attending Staff, University Hospital, and Senior Staff, Children's Hospital and Health Center, San Diego, California
Age-Specific Urinary Problems: Pediatric

HERBERT J. BUCHSBAUM, M.D.
Professor of Obstetrics and Gynecology and Director, Division of Gynecologic Oncology, University of Texas-Southwestern Medical School, Dallas, Texas
Office and Gynecologic Surgery; The Urinary Tract and Radical Hysterectomy; Urinary Diversion in Pelvic Exenteration; Urinary Tract Involvement by Benign and Malignant Gynecologic Disease; Clinical and Operative Obstetrics; Radiation Cystitis, Fistulas, and Fibrosis

FREDERICK KEITH CHAPLER, M.D.
Professor, Obstetrics and Gynecology; Director, Division of Reproductive Endocrinology, University of Iowa College of Medicine; Attending Staff, University of Iowa Hospital, Iowa City, Iowa
Clinical Aspects of Genital and Urinary Tract Anomalies

ROBERT C. CORLETT, M.D.
Assistant Clinical Professor, Department of Obstetrics and Gynecology, Los Angeles County–University of Southern California Medical Center, Los Angeles; Staff, Goleta Valley Community Hospital, Santa Barbara, California
Age-Specific Urinary Problems: Postmenopausal

DAVID A. CULP, M.D.
Professor and Head, Department of Urology, University of Iowa College of Medicine; Attending Urologist, University of Iowa Hospitals and Clinics, Iowa City, Iowa
The Urologic Examination; Incontinence Secondary to Neurogenic Bladder, Anatomic Defects and Urgency

F. GARY CUNNINGHAM, M.D.
Professor of Obstetrics and Gynecology, University of Texas Health Sciences Center, Southwestern Medical School; Chief of Obstetrics, Parkland Memorial Hospital; Consultant in Maternal-Fetal Medicine, St. Paul Hospital, Methodist Hospital, and Presbyterian Medical Center, Dallas, Texas
Asymptomatic Bacteriuria During Pregnancy

ANANIAS C. DIOKNO, M.D.
Associate Professor of Surgery, University of Michigan Medical Center; Staff Urologist, University Hospital, Ann Arbor, Michigan
Physiology of Micturition

E. S. DONALDSON, M.D.
Associate Professor, Division of Gynecologic Oncology, University of Kentucky School of Medicine; Associate Director, Gynecologic Oncology, University of Kentucky Medical Center, Lexington, Kentucky
Invasive Cervical Carcinoma

BRUCE H. DRUKKER, M.D.
Clinical Professor of Obstetrics and Gynecology, University of Michigan Medical School, Ann Arbor; Chairman, Department of Gynecology-Obstetrics, Henry Ford Hospital, and Head, Division of Gynecologic Oncology, Henry Ford Hospital, Detroit, Michigan
Anterior Colporrhaphy

BERNARD FALLON, M.D.
Associate Professor, Department of Urology, University of Iowa College of Medicine; University of Iowa Hospitals and Clinics, Iowa City, Iowa
The Urologic Examination

E. C. GAY
Research Associate, Division of Gynecologic Oncology, University of Kentucky School of Medicine, Lexington, Kentucky
Invasive Cervical Carcinoma

LARRY C. GILSTRAP III, M.D., Lt.Col. USAF MC
Chief Obstetrical Service, Department of Obstetrics and Gynecology, Wilford Hall USAF Medical Center, Lackland Air Force Base; Clinical Assistant Professor, Department of Obstetrics and Gynecology, University of Texas Health Science Center at San Antonio, Texas
Urinary Infections, Including Pyelonephritis

THOMAS H. GREEN, Jr., M.D.
Late Associate Clinical Professor of Gynecology, Harvard Medical School, Boston; Late Gynecologist, Senior Staff, Deaconess Hospital, Boston, and Chief of Gynecology, Massachusetts State Cancer Hospital, Pondville, Massachusetts
Urinary Stress Incontinence: Historical Review, Pathophysiology, and Classification

LAURENCE F. GREENE, M.D., Ph.D.
Anson L. Clark Professor of Urology, Emeritus, Mayo Medical School, Rochester, Minnesota; Clinical Professor of Surgery/Urology, University of California, San Diego, School of Medicine; Consultant in Urology, Veterans Administration Medical Center, San Diego, California
Diseases of the Urethra

C. E. HAWTREY, M.D.
Professor of Urology, University of Iowa College of Medicine; Staff Urologist, University Hospitals; Urologic Consultant, Iowa City Veterans Administration Hospital, Iowa City, Iowa
Surgical Anatomy

E. C. JACOBO, M.D.
Assistant Clinical Professor of Urology, University of Iowa School of Medicine; Staff Urologist, Schoitz Memorial Hospital, and St. Francis Hospital, Waterloo, Iowa
Diseases of the Urethra

GEORGE W. KAPLAN, M.D., M.S., F.A.A.P., and F.A.C.S.
Clinical Professor of Surgery/Urology and Chief, Pediatric Urology, University of California, San Diego, School of Medicine; Attending Staff, University Hospital, and Senior Staff, Children's Hospital, San Diego, California
Age-Specific Urinary Problems: Pediatric

WILLIAM C. KEETTEL, M.D.
Late Professor Emeritus, Department of Obstetrics and Gynecology, University of Iowa College of Medicine, Iowa City, Iowa
Vaginal Repair of Vesicovaginal and Urethrovaginal Fistulas

SUSHIL S. LACY, M.D., F.A.C.S.
Clinical Associate Professor of Urology, The University of Nebraska College of Medicine; Attending Staff, Bryan Memorial Hospital, St. Elizabeth Community Hospital, and Lincoln General Hospital, Lincoln; Consulting Staff, University of Nebraska Hospital and Omaha Veterans Administration Hospital, Omaha, Nebraska
Urinary Tract Infections

JACK LAPIDES, M.D., M.A.
Professor of Surgery, University of Michigan Medical School; Head, Section of Urology, University of Michigan Medical School, and Hospital, Ann Arbor, Michigan
Physiology of Micturition

DOUGLAS W. LAUBE, M.D.
Assistant Professor, Department of Obstetrics and Gynecology, University of Iowa College of Medicine; University of Iowa Hospitals and Clinics, Iowa City, Iowa
Vaginal Repair of Vesicovaginal and Urethrovaginal Fistulas

T. B. LEBHERZ, M.D., F.A.C.O.G.
Professor of Obstetrics and Gynecology, University of California at Los Angeles; Health Science Center, University of California at Los Angeles Medical School, Los Angeles, California
The Modified Pereyra Procedure

RAYMOND A. LEE, M.D.
Professor of Obstetrics and Gynecology, Mayo Medical School; Consultant, Division of Gynecologic Surgery, Mayo Clinic and Mayo Foundation; St. Marys Hospital and Rochester Methodist Hospital, Rochester, Minnesota
The Modified Marshall-Marchetti-Krantz Operation as a Primary Procedure in Urinary Stress Incontinence; Surgical Procedures for Recurrent Stress Incontinence

SAMUEL LIFSHITZ, M.D., F.A.C.O.G., F.A.C.S.
Associate Professor of Obstetrics and Gynecology, University of Texas Southwestern Medical School at Dallas; Attending Staff, Parkland Memorial Hospital, St. Paul Hospital, Presbyterian Hospital, and Baylor University Medical Center, Dallas, Texas
Urinary Tract Involvement by Benign and Malignant Gynecologic Disease

S. A. H. LOENING, M.D.
Associate Professor of Urology, University of Iowa College of Medicine; Attending Urologist, University of Iowa Hospitals and Clinics, Iowa City, Iowa
Incontinence Secondary to Neurogenic Bladder, Anatomic Defects, and Urgency

THOMAS A. McCARTHY, M.D.
Assistant Professor, Department of Obstetrics and Gynecology, University of California at Los Angeles School of Medicine; Harbor/UCLA Medical Center, Los Angeles, California
Office Cystourethroscopy

DANIEL A. NACHTSHEIM, M.D., F.A.C.S.
Assistant Clinical Professor of Surgery/Urology, University of California, San Diego, School of Medicine; Staff Physician, Veterans Administration Medical Center, San Diego, California
Endoscopically Controlled Urethropexy

JOHN B. NANNINGA, M.D.
Associate Professor of Urology, Northwestern University Medical School; Associate Attending Urologist, Northwestern Memorial Hospital, Chicago, Illinois
Suprapubic Transvesical Closure of Vesicovaginal Fistula

VINCENT J. O'CONOR, Jr., M.D.
Professor of Urology, Northwestern University Medical School; Chief of Urology, Northwestern Memorial Hospital, Chicago, Illinois
Suprapubic Transvesical Closure of Vesicovaginal Fistula

DONALD R. OSTERGARD, M.D.
Professor of Gynecology, University of California, Irvine, California College of Medicine, Irvine; Associate Medical Director for Gynecology and Chief, Division of Gynecologic Urology, Women's Hospital and Memorial Hospital Medical Center of Long Beach, Long Beach, California
Office Cystourethroscopy

C. LOWELL PARSONS, M.D.
Associate Professor of Surgery/Urology, University of California, San Diego, School of Medicine; Chief, Urology Section, Veterans Administration Medical Center, San Diego, California
Urinary Tract Infections

ARMAND J. PEREYRA, M.D. F.A.C.S., F.A.C.O.G.
Clinical Professor, Obstetrics and Gynecology, University of California at Los Angeles; Consultant, Gynecologic Urology, Harbor General Hospital, Los Angeles, and San Bernardino County Hospital, San Bernardino, California
The Modified Pereyra Procedure

PAUL C. PETERS, M.D.
Professor and Chairman, Division of Urology, The University of Texas Health Science Center at Dallas; Chief of Urology, Parkland Memorial Hospital; Chief, Urologic Services, Children's Medical Center; Consultant in Urology, Veterans Administration Hospital, Baylor University Medical Center, Dallas, and John Peter Smith Hospital, Fort Worth, Texas
Postoperative Bladder Drainage

ROY M. PITKIN, M.D.
Professor and Chairman, Department of Obstetrics and Gynecology, The University of Iowa; Chief of Obstetrics and Gynecology, The University of Iowa Hospitals and Clinics, Iowa City, Iowa
Morphologic Changes in Pregnancy

CHARLES E. PLATZ, M.D.
Professor, Department of Pathology, University of Iowa College of Medicine; University of Iowa Hospitals and Clinics, Iowa City, Iowa
Radiation Cystitis, Fistula, and Fibrosis

SHLOMO RAZ, M.D.
Associate Professor of Surgery/Urology, University of California at Los Angeles School of Medicine, Los Angeles; Co-Chief of Urology, Veterans Administration Medical Center, Sepulveda, California
Urodynamics; Urodynamic Evaluation

EUAN G. ROBERTSON, M.D., F.A.C.O.G., F.R.C.O.G.
Professor of Obstetrics and Gynecology, and Director, Perinatal Metabolic Unit, University of Miami School of Medicine; Attending Obstetrician-Gynecologist, University of Miami and Jackson Memorial Hospitals, Miami, Florida
Alterations in Renal Function During Pregnancy; Renal Changes in Toxemia

RIGOBERTO SANTOS-RAMOS, M.D., F.A.C.O.G.
Associate Professor, Obstetrics and Gynecology, Division of Maternal-Fetal Medicine, University of Texas Southwestern Medical School at Dallas; Teaching and Faculty, Parkland Memorial Hospital; Consulting Staff, St. Paul Hospital and Presbyterian Hospital, Dallas, Texas
Ultrasound in Intrauterine Diagnosis

JOSEPH D. SCHMIDT, M.D.
Professor of Surgery/Urology and Head, Division of Urology, University of California, San Diego, School of Medicine; Consultant, Urology Section, Veterans Administration Medical Center; Consultant Urologist, Naval Regional Medical Center; Consulting Staff, Department of Surgery (Urology), Mercy Hospital and Medical Center, San Diego, California
Management of Urinary Tract Injuries; Urinary Diversion in Pelvic Exenteration; Radiation Cystitis, Fistula, and Fibrosis; Urinary Calculi in Pregnancy

JAMES R. SCOTT, M.D.
Professor and Chairman, Department of Obstetrics and Gynecology, University of Utah School of Medicine; Chairman, Department of Obstetrics and Gynecology, University of Utah Medical Center, Salt Lake City, Utah
Gynecologic and Obstetric Problems in Renal Allograft Patients

J. R. van NAGELL, Jr., M.D.
Professor and Director, Gynecologic Oncology, University of Kentucky School of Medicine; Director of Gynecologic Oncology, University of Kentucky Medical Center; American Cancer Society Professor of Clinical Oncology, University of Kentucky Medical Center, Lexington, Kentucky
Invasive Cervical Carcinoma

PEGGY J. WHALLEY, M.D.
Jack A. Pritchard Professor of Obstetrics, University of Texas Southwestern Medical School at Dallas; Parkland Memorial Hospital, St. Paul Hospital, and Presbyterian Hospital, Dallas, Texas
Asymptomatic Bacteriuria During Pregnancy

A. J. WHITE, M.D.
Clinical Assistant Professor, Department of Obstetrics and Gynecology, University of Texas Health Science Center, San Antonio, Texas
Radiation Cystitis, Fistula, and Fibrosis

PREFACE

In preparing the second edition of *Gynecologic and Obstetric Urology,* we have expanded the text from 28 to 38 chapters. The reader will find new chapters reflecting technologic advances, including urodynamics and ultrasonography, and extended descriptions of surgical procedures such as endoscopically controlled urethropexy for the relief of stress incontinence and transvesical repair of vesicovaginal fistulas. A new three-section chapter addresses the age-specific and sometimes unique urinary problems of the child, the adolescent, and the postmenopausal woman. Another new chapter deals with office cystourethroscopy utilizing carbon dioxide, a technique finding increased popularity with gynecologists.

It is not our intent to take sides on issues of territoriality, such as the current controversies over endoscopy in the female patient or the entire subject of female urology. Rather, we wish to present to the interested reader all techniques currently available for diagnosis and treatment in the female patient. We have again tried to avoid overlap and duplication, but have not hesitated to present divergent surgical solutions to gynecologic and obstetric problems, as presented by authors from the disciplines of gynecology and urology.

We wish to express our thanks for the continued effort and devotion of our editorial assistants, Bette Jo Garrett (San Diego) and Joyce Perry (Dallas), as well as for the support of Carroll Cann, Medical Editor at W. B. Saunders Company.

Lastly, it is with deep regret that we acknowledge the death of two contributors, Drs. William C. Keettel and Thomas H. Green, Jr.

HERBERT J. BUCHSBAUM
JOSEPH D. SCHMIDT

CONTENTS

SECTION

1

ANATOMY, PHYSIOLOGY AND EXAMINATION

1

DEVELOPMENTAL ANATOMY

MARGARET B. AYDELOTTE, Ph.D.

During embryonic development there is a close association between the urinary and genital systems, especially in the early stages. Both systems develop largely from the urogenital ridges, bilateral thickenings of intermediate mesoderm with overlying coelomic epithelium, which lie along the dorsal wall of the abdominal cavity. In the male the close connection between the two systems is retained in the adult, but in the female this early association is lost with the development of separate müllerian (paramesonephric) ducts, which give rise to the uterus, fallopian tubes, and part of the vagina. Although the urinary and genital systems are closely linked in development, it is easier to describe their formation separately, after first reviewing some aspects of early embryology.

EARLY DEVELOPMENT

Two weeks after fertilization, the implanted human embryo consists of a flat disc with two layers of cells, a columnar ectoderm forming the floor of the amniotic cavity, and a layer of flattened endodermal cells constituting the roof of the yolk sac (Figure 1–1). Both layers of the embryonic disc are continuous at their edges with tissue that will form the extraembryonic membranes.

The third germ layer, the mesoderm, from which the urogenital system largely develops, begins to segregate during the early part of the third week of development (Figure 1–2). Cells of the primitive streak (i.e., in the midline at the future caudal end of the embryo) leave the upper ectodermal layer, sink below the surface, and migrate laterally, spreading out between the ectoderm and endoderm to form the embryonic mesoderm, the middle layer of the trilaminar embryonic disc. At two sites in the midline of the embryo, this mesoderm fails to separate the ectoderm from the adhering, underlying endoderm. One of these two remaining bilaminar regions is found cranial to the developing notochord, and is destined to become the oropharyngeal (or buccopharyngeal) membrane; the other region lacking mesoderm lies caudal to the primitive streak, and will form the cloacal membrane (Figure 1–2). Mesodermal cells continue to migrate around the edges of both of these membranes to meet in the midline. That mesoderm which comes to lie lateral to the cloacal membrane contributes to the external genitalia, and that which migrates to the midline, initially caudal to the cloacal membrane, helps to form the phallus and the infraumbilical part of the body wall (Patten and Barry, 1952).

The intraembryonic mesoderm differentiates as shown in Figure 1–3. On each side of the developing notochord and neural tube the paraxial mesoderm forms segmentally arranged blocks of tissue, the somites. The columns of intermediate mesoderm adjacent to the somites show segmentation only at the cranial end of the embryo. Lateral to the intermediate mesoderm, the coelomic cavity forms as the lateral plate mesoderm splits into the outer somatic and inner splanchnic layers. Both the inter-

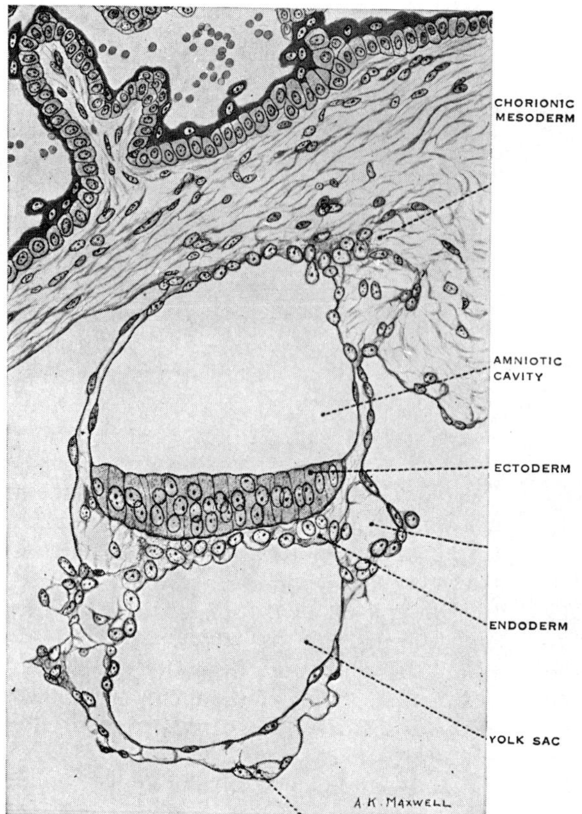

Figure 1–1. Transverse section through the anterior part of the bilaminar embryonic disc and chorionic vesicle of a 15-day-old human embryo. (From Hamilton, W. J., and Mossman, H. W.: Human Embryology. 4th Ed. © 1972 The Williams & Wilkins Co., Baltimore.)

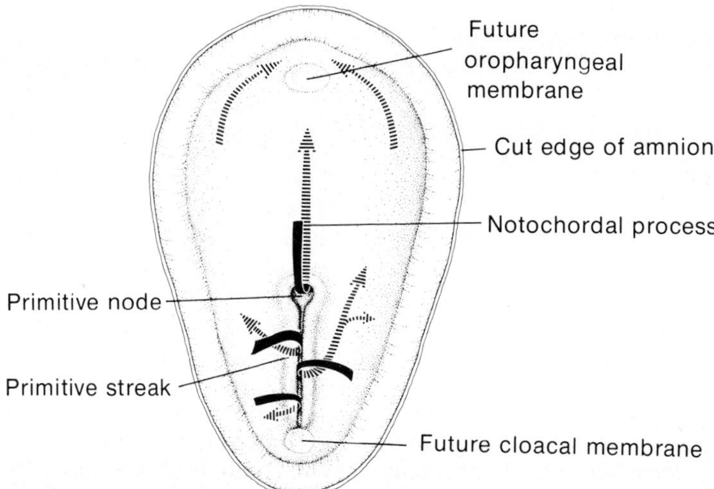

Figure 1–2. Dorsal side of the embryonic disc during the third week, indicating movement of superficial cells (solid black lines) towards the primitive streak and node, and subsequent migration of mesodermal cells (broken lines) away from the primitive streak between the ectodermal and endodermal germ layers. (From Langman, J.: Medical Embryology. 4th Ed., © 1981 The Williams & Wilkins Co., Baltimore.)

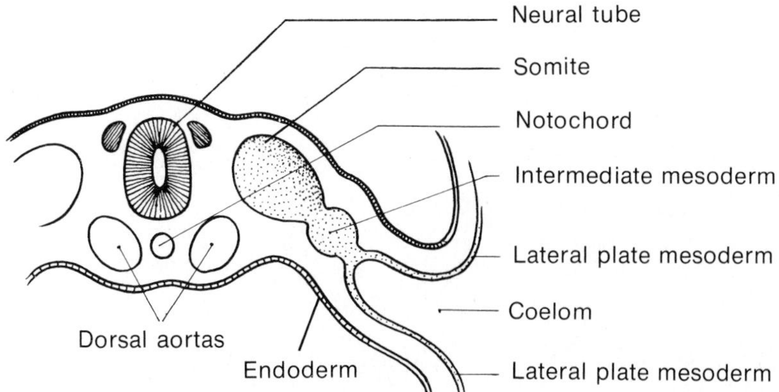

Figure 1–3. Diagrammatic cross-section of a 3-week embryo, showing development of the mesoderm. (From Tuchmann-Duplessis, H., David, G., and Haegel, P.: Illustrated Human Embryology. Vol. 1, 1972. Courtesy Springer-Verlag, New York, and Masson, Editeurs, Paris.)

mediate mesoderm and a portion of the coelomic lining, the superficial layer of lateral plate mesoderm, contribute to the urogenital system.

DEVELOPMENT OF THE URINARY SYSTEM

The Kidney and Ureter

Below the mesothelium along the dorsal wall of the coelomic cavity, the intermediate mesoderm on each side of the embryo forms a longitudinal ridge, the nephrogenic cord. Each nephrogenic cord shows a craniocaudal sequence in its development. The most cranial portion differentiates before the more caudal regions, and according to the classic view, the ridge gives rise successively to three kidneys: the pronephros, the mesonephros, and the metanephros, or definitive kidney (Figure 1–4). The first two are not completely distinct in the human being, the caudal end of the pronephros merging with the cranial end of the mesonephros. There is probably little reason to regard them as separate entities, but for convenience their names are retained (Potter, 1972).

Pronephros

The pronephros is a transitory, nonfunctional structure in the human being. It consists of a few nephrotomes, small clumps of cells or vesicles which begin to form late in the third week of development from the cervical segmented intermediate mesoderm. These vesicles or tubules have no glomeruli, do not connect with the pronephric duct, and regress by the end of the fourth week. The pronephric duct is independent in origin from the pronephric vesicles (Torrey, 1954), and first appears as a solid cord of cells in the dorsal part of the nephrogenic cord. The duct acquires a lumen progressively from its cranial end, and gradually grows in a caudal and then a ventral direction. It opens into the dorsolateral part of the cloaca early in the fifth week of development (Figure 1–4).

Mesonephros

As the pronephros regresses, the nephrogenic cord in the thoracic and lumbar regions gives rise to tubules of the mesonephros. These tubules become S-shaped and open laterally into the adjacent portion of the pronephric duct, called at this point in development the mesonephric (or wolffian) duct. The medial end of each mesonephric tubule enlarges and invaginates to form a Bowman's capsule in association with a developing knot of capillaries, the glomerulus (Figure 1–5*A*). The S-shaped mesonephric tubule lengthens rapidly and becomes highly coiled, but no loop of Henle develops. Since the most cranial

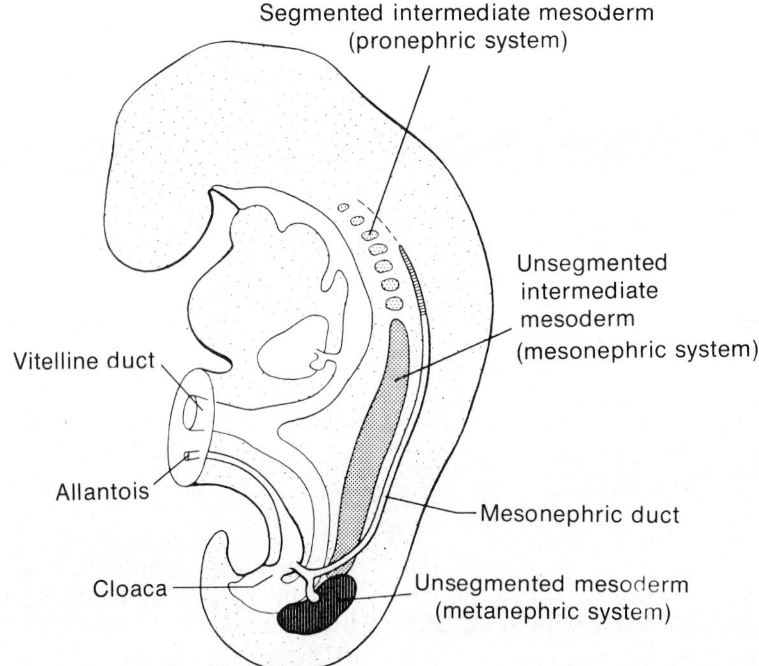

Figure 1–4. Relative positions of the pronephros, mesonephros and metanephros and associated mesonephric duct. (From Langman, J.: Medical Embryology. 4th Ed. © 1981 The Williams & Wilkins Co., Baltimore.)

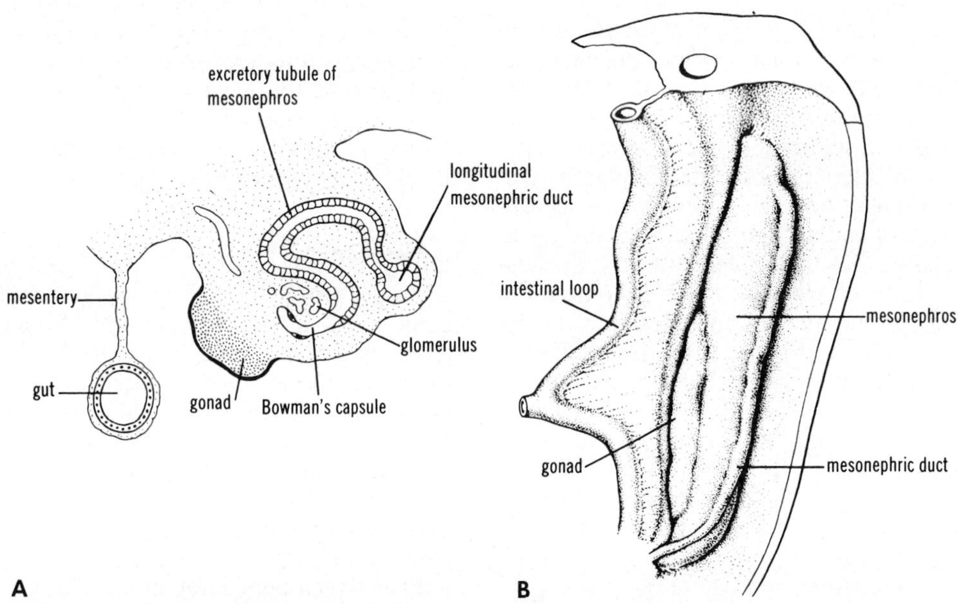

Figure 1–5. *A,* Transverse section through the lower thoracic region of a 5-week embryo, showing a mesonephric excretory tubule. Note the Bowman's capsule and developing glomerulus at the medial end of the tubule and the opening laterally to the mesonephric duct. The gonad is beginning to form on the medial side of the mesonephros.

B, The relationship between the left mesonephros and developing gonad. (From Langman, J.: Medical Embryology. 4th Ed. © 1981 The Williams & Wilkins Co., Baltimore.)

mesonephric tubules degenerate before the more caudal ones differentiate, the full extent of the mesonephros cannot be appreciated by examining only one stage. At its peak of development, towards the end of the second month, the mesonephros forms a prominent oval swelling on each side of the dorsal mesentery, suspended from the abdominal wall by a thick mesonephric mesentery (Figure 1–5*B*).

Structural differences have been observed between the functional units of the mesonephros and metanephros: (1) the epithelium of distal tubules, (2) the absence of the loops of Henle from the mesonephric nephrons, and (3) the arrangement of glomerular arterioles (de Martino and Zamboni, 1966). However, because of clear similarities between the nephrons of the meso- and metanephroi, notably in the structure of the Bowman's capsules and proximal tubules, it is likely that during the third and fourth months of fetal life the mesonephros excretes small quantities of dilute urine (Leeson, 1957; de Martino and Zamboni, 1966). With its gradual recession the mesonephros is nonfunctional by the end of the fourth month, and the definitive kidney has progressively taken over the role of urine production. The mesonephric glomeruli all disappear, but a few tubules that fail to degenerate at this stage in the female remain associated with the ovaries as vestigial structures, the epoophoron and paroophoron (see p. 15).

Metanephros

The permanent kidney or metanephros has a dual origin: the metanephric blastema gives rise to the nephrons, or excretory units of the kidney, while the ureteric bud forms the system of collecting ducts, calyces, pelvis of the kidney, and the ureter. Renal agenesis can, therefore, result from failure of normal development or normal interactions of these two primordia (Davidson and Ross, 1954; Magee et al., 1979). During the fifth week of development, the ureteric bud develops as a hollow outgrowth from the caudal end of each mesonephric duct, close to its opening into the cloaca (Figure 1–6). The bud grows dorsocranially, its tip pushing into the most caudal portion of the nephrogenic cord in the lower lumbar and sacral segments. This part of the nephrogenic cord then condenses to form a cap of tissue, the metanephric blastema, around the tip of the ureteric bud.

Mutual inductive influences have been demonstrated between these two components: a specific stimulus from the metanephric blastema induces the ureteric bud to enlarge, form an ampulla, and undergo a series of dichotomous branchings, while differentiation of normal nephrons from the nephrogenic blastema occurs only in response to an inductive stimulus from the ampullae of the ureteric bud (Grobstein, 1955; Potter, 1972). Experimental studies in

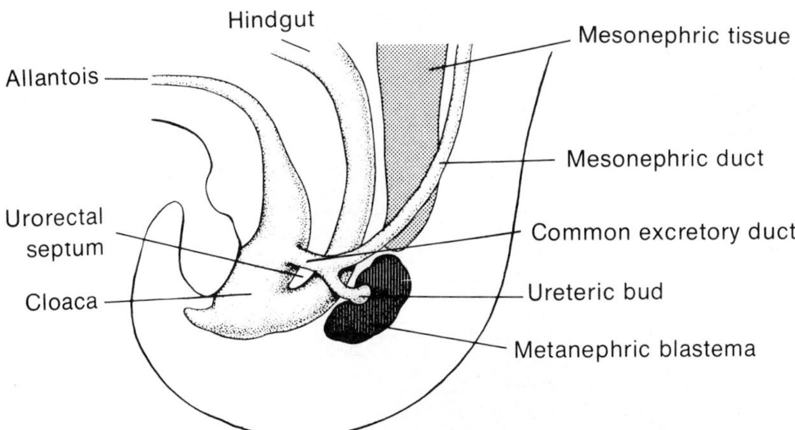

Figure 1–6. Caudal end of a 5-week embryo, showing the relationship between the mesonephric duct, its outgrowth, the ureteric bud, and the cloaca. Note that the urorectal septum is beginning to divide the cloaca. (From Langman, J.: Medical Embryology. 4th Ed. © 1981 The Williams & Wilkins Co., Baltimore.)

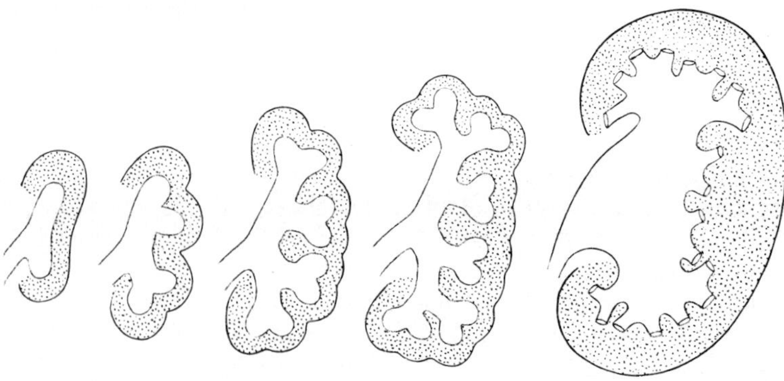

Figure 1–7. The early divisions of the ureteric bud to form the pelvis and major and minor calyces of the kidney. (From Hamilton, W. J., and Mossman, H. W.: Human Embryology. 4th Ed. © 1972 The Williams & Wilkins Co., Baltimore.)

the mouse indicate that differentiation of the specific segments of the nephron is programmed during an initial brief period of induction; close contact between the interacting tissues and formation of a glycoprotein are necessary during this induction (Ekblom et al., 1979 *a, b*; Ekblom et al., 1980).

Following each division of the ureteric bud, new ampullae form at the tips of the branches; these are surrounded by tissue of the metanephric blastema. The first division is symmetrical and produces a cranial and a caudal branch, but thereafter division is both asymmetrical and asynchronous. It proceeds more rapidly cranially and caudal-

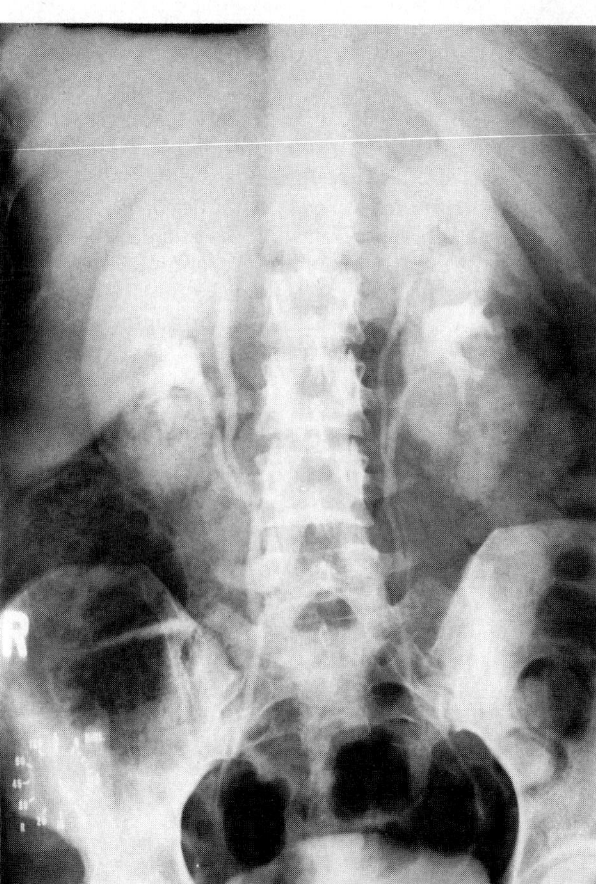

Figure 1–8. Intravenous pyelogram showing duplication of both ureters.

ly at the future poles of the kidney than in the developing interpolar region, so that the characteristic kidney shape develops rapidly (Figure 1–7). Towards the end of the third month, the renal pelvis has formed by dilatation of the first five polar and three to four interpolar branches of the ureteric bud (Osathanondh and Potter, 1963). The next generations of branches become only slightly dilated to form the major and minor calyces, and successive branches give rise to generations of collecting ducts. The lengthening unbranched part of the ureteric bud is the metanephric duct, which forms the ureter, linking the future pelvis of the kidney with that region of the cloaca that develops into the urinary bladder. Premature division of the ureteric bud results in doubling of the ureters on that side. These double ureters may be associated with one kidney, or if the division includes the metanephric blastema, both the ureter and kidney are duplicated (Figure 1–8).

Induction of Nephrons. Only that tissue of the metanephric blastema which surrounds the ampullae differentiates into nephrons, while the remaining tissue around the interstitial portions of branches of the ureteric bud forms the renal connective tissue (Potter, 1972). The first nephrons and their glomeruli develop in what will become the juxtamedullary region, and later nephrons form progressively further from the future hilum of the kidney. During the early stages of nephron formation, beginning about the seventh week, each ampulla divides, then one branch induces the formation of a nephron while the other branch divides again, and the process is repeated many times. When the ampullae have ceased to divide, nephron arcades form (from the fourteenth to the twenty-second week), each ampulla inducing the formation of several nephrons all attached to one another by connecting tubules and sharing a common junction with the collecting duct (Figure 1–9) (Osathanondh and Potter, 1963). In the last period of nephron induction, from the twentieth to the thirty-sixth week, each ampulla continues to advance cortically, beyond the point of attachment of the arcade, and induces from four to seven nephrons in the peripheral part of the cortex, each one being attached separately to the collecting duct (Figure 1–9).

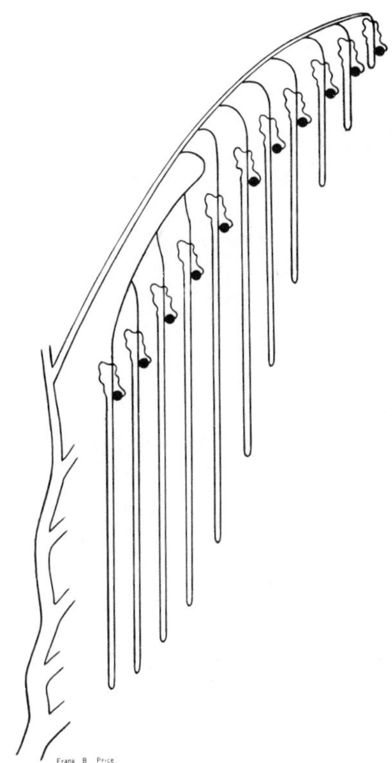

Figure 1–9. Arrangement of nephrons at the time of birth. (From Hamilton, W. J., and Mossman, H. W.: Human Embryology. 4th Ed. © 1972 The Williams & Wilkins Co., Baltimore.)

Differentiation of Nephrons. Differentiation of nephrons at first resembles the development of mesonephric tubules: a hollow, pear-shaped vesicle forms, this lengthens to an S-shaped tube (Figure 1–10*A*), and a glomerulus develops in association with the end farthest from the ampulla. As the tubule continues to lengthen it becomes convoluted; then, unlike the mesonephric tubule, a loop of Henle also develops (Figure 1–10*B*). The lumen of the nephron becomes confluent with that of the adjacent developing collecting duct derived from the ampulla. Failure to establish continuity between the nephron and collecting duct — tubules of different origins — was for a long time regarded as the cause of congenital polycystic kidney. However, more recent microdissection studies of polycystic kidneys suggest that failure of union is not the cause of cyst formation (Osathanondh and Potter, 1964). Cysts apparently develop when collecting tubules become secondarily enlarged, when neph-

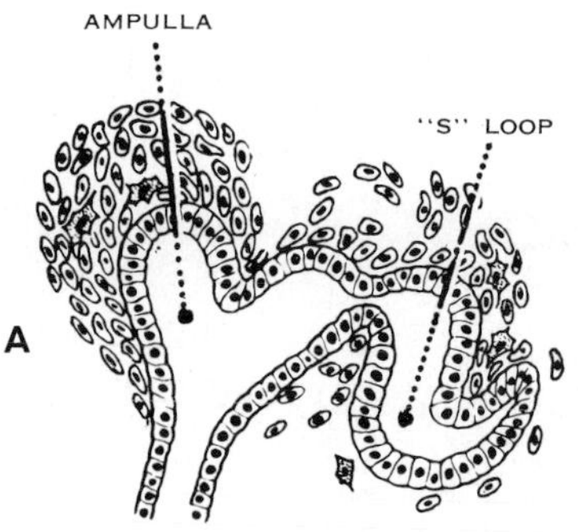

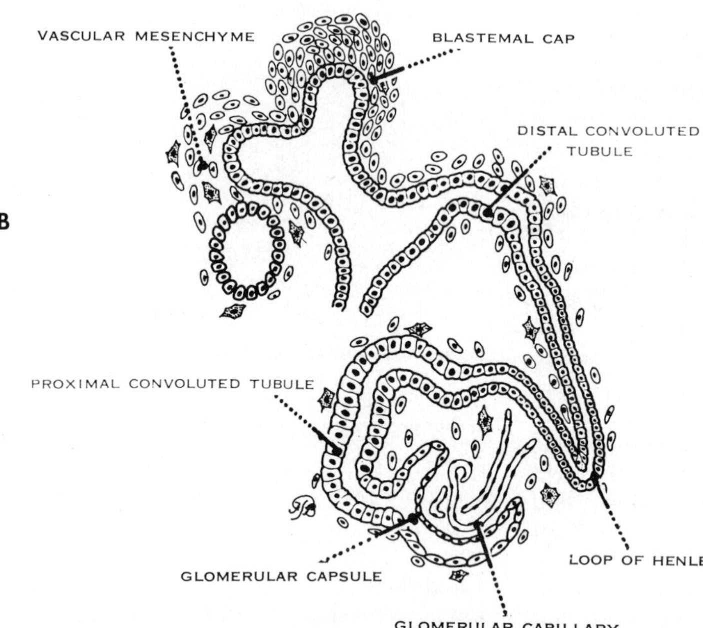

Figure 1–10. Two stages in the development of the metanephric nephrons. Note in *B* the early stage of a nephrogenic vesicle, induced by one branch of the divided ampulla. (From Hamilton, W. J., and Mossman, H. W.: Human Embryology. 4th Ed. © 1972 The Williams & Wilkins Co., Baltimore.)

rons in the S-stage of development become distended, or when ampullae are unable to induce differentiation of nephrons.

During the last month of gestation the ampullae disappear and no new nephrons form, but interstitial growth of the kidney continues as the convoluted tubules and loops of Henle lengthen. At term, some of the loops of Henle are still confined to the renal cortex, and the proximal tubules in particular are small and short (Fetterman et al., 1965; Osathanondh and Potter, 1966). Growth and differentiation continue postnatally.

"Ascent" of Kidney. The metanephros starts to develop at the level of the upper sacral segments, but during the sixth and seventh weeks the kidney "ascends" from the pelvis to its final lumbar position (Figure 1–11). Most of this apparent ascent is caused by straightening of the embryo and rapid growth of the regions of the body caudal to the developing kidneys (Gruenwald, 1943). The kidney also rotates during this ascent so that the hilum, originally directed ventrally, comes to a medial position. Initially the kidney receives its blood supply from sacral branches of the aorta, but as it ascends out of the pelvis it is supplied by arteries at successively higher levels. The definitive renal artery is at the second lumbar level. Aberrant renal arte-

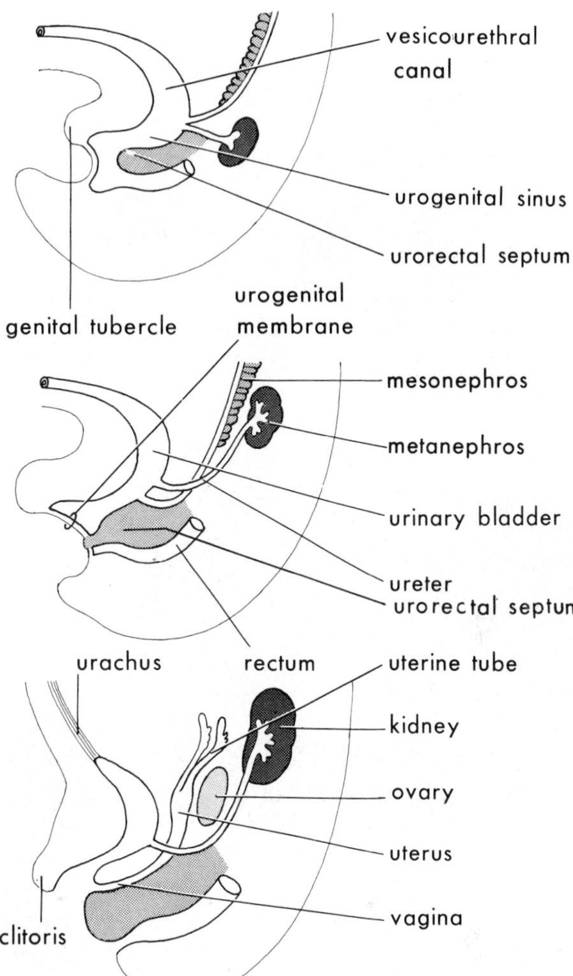

Figure 1–11. The gradual division of the cloaca by the urorectal septum, and the ascent of the kidney from the sixth through the twelfth weeks of development. (From Moore, K. L.: The Developing Human. 2nd Ed. W. B. Saunders Co., Philadelphia, 1977.)

ries represent retained vessels from the lower levels which failed to regress during the ascent. If a kidney fails to ascend normally it may remain in the pelvis. Fusion of the two kidneys during the early stages of ascent results in a single malformed organ that may be horseshoe- or rosette-shaped. A horseshoe kidney, formed by fusion of the lower poles of the two kidneys, remains in a low lumbar position, being prevented from further ascent by the root of the inferior mesenteric artery (Figure 1–12).

During the fourth month of fetal life the metanephros is gradually taking over the function of urine formation from the regressing mesonephros. Urine is passed into the amniotic cavity, and the kidneys may thus help to regulate the volume of the amniotic fluid.

The Bladder and Urethra

The cloaca, the expanded terminal portion of the hindgut, receives the allantois ventrally and the two mesonephric ducts laterally. The thin cloacal membrane composed of ectoderm and endoderm closes this cavity (see Figure 1–6). The cloaca gradually becomes divided into a ventral urogenital sinus and a dorsal anorectal canal by the urorectal septum, a coronal wedge of tissue that grows caudad in the angle between the allantois and the hindgut (see Figure 1–11). The urorectal septum

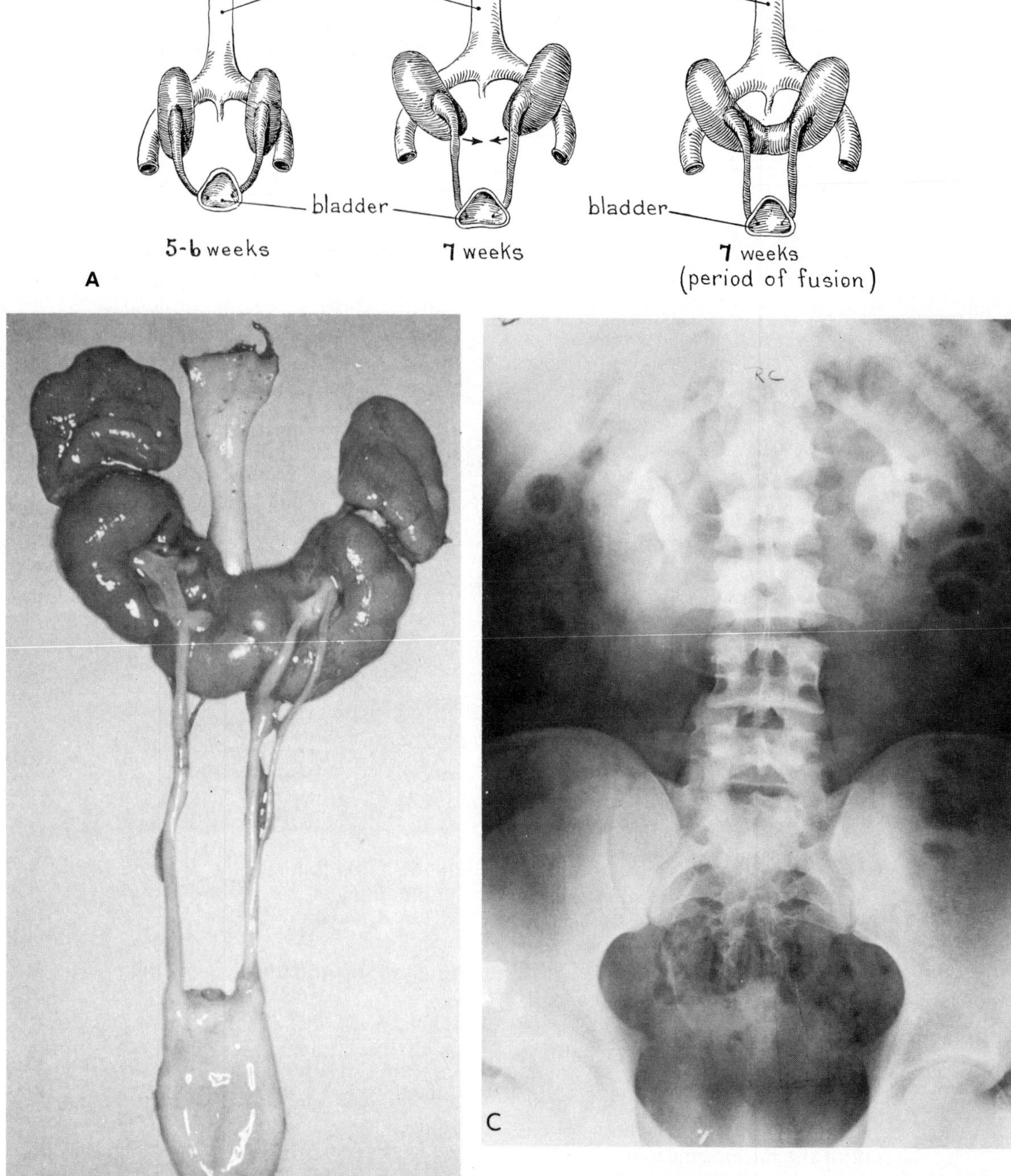

Figure 1–12. Horseshoe kidney. *A,* Schematic diagram indicating the embryologic etiology; lower polar fusion is shown. *B,* Gross specimen showing lower polar fusion. *C,* Radiogram of a horseshoe kidney. (*A, B,* From Perlmutter, A. D., Retek, A. B., and Bauer, S. B.: *In* Campbell, M. F., and Harrison, J. H.: Urology, Vol. 2. 4th Ed. W. B. Saunders, Philadelphia, 1977.)

eventually fuses with the cloacal membrane, dividing the latter into a ventral urogenital membrane and dorsal anal membrane, with the primitive perineal body being formed at the point of fusion.

The urogenital membrane disintegrates at about the end of the sixth week, opening the urogenital sinus to the amniotic cavity. That portion of the sinus above the level of entry of the mesonephric ducts communicates at its cranial end with the allantois and is called the vesicourethral canal. The upper part of this canal expands to form the urinary bladder, and the lower part lengthens and becomes the major part of the urethra in the female. The part of the sinus caudal to the mesonephric ducts is the definitive urogenital sinus. Its further development to form the vestibule is described below (p. 21).

Epithelial Structures

Although the mesonephric ducts begin to degenerate in the female during the early fetal period, they first give rise to the ureteric buds, and also contribute to the bladder and urethra. The common excretory ducts (i.e., the mesonephric ducts below the junction with the metanephric ducts or developing ureters) (see Figure 1–6) gradually become absorbed into the dorsal wall of the expanding urinary bladder. By differential growth the ureters then come to open laterally into the bladder, independently of the openings of the mesonephric ducts, which migrate caudally with respect to the ureteric orifices and remain relatively close to the middorsal line (Figure 1–13). The vesicourethral canal, derived from the cloaca, is lined by endoderm, whereas the mesonephric ducts are of mesodermal origin. With incorporation of the terminal parts of the mesonephric ducts into the walls of the developing bladder and urethra, the linings of these two organs are of dual origin (Gyllensten, 1949). As far as can be determined, the trigone of the bladder, in the dorsal wall, demarcated by the openings of the two ureters and the internal urethral orifice, and also some tissue in the dorsal wall of the primitive urethra as far caudal as the openings of the mesonephric ducts are originally derived from mesoderm. However, since endodermal epithelium may later extend into these regions, the different epithelial contributions in the adult are not known with certainty. Some fairly common urologic problems, such as ureteroceles, megaureters, and vesicoureteral reflux, may arise by malformation of this complex trigonal region (Muecke, 1975). Epithelial buds that arise from the lining of the urethra and upper part of the urogenital sinus form the urethral glands and paraurethral glands of Skene, respectively; these are homologous with the glands of the prostate in the male (Glenister, 1962).

Muscle and Connective Tissue

The connective tissue and muscular coats of the bladder and urethra are derived from mesoderm of the lateral plate that surrounds the endodermal vesicourethral canal. The bladder normally receives a secondary reinforcement of muscle on its ventral side (Glenister, 1958). Extrophy of the bladder, a rare condition, results from a lack of normal development of this ventral musculature of the bladder and of the overlying ventral body wall. At the primitive streak stage, if mesoderm fails to migrate caudal to the cloacal membrane, this region remains as a thin extension of the cloacal membrane. Later, by folding of the embryonic body, it comes to a midventral position between the umbilicus and the cloacal membrane, but it lacks the muscle and connective tissue that normally develop from the invading mesoderm (Patten and Barry, 1952). This thin sheet of ectoderm and endoderm later ruptures under tension when the urogenital membrane breaks down, consequently exposing the posterior wall of the bladder (Muecke, 1964). Frequently this condition is accompanied by other midline defects, such as division of the clitoris and separation of the pubic bones, and anomalies of the genital tract (see Chapter 5).

Urachus

At the cranial end of the vesicourethral canal, the lumen of the allantois is gradually reduced or obliterated (see Figure 1–11), but its connective tissue remains as the urachus, or median umbilical ligament. In

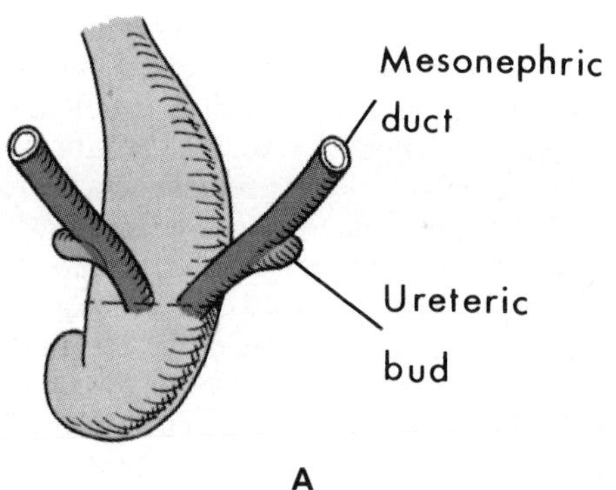

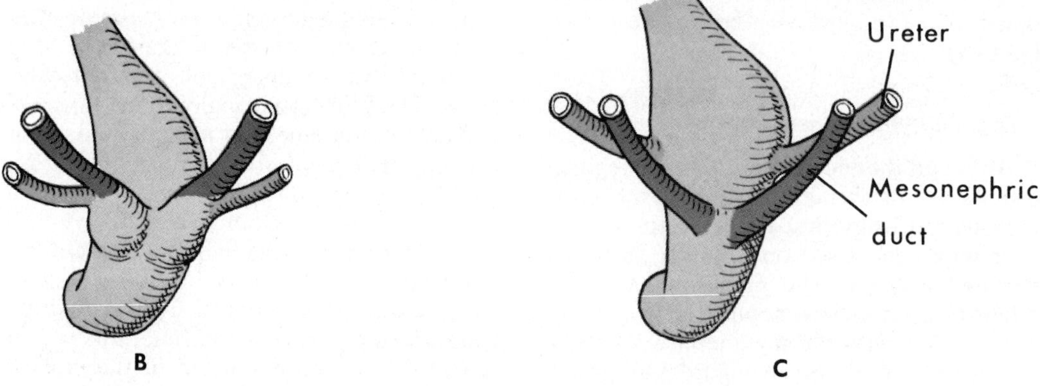

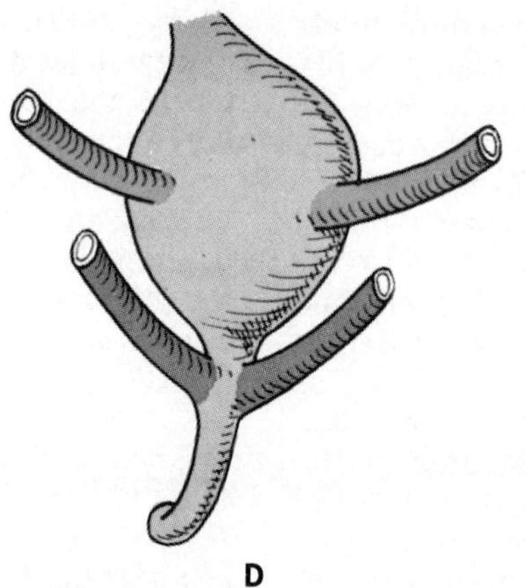

Figure 1–13. Schematic drawings of the dorsal side of the vesicourethral canal, showing the relationship between the mesonephric ducts and ureters during development of the urinary bladder and urethra. (From Tuchmann-Duplessis, H., and Haegel, P.: Illustrated Human Embryology. Vol. 12, 1972. Courtesy Springer-Verlag, New York, and Masson, Editeurs, Paris.)

the adult this is a fibrous strand extending from the apex of the bladder to the umbilicus, and containing a central cord or narrow tubular remnant of epithelium. Failure of the allantois to close may result in a urachal fistula from the bladder to the umbilicus, a urachal sinus opening either to the bladder or the umbilicus, or more commonly, small urachal cysts.

DEVELOPMENT OF THE GENITAL SYSTEM

Although the genetic sex of an individual is established at fertilization, development of the genital system proceeds through an indifferent stage during which both male and female are anatomically identical. The gonads at first show no evidence of whether they will become testes or ovaries, and a double set of ducts forms. It is not until late in the sixth week of development that the gonads begin to show sexual differentiation. Male and female individuals are identical externally for an even longer period, since it is not until the fetus is nearly 3 months old that sex can be determined with certainty by examining the external genitalia. Thus in describing the development of each portion of the female genital system it is necessary to consider first the indifferent stage.

The Ovary

The gonads are derived from three components: the coelomic epithelium, the underlying mesenchyme, and the primordial germ cells. During the fifth week, genital ridges, thickenings of coelomic epithelium, appear on the medial side of each mesonephros (see Figure 1–5, *A*,*B*). This coelomic epithelium proliferates, forming the primitive sex cords, which begin to invade the underlying mesenchyme and mingle with the immigrating primordial germ cells. The mesonephros, developing gonad, and supporting mesentery together constitute the urogenital ridge.

Primordial Germ Cells

The primordial germ cells, which are the source of all the gametes, are probably segregated at an early stage in the presomite embryo, but can first be identified in a 4-week embryo some distance away from the genital ridges. The primordial germ cells, distinguished by their large size relative to that of the surrounding somatic cells, are found in the endoderm of the allantois and adjacent parts of the yolk sac (Witschi, 1948; Jirasek, 1977). From here they are believed to pass to the wall of the hindgut and then to migrate cranially by ameboid movement along the dorsal mesentery (Figure 1–14). The germ cells reach the genital ridges during the sixth week of development (Witschi, 1948; Pinkerton et al., 1961). The primordial germ cells can multiply and mature normally only in the genital ridge, where they become associated with the developing primitive sex cords of the indifferent gonad (Figure 1–15*A*). Therefore, failure of the primordial germ cells to reach the genital ridges is one cause of gonadal dysgenesis.

Further Differentiation

In developing from the indifferent gonad, the ovary acquires its characteristic features more slowly than does the testis. The primordial germ cells remain in a cortical position close to the overlying coelomic epithelium. The primitive sex cords largely degenerate, but they first give rise to the rete ovarii in the medullary part of the developing ovary (Figure 1–15*B*). The mesonephric tubules that are closely associated with the rete, but not usually continuous with it, also mostly regress in the female, leaving remnants, the epoophoron and paroophoron. The coelomic (or germinal) epithelium proliferates and forms cortical cords. These cords become broken up by invasion of medullary mesenchyme into cell clusters surrounding one or more of the primordial germ cells (Figure 1–15*B*). Since a distinct tunica albuginea does not develop under the coelomic epithelium of the ovary (as it does in the testis at this stage), the epithelium may continue to contribute to the cords and clusters throughout fetal life.

During the late embryonic and early fetal periods, especially from the eighth to the twentieth weeks (Pinkerton et al., 1961), the primordial germ cells undergo repeated mitotic divisions to provide all of the oo-

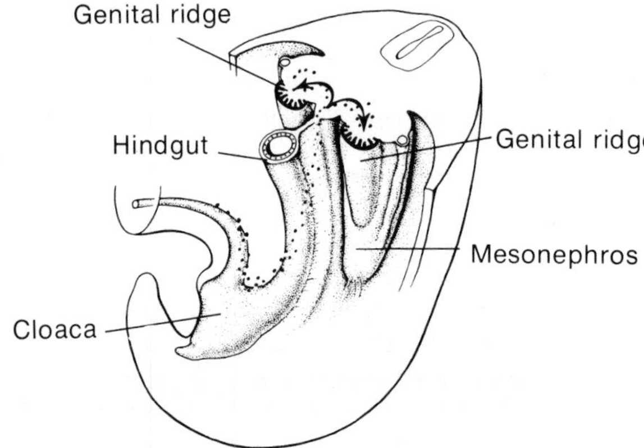

Figure 1–14. The pathway taken *(arrows)* by primordial germ cells along the wall of the hindgut and dorsal mesentery to the genital ridges. (From Langman, J.: Medical Embryology. 4th Ed. © 1981 The Williams & Wilkins Co., Baltimore.)

gonia for later life. The surrounding cells derived from coelomic epithelium become follicular cells, and mesenchyme between the follicles forms the ovarian stroma. During the late fetal stage (sixteenth week until shortly after birth), meiotic division of the oocytes is suspended in prophase, and either the oocytes become completely surrounded by follicle cells, forming primary follicles, or they degenerate (Jirasek, 1977). The primary follicles become separated from each other by ovarian stroma. This differentiation of primary follicles requires the presence of two normal X chromosomes (46,XX fetuses). In individuals with Turner's syndrome (45,X), in whom there is only a single dose of feminizing determinants (genes carried on the short arm of the X chromosome), the early stages of ovarian development and meiosis occur normally, but the oocytes degenerate when the follicular envelopes fail to surround them completely (Jirasek, 1977). Differentiation of the ovary is thus determined by the 46,XX chromosomal constitution of the fetus, and it establishes the gonadal sex of the individual.

During this differentiation and growth,

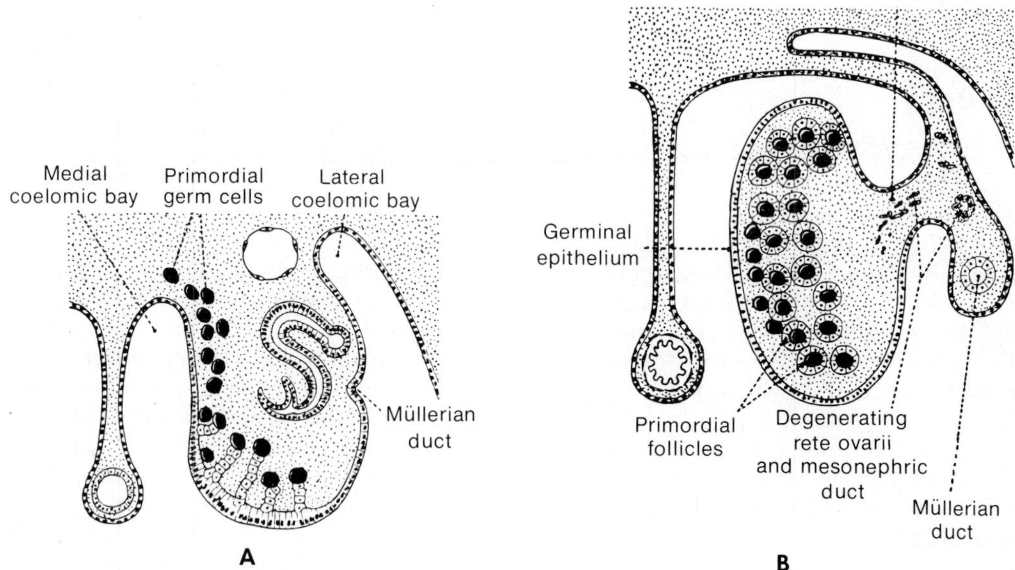

Figure 1–15. Development of the ovary. *A,* Indifferent stage. Note the site of origin of the opening of the müllerian duct.

B, Ovary with primordial follicles and degenerating rete in the mesovarium. (From Hamilton, W. J., and Mossman, H. W.: Human Embryology. 4th Ed. © 1972 The Williams & Wilkins Co., Baltimore.)

the ovary gradually projects further into the coelomic cavity and displaces the regressing mesonephros in a dorsolateral direction, while the originally broad attachment of the gonad to the mesonephros becomes reduced to a mesentery, the mesovarium (Figure 1–15*B*). The displaced mesonephros consists of a dorsal portion with regressing tubules and a more ventral tubal part containing the mesonephric and müllerian (paramesonephric) ducts.

The Genital Ducts

During the sixth week, the müllerian ducts begin to develop in both sexes as groove-like invaginations of the coelomic epithelium lateral to the cranial tip of each mesonephric duct (Figure 1–15*A*), and apparently induced by the adjacent mesonephric duct. Each invagination pushes caudally as a solid bud growing at first parallel to the mesonephric duct in the tubal portion of the mesonephros (Figure 1–16; see also Figure 1–21*B*, p. 22). As the epithelial cord extends further caudally, it progressively acquires a lumen from its cranial end.

Opposite the caudal end of the mesonephros each müllerian duct crosses toward the midline, passing ventral to the mesonephric duct and then growing in a caudomedial direction to join and fuse with its counterpart from the opposite side (Figure 1–16; see also Figure 1–21*C*). At the caudal end the solid epithelial tip of the fused müllerian ducts becomes continuous with an endodermal epithelial proliferation from the dorsal wall of the urogenital sinus. Together these form an elevation, the sinus or müllerian tubercle, between the openings of the mesonephric ducts (Figure 1–17). Development of the dual duct system up to this indifferent stage of about 8 weeks is the same in both sexes.

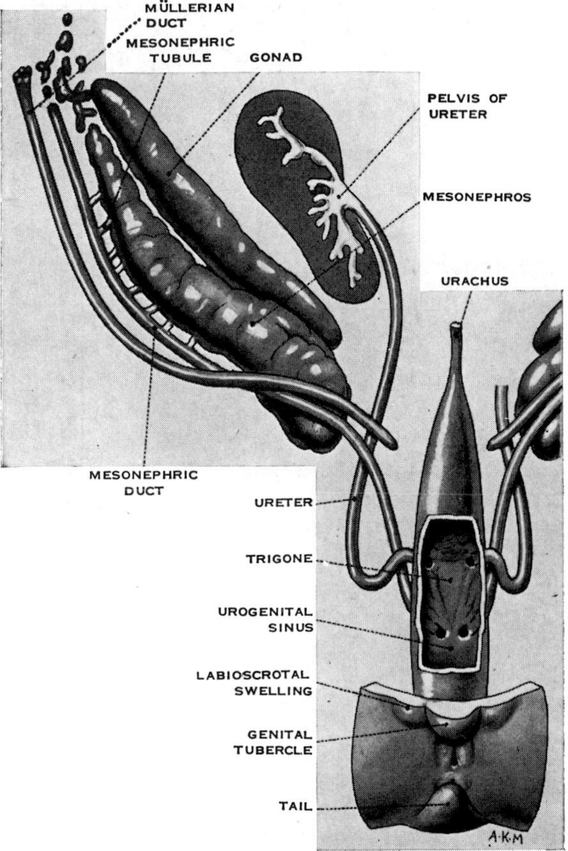

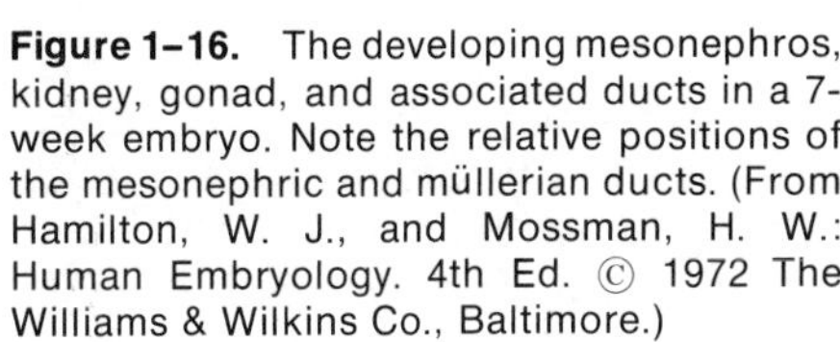

Figure 1–16. The developing mesonephros, kidney, gonad, and associated ducts in a 7-week embryo. Note the relative positions of the mesonephric and müllerian ducts. (From Hamilton, W. J., and Mossman, H. W.: Human Embryology. 4th Ed. © 1972 The Williams & Wilkins Co., Baltimore.)

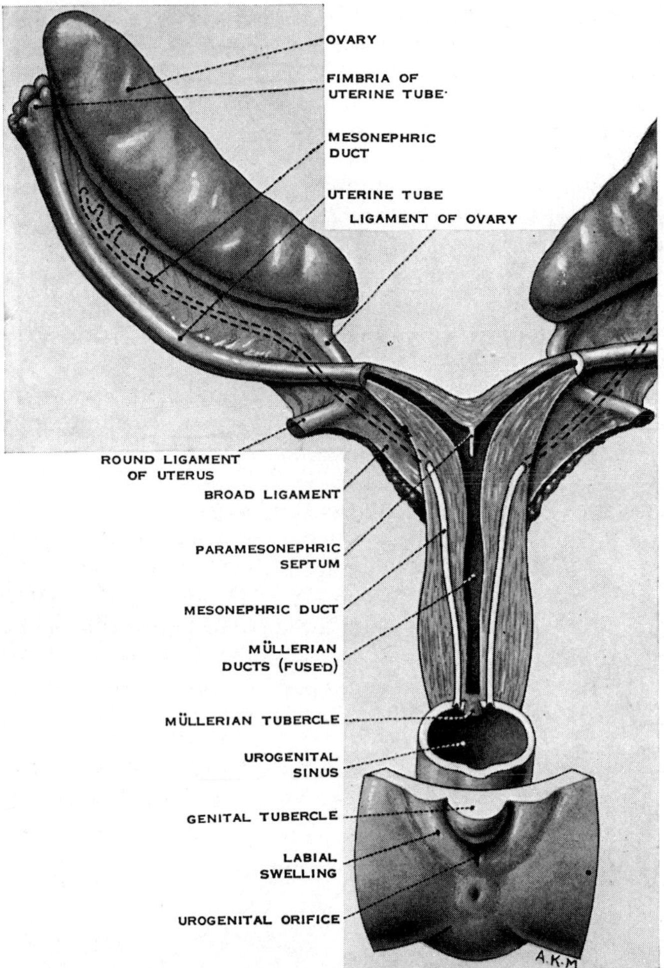

Figure 1–17. The genital ducts in a 10-week fetus. The anterior half of the uterus has been removed. The regressing mesonephros and its duct are shown by broken lines. (From Hamilton, W. J., and Mossman, H. W.: Human Embryology. 4th Ed. © 1972 The Williams & Wilkins Co., Baltimore.)

Hormonal Influences on Development

Beyond the indifferent stage, development of the male genital system is determined by hormonal influences from the gonads. As the testes differentiate, they begin to elaborate and secrete androgens, and an anti-müllerian hormone (Blanchard and Josso, 1974; Josso et al., 1977). The androgens stimulate further development of the mesonephric ducts to form the internal genital ducts, and cause the external genitalia to become masculine. The anti-müllerian hormone, a protein secreted by the Sertoli cells, suppresses development of the müllerian ducts beyond the indifferent stage (Jost, 1971; Josso, 1972; Josso et al., 1977).

In the female, in the absence of these testicular hormones, the mesonephric ducts remain rudimentary and later regress, but the müllerian ducts continue to develop and form the fallopian tubes, uterus, and cranial part of the vagina. Fetal ovaries are much less active in hormone production than are the testes (Block, 1964; Winter et al., 1977); indeed, there is no evidence that the fetal ovaries play any morphogenetic role in the development of the female genital ducts and external genitalia (Jirasek, 1977). Embryos of both sexes develop within an environment containing hormones from the maternal circulation and placenta, and these extraembryonic hormones may influence the genitalia to develop into the female type. Thus, a female phenotype develops in the absence of actively secreting testes, even without the presence of normal ovaries. Individuals with Turner's syndrome (45,X chromosomes), for example, have ovarian dysgenesis accompanied by otherwise normal internal and external genitalia (Carr et al., 1968) (see also Chapter 5). One exception is in individuals with testicular feminization, or androgen-insensitive syndrome (see Chapter 5). In these patients, who have 46,XY genotype but a female phenotype, testes develop and secrete androgens, but the mesonephric ducts and external genitalia fail to show characteristic masculine development because of congenital insensitivity of the target cells to androgens (O and Short, 1977). On the other hand, in patients with congenital adrenal hyperplasia, in the absence of testicular tissue, but in spite of normal ovarian development (46,XX chromosomes), increased quantities of circulating androgens from the hyperplastic fetal adrenal glands cause varying degrees of masculinization of the external genitalia. In these examples of female intersex, the gonads and upper part of the internal genital tract are usually normal, since no testes are present to secrete the anti-müllerian hormone (Dewhurst, 1970). However, the clitoris may be enlarged and the labia majora partially fused, giving the appearance of a scrotum (see Chapter 5). Thus, because of complex endocrine and genetic influences, the type of genital ducts and external genitalia may not always coincide with the genetic and gonadal sex of the individual.

Fallopian Tubes and Uterus

In the normal female, fusion of the müllerian ducts to form the uterovaginal canal begins at the caudal end and progresses cranially. The lumen of the canal is at first divided by a septum, which normally disappears by the end of the third month (Figure 1–17). The fused vertical parts of the müllerian ducts form the lower portion of the uterus. As the uterus grows, the horizontal regions of the müllerian ducts become incorporated into the corpus and fundus. The cranial limit of fusion of the ducts marks the fundus of the uterus (Figure 1–17).

The remaining unfused portions of the müllerian ducts become the epithelial lining of the fallopian tubes. Fimbriae develop around the openings into the coelomic cavity, which remain as the abdominal ostia of the tubes. The extreme cranial tip of the müllerian duct may not contribute to the infundibulum of the fallopian tube but remain as a vesicular appendage, the hydatid of Morgagni (see Figure 1–22, p. 23). The mesenchyme surrounding the müllerian ducts condenses to form the connective tissue and muscular coats of the fallopian tubes and uterus.

Since the uterus is formed from paired ducts that fuse progressively from their caudal ends, many uterine abnormalities can be explained in terms of incomplete fusion of varying degrees (see Chapter 5).

The Vagina

Normal vaginal development in the human depends on contact being established between one or both müllerian ducts and the endodermal epithelium of the urogenital sinus (Sarto and Simpson, 1978). Therefore, the vagina is most likely an organ of composite origin, although its development is still a controversial topic (O'Rahilly, 1977). The müllerian ducts probably give rise to the cranial three fifths of the vagina, while the caudal two fifths are derived from the urogenital sinus (Cunha, 1975). When the caudal tip of the fused müllerian ducts contacts the dorsal wall of the urogenital sinus, the latter proliferates to form bilateral evaginations, the sinovaginal bulbs. These give rise to a thick vaginal plate of endoderm, flattened in an anteroposterior direction, between the sinus and the lumen of the uterovaginal canal. This vaginal plate expands around the closed tip of the canal and also elongates, pushing the uterovaginal lumen farther away from the urogenital sinus (Figure 1–18). The tip of the uterovaginal canal also proliferates and adds to the distance between the sinus and the canal.

Later the vaginal plate becomes vacuolated. Gradually the lumen of the vagina appears and becomes continuous with that of the uterovaginal canal, while the peripheral cells of the plate form the epithelial lining of the vagina (Figure 1–19). By the fifth month the whole vagina is a hollow canal with expansions, the vaginal fornices, around the uterine cervix. Until late in fetal life the caudal end of the vagina remains closed from the urogenital sinus by a thin

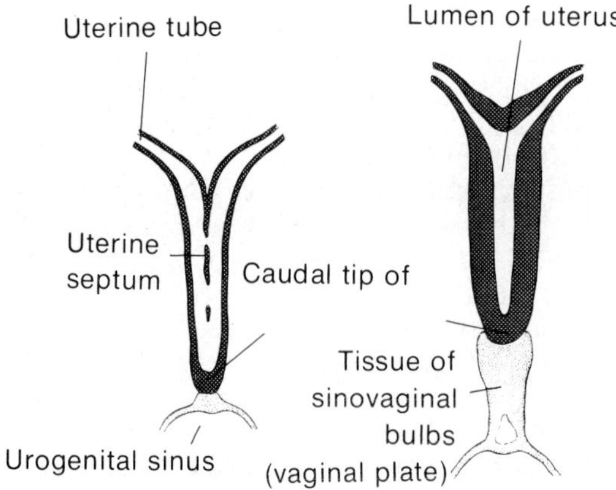

Figure 1–18. The formation of the uterus and vagina at 9 weeks and 3 months of age. (From Langman, J.: Medical Embryology. 4th Ed. © 1981 The Williams & Wilkins Co., Baltimore.)

membrane, the hymen, formed from the vaginal plate and the urogenital sinus (Figure 1–19). The mesenchyme surrounding the developing vagina evidently plays an important role in induction and maintenance of differentiation of the adjacent epithelium, in addition to forming the connective tissue and muscular coats of the organ (Cunha and Lung, 1979).

Many vaginal malformations in the human seem to fall into two distinct groups that can be best explained by the dual embryologic origin of the vagina. Absence of most of the vagina (all except the most caudal part) accompanied by absence of most of the uterus may be caused by müllerian aplasia, a condition which may be transmitted as an X-linked, autosomal dominant trait (Sarto and Simpson, 1978; Shokeir, 1978). A much less common condition is vaginal atresia, in which the uterus is normal and only the lower part of the vagina is absent. Vaginal atresia can result from failure of development of that part of the vagina normally derived from the urogenital sinus (Sarto and Simpson, 1978; Ingerslev, 1979). When both primordia develop, but fail to unite normally, a transverse vaginal septum may remain (Sarto and Simpson, 1978) (see Chapter 5).

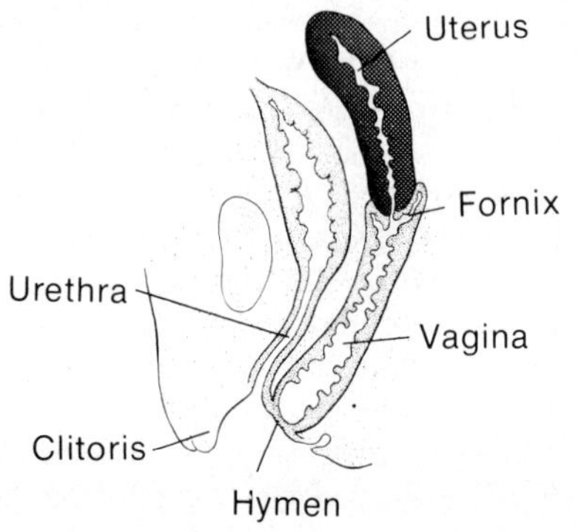

Figure 1–19. Diagrammatic sagittal section of the uterus and vagina in a newborn infant. (From Langman, J.: Medical Embryology. 4th Ed. © 1981 The Williams & Wilkins Co., Baltimore.)

Associated Genital and Urinary Malformations

The close relationship between the urinary and genital tracts during early embryogenesis accounts for the high incidence of associated anomalies in the two systems. Since development of the müllerian duct is normally induced by an adjacent mesonephric duct, faulty differentiation of the mesonephric duct and ureteric bud, leading to renal agenesis, is very frequently accompanied by gynecologic malformations. For example, individuals with a hemiuterus (of single müllerian origin) frequently have contralateral renal agenesis, while bilateral renal agenesis (incompatible with postnatal life) may be associated with complete absence of the uterus and fallopian tubes (Magee et al., 1979; Sarto and Simpson, 1978) (see Chapter 5). There also seems to be a nonrandom association between certain cervical vertebral anomalies and renal and müllerian aplasia. These syndromes may result from alterations in the primordia of all of these structures while they are in very close spatial relationship, during the fourth and fifth weeks of development (Duncan et al., 1979). On the other hand, renal agenesis that results from absence of the metanephric blastema probably arises later in development and does not necessarily occur with genital tract anomalies (Magee et al., 1979).

The External Genitalia

During the third week of development embryonic mesoderm from the primitive streak begins to migrate between the ectoderm and endoderm around the edges of the cloacal membrane (see Figure 1–2). It forms a series of swellings: the genital tubercle in the midline between the cloacal membrane and the umbilical cord, and the genital or labioscrotal swellings on each side of the cloacal membrane (Figure 1–20*A*). Endoderm lining the anterior part of the cloaca at the base of the genital tubercle proliferates to form a urethral plate. The plate grows forward into the mesenchyme in contact with the ectoderm on the underside of the lengthening genital tubercle or phallus. In effect, this urethral plate extends the ectodermal-endodermal cloacal membrane in a cranial direction. Mesenchyme along the edges of the cloacal membrane meanwhile proliferates, with the result that the cloacal membrane and urethral plate lie at the bottom of a shallow groove bordered by folds (Figure 1–20*B*).

During this period of development, the urorectal septum grows down internally to divide the cloaca and its membrane (see Figure 1–11). The surrounding folds also become divided into anal folds around the anal membrane and urethral folds around the urogenital membrane and at the base of the phallus (Figure 1–20*B*). At about 6 weeks of gestation the urogenital membrane ruptures, opening the urogenital sinus (Figure 1–20*C*). The urethral plate also begins to break down, leaving an endodermally lined groove continuous with the urogenital sinus in the proximal part of the genital tubercle. Up to this stage of about 9 weeks the external genitalia are very similar in both sexes.

In the female, in whom testicular an-

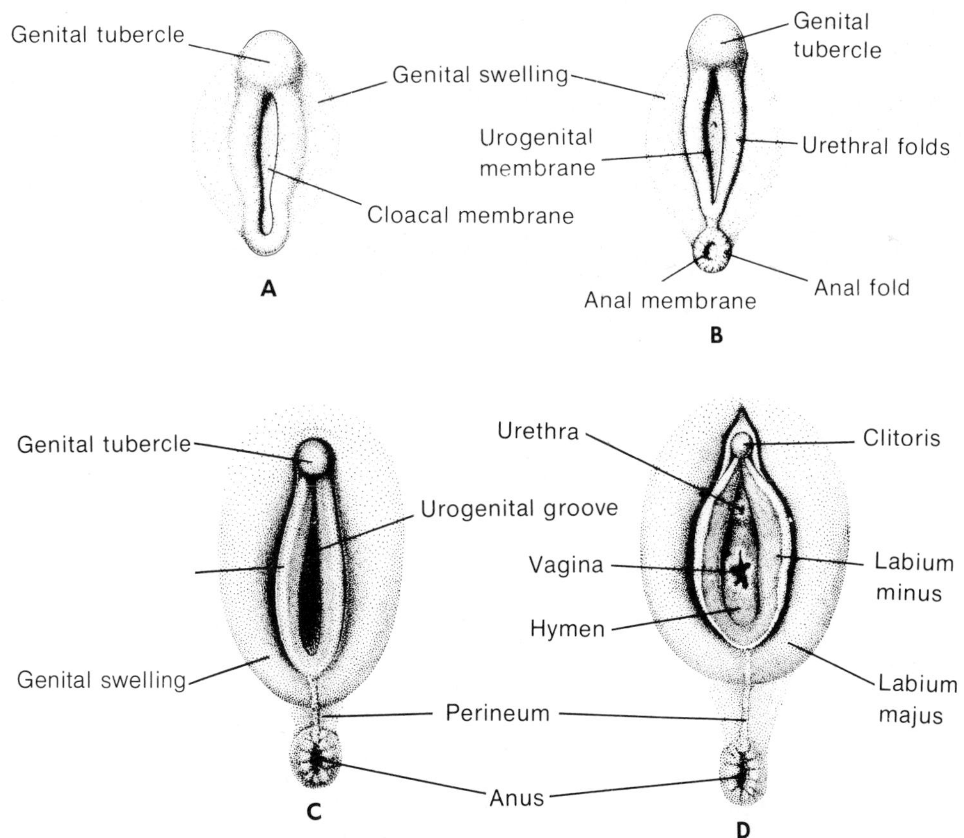

Figure 1–20. Development of the external genitalia. *A*, Indifferent stage in a 4-week embryo. *B*, Indifferent stage in a 6-week embryo. *C*, Female fetus at 5 months. *D*, Newborn female. (From Langman, J.: Medical Embryology. 4th Ed. © 1981 The Williams & Wilkins Co., Baltimore.)

drogens are absent, the portions of the urethral folds on the underside of the genital tubercle soon regress. The phallus fails to grow much more in length and bends caudally to become the clitoris. That part of the urogenital sinus distal to the hymen extends in a dorsoventral direction and becomes relatively shallow (see Figure 1–11). The urethral folds (which in the male close to form the penile urethra) remain unfused in the female fetus and form the labia minora. The urogenital sinus remains open permanently as the vestibule, into which open both the urethra and the vagina (Figure 1–20*D*).

Two pairs of glands, the greater vestibular glands of Bartholin and the lesser vestibular glands, arise from the vestibular endoderm. The labial swellings fuse in front of the anus to form the posterior commissure, and laterally they enlarge to become the labia majora (Figure 1–20*D*). Later another swelling cranial to the clitoris gives rise to the mons pubis.

Ovarian Ligaments and Ovarian Descent

Ovarian Ligaments

Since the gonad develops only in the middle part of the urogenital ridge, the cranial and caudal portions of the ridge gradually degenerate with decline of the mesonephros, and are replaced by fibrous strands that become the ovarian ligaments. The cranial part of the urogenital ridge thus gives rise to the suspensory ligament of the ovary. At its caudal end the gonad is attached to a band of mesenchyme that is continuous with the urogenital ridge and then crosses around the abdominal wall to end in the inguinal region. This mesenchyme, which in turn passes into the me-

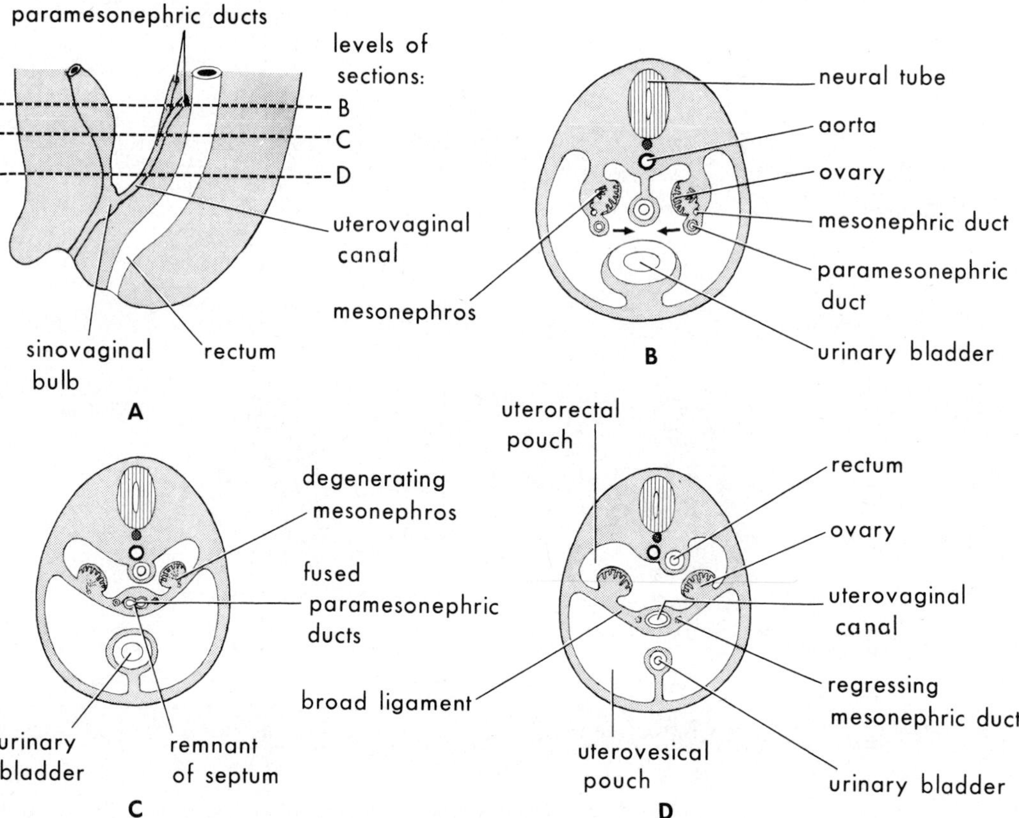

Figure 1–21. *A,* Sagittal section of the caudal region of a 9-week female fetus. *B, C, D,* Transverse sections taken at levels indicated on *A* to illustrate the formation of the broad ligament and pouches in the pelvic cavity. (From Moore, K. L.: The Developing Human. 2nd Ed. W. B. Saunders Co., Philadelphia, 1977.)

senchyme of the labioscrotal swelling, marks the future inguinal canal. Thus, a continuous strand of mesenchyme, the gubernaculum, extends from the caudal pole of each developing gonad to the ipsilateral labioscrotal swelling. At the point where the two müllerian ducts swing in a medial direction to fuse in the midline, the urogenital ridges are brought into a transverse plane. These ridges form a broad transverse pelvic fold extending from the sides of the fused uterovaginal canal to the abdominal wall (Figure 1–21). This fold becomes the broad ligament of the uterus, with the uterine tubes lying at its superior edge and remnants of the regressing mesonephroi between its leaves. The broad ligament divides the pelvic cavity into the uterorectal pouch (of Douglas) and the uterovesical pouch (Fig. 1–21*D*). As the uterus develops, the gubernaculum becomes attached close to its junction with the uterine tube. The cranial portion of the gubernaculum then forms the ovarian ligament (Figure 1–22). The caudal part, running from the uterus through the inguinal canal to the developing labium majus, becomes the round ligament of the uterus (Figure 1–22).

Ovarian Descent

By the end of the third month, the ovary descends from its original position on the dorsal abdominal wall to reach the brim of the pelvis. Most of this apparent descent is the result of rapid growth of the trunk relative to growth of the gonad and gubernaculum. Later the ovary rotates to its final position, with the original caudal pole directed medially. It comes to lie dorsal to the end of the fallopian tube on the posterior surface of the broad ligament. A small processus vaginalis (canal of Nuck) develops in the female. This is a diverticulum of the coelomic cavity through the inguinal canal towards the genital swelling. It is normally obliterated before birth. Very rarely does the ovary descend to the inguinal canal or labium majus. It is normally prevented from descending to an extra-abdominal site by the attachment of the gubernaculum to the uterus.

The mesonephric duct does not degenerate completely in the female. It leaves remnants: the duct of the epoophoron in the mesosalpinx, and Gartner's duct in the broad ligament and lateral walls of the uterus and vagina (Figure 1–22). Remnants of two groups of mesonephric tubules also remain: as the epoophoron between the ovary and the uterine tube in the mesosalpinx, and as the paroophoron caudal to the ovary in the broad ligament (Figure 1–22). These remnants of the mesonephroi and their ducts are nonfunctional and are not usually detected unless they become cystic later in life.

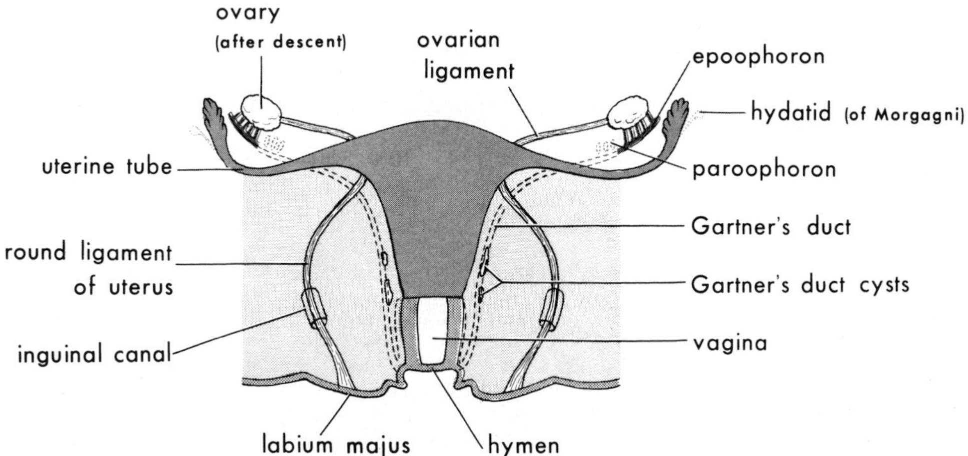

Figure 1–22. Ventral aspect of the reproductive system in a newborn female. (From Moore, K. L.: The Developing Human. 2nd Ed. W. B. Saunders Co., Philadelphia, 1977.)

REFERENCES

Blanchard, M-G., and Josso, N.: Source of the anti-müllerian hormone synthesized by the fetal testis: müllerian-inhibiting activity of fetal bovine Sertoli cells in tissue culture. Pediatr. Res. *8*:968, 1974.

Block, E.: Metabolism of 4-^{14}C-progesterone by human fetal testis and ovaries. Endocrinology *74*:833, 1964.

Carr, D. H., Haggar, R. A., and Hart, A. G.: Germ cells in the ovaries of XO female infants. Am. J. Clin. Pathol. *49*:521, 1968.

Cunha, G. R.: The dual origin of vaginal epithelium. Am. J. Anat. *143*:387, 1975.

Cunha, G. R., and Lung, B.: The importance of stroma in morphogenesis and functional activity of urogenital epithelium. In Vitro *15*:50, 1979.

Davidson, W. M., and Ross, G. I. M.: Bilateral absence of the kidneys and related congenital anomalies. J. Pathol. Bacteriol. *68*:459, 1954.

Dewhurst, C. J.: Foetal sex and development of genitalia. *In* Philipp, E. E., Barnes, J., and Newton, M. (Eds.): Scientific Foundations of Obstetrics and Gynecology. London, William Heinemann, Ltd., 1970, pp. 173–181.

Duncan, P. A., Shapiro, L. R., Stangel, J. J., Klein, R. M., and Addonizio, J. C.: The MURCS association: müllerian duct aplasia, renal aplasia, and cervicothoracic somite dysplasia. J. Pediatr. *95*:399, 1979.

Ekblom, P., Miettinen, A., and Saxen, L.: Induction of brush border antigens of the proximal tubule in the developing kidney. Dev. Biol. *74*:263, 1979*a*.

Ekblom, P., Nordling, S., Saxen, L., Rasilo, M. L., and Renkonen, O.: Cell interactions leading to kidney tubule determination are tunicamycin sensitive. Cell Differ. *8*:347, 1979*b*.

Ekblom, P., Alitalo, K., Vaheri, A., Timpl, R., and Saxen, L.: Induction of a basement membrane glycoprotein in embryonic kidney: possible role of laminin in morphogenesis. Proc. Natl. Acad. Sci. USA *77*:485, 1980.

Fetterman, G. H., Shuplock, N. A., Philipp, F. J., and Gregg, H. S.: The growth and maturation of human glomeruli and proximal convolutions from term to adulthood. Pediatrics *35*:601, 1965.

Glenister, T. W.: A correlation of the normal and abnormal development of the penile urethra and of the infra-umbilical abdominal wall. Br. J. Urol. *30*:117, 1958.

Glenister, T. W.: The development of the utricle and the so-called "middle" or "median" lobe of the human prostate. J. Anat. *96*:443, 1962.

Grobstein, C.: Inductive interaction in the development of the mouse metanephros. J. Exp. Zool. *130*:319, 1955.

Gruenwald, P.: The normal changes in position of the embryonic kidney. Anat. Rec. *85*:163, 1943.

Gyllensten, L.: Contributions to the embryology of the urinary bladder: Part 1. The development of the definitive relations between the openings of the Wolffian ducts and the ureters. Acta Anat. *7*:305, 1949.

Ingerslev, M.: Failure of fusion between an upper and a lower segment of the vagina. Acta Obstet. Gynecol. Scand. *58*:215, 1979.

Jirasek, J. E.: Morphogenesis of the genital system in the human. Birth Defects — Original Article Series, Vol. 13, No. 2. New York, Alan R. Liss, 1977, pp. 13–39.

Josso, N.: Permeability of membranes to the Müllerian-inhibiting substance synthesized by the human fetal testis *in vitro*: a clue to its biochemical nature. J. Clin. Endocrinol. *34*:265, 1972.

Josso, N., Picard, J-Y., and Tran, D.: The anti-müllerian hormone. Birth Defects — Original Article Series, Vol. 13, No. 2. New York, Alan R. Liss, 1977, pp. 59–84.

Jost, A.: Embryonic sexual differentiation. *In* Jones, H. W., and Scott, W. W. (Eds.): Hermaphroditism, Genital Anomalies and Related Endocrine Disorders. Baltimore, Williams & Wilkins Co., 1971, pp. 16–64.

Leeson, T. S.: The fine structure of the mesonephros of the 17-day rabbit embryo. Exp. Cell Res. *12*:670, 1957.

Magee, M. C., Lucey, D. T., and Fried, F. A.: A new embryologic classification for uro-gynecologic malformations: the syndromes of mesonephric duct–induced müllerian deformities. J. Urol. *121*:265, 1979.

de Martino, C., and Zamboni, L.: A morphological study of the mesonephros of the human embryo. J. Ultrastruct. Res. *16*:399, 1966.

Muecke, E. C.: The role of the cloacal membrane in extrophy: the first successful experimental study. J. Urol. *92*:659, 1964.

Muecke, E. C.: Embryology of common urologic problems in children. Pediatr. Ann. *4*:498, 1975.

O, W., and Short, R. V.: Sex determination and differentiation in mammalian germ cells. Birth Defects — Original Article Series, Vol. 13, No. 2. New York, Alan R. Liss, 1977, pp. 1–12.

O'Rahilly, R.: The development of the vagina in the human. Birth Defects — Original Article Series, Vol. 13, No. 2. New York, Alan R. Liss, 1977, pp. 123–136.

Osathanondh, V., and Potter, E. L.: Development of human kidney as shown by microdissection. I, II, III. Arch. Pathol. *76*:271, 277, 290, 1963.

Osathanondh, V., and Potter, E. L.: Pathogenesis of polycystic kidneys, I, II, III, IV. Arch. Pathol. *77*:466, 474, 485, 502, 1964.

Osathanondh, V., and Potter, E. L.: Development of human kidney as shown by microdissection. IV, V. Arch. Pathol. *82*:391, 403, 1966.

Patten, B. M., and Barry, A.: Genesis of extrophy of the bladder and epispadias. Am. J. Anat. *90*:35, 1952.

Pinkerton, J. H. M., McKay, D. G., Adams, E. C., and Hertig, A. T.: Development of the human ovary — a study using histochemical techniques. Obstet. Gynecol. *18*:152, 1961.

Potter, E. L.: Normal and Abnormal Development of the Kidney. Chicago, Year Book Medical Publishers, Inc., 1972, pp. 3–79.

Sarto, G. E., and Simpson, J. L.: Abnormalities of the müllerian and wolffian duct systems. Birth Defects — Original Article Series, Vol. 14, No. 6c. New York, Alan R. Liss, 1978, pp. 37–55.

Shokeir, M. H. K.: Aplasia of the müllerian system: evidence for probable sex-linked autosomal dominant inheritance. Birth Defects — Original Article Series, Vol. 14, No. 6c. New York, Alan R. Liss, 1978, pp. 147–165.

Torrey, T. W.: The early development of the human nephros. Contr. Embryol. Carneg. Instn. *35*:175, 1954.

Winter, J. S. D., Faiman, C., and Reyes, F. I.: Sex steroid production by the human fetus: its role in morphogenesis and control by gonadotropins. Birth Defects — Original Article Series, Vol. 13, No. 2. New York, Alan R. Liss, 1977, pp. 41–58.

Witschi, E.: Migrations of the germ cells of human embryos from the yolk sac to the primitive gonadal folds. Contr. Embryol. Carneg. Instn. *32*:67, 1948.

FURTHER READING

Corliss, C. E.: Patten's Human Embryology: Elements of Clinical Development. New York, McGraw-Hill Book Co., 1976.

Gray, S. W., and Skandalakis, J. E.: Embryology for Surgeons: The Embryological Basis for the Treatment of Congenital Defects. Philadelphia, W. B. Saunders Co., 1972, pp. 443–552, 563–593, 633–664.

Hamilton, W. J., and Mossman, H. W.: Human Embryology. 4th Ed. Baltimore, Williams & Wilkins Co., 1972.

Langman, J.: Medical Embryology. Human Development — Normal and Abnormal. 4th Ed. Baltimore, Williams and Wilkins Co., 1981.

Moore, K. L.: The Developing Human: Clinically Oriented Embryology. 2nd Ed. Philadelphia, W. B. Saunders Co., 1977.

Page, E. W., Villee, C. A., and Villee, D. B.: Human Reproduction. The Core Content of Obstetrics, Gynecology and Perinatal Medicine. 2nd Ed. Philadelphia, W. B. Saunders Co., 1976.

Williams, P. L., and Warwick, R. (Eds.): Gray's Anatomy. 36th British Ed. Philadelphia, W. B. Saunders Co., 1980.

2

SURGICAL ANATOMY

C. E. HAWTREY, M.D.

The anatomy and relationships of urogenital structures are exhaustively analyzed in several authoritative texts (e.g., Brenner and Rector, 1981). This chapter emphasizes the experience of operating physicians who are confronted with distorted anatomy daily. The anatomic drawings illustrating this chapter depict the problems of surgery concerning fascial planes, organ blood supply and distortion from disease.

THE KIDNEY

The kidney infrequently concerns the operating obstetrician or gynecologist except for a few important anatomic variations. The most significant of these are the unilateral pelvic kidney and the pancake kidney or fused pelvic disk kidney. These anomalies result from fusion of the metanephric blastema in the midline or failure of ascent to the usual flank location. Other variations include the crossed ectopic kidney, with or without fusion, and the horseshoe kidney, resulting from a fused isthmus of renal tissue anterior to the distal aorta and inferior vena cava. The blood flow to the kidney may arise from the aorta or internal iliac, common iliac, or sacral artery.

Identification of these variations is difficult at times. Preoperative excretory urograms are indicated but may be obscured if the renal mass overlies a bony structure so that it cannot be identified. In addition, during surgical procedures a pelvic kidney may be mistaken for a retroperitoneal tumor. Excision of solitary pelvic kidneys with resultant anuria has been reported (Anderson and Harrison, 1965).

THE URETER

The ureter functions as a muscular tube conveying urine over a distensible urothelial lining from the renal pelvis to the bladder. The ureter, with its spirally arranged double layer of smooth muscle, moves freely in the retroperitoneal space. Proximally the ureter is surrounded by a thin delicate condensation of the perinephric fascia (Gerota's fascia) extending inferiorly from the kidney.

The ureter lies in a bed of loose areolar connective tissue containing a variable amount of fat. That the ureter is not fixed to any great degree is exemplified by the active peristalsis observed under normal circumstances. The loose periureteral tissue becomes important as a boundary for infiltration by disease, e.g., retroperitoneal fibrosis or cervical or vesical neoplasia. These infiltrative processes entrap the ureter, fixing it in the retroperitoneal space, and result in functional and anatomic obstruction. Aneurysmal dilatation of the aorta or retroperitoneal lymph node enlargement may displace the ureter laterally and anteriorly.

Fascial Envelopment

The perinephric fascia envelops the kidney and ureter cephalad but becomes indistinct as the ureter courses anterior to the common iliac artery. The anterior layer of Gerota's fascia is evident as a well-developed structure seen after the adjacent colon and mesocolon are mobilized medially. The posterior fascial layer is encountered in flank or extraperitoneal approaches to the proximal ureter. Lymphatic channels course with the ureter and major vessels along the pelvic wall. The periureteral areolar tissue blends with the adventitial fascia of the bladder and uterus.

The ureter may be displaced in its pelvic portion by masses in adjacent pelvic organs, e.g., laterally by uterine myomas or medially by bladder diverticula. The ureter becomes a relatively more fixed structure in the true pelvis, particularly distal to the internal iliac artery. This fixation results primarily from the arterial and venous network supplying the uterus and bladder (Figure 2–1).

The ureter has a remarkable capacity for elongation within its fascial envelope. For example, the ureter may be prolapsed through the introitus by an extensive cystocele (Figure 2–2). Ureteral elongation and tortuosity are seen with obstructive hydroureteronephrosis from any cause. As the ureter dilates, it also elongates between its segmental blood supply, producing obvious changes in course on intravenous or retrograde pyelograms. The ureter is not obstructed at these kinks, but must carry its urine bolus past these areas of relative fixation. The perinephric (Gerota's) fascia, enveloping the ureter anteriorly and posteriorly, confines most elongation in a medial-lateral plane until the ureter enters the true pelvis. There the peritoneum covers the anterior aspect of the ureter.

Blood Supply

The ureter receives a delicate blood supply from several sources: the renal artery, aorta, and common iliac, internal iliac, and vesical arteries (Figure 2–3). Anastomosing networks of vessels appear in the adventitia and between the spiraling circular and longitudinal muscle bundles in the ureteral wall. The midureteral adventitial vessels connect with tributaries from the renal artery supplying the renal pelvis. Venous outflow from the ureter also includes a plexus that anastomoses with renal pelvic vessels, ovarian veins, and lumbar veins on the left and with the inferior vena cava on the right. All these vessels course from medial to lateral between the layers of perinephric fascia in the proximal ureter. These vessels may be encountered in retroperitoneal

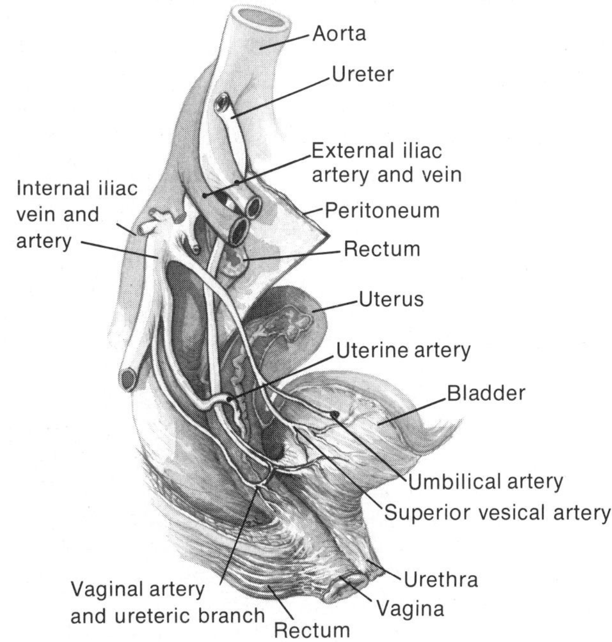

Figure 2–1. Anatomic relationship of ureter to arterial vessels supplying major pelvic viscera. Note the course of ureter lateral to the uterine body and posterior to the uterine artery. The relative fixation of the pelvic ureter by vascular structures is evident.

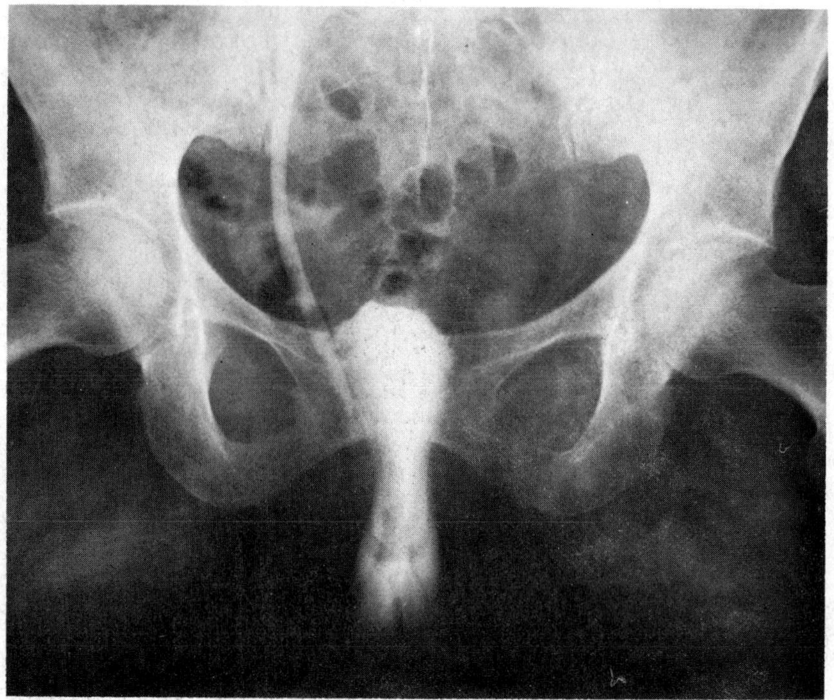

Figure 2–2. Excretory urogram demonstrating anatomic distortion of the right ureter carried out the introitus by vaginal prolapse.

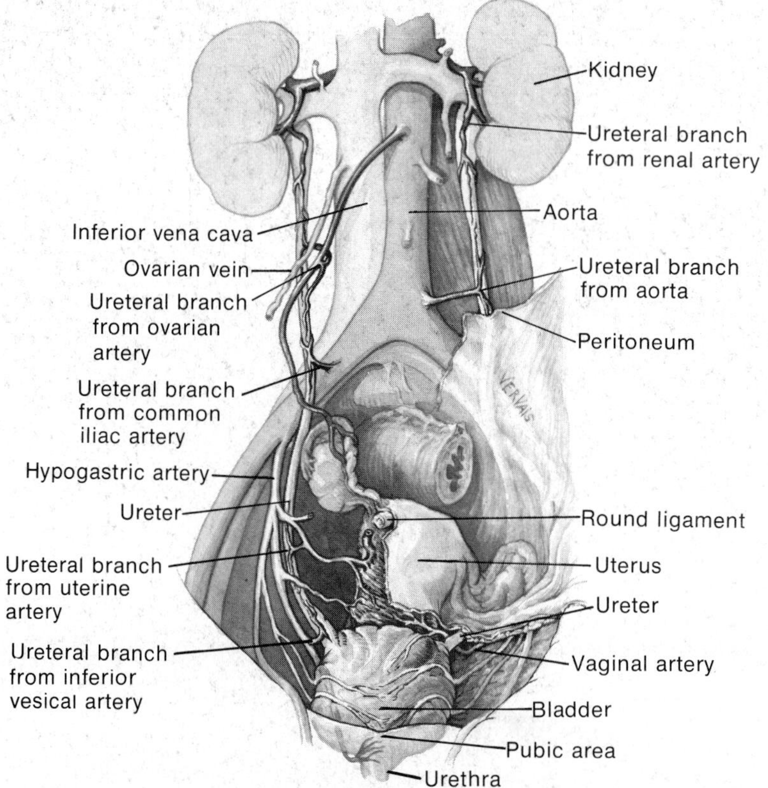

Figure 2–3. Arterial blood supply of the ureter.

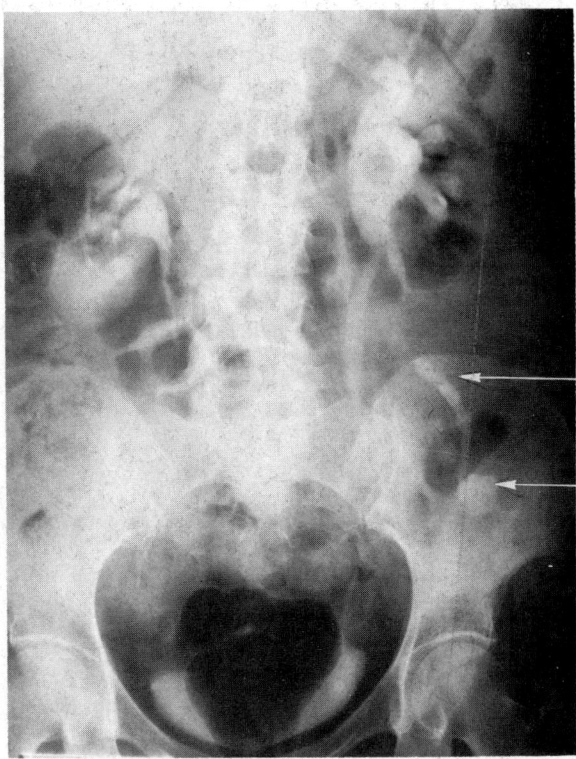

Figure 2–4. Intravenous pyelogram revealing urine extravasation into the colon (*upper arrow*) and to the skin (*lower arrow*), following suture ligation of the ovarian vascular plexus during an ovarian cystectomy.

lymph node surgery, where ligatures to control bleeding can be placed too close to the ureter. Under such circumstances ureteral peristalsis may be inhibited, leading to obstruction (Figure 2–4).

As the ureter courses over the pelvic brim the nutrient vessels arise from the internal iliac and superior vesical arteries. The ureter passes medial deep to the obliterated umbilical artery and the uterine artery. These arteries fix the free movement of the distal ureter, thus accounting for the entrapment injuries associated with mass ligation of the uterine vascular pedicle. The ureter then courses medially into the vesical hiatus.

Several small perforating vessels are seen in the lateral aspect of the muscular portion of the ureteral tunnel. Additional vessels enter into the submucosa from lateral and medial plexuses. Again the ureter is relatively fixed in position in this hiatus, but there is some free movement with peristalsis toward the bladder lumen in systole and with relaxation in the opposite direction in diastole.

Anatomic Variations. The ureteral blood supply may have considerable variation. In particular there may be a paucity of nutrient vessels in the upper and middle thirds. These anatomic variations are of practical significance when large segments of the pelvic ureter are skeletonized, as occurs during the removal of large uterine or ovarian masses. This skeletonization causes ureteral devascularization.

An "adding of insult to injury" can result from the placement of large rubber ureteral catheters within the ureter. Such catheters distend the lumen of the ureter and stretch the small intramural vessels, resulting in impaired blood flow. Edema arising from surgery may further compromise ureteral blood supply, leading to necrosis. Small polyethylene feeding tubes (No. 5 French) provide the least embarrassment of ureteral blood supply while diverting urine flow adequately.

Special Considerations

Two special anatomic variations that are of clinical concern are ureteral duplication and the ectopic ureteral orifice.

Ureteral Duplication. Duplicated or double ureters lie within a common vascular

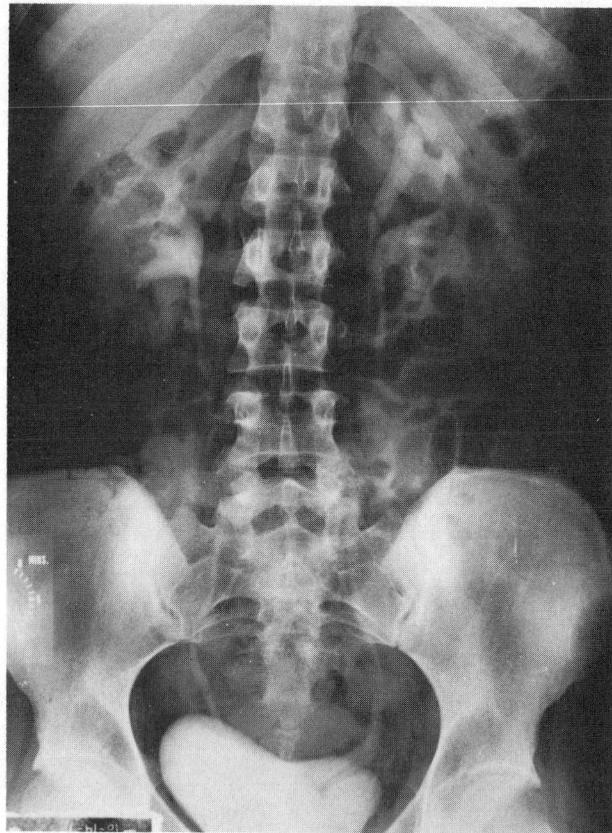

Figure 2–5. Intravenous pyelogram demonstrating a duplex left ureter entering the bladder in a common sheath. This patient has had a uretero-neocystostomy on the left, correcting both ureteral reflux and a ureterocele.

sheath and entwine around each other as they course from the renal pelvis to the vesical hiatus. At the level of the uterine artery this common sheath becomes a more prominent investing fascia, with more intimate fixation of the ureter and its blood supply (Figure 2–5). Ureteral separation during dissection at this level may lead to devascularization.

Following the Meyer-Weigert law, the more medial and distal ureteral orifice in the bladder drains the superior segment of the kidney. The more lateral and proximal ureteral orifice drains urine from the inferior renal segment. Vesicoureteral reflux is demonstrated more commonly in the inferior segment of such a duplex collecting system, since the submucosal tunnel in this segment is shorter. If one of the duplicated ureters becomes dilated, a disproportionate elongation also occurs. This elongation is limited by the nutrient vessels supplying the ureter. If the dilated ureter is not visualized on urography, the "normal" ureter may appear scalloped.

Ectopic Ureteral Orifice. The ectopic ureter maintains the orientation of spiral smooth muscle bundles until reaching the trigone. The portion of ureter coursing deep to the trigone into the vagina, urethra, or introitus maintains only a haphazard array of smooth muscle bundles, and thus may appear irregular on contrast studies (Figure 2–6). Radiographic studies reveal a variously distensible tubular structure that may passively transport urine or become obstructive, producing dilatation in the proximal portion of the ureter. Because of its terminus distal to normal sphincteric mechanisms, the ectopic ureter presents clinically as continual incontinence (Figure 2–7). Attempts to remove the ectopic ureter distal to the trigone can cause neuromuscular damage to the bladder or urethra, or both. Such extensive dissection is seldom justified, since ipsilateral ureteroureterostomy can resolve the patient's incontinence.

Other Anatomic Variations. Anatomic distortion occurs when adjacent structures

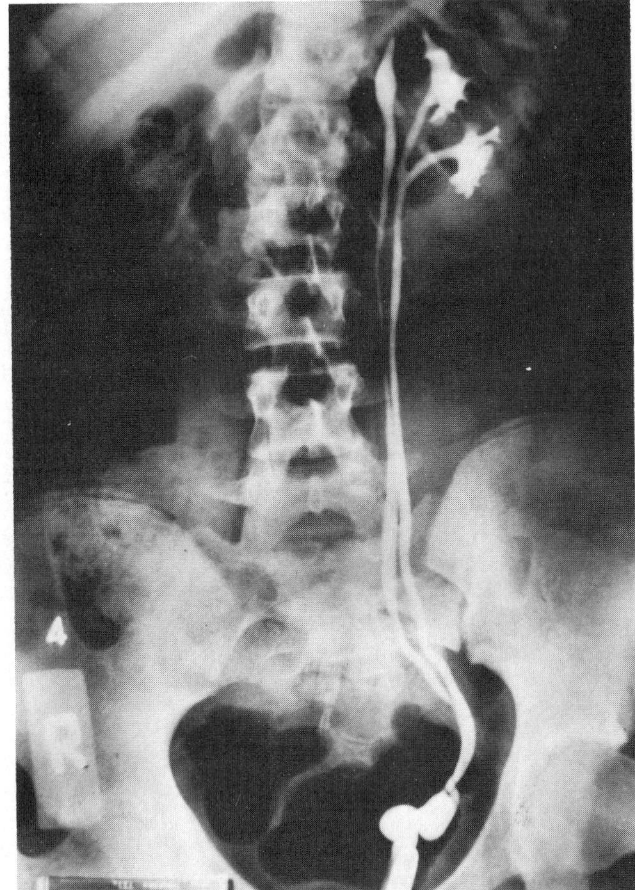

Figure 2–6. Retrograde pyelogram demonstrating the dilated distal portion of an ectopic ureter coursing under the trigone. The ureteral common sheath in the true pelvis is also evident. The ectopic ureter drains the much smaller superior renal segment.

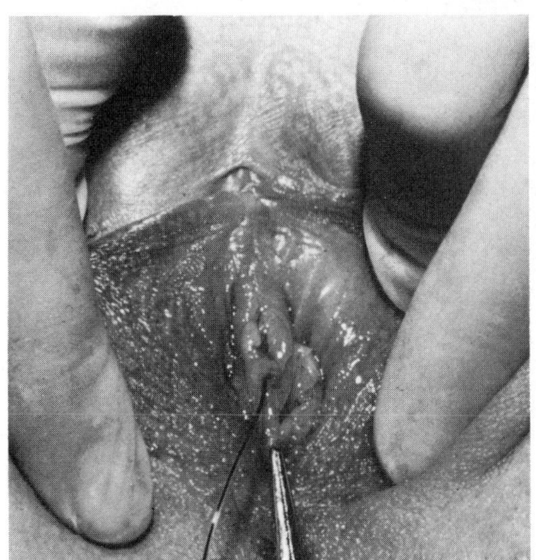

Figure 2–7. A left upper pole ectopic ureter, emptying into the vestibule at the urethral meatus level, catheterized with a polyethylene feeding tube filled with indigo carmine.

enlarge, displacing the ureter laterally against the pelvic wall. A variety of pathologic processes involving pelvic lymph nodes displace the ureter medially. Similarly, as the endopelvic fascia (cardinal ligaments and the urethrovaginal septum) elongates and thins from age or multiparity, the pelvic ureter elongates laterally and develops a J-shaped deformity. Any anatomic distortion thus can increase the risk of surgical injury to the ureter.

THE URINARY BLADDER

The female bladder maintains a roughly crescent shape owing to posterior uterine "compression." As the bladder distends with urine, the basketweave interdigitation of smooth muscle fascicles allows for a more ovoid shape. The relatively immobile trigone participates only to a limited degree, forming the bladder base overlying the cervix uteri.

Bladder Musculature

The trigonal musculature decussates across the midline, forming the more or less prominent interureteric ridge (Figure 2–8). Additional long fascicles of smooth muscle course from the ureter in its submucosal tunnel along the lateral border of the trigone, inserting into the distal third of the urethra (Wesson, 1920; Woodburne, 1967). These longitudinal fascicles open the bladder neck and shorten the urethra during voiding. Their contraction funnels the bladder neck and decreases urethral resistance, allowing urine outflow in a lamellar stream.

Coursing deep to the superficial trigone is a U-shaped bundle of smooth muscle cells described by Wesson (1920) and Woodburne (1967) and illustrated by Brodel (Kelly, 1922). This muscle bundle courses from a posterolateral position around the bladder neck anteriorly and then inserts posterolaterally again. The fascicles do not form a true circle, but do compress the urethra against the urethrovaginal septum, forming a portion of the continence mechanism. Functional proof of internal sphincter integrity is obtained by pudendal block, which paralyzes the external sphincter while allowing the internal bladder neck smooth muscle to maintain continence of urine. The patient may still void on request but cannot start or stop urine flow as precisely as before the pudendal block. The neural innervation to the blad-

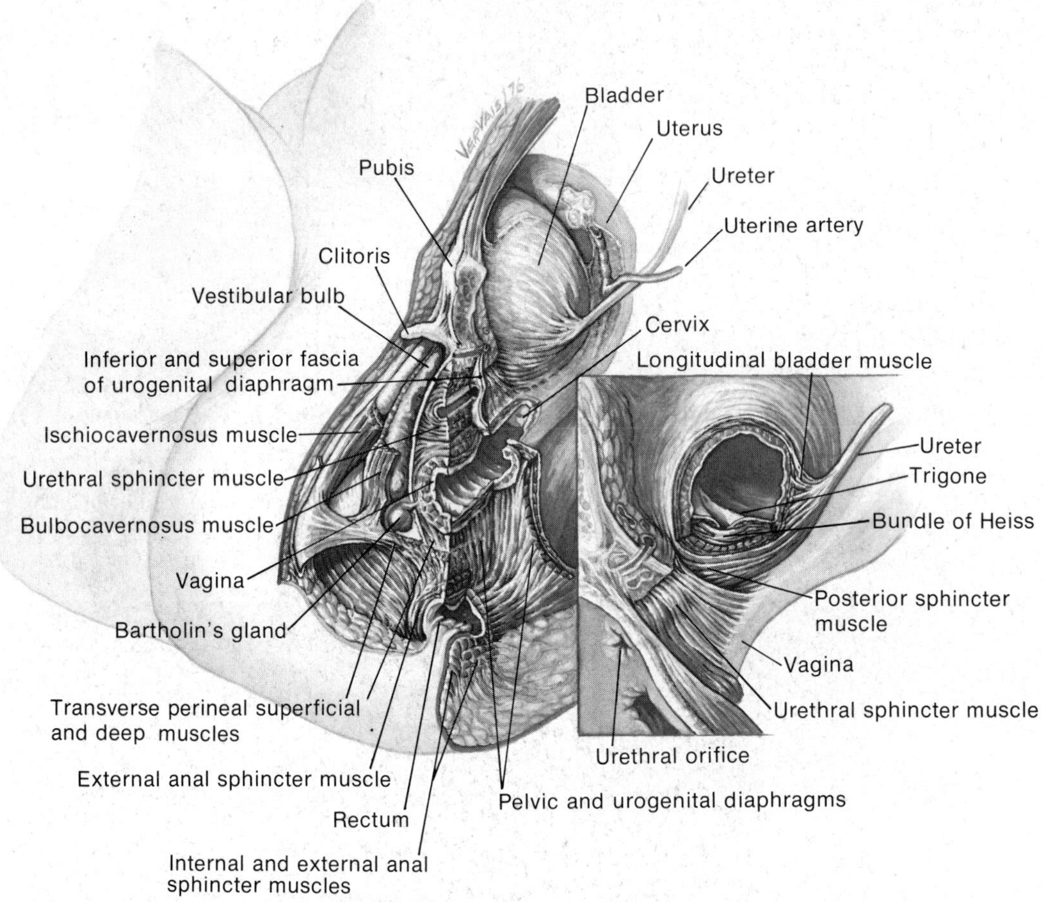

Figure 2–8. The relationship of bladder to vagina and uterine body, sagittal view.

der accompanies the vascular supply. Consequently, extensive dissection around the bladder base may cause denervation, resulting in a neurogenic bladder.

Mucosal Lining

The bladder musculature is surrounded by a loose areolar connective tissue and is lined by a transitional cell mucosa. The transitional cells, which are usually three layers in thickness, possess a corrugated cell membrane. Upon distention, the corrugations flatten out, allowing the remarkable distensibility of the vesical reservoir without significant mucosal permeability.

Related Anatomy

The infant bladder maintains an intra-abdominal position and thus has a larger peritoneal surface than does the adult bladder. The peritoneal reflection over the bladder may extend down to the junction of the bladder with the distal one third of the uterine body. The bladder is separated from the uterus by an avascular plane of connective tissue that extends distally into the urethrovaginal septum. This plane extends laterally from the midline to the four and eight o'clock positions, at which level vascular, lymphatic, and neural structures enter the bladder wall. Surgical manipulations in this midline plane represent little hazard to the bladder. Unilateral manipulations of the neurovascular pedicle are also relatively safe, since the bladder has lush anastomotic vascular channels in its adventitia, muscularis, and submucosa. Multiple or sequential operative distortion of neurovascular structures, however, may impair bladder neurologic function (Chapter 10).

Blood Supply

The obliterated umbilical artery is the first anterior branch from the internal iliac artery and courses medially over the lateral wall of the bladder. Since the infant bladder extends intra-abdominally, a distinct lateral indentation on cystography represents the obliterated umbilical artery. Just caudad to this structure, the superior vesical artery courses anterior to the ureter; progressing inferiorly, the middle and inferior vesical branches enter the bladder wall. The inferior vesical artery gives off branches supplying the upper third of the urethra.

Surrounding the vesical arteries is a broad sheath of veins. The endopelvic fascia covers these vessels anteriorly and posteriorly. This lateral fibrovascular pedicle

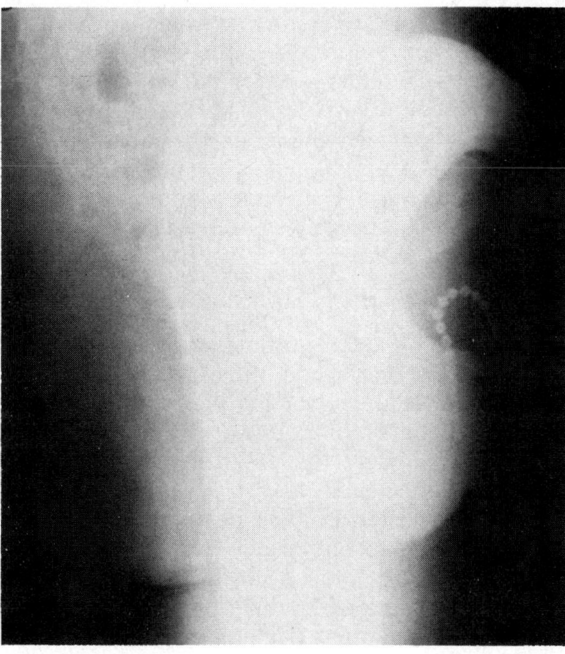

Figure 2–9. Beadchain cystogram demonstrating marked bladder descensus through the introitus from anterior vaginal prolapse.

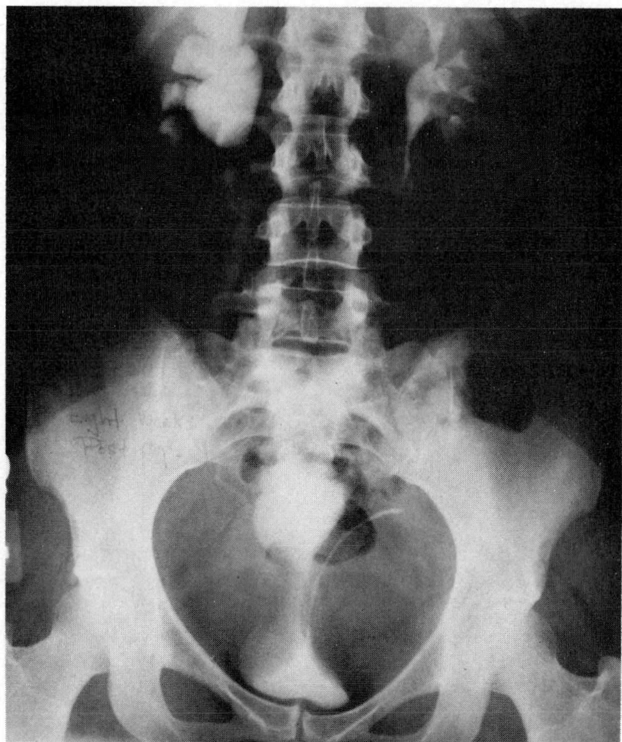

Figure 2–10. Intravenous pyelogram demonstrating bilateral lymphoceles resulting from a radical hysterectomy. The medial displacement occurs as the ureter enters the true pelvis, coursing distally into the goblet-shaped bladder.

supports the bladder in its anterior position and allows cephalad distention into the abdominal cavity.

Vascular compromise from surgical trauma is frequent, since anastomoses from the pudendal artery and the middle vaginal artery supplying the urethra provide vesical perfusion (see Figure 2–1). These vessels account for the failure of internal pudendal ligation to control vesical hemorrhage. Anastomoses between the internal pudendal and vaginal artery branches via the hemorrhoidal vessels also provide blood flow to the bladder.

Anatomic Variation and Distortion

Anatomic bladder variations are rare. Occasionally, unsuspected urachal prolongation may lead to bladder injury during anterior abdominal incisions.

During delivery, the endopelvic fascia becomes thinned out, allowing descent of the bladder posteriorly and inferiorly (Figure 2–9). As relaxation occurs, the vascular pedicles and ureters elongate. Such distortion can lead to bladder injury during corrective pelvic surgery. Extensive perivesical lymphatic disruption resulting in a lymphocele may displace the bladder and ureters medially (Figure 2–10).

THE URETHRA

The normal urethra, 3 to 5 cm. in length, develops a roughly conical shape during voiding. This cone is broader at the bladder neck than at the external meatus. Urethral caliber at the bladder neck may approach 35 French, while the external meatus may measure 26 to 30 French in adult patients. In the nondistended state, the mucosa and submucosa are thrown into circumferential corrugated folds. These folds are supported by elastic connective tissue, which increase urethral resistance in the resting state, thus contributing to continence. During voiding the flow pattern is lamellar, but it can be distorted by a fibrous ring in the middle third of the urethra or by stenosis at the external meatus. Since bacteria colonize the distal half of the urethra, irregular flow patterns caused by urethral stenosis enhance retrograde bacterial migration into the bladder.

Anatomic Function of the Bladder Sphincter Mechanism

The continence mechanisms of the detrusor, trigone, and urethra were investigated by Kelly (1922), Wesson (1920), and Woodburne (1960). The anatomic integrity of bladder function implies intact neurologic sensory and motor arcs modified by spinothalamic tracts and cerebral control. For comprehensive detail about neurogenic dysfunction, the reader should consult Chapter 23.

Urinary Incontinence. Anatomically the sphincter mechanism consists of a smooth muscle internal sphincter coursing around the bladder neck deep to the superficial trigone. The muscle bundles surround the bladder laterally and anteriorly, compressing the proximal urethra against the urethrovaginal septum much as a horse's bridle girds the jaw and neck of the animal. The second region governing urinary continence is maintained by the elastic tissue urethra that supports the intrinsic length of the proximal two thirds of the urethra. The resistance to outflow through the rugated tube is sustained by the circular elastic tissue. The external sphincter, which is striated voluntary muscle, surrounds the urethra in its middle third. Anatomic dissections demonstrate insertion of these striated fibers into the urethrovaginal septum, and some fibers condense around the urethra as high as the bladder neck in a roughly triangular fashion. The triangular muscle tissue rests its base on the genitourinary diaphragm and courses around the urethra anteriorly and laterally. When the striated muscle is voluntarily activated, the midportion is compressed against the urethrovaginal septum. The distal third of the urethra does not participate in continence mechanisms.

Functional bladder control represents a balance between these resistance factors and the intrinsic tone of the bladder detrusor mechanism. This dynamic process varies during the phase of bladder filling. Resistance is maintained against progressively increasing bladder tone measured as 10 to 25 cm. of water pressure. Factors of cerebral inhibition may vary the pressure relationships, but as capacity (400 to 450 ml) is reached, the mechanisms of voiding ensue.

Anatomic Mechanisms of Voiding. Stretch receptors within the superficial trigone stimulate the motor contraction of its smooth muscle. The superficial trigone originates as longitudinal smooth muscle bundles as the ureteral orifice empties into the bladder. A portion of these bundles decussates medially, forming the interureteric ridge. The lateral longitudinal fibers spread through the bladder neck and insert in the region of the genitourinary diaphragm in the middle third of the urethra. Contraction of the superficial trigone opens the internal sphincter and shortens the urethral length. During the longitudinal contraction, the ureteral orifice migrates medially toward the bladder neck, thus effectively elongating the submucosal tunnel of the ureter. The increased tunnel length protects the kidney from ureteral reflux during periods of augmented intravesical pressures associated with voiding. As the bladder neck opens, the contraction phase of detrusor activity accelerates, rising to 40 to 60 cm. of water pressure. Finally, the external striated sphincter, which has initiated tonus at the beginning of this sequence of voiding events, relaxes, and urine flow is directed through the passive distal third of the urethra. This urethral segment directs urine flow away from the perineum. Cinecystograms in prepubertal girls with an intact hymeneal ring demonstrate vaginal reflux of urine during voiding. This anatomic phenomenon accounts for the finding of micropyuria and bacteriuria in some voided urine specimens.

Upon completion of the voiding act, tonus returns to the external sphincter, stopping urine flow. The superficial trigone relaxes and the elastic tissue collapses the urethral lumen upon itself from the genitourinary diaphragm ascending to the bladder neck. Contraction of the internal sphincter closes the bladder neck. Finally, the detrusor muscle relaxes, returning to intravesical resting pressures of 0 to 5 cm. of water. Should a woman arise quickly following voiding prior to detrusor relaxation, she may lose a few drops of urine. A simple explanation of anatomic functional dynamics or Kegel exercises resolve the problem.

Anatomic Variation and Distortion. Occasionally a patient with incomplete formation of a urethrovaginal septum, the so-called female hypospadias, is observed. Characteristically, the patient has a lifelong history of stress incontinence, and physical examination reveals a conal urethra based on the perineum. Electromyography demonstrates striated muscle activity anteriorly, but contractile activity is ineffective, since there is no insertion into the urethrovaginal septum. Urethral resistance is not effective, and urinary control depends upon internal sphincter control alone.

Persons with neurogenic dysfunction from meningomyelocele may have impaired internal sphincter closure or external sphincter paralysis. The urinary control that they have is related to the fibroelastic resistance of the urethra. Fortunately, modern pharmaceutics may resolve internal sphincter incompetence and detrusor hyperactivity, granting continence to the patient.

Patients who suffer from cystocele have progressive dilatation of the bladder neck, since descensus of the trigone pulls the bladder neck open. The resulting shortening of the urethra impairs elastic tissue closure of the urethra, resulting in stress incontinence. Resupport of the urethrovesical angle or bladder neck position allows return of urinary control.

Paraurethral Glands

The paraurethral adnexal glands enter the urethral lumen at multiple levels and are developed to varying degrees. The paraurethral Skene's glands lie at five and seven o'clock positions along the urethra. Their acini extend into the urethrovaginal septum toward the bladder neck.

Blood Supply

The urethral vasculature is divided into three segments, extending toward the urethral orifice in the five and seven o'clock positions. At the bladder neck, branches of the inferior vesical artery perfuse the upper third of the urethra. The middle third receives supply from the middle vaginal artery and the distal third from branches of the pudendal artery. Anastomotic branches occur between all segments. Venous outflow is located throughout the periurethral plexus, which communicates with the perivesical system.

THE OVARY

The special anatomic considerations of the ovary are related to its position in the true pelvis and its close proximity to the ureter. The ovary is supported on a freely movable mesovarian pedicle that follows the ureter, coursing in the retroperitoneal space. On the right, the ovarian vessels are outlined by a prominent mesentery as they course over the ureter at the pelvic brim. A thrombosed ovarian vein or a hypertrophied vessel after multiple pregnancies may be mistaken for a ureter. The observation of peristalsis, occurring spontaneously or on gentle stimulation, usually will identify the ureter; however, previous surgery or retroperitoneal inflammation may diminish the effectiveness of this test. On the left pelvic wall, the ureteral and ovarian vessel relationships are obscured by the sigmoid mesentery. Disease in the ovary, ureter, or sigmoid colon may increase the risk of surgical trauma to one or more of these structures.

Expanding lesions within the ovary may incorporate the ureter into its common wall. This usually displaces the ureter laterally. Inflammatory lesions that dissect into the infundibulopelvic ligaments may fix the ureter, making it more susceptible to injury (see Figure 2–4). The fallopian tubes course from the uterine body laterally and posteriorly, surrounding the ovary superiorly and laterally. The visceral peritoneal surfaces of the ovary allow relatively free movement in the true pelvis, thus involving the relatively fixed retroperitoneal structures to a limited degree.

THE UTERUS

The laterally placed broad and round ligaments course medially and support the uterine body. The broad ligament provides the lateral support of the uterus. A posterior condensation of two layers of peritoneum overlying the ovarian vessels represents the mesovarium. The cephalic margin surrounds the fallopian tube as it courses laterally, surrounding the ovary. At its lateral margin, the fimbriated end of the oviduct drapes over the lateral margin of the ovary.

Coursing from its inguinal ligament condensation, the round ligament blends over the anterior surface of the broad ligament. The broad ligament thickens as it approaches the pelvic floor and the supravaginal portion of the cervix. The ureter courses obliquely from a lateral-posterior position to its anterior-medial hiatus in the bladder. The uterine arteries course anterior to the ureter. The deeper extension of the parametrium becomes the anterior and posterior leaves of the cardinal ligaments surrounding the vagina. The round ligament courses out through the canal of Nuck. This area is of significance in that an inguinal hernia may suggest the diagnosis of female intersexuality.

The helically arranged smooth muscle of the uterine body maintains considerable flexibility in the anteroposterior plane. The cervix, surrounded by the cardinal ligaments, which course anteriorly and posteriorly, maintains a more fixed position. The peritoneal reflection extends down over the posterior bladder wall onto the lower uterine segment. Laterally, the lush plexi of uterine arteries anastomose with the more cephalad ovarian vessels. Those vessels lie superficial (anterior) to the ureter, which courses from a lateral position at the level of the lower uterine segment and cervix to insert into the vesical hiatus. The firm fascial attachments of the uterus account for the frequent distortion of the bladder in uterine disease.

The uterine body and cervix maintain a fixed intrapelvic relationship to the bladder base and trigone. The plane of dissection between the bladder and uterus can be developed relatively simply in some situations, e.g., low cervical cesarean section; conversely, cystocele formation may thin out layers, making fascial planes undefinable. Intrauterine masses such as fibromyomas may indent the posterolateral bladder wall, causing intravesical filling defects.

Lymphatics

The lymphatics draining the uterine cervix and body have special significance as they course laterally around the uterine vessels and surround the ureter. This intimate relationship of entwining lymph vessels and the obliquely coursing ureter accounts for the high incidence of ureteral obstruction by direct extension and nodal metastases in cervical neoplasia. Postoperative lymph collections also may distort the ureter and bladder.

THE VAGINA

The proximity of the vagina to three major portions of the urinary tract accounts for its involvement in many pathologic processes affecting the latter. The urethra, bladder trigone, and distal ureters are all supported by the relatively nondistensible anterior vaginal wall. The distal ureteral segments cross obliquely just anterior to the lateral fornices of the vagina as they surround the cervix. In fact, a distal ureteral calculus may be palpable through the vagina and be potentially removable via this route. Occasionally, vaginal repair sutures placed after hysterectomy may distort or incorporate a portion of the periureteral fascia, resulting in a ureterovaginal fistula.

The trigone overlies the cervix and upper one third of the vaginal wall, representing a fixed lateral plane in the pelvis because of the pelvic cardinal ligaments. Because of this fixed position, surgical manipulation of the uterine body and cervix may be associated with neurologic injury to the bladder. The replacement fibrosis occurring when uterine or cervical neoplasia is treated with radiation also affects the adjacent trigone, resulting in necrosis and vesicovaginal fistula.

In multiparous individuals, the cardinal ligaments and anterior vaginal wall musculature may be attenuated and thinned, resulting in bladder descent into the vagina. Trigonal displacement may be so severe that intra-abdominal pressure during voiding is directed against the posterior bladder wall instead of the urethra, resulting in residual urine. These features suggest an anatomic cause for the recurring urinary infections observed in women with cystocele.

The urethra is supported by the condensation of the cardinal ligaments and the anterior vaginal wall musculature, which form a fixed plane, allowing sphincteric function (see Figure 2–8). The internal sling of smooth muscle at the bladder neck must contract against this plane, providing adequate bladder neck closure for continence. The bandana-like external sphincter also contracts against the urethrovaginal septum, providing urinary control. The length of the anterior vaginal wall may contribute in part to urethral length and represents the third factor influencing urinary control. Thinning and relaxation of the anterior vaginal wall result in incontinence, varying from occurring only on stress to total.

REFERENCES

Anderson, E. E., and Harrison, J. H.: Surgical importance of the solitary kidney. N. Engl. J. Med. *273*:683, 1965.

Brenner, B. M., and Rector, F. C.: The Kidney. 2nd Ed. Philadelphia, W. B. Saunders Co., 1981.

Flocks, R. H., and Boldus, R.: The surgical treatment and prevention of urinary incontinence associated with disturbances of the internal urethral sphincteric mechanism. J. Urol. *109*:279, 1973.

Goss, C. M.: Gray's Anatomy. 29th American Ed. Philadelphia, Lea and Febiger, 1973.

Wesson, M. B.: Anatomical, embryological and physiological studies of the trigone and neck of the bladder. J. Urol. *4*:279, 1920.

Woodburne, R. T.: Structure and function of the urinary bladder. J. Urol., *84*:79, 1960.

Woodburne, R. T.: Anatomy of the urinary system. *In* Ureteral Reflux in Children. Washington, D.C., National Academy of Sciences, 1967, pp. 67–87.

3

PHYSIOLOGY OF MICTURITION

JACK LAPIDES, M.D.
ANANIAS C. DIOKNO, M.D.

Although most individuals visualize the urinary bladder as a ball-shaped organ, its configuration is (when it is distended with urine) actually that of a round-bottomed flask composed of a spherical portion called the fundus and a cylindrical part commonly known as the posterior urethra (Figure 3–1). In the young adult, the posterior urethra is approximately 3.0 cm. long. The male posterior urethra includes the prostatic and membranous portions, whereas in the female, it is the proximal three fourths of the entire urethral length (Figure 3–2).

PHYSIOLOGIC ASPECTS OF BLADDER ANATOMY

The fundus and posterior urethra should be considered as one unit both anatomically and functionally (Lapides, 1958; Woodburne, 1960). Embryologically, both are derived from the vesicourethral sac of the urogenital sinus and both possess smooth muscle and elastic tissue in their walls. Parasympathetic fibers coursing in the pelvic nerve supply identical motor impulses to the fundus and urethra. The smooth muscle of the bladder can be considered as a sheet of muscle in the form of a reticulum, or webwork, that extends without interruption down into the urethra as the muscular wall. There is a particularly heavy concentration of elastic connective tissue fibers in the wall of the urethra (Figure 3–3).

This bladder unit, consisting of a sphere and a cylinder, has certain intrinsic properties completely independent of any nervous regulation from the central nervous system. As stated previously, the smooth muscle and elastic tissue exert continuous tension in an autonomous fashion and with a negli-

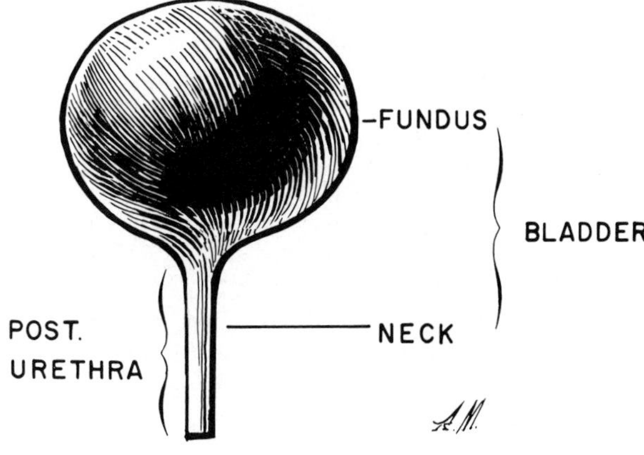

Figure 3–1. The urinary bladder is shaped like a round-bottomed flask.

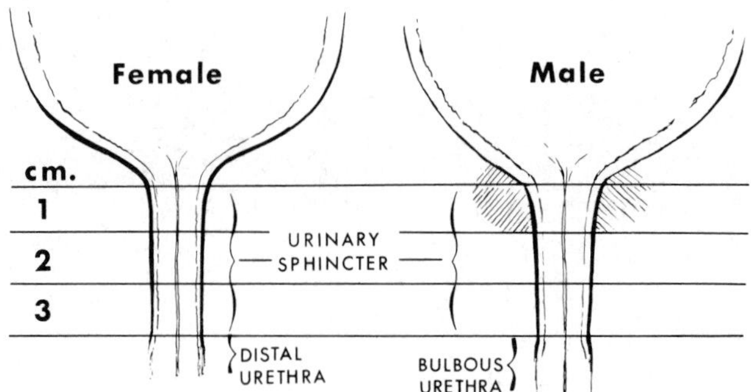

Figure 3–2. The urinary sphincter in both the young adult male and the female is the proximal 3 cm. of the posterior urethra. (From Lapides, J.: Fundamentals of Urology. Philadelphia, W. B. Saunders Co., 1976.)

gible expenditure of energy. When the bladder fundus is distended with fluid, the smooth muscle fibers of the bladder wall are first stretched and caused in turn to contract and increase their tension. Thus, measurement of intravesical pressure will demonstrate an initial increase on filling of the bladder with fluid, but then, as filling continues, the intravesical pressure will remain approximately constant until bladder capacity is reached (Figure 3–4). At capacity, the intravesical pressure will start to rise sharply in the form of a straight-line relationship.

The ability of the bladder fundus to maintain a relatively low intravesical pressure with distention is due to its vesicoelastic properties and is called accommodation. Accommodation serves an important function in that it permits the ureters to pump urine into the bladder without excessive effort. The sharp rise in pressure at capacity is believed to be caused by stretching of connective tissue in the bladder wall.

Urine present in the bladder fundus is prevented from leaking out through the urethra by the proximal 3.0 cm. of urethra or tubular part of the bladder unit. The urethra accomplishes this by virtue of the continuous intrinsic autonomous tension exerted by the smooth muscle and connective tissue in its wall. These tissues keep the urethra compressed so that its lumen is sufficiently obliterated to prevent urine from flowing out of the bladder fundus under low or moderate pressures.

Periurethral Striated Muscle

When high intravesical pressures occur as a result of increased intra-abdominal pressure, such as in coughing, straining, or exercising, urinary incontinence would ensue if only the proximal urethra or uri-

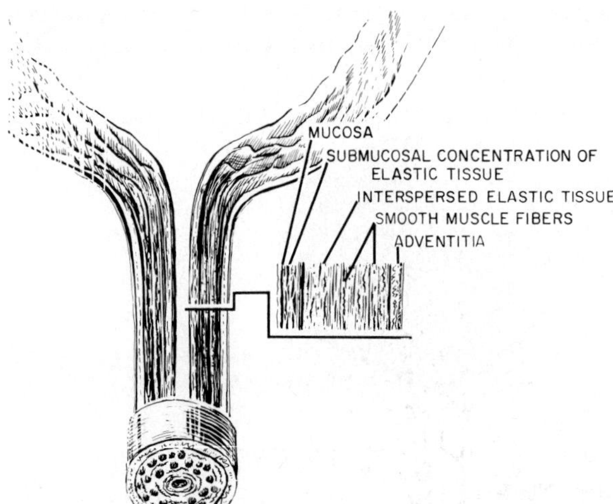

Figure 3–3. The urinary sphincter, or posterior urethral wall, has a particularly heavy concentration of elastic fibers in the submucosal layer and interspersed among the smooth muscle fibers. (From Lapides, J.: Fundamentals of Urology. Philadelphia, W. B. Saunders Co., 1976.)

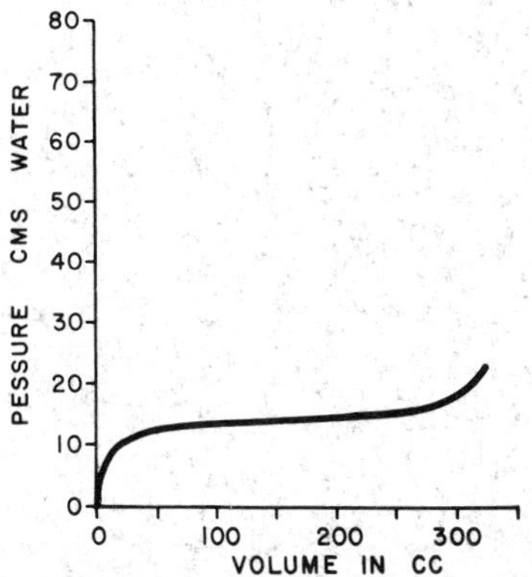

Figure 3–4. Intravesical pressure. When the bladder is filling with urine, the intravesical pressure remains constant until bladder capacity is reached. Distending the bladder beyond capacity results in a marked increase in intravesical pressure. (From Lapides, J.: Fundamentals of Urology. Philadelphia, W. B. Saunders Co., 1976.)

nary sphincter per se existed to stop it. Under conditions of high intravesical pressure, the efficiency of the urinary sphincter must be enhanced to maintain continence. This feat is accomplished with the aid of the voluntary striated muscle surrounding the posterior urethra.

The muscle of the urogenital diaphragm and the levator ani muscle surround the urethra and are in contact with it for about 2.0 cm. In the female, it is the middle 2.0 cm. of urethra that is contiguous with the periurethral striated muscle (Figure 3–5). These muscles increase the efficiency of the urinary sphincter by compressing the urethra circumferentially and elongating it by pulling it cephalad. The striated muscle can act either on a voluntary basis or reflexly: The urethra can be compressed in a conscious act to prevent urinary incontinence when the bladder is full and there is an urgent desire to urinate. The muscle also can contract reflexly to compress and elongate the urinary sphincter, as in conditions of increased intra-abdominal pressure such as coughing and straining, when the erect posture is assumed, and in filling of the bladder (Figure 3–6).

The striated muscle is supplied by motor fibers emanating from motor neurons in the ventral horn of the upper sacral segments and carried in the pudendal nerve. It is important to note that the urinary sphincter is the intact urethra and that the striated muscles surrounding the urethra are of

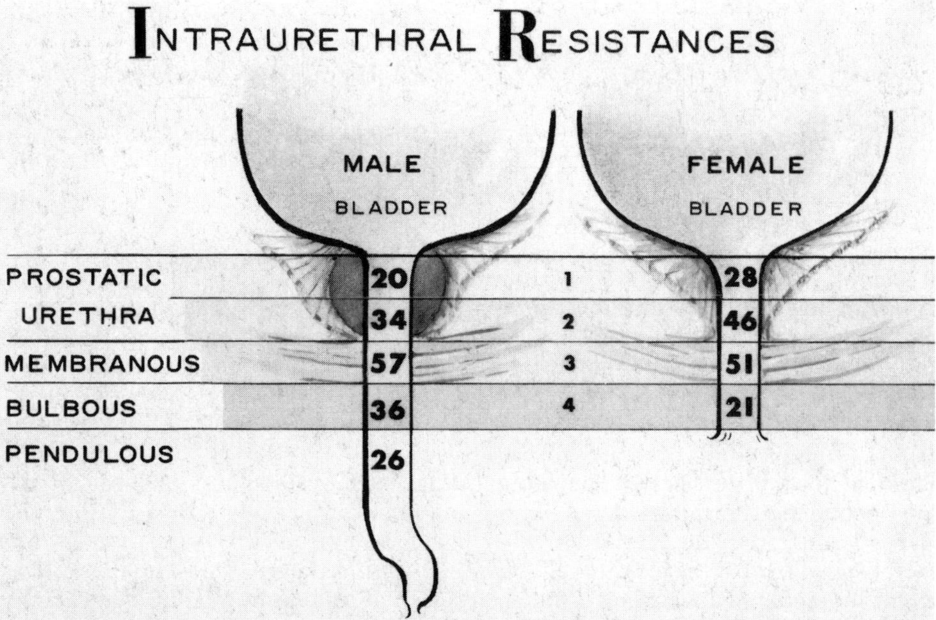

Figure 3–5. The periurethral striated muscle (levator ani and muscle of the urogenital diaphragm) is contiguous with the middle 2 cm. of the female urethra and its counterpart in the male—the distal part of the prostate and membranous portions of urethra. (From Lapides, J.: Fundamentals of Urology. Philadelphia, W. B. Saunders Co., 1976.)

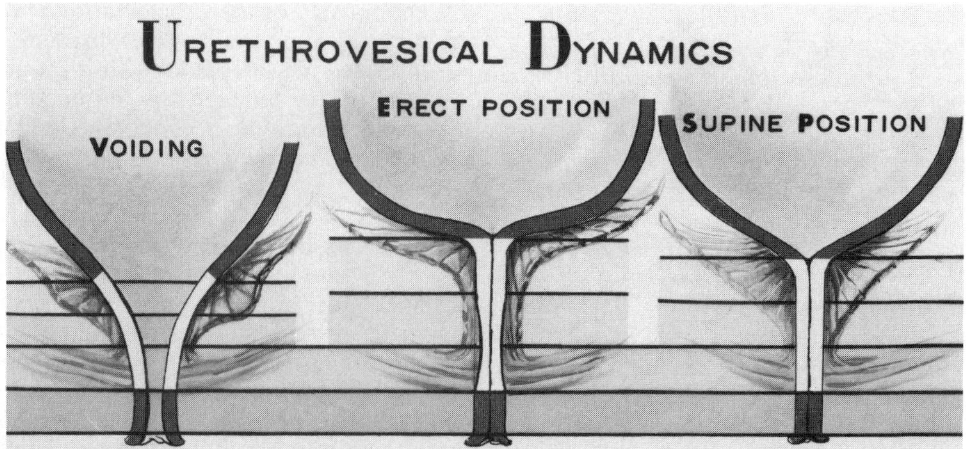

Figure 3–6. When the patient assumes the erect position or contracts the periurethral striated muscle, the urethra is elongated and compressed. During micturition the periurethral striated muscle is relaxed. In addition, the urethrovesical junction is pulled open into a funnel-shaped structure by active contraction of the vesicourethral smooth muscle sheet. The net result is a functional shortening and widening of the posterior urethra. (From Lapides, J.: Fundamentals of Urology. Philadelphia, W. B. Saunders Co., 1976.)

secondary importance in that they can increase the efficiency of the urinary sphincter but cannot substitute for it. The striated muscles serve also to interrupt urination rapidly (1 to 2 seconds) when there is an urgent need by compressing and elongating the urinary sphincter until the vesical smooth muscle stops contracting (10 to 20 seconds).

NEUROPHYSIOLOGY

Innervation of the Bladder

The basic bladder unit can store urine under moderate pressure autonomously, but it cannot evacuate its contents without the aid of motor impulses from the central nervous system. The bladder (fundus and urethra) is supplied by sensory and motor fibers. The afferent fibers carry pain, temperature, and proprioceptive (desire to void and fullness) sensations and are located primarily in the pelvic nerve. The motor neurons supplying the musculature of the bladder are situated in the lateral horns of the sacral spinal cord at the levels of S2, S3, and S4. The motor fibers extend from the motor neuron to the wall of the bladder and posterior urethra, where ganglionic synapses and postganglionic fibers are situated. The motor pathways are parasympathetic in nature and also form part of the pelvic nerve (Figure 3–7) (Bradley et al., 1974).

Bradley and co-workers (1974) and DeGroat (1975) suggest that the normal micturition reflex arc is supraspinal in nature, with the supraspinal reflex neuron being located in the pontine mesencephalic area. DeGroat (1975) believes that impulses travel through the pelvic afferent nerves and ascending pathways to the brain stem and then descend to synapse with parasympathetic neurons at the sacral cord level. This may help to explain the various abnormally functioning bladders occurring with spinal transection.

Initiation of Micturition

In the infant, micturition occurs in an uncontrolled fashion, by virtue of a simple spinal reflex arc synapsing in the sacral spinal cord. The limbs of the reflex arc were described previously. Although the motor side of the reflex is part of the autonomic nervous system and has ganglionic synapses, for purposes of clarity the reflex arc can be considered to function in the same fashion as does the simple, skeletal segmental reflex arc. As the bladder fills with urine and is stretched, proprioceptive endings in the wall are stimulated to send sensory impulses to the sacral spinal cord. In the infant spinal cord, the motor neurons

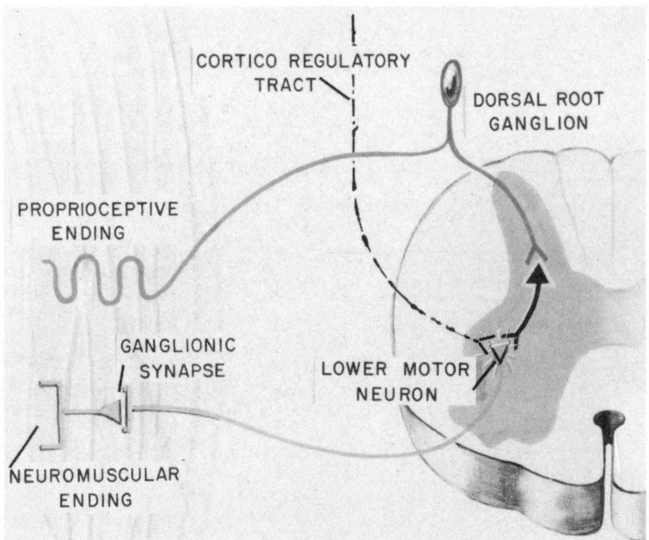

Figure 3–7. The spinal reflex arc concerned with micturition is found at the level of sacral spinal cord segments, 2, 3, and 4. (From Lapides, J.: Fundamentals of Urology. Philadelphia, W. B. Saunders Co., 1976.)

to the bladder are activated by the proprioceptive impulses, and motor impulses are transmitted to the bladder muscle to cause it to contract. With small volumes of urine, the bladder may exhibit several weak contractions without expelling any urine, but then with increased stretching a strong detrusor contraction will occur, with resultant emptying of the bladder.

Measurement of intravesical pressure during normal micturition indicates that pressures varying between 25 and 50 cm. of water obtain when the urinary stream is most forceful. Yet, when the bladder is at rest and storing urine, it may require intravesical pressures of greater than 150 to 250 cm. of water to overcome the resistance of the posterior urethra or urinary sphincter so that urinary flow occurs. We have already discussed the fact that the urinary sphincter maintains continence during stress by action of the periurethral striated muscle. During urination, it is preferable for intravesical pressures to be low since high pressures, as seen in obstructive uropathy, predispose to infection, dilatation of the urinary tract, and renal deterioration.

Function of the Urinary Sphincter

How does the urinary sphincter decrease its resistance during urination? The posterior urethra accomplishes this in a most simple fashion. First, there is relaxation of the periurethral striated muscle either reflexly or voluntarily. This results in some decrease in length of the urethra and tension of the urethral wall against its lumen. *A further decrease in length of the urethra and increase in caliber of the urethral lumen is effected by active contractions of the smooth muscle of the bladder and urethra.* When the bladder begins to contract down upon a volume of urine, the urethrovesical junction and proximal portion of the urinary sphincter are pulled open by active contraction of the muscle sheet that is continuous from bladder into posterior urethra (Figure 3–8). The urinary sphincter opens not by passive relaxation but by active contraction of the vesicourethral muscle fibers.

The urinary sphincter is a tube, not a ring, with its greatest resistance in the midposterior urethra and its least resistance at the vesical outlet or urethrovesical junction. It can readily be discerned that any pathologic entity that prevents a widening of the urethral lumen, a shortening of the urethra, and a decrease in tension of the urethral walls against the lumen during initiation of urination will lead to the complications of obstructive uropathy just as certainly as will an obstructing neoplasm, occluding calculus, or pinpoint stricture. A urethrovesical junction that appears quite adequate on urethroscopy during the stor-

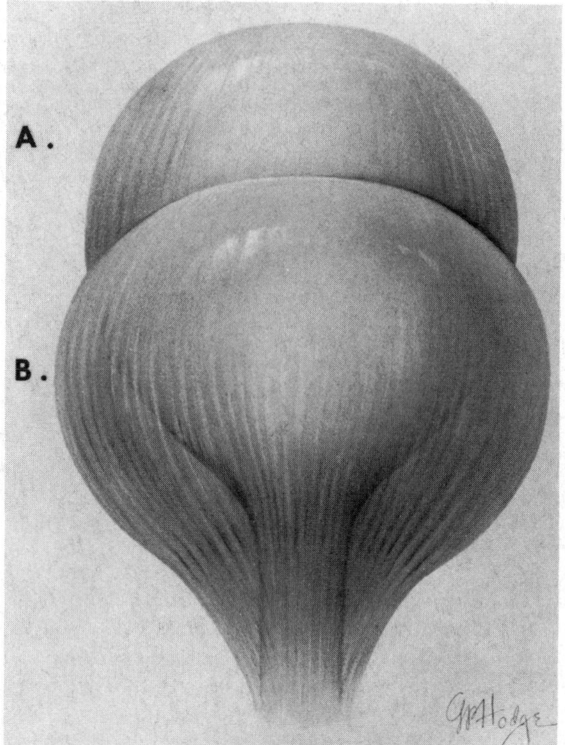

Figure 3–8. When the detrusor muscle contracts down upon a volume of urine, the urethrovesical junction is pulled open by the muscle sheet, and the vesicourethral configuration changes from a flask with a long, narrow neck (*A*) to a squat bottle with a short, wide neck (*B*). (From Lapides, J.: Fundamentals of Urology. Philadelphia, W. B. Saunders Co., 1976.)

ing phase of the bladder may be entirely inadequate during micturition if a wide-caliber rigid ring is present at the urethrovesical junction. Such a stricture will prevent the pulling-open of the vesical outlet, shortening of the urethra, and increase in its caliber. Similarly, a bladder with involvement of its lower motor neurons, with a resultant inability to contract fully its muscle sheet, will be unable to open the urinary sphincter and permit voiding at low intravesical pressures.

Studies of the mechanics of the normal urinary sphincter in women (Lapides, 1960) reveal that the urinary sphincter or urethra is a mobile structure whose length varies with the type of activity. A young, nulliparous woman under spinal anesthesia may demonstrate a urethral length of 3.8 cm. If she is perfectly relaxed in the supine position, the urethral length will still be 3.8 cm. without anesthesia. Voluntary contraction of the levator ani muscles will lengthen the urethra to 4.3 cm. Reflex contraction of the levator ani, as in changing from the supine to the erect position, will also increase urethral length to 4.3 cm. The urethral length in 35 normal women without urinary incontinence varied from 3.0 to 4.5 cm., with an average of 3.8 cm. in both the supine and the standing positions.

It is interesting to note that intraurethral resistance to retrograde flow of urine is increased every time the urethra is lengthened; and the urethra is elongated when the periurethral striated muscles are stimulated to contract, as in coughing, straining, sneezing, and sudden voluntary interruption of urination.

Intravesical pressure in the normal individual varies also with the type of activity. In the supine position, the average intravesical pressure in the female is approximately 17 cm. of water. On standing, the pressure is increased to 32 cm., and on straining it is elevated to 60 cm. A portion of the intravesical pressure in the relaxed, supine position and the increases beyond that pressure observed on standing, straining, or coughing are due entirely to contraction of the striated muscle surrounding the body cavities.

When normal females cough or strain, a "beak" or infundibulum of urine from the bladder enters the proximal third of the urethra and then returns to the bladder after cessation of exertion. Apparently the urinary sphincter cannot keep the urine confined entirely to the fundus of the bladder when intravesical pressure is increased abruptly; urine is pushed through the lumen into a portion of the urethra.

At this point it should be emphasized that competence of the urinary sphincter can be impaired by an abnormality of the smooth muscle or elastic tissue of the urethral wall, as in excision or necrosis with replacement by fibrous tissue; by stretching of the musculofascial elements supporting the urethrovesical junction, as in the garden variety of stress incontinence; and by paralysis of periurethral striated muscles, as in myelomeningocele, herniated nucleus pulposus, and other sacral cord lesions.

Function of the Corticoregulatory and Other Sensory Tracts

The normal urinary sphincter can maintain continence in the infant between voidings, but it cannot inhibit reflex voiding contractions. Thus, the normal baby will not dribble urine continuously but will wet at intervals during forceful bladder contractions. Voluntary control of urination is gained, or the child becomes "house-broken," as soon as the corticoregulatory tract begins to function (Bradley et al., 1974). The corticoregulatory tract (Figure 3–9) runs from the motor cortex to the lower motor neurons. It can either stimulate the lower motor neurons to discharge motor impulses or inhibit the lower motor neurons from discharging in response to afferent impulses from the bladder and elsewhere. Thus, the individual having normal voluntary control can urinate with only a small volume of urine in the bladder because of the ability of the higher centers to stimulate the lower motor neurons. When there is a large volume of urine in the bladder, urination is accomplished by removing the inhibitory influence from the higher centers and permitting the lower motor neurons to become activated by proprioceptive impulses from the stretched bladder wall.

In addition to the descending corticoregulatory tract, there are sensory tracts ascending to the higher centers. Sensations of pain and temperature are carried to the brain via the lateral spinothalamic tracts, whereas proprioceptive sensation ascends by way of the posterior columns.

Function of the Sympathetic Nervous System

The exact function of the sympathetic or adrenergic system in urination is unknown at present (Lapides, 1974*b*). Studies have shown that alpha- and beta-adrenergic receptors are present in both bladder and urethra. The beta-adrenergic receptors are concentrated in the fundus, whereas the alpha-adrenergic receptors are most frequent in the trigone and urethra. When the presacral or hypogastric nerve is stimulated in the male, the urethrovesical junction closes, and the posterior urethra contracts, with resultant seminal emission; during this time the detrusor initially contracts and then relaxes.

It is probable that the sympathetic nervous system relates primarily to sexual function and affects the urinary bladder indirectly in carrying out this activity, i.e., inhibiting detrusor contraction during ejaculation. Since, in the male, urination, continence, and ejaculation all involve the posterior urethra, it is apparent that the several functions must be highly coordinated in order to avoid urinating during intercourse or ejaculation during micturition. This concept is supported by recent studies demonstrating a close relationship among the hypogastric, pelvic, and pudendal nerves to the bladder, urethra, and periurethral striated muscle.

Not only does the urethral wall possess smooth muscle that is a continuation of the detrusor meshwork into the posterior urethra, responsive to cholinergic stimulation, and involved in storage and evacuation of urine; in addition, it also has the smooth muscle layer described previously that is influenced by the sympathetic or adrenergic system and related to sexual function. Although the layer of adrenergic-sensitive smooth muscle is activated primarily during orgasm, it can affect conti-

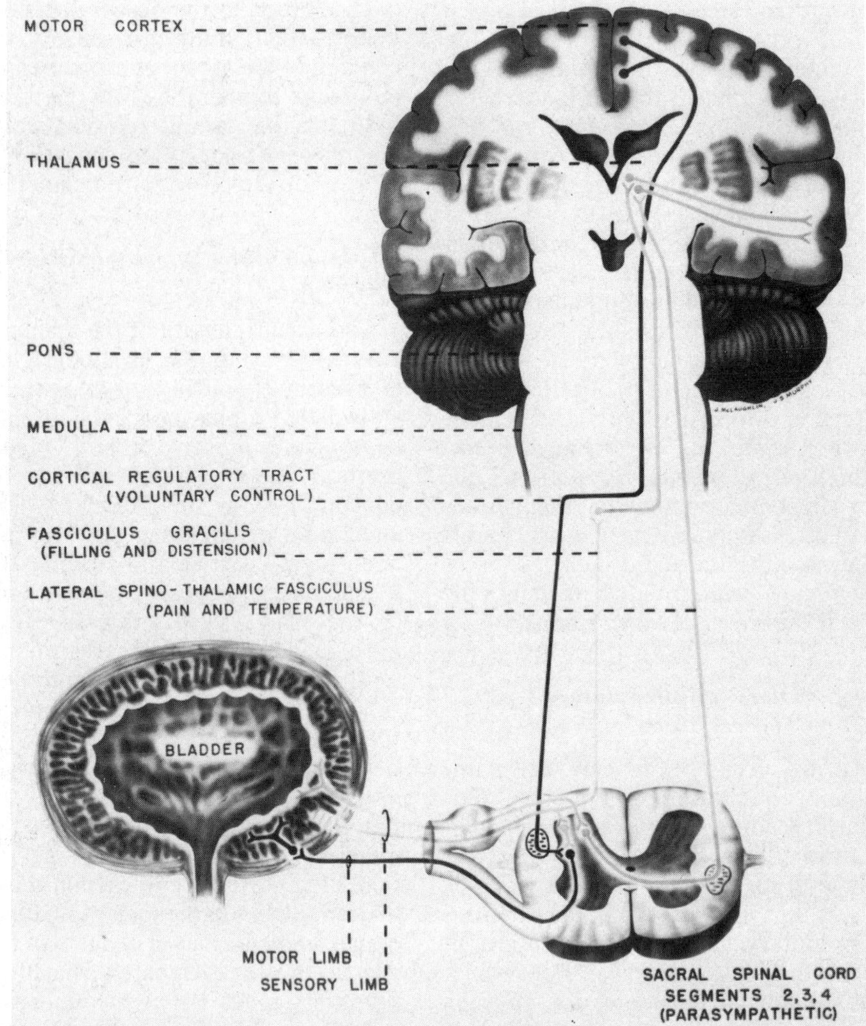

Figure 3–9. The motor neurons to the bladder are controlled by the higher centers via the corticoregulatory tract. (From Lapides, J.: Fundamentals of Urology. Philadelphia, W. B. Saunders Co., 1976.)

nence and micturition in patients with neurogenic bladder and other disorders of the lower urinary tract.

EVALUATION OF BLADDER FUNCTION

Cystometry

Cystometric Apparatus

(Wear, 1974)

Bladder function is evaluated by a series of diagnostic procedures that include endoscopy, urography, cystometry, and electromyography (see Chapters 4 and 5). The instrument used in measuring various modalities of bladder function is called the cystometer. There are various types of cystometers in use, but we prefer the simple, inexpensive water type (Figure 3–10), consisting of a graduated reservoir, a Murphy drip, a screw clamp to regulate the rate of flow of fluid, a water manometer (meter stick with attached glass tubing), rubber tubing to connect the Murphy drip and water manometer to a glass Y tube, and a hemostat to start and stop the flow of fluid.

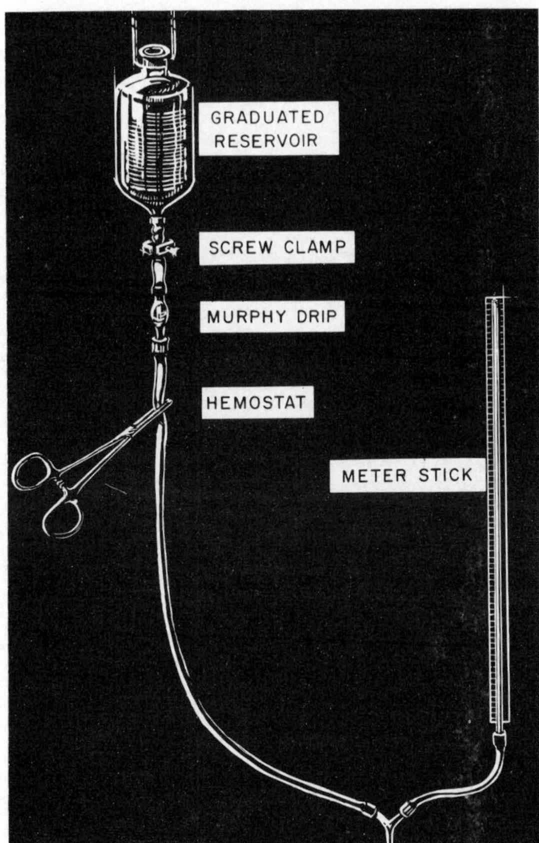

Figure 3–10. The water cystometer is a simple, extremely reliable apparatus for evaluating bladder function. (From Lapides, J.: Fundamentals of Urology. Philadelphia, W. B. Saunders Co., 1976.)

It will be noted in Figure 3–10 that the top of the manometer is made level with the Murphy drip in order to permit the flow of fluid from the reservoir even with high intravesical pressures. The cystometer is made ready for use by filling the reservoir and tubing with sterile water so that all the air bubbles are removed from the system except in the Murphy drip chamber. The zero mark on the manometer is made level with the subject's bladder. The cystometric apparatus can be used most efficiently by being hung on a parenteral fluid stand.

Method of Cystometry

The cystometric examination is initiated by requesting the patient to void and observing the time required to initiate micturition; size, force and continuity of stream; amount of straining during urination; and terminal dribbling. A uroflowmeter apparatus may be used instead of direct observation. The female patient is requested to void in the erect or sitting posture. After the patient has completed voiding and assumed the lithotomy position, a No. 16 or No. 18 French retention catheter is passed through the urethra into the bladder and left in place. The volume of residual urine is measured. Through the catheter 60 ml. of cold and then 60 ml. of warm water are instilled to test exteroceptive sensation.

The urethral catheter is then connected to the water manometric cystometer, and water is instilled into the bladder at a rate of about 1 ml. per second; this rate is obtained by adjusting the screw clamp so that the flow of fluid is just beyond the drop stage or a slow stream. The patient is requested to inform the examiner when the first desire to urinate occurs and again when the bladder feels quite full. The intravesical pressures and volumes are plotted on a cystometrographic sheet.

When the subject's bladder is full, the

urethral catheter is removed. First the patient is requested to cough in the lithotomy position and is observed for evidences of stress incontinence. The patient is then requested to void and the micturition pattern noted.

When a patient is being investigated for urinary incontinence, a No. 18 French *calibrated* retention catheter with a 5 ml. balloon is used instead of the unmarked Foley catheter. These calibrated catheters* are graduated in centimeters for a distance of 5 cm. from the balloon. The catheter balloon is inflated and gently snugged against the vesical outlet; the urethral length is measured; the residual urine is checked and then the cystometric examination performed. After the bladder is distended to capacity, the patient assumes the standing position with the catheter clamped and still in place, and the urethral length is again measured.

The urethral length in the erect position is obtained by sliding the thumb and index finger of the ungloved hand along the calibrated catheter until both fingers touch the unseen urethral meatus. The catheter is then grasped at that point with the two fingers to mark the urethral length as an assistant deflates the balloon and removes the catheter.

After the catheter is removed, the patient is requested to cough or strain, and any urinary leakage is observed. She is asked to empty her bladder and then resumes the lithotomy or supine position and is recatheterized. A second volume of residual urine is obtained and the *Urecholine (bethanechol chloride) supersensitivity test* performed. Fluid is instilled into the bladder from the cystometric apparatus at a rate of 1 ml. per second. When the volume of fluid in the bladder reaches 100 ml., the intravesical pressure is recorded and the flow of fluid stopped. After repeating the control run several times, the adult patient is given 2.5 mg. of Urecholine subcutaneously, and the cystometric runs are repeated 20 and 30 minutes after Urecholine administration.

In children, the Urecholine dosage is calculated according to weight, assuming the average adult to weigh 150 pounds. Thus, a 25-pound child would receive 25/150 or 1/6 of 2.5 mg. Urecholine, or 0.4 mg.; a 50-pound child 50/150, 1/3 of 2.5 mg. or 0.8 mg.; a 75-pound child 75/150, 1/2 of 2.5 mg. or 1.25 mg.

Interpretation of Cystometric Examination

An individual with normal micturition starts voiding within seconds after request if the bladder is full and the patient has an intense desire to urinate. On the other hand, if the bladder contains a small volume of urine, it may take 20 to 30 seconds before micturition is initiated; some individuals may be unable to begin urination at all in the presence of the examiner. The urinary stream is of good caliber and force and uninterrupted. At the termination of urination, the stream is interrupted for a short period of time as efforts are made to empty the urethra with forceful contractions of the periurethral striated musculature. On completion of urination, the volume of residual urine is less than 30 ml.

The normal subject is able to perceive cold and hot water, has the first desire to void at a volume of somewhere between 175 and 250 ml., and feels full at a volume of between 350 and 450 ml.

When fluid is first instilled into the bladder, there is a rather sharp rise in intravesical pressure with the first 50 ml. instilled to between 5 and 25 cm. of water, and then the intravesical pressure remains approximately constant until bladder capacity is reached. At a volume of 350 to 450 ml., the patient complains of bladder distention, and the intravesical pressure begins to increase in a straight line relationship with the volume. *No uninhibited voiding contractions of the detrusor are observed at any time during filling of the bladder, even at capacity, when the subject is uncomfortable.* After the bladder has been distended to capacity and the catheter has been removed, no urine is propelled through the urethra on coughing. Micturition with a full bladder conforms to all the characteristics previously outlined.

The intravesical pressure rise in the Urecholine supersensitivity test is less than 15 cm. of water over that of the control in the

*Obtainable from C.R. Bard, Inc., Murray Hill, N.J. 07974.

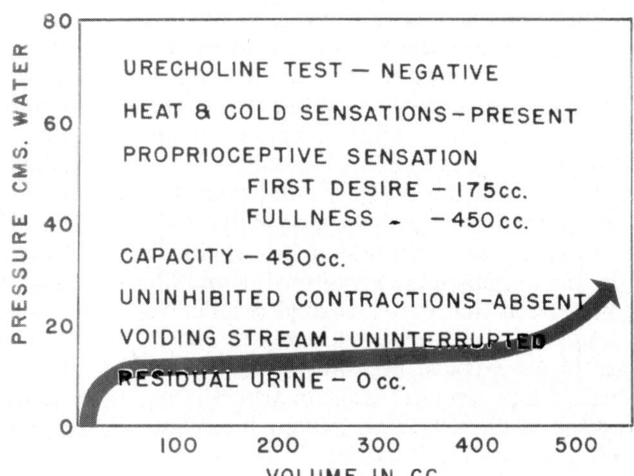

Figure 3–11. Cystometrograph of normal bladder. (From Lapides, J.: Fundamentals of Urology. Philadelphia, W. B. Saunders Co., 1976.)

normal subject. The cystometrograph and cystometric findings of the normal bladder are depicted in Figure 3–11.

Urecholine Supersensitivity Test
(Lapides, 1962)

As stated previously, when bladder muscle is stretched by fluid flowing into the lumen of the bladder, it responds by contracting and increasing the intravesical pressure (Figure 3–12). The stretch response of bladder muscle is a phenomenon localized to the muscle fibers; it is not mediated by acetylcholine, and it is completely independent of the central nervous system. Normal, atonic, and neurogenic bladders demonstrate essentially the same response to stretching; i.e., they all exhibit an intravesical pressure varying from 5 to 18 cm. of water in response to a flow rate of 1 ml. per second at a volume of 100 ml.

When 2.5 mg. of Urecholine is administered subcutaneously to an adult with a

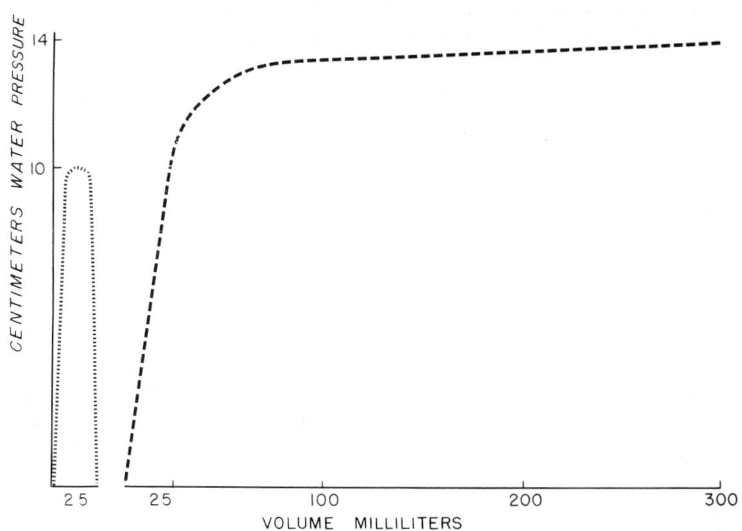

Figure 3–12. When 25 ml. of fluid is instilled into the bladder, the detrusor muscle is stretched and stimulated to contract and produce a rise in intravesical pressure. On cessation of stimulation, the smooth muscle of the bladder resumes its previous resting tension. A continuous flow of fluid into the bladder will result in a sustained increase in intravesical pressure. (From Lapides, J.: Fundamentals of Urology. Philadelphia, W. B. Saunders Co., 1976.)

normal bladder, the intravesical pressure response to stretching is increased by 2 to 15 cm. of water over that of the control. The maximal response is observed usually 20 to 30 minutes after injection of the Urecholine. Differential blocking of the motor limb of the reflex arc indicates that the Urecholine stimulates primarily at the neuromuscular junction and to a slight degree at the ganglionic synapse. It should be emphasized that every normal bladder responds to Urecholine and stretch with a rise in intravesical pressure never greater than 15 cm. over the control with the exception of the uremic or azotemic patient.

If 2.5 mg. of Urecholine is administered subcutaneously to an adult with significant detrusor denervation, the intravesical pressure response to stretch will always be greater than 15 cm. over that of the control. The motor and sensory paralytic bladders show the greatest sensitivity at the neuromuscular junction and the ganglionic synapse, respectively (Figures 3–13 and 3–14).

In the patient with an uninhibited neurogenic bladder, the lower motor neuron is supersensitive, while the ganglionic synapse and neuromuscular junction retain their normal sensitivity (Figure 3–15). Thus, the patient with the upper motor neuron bladder demonstrates supersensitivity to Urecholine by exhibiting an uncontrolled voiding contraction of the bladder at a smaller volume than during the control run. The response to Urecholine is variable in patients with uninhibited neurogenic bladders because not all patients with this type of bladder will exhibit an uninhibited bladder contraction at a bladder volume of 100 ml. with 2.5 mg. Urecholine.

In clinical practice, one uses the stretch response test according to the following regimen: The usual cystometric examination is performed. Several control bladder stretch response tests are obtained, using a flow rate of 1 ml. per second and recording the intravesical pressure at a 100 ml. volume. The adult patient is given 2.5 mg of Urecholine subcutaneously and stretch response tests are obtained at 10, 20, and 30 minutes after administration. If the greatest intravesical pressure rise over that of the control is less than 15 cm. of water, the patient does not have significant chronic neurogenic disease in the sacral spinal cord area or the lower reflex arc. A pressure response greater than 15 cm. over that of

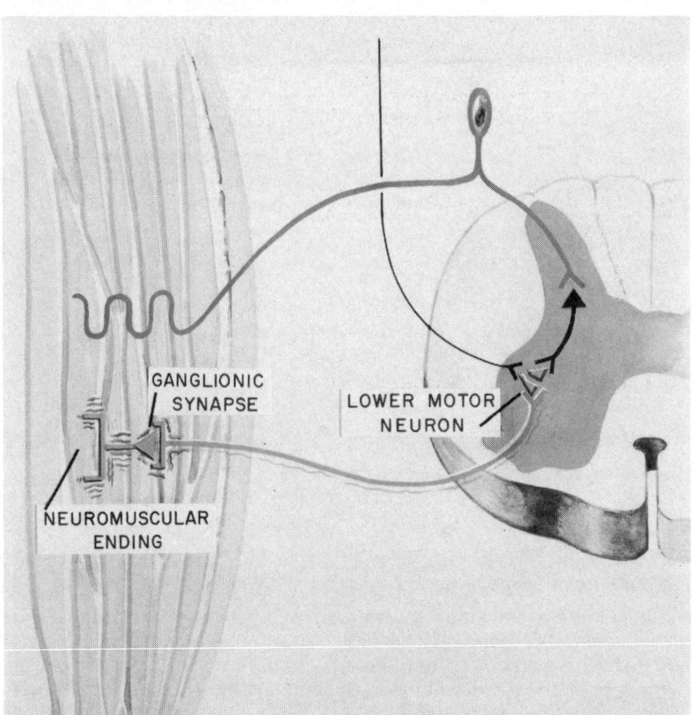

Figure 3–13. A chronic impairment of the lower motor neuron or nerve fiber will result in denervation supersensitivity of the neuromuscular ending and ganglionic synapse. (From Lapides, J.: Fundamentals of Urology. Philadelphia, W. B. Saunders Co., 1976.)

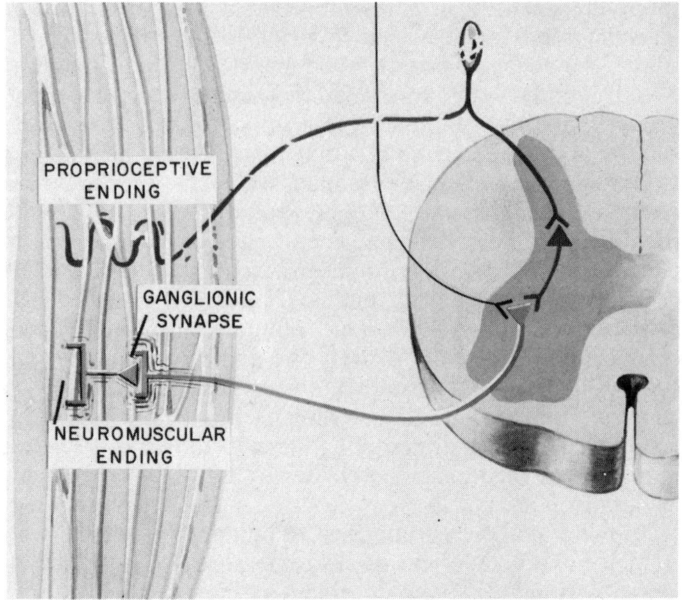

Figure 3–14. Chronic denervation of the sensory limb of the reflex arc results in supersensitivity, primarily of the ganglionic synapse and, to a lesser degree, of the neuromuscular ending. (From Lapides, J.: Fundamentals of Urology. Philadelphia, W. B. Saunders Co., 1976.)

the control, in the absence of uremia, is positive diagnosis of a neurogenic bladder, which may be due to chronic involvement of the corticoregulatory tract, the sensory limb of the lower reflex arc, the motor limb of the segmental reflex arc, or any combination of the three (See Chapter 23).

Evaluation of Cystometric Examination

It should be borne in mind that the cystometric examination is a diagnostic procedure in conjunction with other methods, e.g., pyelography, cineradiography, voiding cystourethrography, endoscopy, and urethral resistance measurements. It cannot and should not be used in a manner similar to that employed by the cardiologist in reading an ECG. The electrocardiogram is entirely objective in nature, whereas the cystometric examination is both subjective and objective. Furthermore, the cystometrograph in a particular type of neurogenic bladder may vary, depending upon existing conditions. For example, the motor paralytic bladder may show a capacity of 450 ml. if the patient is catheterized shortly

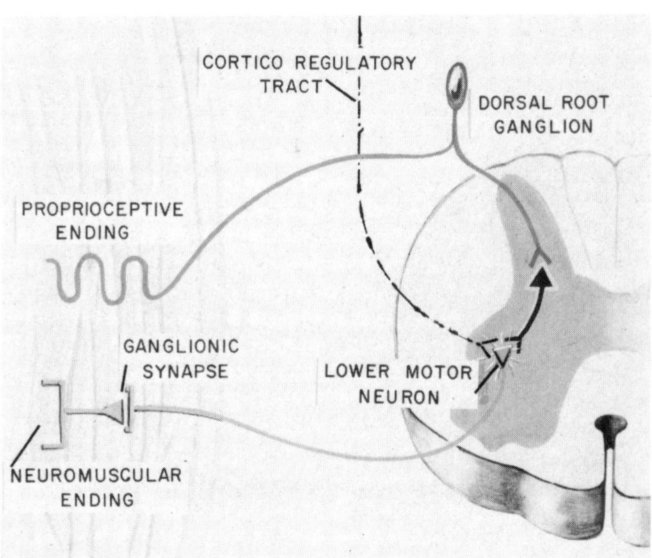

Figure 3–15. Destruction of the corticoregulatory tract leads to denervation supersensitivity of the lower motor neuron. (From Lapides, J.: Fundamentals of Urology. Philadelphia, W. B. Saunders Co., 1976.)

after the onset of urinary retention; if the patient is not catheterized for a period of days, the capacity may be 1000 ml.

Frequently, one must perform endoscopy in addition to the cystometric examination in order to arrive at a diagnosis. For example, a middle-aged female with undiagnosed poliomyelitis may present with a complaint of acute urinary retention. Cystometry may disclose normal sensation and normal bladder capacity but no evidences of bladder contraction, either voluntary or involuntary. These are exactly the findings observed in patients with acute urinary retention due to obstruction. Thus, urethroscopy must be performed in addition to the cystometric examination in order to arrive at a correct diagnosis.

However, the cystometric examination, which now includes the Urecholine supersensitivity test, is the only objective method for specifically pinpointing a lesion of the corticoregulatory tract or the lower segmental reflex arc involving bladder function. All other tests are suggestive in that lesions of the sacral cord or corticoregulatory tract may be diagnosed, but it is the cystometric examination that shows that the bladder per se is involved. For example, the presence of hyperactive reflexes, ankle clonus, and Babinski signs is not an absolute indication of an uninhibited neurogenic bladder unless the cystometrograph denotes uncontrolled contractions of the bladder. On the other hand, a positive diagnosis of uninhibited neurogenic bladder can be made on cystometrography alone — irrespective of the absence or presence of any other neurologic deficits.

This diagnostic specificity is also true for the Urecholine supersensitivity test: When there is a positive response, the patient has a lesion of the lower segmental reflex arc regardless of any other findings. It is extremely important to comprehend these concepts, for we have found a number of patients with neurogenic bladder but with absolutely no other sign of neurologic deficit. These abnormalities would in all probability have remained undiagnosed if complete neurologic and electromyographic examinations had been employed as the only diagnostic procedures.

Electromyography of the Urogenital Diaphragm

(Diokno, 1974)

Because micturition and continence depend upon the closely coordinated activity of the bladder, urethra, and periurethral striated muscle, it is essential to know the dynamics of the levator ani and especially of the muscle of the urogenital diaphragm during the storage and evacuation phases of the bladder. A large share of the urinary

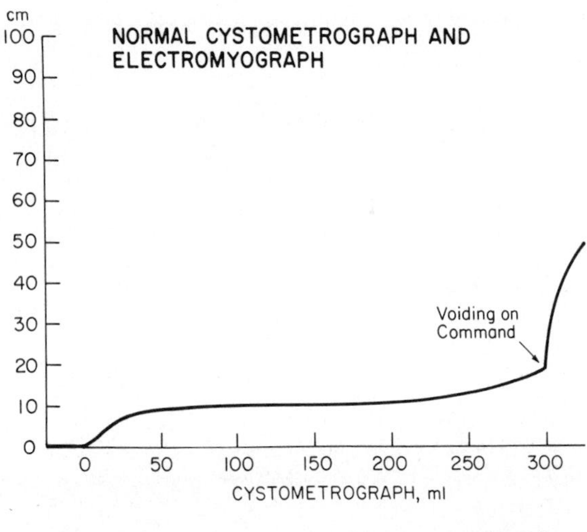

Figure 3–16. The motor impulses to the urogenital diaphragm (UGD) increase as the bladder reaches capacity and stop abruptly when urination is considered or performed. (From Lapides, J.: Fundamentals of Urology. Philadelphia, W. B. Saunders Co., 1976.)

difficulties encountered by the patient with spinal cord disturbances stem from a lack of coordination between the detrusor and the periurethral striated muscle.

Measurement of striated muscle contraction or relaxation can be readily accomplished by inserting an electrode into the urogenital diaphragm and observing the action potentials via an electromyographic machine; the examination is performed in conjunction with the cystometric study. The technique for proper placement of the electrode is relatively simple, but does require some experience. With the female in the lithotomy position and a guiding index finger in the vagina, the fine needle electrode is pushed gently through the epithelium of the periurethral tissue at approximately the ten to twelve o'clock positions and about 3 to 5 mm. lateral to the meatus. The needle point is moved deeper in 1 millimeter steps, for the muscle is often quite superficial. Proper placement is indicated by the appearance of discrete action potentials on the machine's sound system and the oscilloscope screen.

The normal individual, tense because of the test situation, will demonstrate a barrage of motor impulses as the electrode needle is first inserted into the muscle. As the patient relaxes, the tempo of the electrical activity will gradually subside to a slow discharge of one to two motor units or complete absence. Upon request to "tighten her bottom" the normal subject can contract the striated muscle surrounding the urethra, as indicated by a burst of sustained action potentials.

During cystometry the continuous filling of the bladder with fluid or air will stimulate a progressive increase in the number of motor units firing until capacity is reached (Figure 3–16). If the patient attempts to void, the electrical activity will disappear despite the lack of onset of an actual detrusor contraction; i.e., just thinking of voiding, without having the bladder contract, will silence the muscle of the urogenital diaphragm. Motor impulses will return as soon as the patient ceases either thinking of urinating or actual urination.

Special Considerations

Neurogenic Bladder

(Langworthy et al., 1940; Bors and Comarr, 1971; Lapides, 1974*c*)

Interference with normal conduction of nerve impulses over one or more of the nerve tracts concerned with urination produces dysfunction of the bladder. Bladders so affected are called neurogenic bladders and can be one of several different types or combinations. (See Chapter 23.)

Urinary Infection

(Lapides, 1975)

The most common cause of lower and upper urinary tract infections are entities that lead to marked increases in intravesical pressure or vesical overdistention with resultant decreased blood flow through the bladder wall. The impairment of circulation lessens host resistance to bacterial invasion because of decrease in available hematogenous antibacterial elements and deterioration of local tissue immunity provided by structural integrity. (See Chapter 24.)

REFERENCES

Bors, E., and Comarr, A. E.: Neurological Urology. Baltimore, University Park Press, 1971.

Bradley, W. E., Timm, G. W., and Scott, F. B.: Innervation of the detrusor muscle and urethra. Urol. Clin. North Am., *1*:3, 1974.

DeGroat, W. C.: Nervous control of the urinary bladder of the cat. Brain Res. *87*:201, 1975.

Diokno, A. C., Koff, S. A., and Bender, L. F.: Periurethral striated muscle activity in neurogenic bladder dysfunction. J. Urol. *112*:743, 1974.

Langworthy, O. R., Kolb, L. C., and Lewis, L. G.: Physiology of Micturition. Baltimore, Williams & Wilkins Co., 1940.

Lapides, J.: Structure and function of the internal vesical sphincter. J. Urol. *80*:341, 1958.

Lapides, J., Ajemian, E. P., Stewart, B. H., et al.: Physiopathology of stress incontinence. Surg. Gynecol. Obstet. *111*:224, 1960.

Lapides, J., Friend, C. R., Ajemian, E. P., and Reus, W. F.: Denervation supersensitivity as a test for neurogenic bladder. Surg. Gynecol. Obstet. *114*:241, 1962.
Lapides, J.: Neurogenic bladder: Principles of treatment. Urol. Clin. North Am. *1*:81, 1974*a*.
Lapides, J.: Micturition and the adrenergic system. Urologists' Letter Club *32*:48, 1974*b*.
Lapides, J.: Symposium on Neurogenic Bladder. Urol. Clin. North Am. *1*:1, 1974*c*.
Lapides, J.: Urinary tract infection in women. J. Pract. Nursing *25*:19, 1975.
Wear, J. B., Jr.: Cystometry. Urol. Clin. North Am. *1*:45, 1974.
Woodburne, R. T.: Structure and function of the urinary bladder. J. Urol. *84*:79, 1960.

4

URODYNAMICS

SHLOMO RAZ, M.D.

The introduction of urodynamic assessment into the clinical routine has resulted in an overdue appraisal of many of our urologic concepts. But surely none were more in need of reappraisal than those relating to urinary incontinence in the female (Turner-Warwick, 1979). I feel that it would be useful first to offer an overview of the type of evaluation that not only includes many of our own diagnostic procedures but which has also been one of the most successful in diagnosing and determining treatment for female urinary incontinence.

In addition to the routine general examination, a full basic urologic examination, gynecologic examination, and, in cases where neurogenic bladder is suspected, neurologic examination should be undertaken (Chapter 14).

A number of tests must be considered in a urodynamic assessment.

Residual Urine

In urology, the most commonly performed diagnostic test is a measurement of residual urine. It is important to rule out postvoid residual, which indicates an associated outflow impairment. Patients with lower urinary tract dysfunction display two types of residuals. One, *significant,* is accompanied by urinary symptoms (frequency, urgency, poor urinary stream) and by objective urologic findings, such as trabeculation, diverticula, vesicoureteric reflux, and upper tract dilatation. The second type, *insignificant,* occurs without urinary tract symptoms, abnormal cystographic findings, or urinary tract infection. This latter type of residual urine should not be treated in the same fashion as symptomatic or otherwise significant residual urine, which poses a threat to lower urinary tract functioning.

Voided Volume Chart

The record of consecutive maximum voided volumes over a period of 48 hours is sometimes helpful in making the clinical distinction between bladder stability (Turner-Warwick, 1979) and instability.

Endoscopy

Expert diagnostic cystourethroscopy is essential to the evaluation of all voiding disorders to rule out relevant or incidental abnormalities, such as tumor or trigonitis. Cystourethroscopy may identify urethral abnormalities, e.g., urethral or bladder neck hypermobility, diverticula, but there is no way in which it can contribute to the evaluation of sphincter function or to the identification of detrusor dysfunction. Endoscopy is discussed in detail in other sections of this book (Chapters 6 and 29).

Cystometry (CMG)

Simple single-channel cystometry performed with the patient in the supine position reveals only about 50 per cent of unstable bladders. However, it is a simple test during the performance of which the revelation of unexpected instability may be clinically significant. *Provocation cystometry* may be attempted with a single-channel instrument with the patient in the erect position, but accurate interpretation of the record often requires special experience. This is because in women many times the bladder will develop only low-pressure detrusor contractions, which tend to be masked by the abdominal pressure changes included in the total bladder pressure record.

Subtracted Detrusor Pressure Dystometry

The electronic subtraction of the intrarectal pressure (approximating the intra-abdominal pressure) from the intravesical pressure provides a record of true detrusor pressure that is sufficiently accurate to identify unstable detrusor contractions by provocation in any position.

Micturating Cystography

Static-film lateral cystography has long been a standard investigative technique in the evaluation of voiding dysfunction. However, it simply demonstrates the anatomic situation; the functional information that it provides is limited.

Urethral Pressure Profile

Opinions differ as to the value of urethral pressure profile measurements in assessing urethral function in clinical practice. But appreciation of its limitations and the need for expert interpretation are essential to its reliability. A particular shortcoming is the impossibility of assessing bladder neck dysfunction.

Synchronous Video-Flow-Pressure Cystourethrography

Simultaneous combined studies undoubtedly provide the best method of evaluating both detrusor and urethral dysfunction during the phases of the normal voiding cycle. This procedure is by far the best method for evaluating individual sphincter mechanisms, and an appropriate adaptation of the technique may be useful whenever information must be obtained from patients unable to void in front of the screen.

CYSTOMETRY

History

In 1872, Schatz accidentally punctured a patient's bladder while trying to measure intra-abdominal pressure, out of which occurrence developed the technique for measuring intravesical pressure.

Dubois (1876) studied the effects of position on intravesical and intra-abdominal pressure. He learned that the desire to void is often associated with a rise in intravesical pressure. When Lewis (1939) introduced the motor-driven strip chart recorder, cystometry began to be accepted by the urologic community. The advent of air cystometry (Merrill et al., 1971) and carbon dioxide cystometry (Bradley et al., 1975*a*, *b*) simplified the procedure even further.

Description

The principle of all cystometers is the same: a manometer is coupled to the inside of the bladder by means of a catheter. Fluid is instilled into the bladder, and as the bladder fills, intravesical pressure is plotted against volume. The apparatus can be as simple as a water-filled "Y" tube, with a centimeter ruler for a manometer, or as sophisticated as a multichannel microtip transducer catheter capable of simultaneously measuring pressures in the bladder and at several points along the urethra (Blaivas, in press).

There are two types of cystometry: *filling cystometry*, which records intravesical pressures at the time of filling, and *voiding cystometry*, during which intravesical pressures are recorded at the time of voiding, usually in conjunction with measurement of urinary flow.

Ideally, urinary flow rate should be determined just prior to cystometry, before any manipulation takes place, and then compared with the urinary flow which is obtained during voiding cystometry (Blaivas, in press). This will be discussed later.

Filling Cystometry

The bladder is catheterized and the postvoid residual measured. Usually, two catheters are inserted into the bladder: a No. 5 to 8 French catheter to fill the bladder and a second, small catheter to record the pressures. A fluid-filled balloon catheter with zero pressure is inserted into the rectum to record intra-abdominal pressures.

Bladder filling is begun at a predetermined rate, usually 80 to 100 ml. per minute, with the patient in the supine position. If the goal is to determine the absence or presence of uninhibited bladder contractions, a rapid rate of filling (more than 100 ml. CO_2 or H_2O per minute) is sufficient. But on certain occasions, filling should be done very slowly. At these times, the patient is instructed neither to inhibit micturition nor to attempt to void, but simply to report all sensations to the examiner. The bladder volume at which each of the following events occurs is noted: (1) sensation of bladder filling; (2) sensation of fullness; and (3) sensation of imminent micturition. Abnormal sensations, such as suprapubic or back pain, are also noted.

When the patient senses that micturition is imminent, she is asked to try to inhibit voiding. *If she is unable to prevent a bladder contraction at that time, the resulting contraction is considered involuntary.* An involuntary bladder contraction is defined as a sudden, involuntary rise in detrusor pressure. The patient may be aware of the contraction, perceiving it as an urge to void, or she may be unaware of it. If she is aware of the involuntary contraction, she may or may not be able to inhibit it. Pressures in involuntary detrusor contractions usually are greater than 15 cm. of water, but may be of lesser magnitude. They sometimes can be appreciated only by measuring intra-abdominal and intravesical pressures simultaneously. If the patient does not demonstrate involuntary bladder contractions, she is asked to try to void without straining, and her ability to do so is recorded. However, when asked to void, a majority of women exert increased intra-abdominal pressure in trying to initiate a bladder contraction. In such instances, it can be extremely difficult to distinguish a bladder contraction from the effects of straining unless intra-abdominal pressure is being simultaneously recorded (Blaivas, in press).

When the patient begins to feel suprapubic discomfort or pain from filling or from the appearance of an uninhibited bladder contraction, filling is stopped. If uninhibited contractions do not occur, voiding cystometry can be initiated.

Voiding Cystometry

Cystometry can be an uncomfortable and embarrassing procedure for the patient, with consequent suppression of the detrusor reflex. However, this suppression cannot be directly observed on cystometrogram (CMG). Therefore, before concluding that the CMG is areflexic, a detrusor reflex activation procedure can be utilized routinely. This involves postural change from the supine to the sitting or standing position; subcutaneous administration of bethanechol (the reflex triggering precipitated by bethanechol should be differentiated from the elevation of the tonus limb that occurs in response to this drug in patients with detrusor impairment); and urethral or rectal distention.

During voiding cystometry, true detrusor pressures are recorded as well as the pattern of micturition. The objective is to determine whether the patient initiates voiding by abdominal straining or by a good, normal bladder contraction; the amount of pressure developed by the bladder should be recorded. Normal voiding pressures range between 30 and 40 cm. of water.

Commonly used infusates for cystometry include water, carbon dioxide, and radiographic contrast material (Blaivas, in press). (Air should no longer be used, because of the danger of causing air emboli [Summers et al., 1974; Blaivas, in press].) Although the numeric values of cystometric parameters differ when carbon dioxide rather than liquid is used, qualitatively similar information may be obtained from either (Gleason et al., 1977). Carbon dioxide offers the advantages of speed, convenience, and simplicity, because it can be instilled at rates of up to 300 ml./minute. The study can be readily repeated under varying conditions and before and after pharmacologic manipulation. Moreover, with carbon dixoide, the response of the bladder to quick stretch can be evaluated. However, because it is a colorless, odorless gas, carbon dioxide can leak unnoticed through the crevices of the urethra or through the cystometer tubing itself, resulting in crucial artifacts. Further inaccuracies may result from the inherent compressibility of the gas and from the fact that it is often irritating to the bladder mucosa. Both of these factors cause cystometric phenomena to occur at lower volumes than when liquid is used. It should also be noted that simultaneous video-pressure-flow studies cannot be performed with carbon dioxide as the medium.

Water cystometry offers the advantage of being more physiologically consistent than carbon dioxide (Blaivas, in press). Leakage from the urethra or from the cystometer tubing is easily detected, and when radiographic contrast is added, synchronous video-pressure-flow studies can be performed. The major disadvantage of water cystometry is that the apparatus is cumbersome to use, and water cannot be instilled as rapidly as gas.

Propantheline Bromide Test

When involuntary detrusor contractions have been demonstrated, it may be desirable to test the efficacy of anticholinergic agents in abolishing them (Blaivas, in press). Propantheline bromide (Pro-Banthine) (15 mg.) is administered intramuscularly after the baseline cystometrogram has been performed. The CMG is repeated 15 to 20 minutes later or whenever the anticholinergic effects (dry mouth or blurred vision) become apparent. A positive response is defined as the complete abolition of involuntary contractions, or a 200 per cent increase in bladder volume, at which the involuntary contraction occurred. If the parenteral medication works, the orally administered drug will be effective more than 90 per cent of the time, provided that the patient can tolerate the necessary dosage without untoward side effects (Blaivas et al., 1980).

The Bethanechol Denervation Supersensitivity Test

The bethanechol denervation supersensitivity test has been recommended as a diagnostic tool for distinguishing neurogenic from non-neurogenic causes of detrusor areflexia (Glahn, 1970; Melzer, 1972; Merrill and Rotta, 1974). As described by Lapides and co-workers (1962), the test is performed during CMG: at 100 ml. of bladder volume, the intravesical pressure is recorded and the bladder emptied. Bethanechol chloride (Urecholine) (2.5 mg.) is administered subcutaneously and the bladder again filled to 100 ml. The pressure at this volume is recorded 10, 20, and 30 minutes after administration. A positive response is defined as a rise in bladder pressure of greater than 15 cm. of water compared with the initial study. Lapides believes that a positive test is indicative of bladder denervation, but other authors have documented positive results in patients with cystitis, diabetes, emotional stress, and urinary retention of neurogenic origin (Glahn, 1970; Melzer, 1972; Merrill and Rotta, 1974) (Chapter 3).

Interpretation

As mentioned, cystometry can be divided into a filling (storage) phase and an expulsive (voiding) phase. Any interpretation of the CMG should recognize that data obtained during the first phase is of a totally different significance from data obtained during the second.

FILLING CYSTOMETRY

When fluid is introduced slowly into the empty bladder, there is an initial rise in pressure. This is probably a contractile response of the detrusor muscle (Klevmark, 1974). The magnitude of this response is related to the rate of infusion, as discussed later in this chapter. This is the first segment of the cystometric curve, designated T_1 (Merrill et al., 1971; Ruch, 1960). During the second segment, or tonus limb (T_2), the smooth muscle of the bladder wall accommodates to stretch (bladder filling) by a very minimal increase in wall tension (according to the law of Laplace) to become a thin-walled sphere. Laplace's law states that the tension in the wall (*T*) is divided by *r* (radius of the sphere, or bladder); therefore, if the pressure in the bladder is increased, there will also be an increase in tension. When the radius is increased, tension lessens. In practice, intravesical pressure remains unchanged during filling. It is usually between the beginning and the end of filling that the maximum sensation of fullness is observed. However, intravesical pressure will not rise higher than 10 to 15 cm. of water (Merrill et al., 1971; Klevmark, 1974). If the bladder continues to be filled or has been stretched to its physiologic limit, there is a progressive increase in the slope of the cystometric curve, paralleling the change in volume. This is the third segment (T_3), a finding that has been attributed to stretching of the collagenous elements of the bladder wall, thus defining true bladder capacity (Swaiman, 1967) (Figure 4–1).

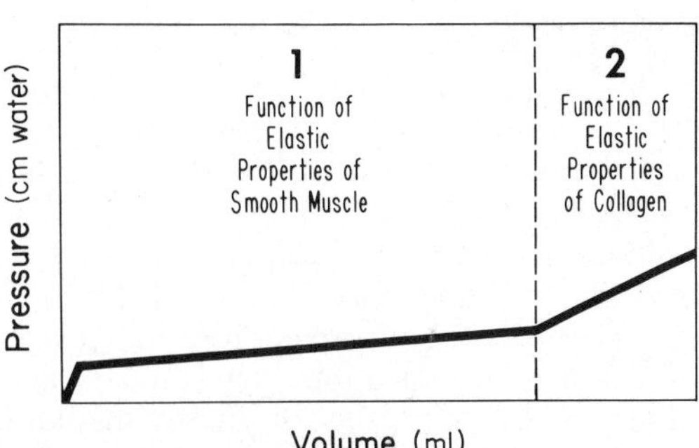

Figure 4–1. Diagram of the two phases of cystometry: (1) related to elastic properties of smooth muscle; (2) related to elastic properties of collagen. During second phase, any volume increase produces parallel increase in pressure. During first phase large volume changes do not produce significant pressure changes. (From Raz, S., and Bradley, W. E.: Neuromuscular dysfunction of the lower urinary tract. *In* Harrison, J. H., et al.: Campbell's Urology. 4th Ed. Philadelphia, W. B. Saunders Co., 1979.)

This adaptability of the bladder to change in volume is a controversial idea. Most probably these changes are due to the viscoelastic properties of smooth muscle and the different components of the bladder wall, independent of innervation, but it is possible also that changes in bladder tonus during bladder filling can be neurogenic in origin and that changes in innervation can alter adaptability to change in volume. This latter theory may explain why patients with preganglionic lesions, as in myelomeningocele, may have poor bladder compliance: partial denervation can alter the bladder's adaptability to changes in volume because of supersensitivity to the neurotransmitter acetylcholine. The origin of the bladder's adaptability to changes in volume is, however, still unsolved (Figure 4–2).

Important information must be extracted from the filling phase of the CMG. I classify this information accordingly: (1) sensations; (2) capacity; (3) changes in bladder compliance and (4) absence or presence of uninhibited bladder contractions.

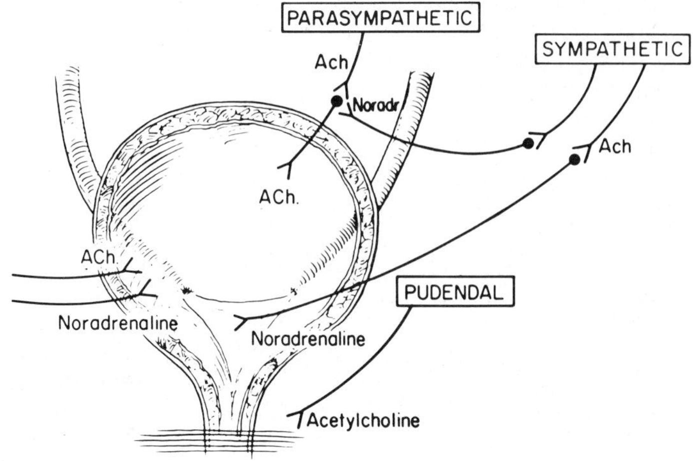

Figure 4–2. Diagram demonstrating integration of lower urinary tract innervation. Parasympathetic fibers from the S_2–S_4 sacral parasympathetic centers have long preganglionic fibers; pelvic ganglia are close to ureters and bladder base; postganglionic fibers discharge acetylcholine (ACh). Sympathetic fibers have long postganglionic fibers, discharge norepinephrine (noradrenaline) to the bladder neck, and also regulate function of pelvic ganglia. (From Raz, S.: Pharmacological treatment of lower urinary tract dysfunction. Urol. Clin. North Am. 5:323, 1978.)

Sensation

It is important to observe the sensations elicited during CMG. The first sensation to void occurs normally during the initial filling with 200 to 250 ml. of water. But initiation of sensation depends as well on the rate of filling. Rapid filling produces an early sensation, whereas slow filling produces a later sensation. Sensation is also affected by the type of filling medium, water or gas. Abnormalities include impairment, pain or discomfort at low filling volumes, and abnormally early or late sensations of filling. Impairment of sensation has been described as an early finding in diabetic autonomic neuropathy. Prolonged overdistention secondary to outlet obstruction can produce a delay in sensation because of damage to the nerve endings that normally produce the sensation to void. Therefore, impairment of bladder sensation may be of both neurogenic and non-neurogenic origin.

Capacity

Cystometric and functional bladder capacity should be sharply differentiated. Functional bladder capacity is the amount of urine the bladder can hold. This can be checked very easily by asking the patient to drink a large amount of water and to hold it until she feels the maximum sensation of filling, and then urinate. One then checks her residual urine. The sum of the urine voided plus the residual urine provides the maximum functional bladder capacity. The artifacts of catheter insertion, the environment of the cystometric examination, and the presence of medical personnel may change the patient's bladder capacity completely, however. These strange nonphysiologic factors often produce an artifactual bladder capacity, making it important to interpret bladder capacity data as derived from CMGs on a comparative basis with the patient's functional capacity. The main aim of the CMG is to determine abnormal sensation and reflexes, rather than bladder capacity. The best way to determine bladder capacity is without simultaneous pressure recording.

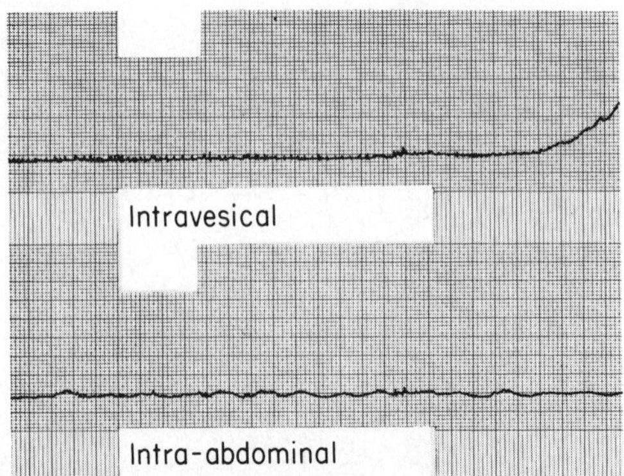

Figure 4–3. Simultaneous recordings of intravesical and intra-abdominal pressures. During prolonged filling, intravesical pressure changes little until the point at which volume increase produces a parallel increase in pressure.

$$C = \frac{\Delta \text{ Vol.}}{\Delta \text{ Press.}} = \frac{300}{60-15} = 6$$

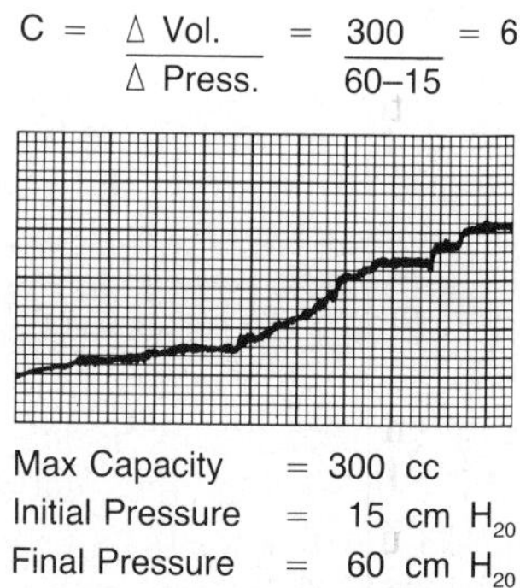

Max Capacity = 300 cc
Initial Pressure = 15 cm H_{20}
Final Pressure = 60 cm H_{20}

Figure 4–4. Filling cystometry in patient with poor bladder compliance secondary to chronic interstitial cystitis. From initial reading of 15 cm. of water, intravesical pressure reaches 60 cm. of water, indicating lack of bladder adaptability to volume change.

Compliance

The adaptability of the bladder to the change in volume was discussed earlier. During bladder filling, there is not much change in intravesical pressure (Figure 4–3). This means that the difference between the initial pressure and terminal pressure is usually no more than 10 to 15 cm. of water during filling. Poor bladder compliance can be defined as the lack of adaptability to the change in volume (Figure 4–4). Disappearance in the adaptability and elasticity of the smooth muscles accounts for poor bladder compliance. Most likely, this occurs any time there is an increase in collagenous deposits in the bladder wall; for example, after chronic interstitial cystitis, urinary tract infection, radiation, che-

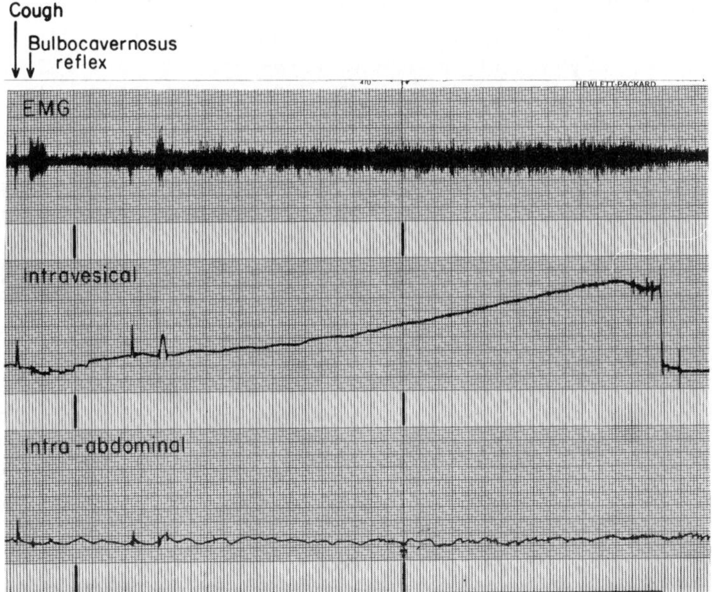

Figure 4–5. Combined study of electromyographic (EMG) activity of the pelvic floor and intravesical and intra-abdominal pressures in patient with neurogenic bladder due to sacral agenesis demonstrates poor bladder compliance. (From Raz, S., and Bradley, W. E.: Neuromuscular dysfunction of the lower urinary tract. *In* Harrison, J. H., et al.: Campbell's Urology. 4th Ed. Philadelphia, W. B. Saunders Co., 1979.)

motherapy, or chronic outlet obstruction with weakening of the bladder wall and chronic bladder distention (Figure 4–5). All of these factors can contribute to lack of bladder compliance. In these cases, there is a clear organic reason for the poor adaptability of the bladder to the change in bladder volume. But there is still some debate surrounding certain types of patients, especially those with myelomeningocele who present with poor bladder compliance. Some authors (Bradley et al., 1975*a, b;* Zinner et al., 1980) believe that changes in bladder tone are dependent only on intrinsic changes in the histologic components of the bladder; these include appearance of collagenous tissue, changes in the elastic tissue, fibrosis, or inflammation. As mentioned previously the question is whether lack of compliance is neurogenic in origin, representing supersensitivity of the smooth muscle to its neurotransmitter acetylcholine. This poor compliance may suggest a preganglionic lesion.

An interesting aspect of poor bladder compliance is its effect on the bladder neck. During the phase of bladder filling, it is possible to see under fluoroscopy that the normal bladder neck remains closed. But when there is a lack of compliance, during bladder filling the tensile forces open the bladder neck, producing funneling. It is for this reason that bladder neck incompetence is seen in patients with interstitial cystitis or after irradiation. In such patients, any diminution of the distal sphincter function may lead to urinary incontinence secondary to high intravesical pressures.

Occasionally difficulty is seen during the filling phase of cystometry, with the curve showing a rapidly ascending loop. This is the problem of differentiating poor compliance from uninhibited bladder contractions. For the purpose of identifying patients with this condition, the propantheline bromide test described earlier is extremely useful. If organic changes in the bladder wall have taken place, Pro-Banthine (15 mg. IM) will do nothing at all to change the filling curve. In patients with neurogenically integrated uninhibited bladder contractions during filling, a flat curve can be demonstrated after the Pro-Banthine injection.

Uninhibited Bladder Contractions (Hyperreflexia)

The main center of reflex micturition is located at the brain stem. Until the age of 3 or 4 years, micturition is achieved by this reflex. With education and maturity, the cortical centers take control, and the appearance of this reflex becomes inhibited. The normal person is able to inhibit this brain stem micturition reflex; therefore, I would expect an adult to be able to inhibit any bladder contraction completely during filling, coughing, or movement. However, this normal inhibition is lacking in some patients. Any bladder contraction that cannot be voluntarily suppressed is defined as an uninhibited contraction, or hyperreflexia.

A few terms need definition: a *stable bladder* is a bladder that functions with normal sensations and ability to suppress any uninhibited contractions. An *unstable bladder* may be defined in two ways; first, in terms of *sensory instability,* and second, in terms of *motor instability*. In the sensory type a patient displays good compliance and no uninhibited bladder contraction (changes in bladder pressure), but develops an early sensation to urinate. This should be differentiated from the motor type, which is indicated by changes in bladder pressure. *Hyperreflexia* is defined as the inability of the patient to suppress the contraction that occurs during filling or under provocation, such as coughing, movement, or postural change.

Three main etiologies of uninhibited bladder contractions can be identified: (1) idiopathic; (2) neurogenic; and (3) vesicogenic, or bladder contractions arising from local problems.

Idiopathic Hyperreflexia. As mentioned previously, a child develops normal control of micturition after the age of 3 or 4 years, and then is capable of inhibiting bladder contractions with cortical control. But in some children this micturition reflex inhibition does not develop, producing a continuation of bladder hyperreflexia. Idiopathic hyperreflexia can present in several ways: a patient can be completely asymptomatic but on CMG develops hyperreflexia. Perhaps 10 to 15 per cent of the female population presents with asymptomatic bladder hyperreflexia. Such patients usually have a history of enuresis. This type of hyperreflexia is significant only when accompanied by neurologic symptoms.

Asymptomatic hyperreflexia occurs in large numbers of patients. But occasionally it is evidenced clinically by the symptoms of urinary frequency, urgency during the day, incontinence, and enuresis. The problem is that during the day there is frequency and urgency because small volumes are voided; at night, when the normal sensation to urinate is suppressed, the patient experiences uninhibited contractions and bedwetting.

In children, bladder hyperreflexia may sometimes seriously affect the urinary tract. During these uninhibited contractions, there is a high level of voluntary sphincter activity (not true dyssynergia). Lack of complete relaxation of the pelvic floor during voiding produces outlet obstruction, trabeculation, and deterioration of the lower urinary tract, along with occasional deterioration of the upper urinary tract, with reflux and hydronephrosis. We define this entity as non-neurogenic neurogenic bladder.

Neurogenic Hyperreflexia. Patients with neurologic disorders very often present with uninhibited contractions. Only the brain stem center is capable of inducing coordinated relaxation of the pelvic floor during bladder contractions. Therefore, lesions above the brain stem will produce bladder hyperreflexia, usually with pre-

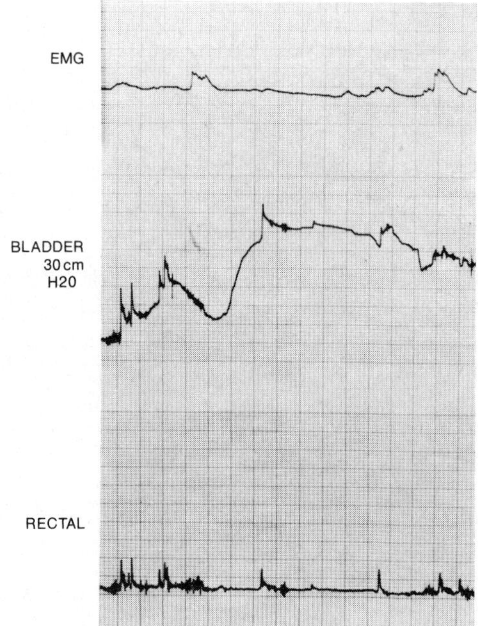

Figure 4–6. Combined recordings of electromyographic (EMG) activity of pelvic floor and intravesical and rectal pressures during filling cystometry. An uninhibited bladder contraction, as evidenced by sudden rise in intravesical pressure without change in intra-abdominal pressure, is evident. The pelvic floor remains "silent." This patient has multiple sclerosis with lesion mainly above brain stem.

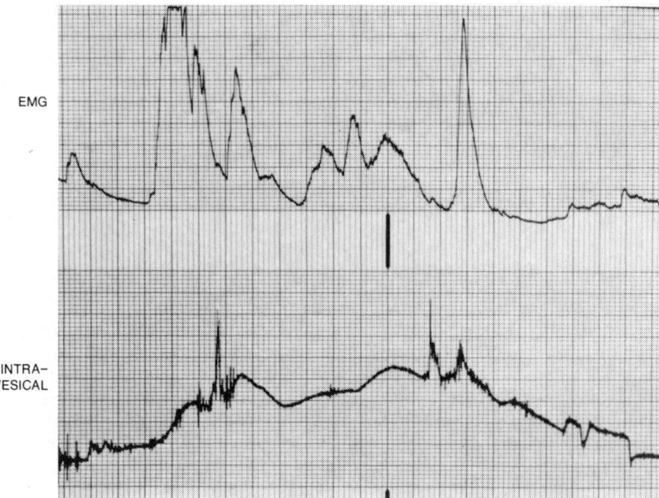

Figure 4–7. Simultaneous recordings of intravesical pressures and electromyographic (EMG) activity show involuntary hyperactivity of external sphincter concomitant to bladder contractions. This is classic pattern of sphincteric dyssynergia in patient with spinal cord lesion.

served bladder-sphincter coordination (Figure 4–6). This type of patient is suffering from a cerebrovascular accident or some other condition above the brain stem; in these patients, hyperreflexia is present, but good coordination between bladder and sphincter is also present. If the fibers connecting the brain stem center to the spinal cord centers are damaged, a very peculiar type of hyperreflexia occurs. This is characterized by lack of bladder-sphincter coordination (bladder-sphincteric dyssynergia) (Figure 4–7). True bladder-sphincteric dyssynergia is defined as the presence of uninhibited bladder contractions with uncoordinated contraction of the pelvic floor, usually with evidence of a spinal cord lesion. Occasionally, in sacral arc lesions, autonomic contractions can be observed. These are small, repetitive, not coordinated, and not capable of producing appropriate bladder emptying (Figure 4–8).

Vesicogenic (Local) Hyperreflexia. This type of hyperreflexia is non-neurogenic and seen mainly in patients with mechanical obstruction and in those with urinary stress incontinence.

Patients with obstruction present with urinary retention deriving from such conditions as stricture or bladder neck contracture with overdistention of the bladder, accompanied by changes in the bladder wall — thickening and hypertrophy of the muscle. Cystometry in these patients can show hyperreflexia. This is more commonly seen in the male, because of the higher incidence of outlet obstruction, but it is also seen in the female.

Another type of hyperreflexia of non-neurogenic origin is seen in females with urinary stress incontinence. Indeed, 30 to 40 per cent of patients complaining of urinary stress incontinence have symptomatic urinary frequency, urgency, urgency incon-

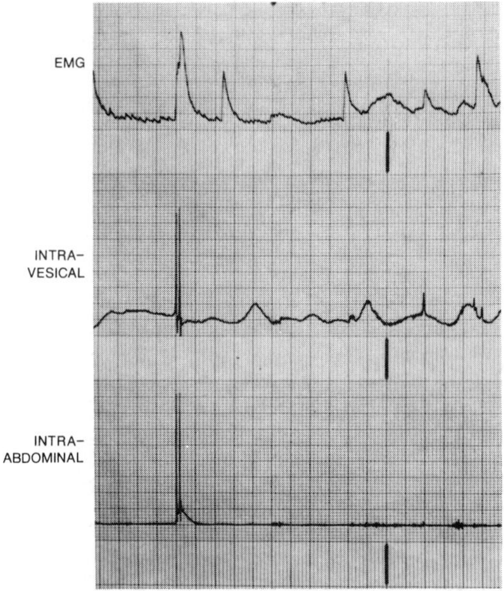

Figure 4–8. Simultaneous recordings of electromyographic (EMG) activity of pelvic floor and intravesical and intra-abdominal pressures in patient with sacral arc lesion (myelomeningocele). Small, ineffective bladder contractions of short duration, with return to baseline pressure (autonomic bladder contractions), are demonstrated.

tinence, and objective demonstration of bladder hyperreflexia on cystometry. It is known, too, that bladder hyperreflexia can disappear with surgery for urinary stress incontinence. However, sometimes only the symptoms of frequency and urgency disappear, and asymptomatic hyperreflexia as demonstrated by cystometrogram persists.

Why does hyperreflexia appear and then disappear? Some suggest that the open bladder neck and constant filling of the posterior urethra, giving an ever-present urge to urinate and sensation of urination, will lead to a tendency toward hyperreflexia. Others believe that these patients are

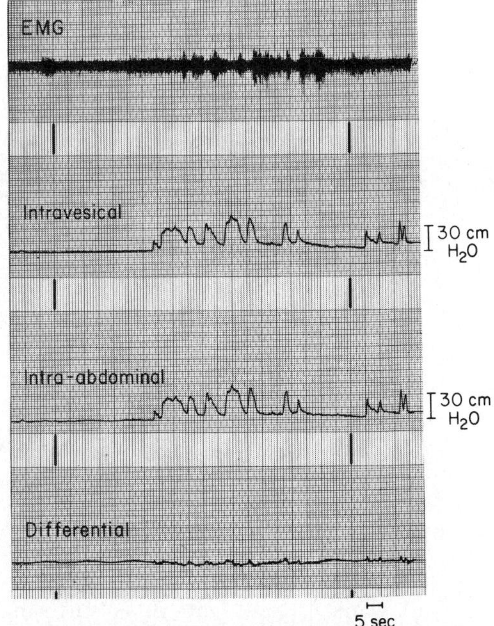

Figure 4–10. Simultaneous recordings of electromyographic (EMG) activity of pelvic floor, intravesical and intra-abdominal pressures, and true detrusor (differential) pressure demonstrate voiding pattern only of abdominal origin with straining. EMG activity of pelvic floor increases without effective bladder contraction.

suffering from idiopathic hyperreflexia in conjunction with sphincteric insufficiency only.

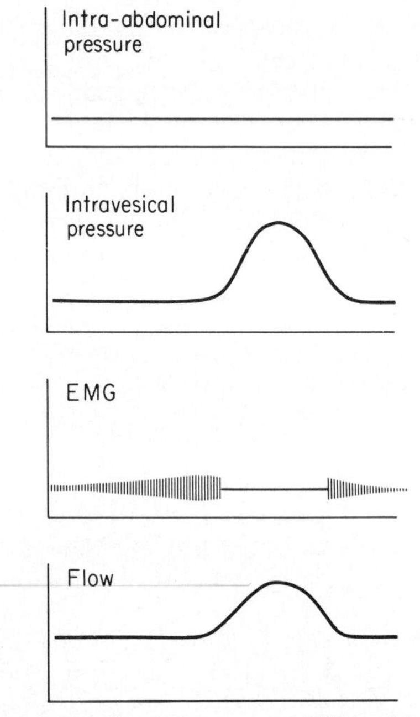

Figure 4–9. Simultaneous recordings of intravesical and intra-abdominal pressures, electromyographic (EMG) activity of pelvic floor, and urinary flow. Normal progressive bladder filling produces increase in the electromyographic activity of the pelvic floor ("holding" pattern). Intravesical pressure is unchanged. During bladder filling, patient is able to abolish any bladder contraction. During voluntary voiding, pelvic floor relaxation occurs 10 to 15 sec. before initiation of bladder contractions. While the bladder contracts, the pelvic floor relaxes (no electromyographic activity or change in intra-abdominal pressure), and excellent urinary flow results. (From Raz, S., and Bradley, W. E.: Neuromuscular dysfunction of the lower urinary tract. *In* Harrision, J. H.: et al.: Campbell's Urology. 4th Ed. Philadelphia, W. B. Saunders Co., 1979.)

VOIDING CYSTOMETRY

When filling cystometry is completed, voiding cystometry is performed. We should remember that filling cystometry tests the ability of the patient to suppress any contractions in the bladder. During voiding cystometry, however, we ask the patient to initiate a bladder contraction. This is done to assess the pattern of micturition, intravesical pressures, and, often, the concomitant urinary flow (Figure 4–9). We also try to determine whether the patient is able to trigger a bladder reflex (Figure 4–10). Again, it should be emphasized that the uncomfortable and embarrassing aspects of cystometry — the instrumentation and unfamiliar environment and personnel — may cause the patient to suppress her detrusor reflex. Therefore, when a patient is asked to urinate under such difficult conditions, sometimes the reflex contraction will not be initiated. This does not mean that the patient has bladder areflexia. On the contrary, in another environment, the patient may be able to produce an excellent urinary stream. For this reason, before we draw any conclusions about the voiding pattern of a particular patient, we should perform a noninvasive urinary flow study under maximal physiologic conditions and assess the comparative curves.

A normal bladder contraction is in the range of 20 to 40 cm of water pressure. At the time of the bladder contraction, there is pelvic floor relaxation and a drop in intraurethral pressure. As soon as the urethra opens widely, the intravesical pressure decreases, because there is equalization between atmospheric and vesical pressure. Patients with severe stress incontinence or incontinence of nonresistance usually present with low vesical pressures, because as soon as the bladder contraction begins, the urethra is wide open and the flow starts immediately. Occasionally, changes in intravesical pressures cannot be recorded (Figure 4–11). This does not mean that the bladder is not contracting. Contractions in the bladder are not detected because the urethra is wide open (funneled) and the patient is contracting her bladder without a measurable change in bladder pressure. Only by occluding the urethra during voiding and stopping micturition in midstream can true intravesical pressures, which cannot be detected on regular voiding cystometry, be recorded.

In the voiding pattern of the female, obstruction produces higher vesical pressures. This signifies outlet obstruction, and it is an attempt to compensate for an obstruction, which is defined as high pressure and low urinary flow. In the female, outlet pressures greater than 50 cm. of water are suggestive of obstruction.

Often, the bladder does not contract during voiding, or the patient is unable to void. If during a noninvasive flow study the patient is also unable to void or has large amounts of retained urine, the pattern of voiding should be observed. Determine if the patient is using abdominal straining (Credé maneuver) to urinate rather than eliciting a true bladder contraction. If the bladder is noncontractile, we try to trigger a bladder contraction by changing the patient's position or by rapid filling. If this is not the case, a denervation supersensitivity test can be performed. The change in intravesical pressure after subcutaneous injection of Urecholine, e.g., an increase in pressure of greater than 15 cm. of water 20 minutes after injection, is suggestive of denervation supersensitivity related to a sacral arc lesion.

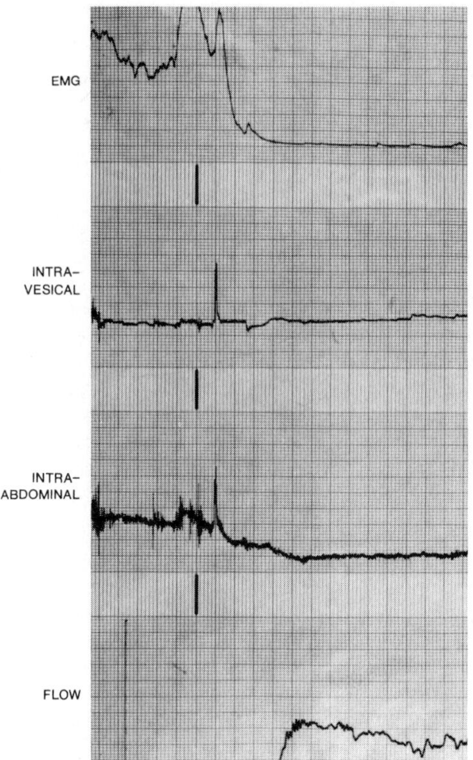

Figure 4–11. Simultaneous recording of electromyographic (EMG) activity of pelvic floor, intravesical and intra-abdominal pressures, and urinary flow in patient with urinary stress incontinence. The pelvic floor relaxes a few seconds before flow starts; there is no detectable change in intravesical pressure.

It is extremely important to record intra-abdominal and intravesical pressures simultaneously. What appears on regular cystometry to be a bladder contraction may be abdominal straining (Figure 4–12). Only by recording true detrusor pressures (subtracting intra-abdominal pressure from total vesical pressure) can this determination be made. Be aware that patients develop changes in intra-abdominal pressure that are reflected in their intravesical pressures.

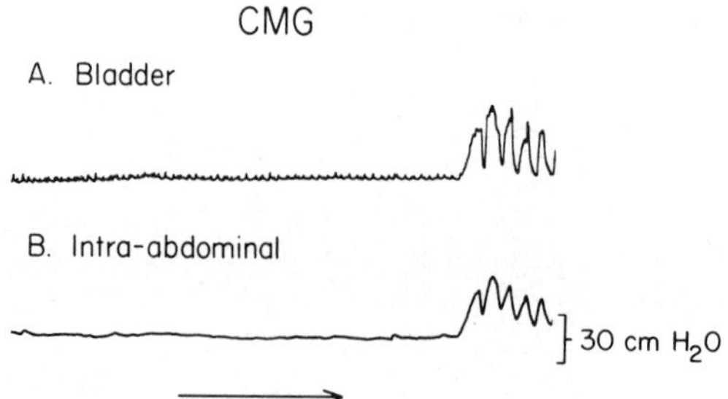

Figure 4–12. Simultaneous recordings of intravesical and intra-abdominal pressures. Attempted voiding with straining is detected by parallel increases in intra-abdominal and intravesical pressures.

These may be falsely detected as bladder contractions when they are really the effects of abdominal straining. Therefore, to define a true bladder contraction, intra-abdominal pressures should be measured and subtracted to obtain true detrusor pressures.

URETHRAL PRESSURE PROFILE

Urethral pressure profile is the measurement of urethral luminal pressures along the length of the urethra while the bladder is noncontractile (Bruskewitz, in press). I will discuss three aspects of this definition: (1) recording of intraluminal pressures; (2) urethral length; and (3) the resting bladder.

Recording Intraluminal Pressures

Several methods have been devised to record pressures: the perfusion method, the balloon method (Einhorning, 1961; Tanagho et al., 1966), and recording of the intraluminal pressure without the use of perfusion by microtip transducers. Each method tests a different aspect of urethral physiology. Although the perfusion method studies the resistance of the urethral wall to the inflow of fluid, pressures as recorded by the balloon or microtip catheter record a different parameter of urethral function — the capability of the urethra to exert intraluminal pressure. Accordingly, there is no one, all-encompassing urethral pressure profile. Each technique provides us with a different parameter of urethral function.

TABLE 4–1. URETHRAL PRESSURE PROFILE

1. Standing and supine position
2. Functional internal outlet
3. Functional length
4. Maximal pressures
5. Active continence
6. Transmission of intra-abdominal pressures to the urethral profile (effect of cough or strain)

Several points are studied during profilometry (Table 4–1).

Urethral Length

The anatomic length of the female urethra is easily measured with a balloon catheter, and it is found to be diminished in patients with sphincteric incompetence. However, urethral pressure profilometry enables us to examine *functional length*, meaning every pressure in the profile curve that is above intravesical pressures. It is this pressure that influences the continence mechanism. As will be discussed below, there can be a great difference between functional length and anatomic length of the urethra.

The Resting Bladder

The third aspect of urethral pressure profilometry is that the bladder should be at rest, especially when carbon dioxide or water perfusion techniques are used with rapid bladder filling. Rapid filling can produce changes in intravesical pressures in patients with bladder neck instability, with every change in intravesical pressure possibly leading to a change in intraurethral pressure and thus a reading that cannot be interpreted. For this reason, it is essential that measurement of urethral pressures be accompanied by a measurement of intravesical pressures. In this way, we can ascertain that there is no artificial change in urethral pressures should the bladder not be at rest during profilometry. Every change in intravesical pressure affects urethral pressure, because during bladder contraction or changes in bladder compliance, stretching forces are exerted on the

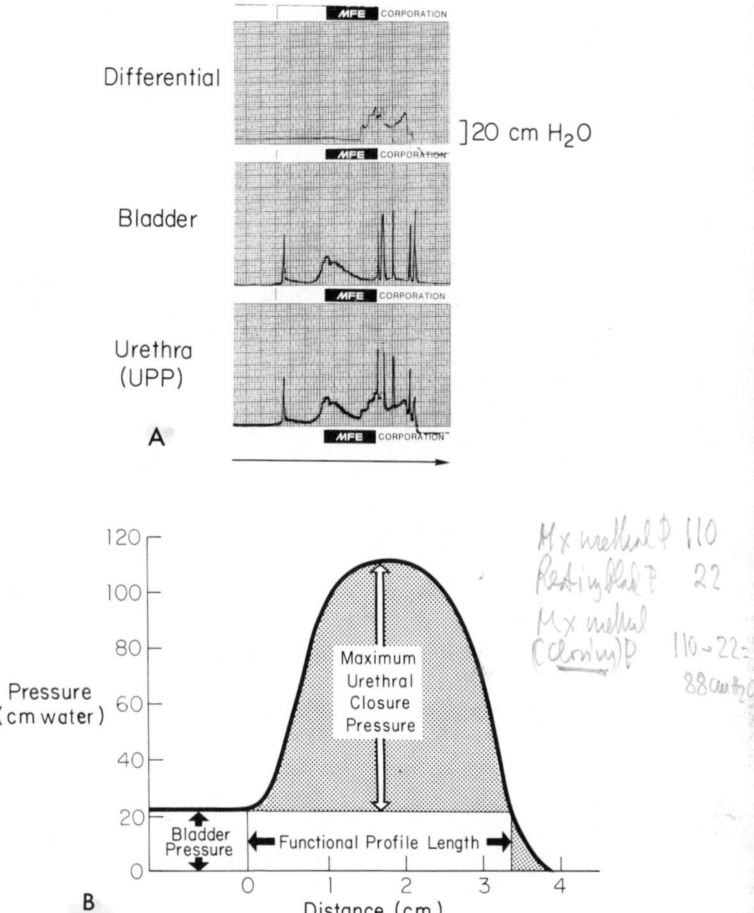

Figure 4–13. *A,* Simultaneous recordings of intravesical and intraurethral (UPP) pressures and the true gradient of pressure between bladder and urethra. Stress hyperreflexia is observed. Immediately after coughing intravesical pressure increases, the same change occurring in the urethra, producing low closing pressure and urinary incontinence. *B,* Diagram showing elements in study of urethral pressure profile. Total profile length is the distance between first increase in pressure at the bladder neck and external meatus, in this case 4 cm. Functional profile length is the distance on the profile curve between two points above intravesical pressure. Total urethral closing pressure is the total pressure from zero line to pressure peak, while the maximal urethral closing pressure is the difference between intravesical pressure and pressure peak of profilometry. (*B,* From Raz, S., and Bradley, W. E.: Neuromuscular dysfunction of the lower urinary tract. *In* Harrison, J. H., et al.: Campbell's Urology. 4th Ed. Philadelphia, W. B. Saunders Co., 1979.)

urethra, as well as funneling and shortening of the urethra (Figure 4–13 *A, B*).

Methodology

The four basic methods for recording urethral pressure are described here.

SPHINCTEROMETRIC STUDY

The sphincterometric study, initially described by Bors (1948), was originally used in males to measure external sphincter function. A modification of the sphincterometric urethral pressure profile was described by Robertson (1974), when he tested the use of carbon dioxide through a urethroscope to measure urethral resistance to the inflow of carbon dioxide.

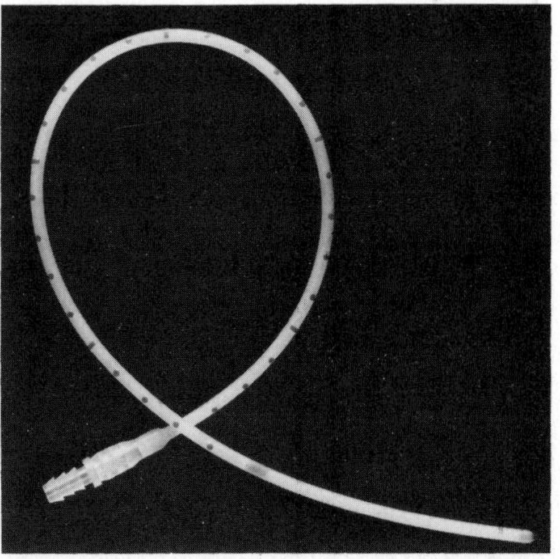

Figure 4–14. Catheter used for perfusion profilometry has a blind tip. Seven to 10 cm. from tip are four to eight small holes per centimeter. Distal to the holes, radiopaque markers are placed to mark centimeters.

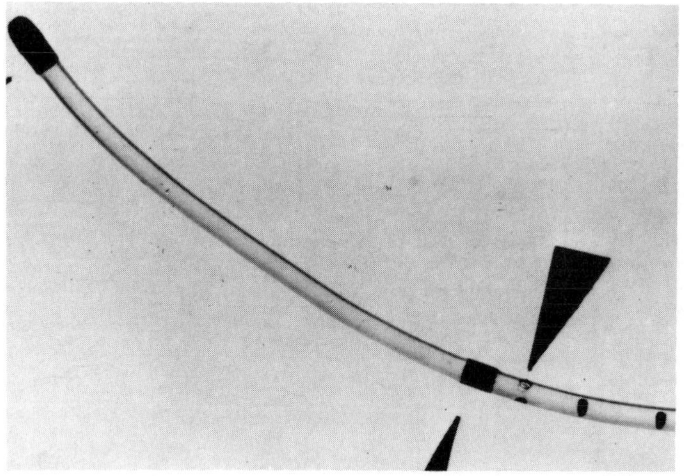

Figure 4–15. Close-up view of the opening of the distal part of perfusion profilometry catheter, showing 1 mm. holes at same level as radiopaque marker, permitting recording of pressures in this area. (From Raz, S., and Bradley, W. E.: Neuromuscular dysfunction of the lower urinary tract. *In* Harrison, J. H., et al.: Campbell's Urology. 4th Ed. Philadelphia, W. B. Saunders Co., 1979.)

BALLOON CATHETER

Urethral pressure profile may also be measured with a balloon catheter (Einhorning, 1961; Tanagho et al., 1966). This method uses a fluid-filled balloon (or balloons) situated near the distal end of the catheter. As the catheter is withdrawn from the urethra, intravesical and intraurethral pressures are recorded via the pressure transducer, which is in communication with the catheter balloons by way of a fluid column. This method measures resistance to urethral distention by a small balloon. Urethral pressure is measured over the entire length of the balloon (Bruskewitz, in press).

PERFUSION TECHNIQUE

The most popular technique for performing urethral pressure profile is the perfusion technique. This method employs a specially adapted catheter with a plugged end and multiple side-facing holes to reduce rotational error (Figures 4–14, 4–15). A continuous flow of either carbon dioxide or water, usually from a perfusion pump, is run through the catheter and exits through the catheter side holes. The catheter is then withdrawn through the urethra, either manually or with a mechanical puller. Urethral resistance to outflow of fluid through the holes is measured (Figures 4–16 to 4–21). Thus, this method has the advantage of localizing changes in urethral pressure (as opposed to the sphincterometric method) at specific points along the urethra. Carbon dioxide is generally perfused at rates of 100 to 150 ml./minute; reliable water perfusion generally employs rates of 2 to 20 ml./minute.

The single channel method relies on initial measurements of bladder pressure, which are assumed to remain constant throughout the study (Bruskewitz, in press). But in situations in which detrusor hyperreflexia is present, the bladder may develop a contraction, and the resultant pressure is transmitted to the urethra, thus

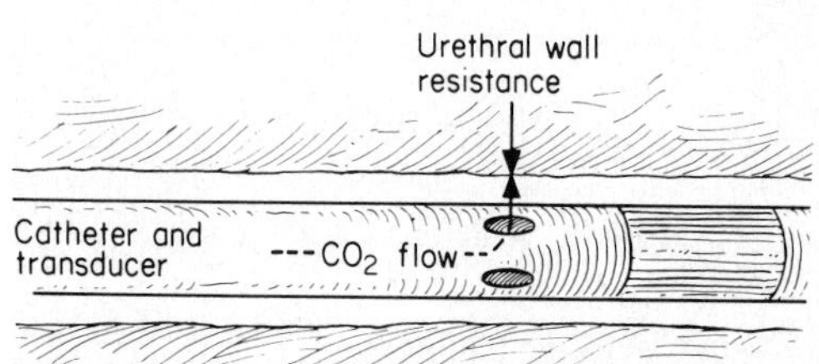

Figure 4–16. Perfusion technique records resistance of urethral wall to perfusion of gas or fluid. Curves obtained will vary depending on size of catheter and rate of perfusion. (From Raz, S.: Diagnosis of urinary incontinence in the male. Urol. Clin. North Am. 5:305, 1978.)

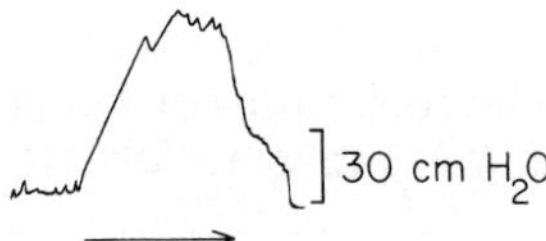

Figure 4–17. Urethral pressure profile in normal young female: functional urethral length of 3 cm. and closing pressure of almost 75 cm. of water.

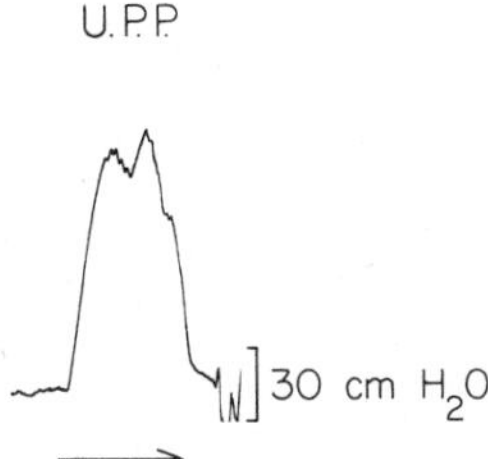

Figure 4–18. Urethral pressure profile (UPP) in patient with very high closing pressure (105 cm. of water).

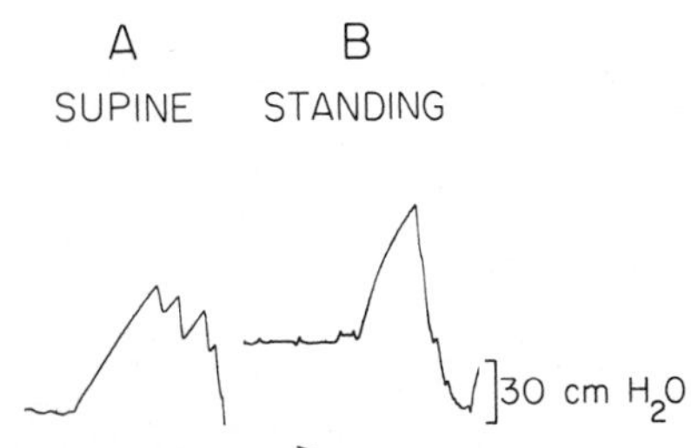

Figure 4–20. Single-channel recordings of urethral pressure profiles in supine *(A)* and standing *(B)* positions. During the study, change in position produces increase in intravesical pressure and parallel increase in (compensation) urethral closing pressure.

producing a change in the urethral pressure profile. This may be erroneously interpreted as true urethral pressure, if bladder pressure is not known at that moment.

The potential for error in balloon and perfusion techniques is manifested when fluid leaks or air bubbles become trapped in the line. There is also an inherent lag time proportional to the connecting catheter and length of tubing (Harrison, 1976). Urethral pressure profiles measured by gas perfusion techniques are also subject to considerable variation with repetitive testing on the same subject, i.e., poor reproducibility (Togure et al., 1979; Wein et al., 1979).

We believe that the most successful method for performing urethral pressure profile on the incontinent female is the one employing the dual channel catheter. A double lumen catheter permits simultaneous recording of bladder and urethral pressures (Glen and Rowan, 1973). Use of x-ray contrast materials for perfusion permits radiographic monitoring (McGuire et al., 1976). Simultaneous recording of intravesical pressures during measurement of the urethral pressure profile allows the operator to note changes occurring in bladder pressure during performance of this study (Bruskewitz, in press). Bladder pressure measurements may be obtained by recording through a suprapubic trocar catheter or by use of a multichannel urethral catheter. In addition to determining urethral closing pressure, defined as bladder pressure subtracted from urethral pressure, bladder pressure may be more accurately recorded at each moment during urethral pressure profilometry.

A variation on the dual channel method is the microtip transducer, which was originally designed to measure intracardiac pressure and subsequently introduced by Asmussen and Ulmsten (1975) for measurements within the lower urinary tract. Side-facing small solid state microtransducers lie within the catheter and allow recording of intraluminal pressures exerted by the urethra on the small catheter membrane. The single side-facing sensor does not result in rotational error. This is a solid state system that does not depend on perfusion of fluid, either through the urethra or through the catheter.

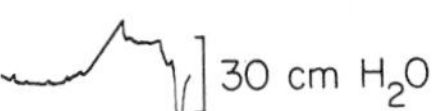

Figure 4–19. Urethral pressure profile in patient with a very short functional urethra and a very low closing pressure (15 cm. of water).

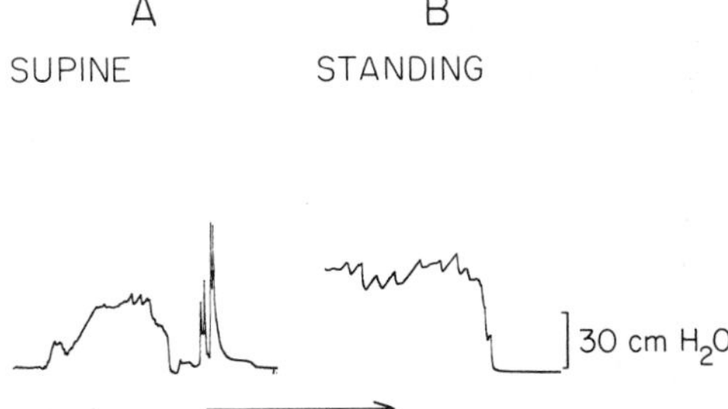

Figure 4–21. Single-channel recordings of urethral pressure profiles in supine *(A)* and standing *(B)* positions. In patients with sphincteric incompetence and urinary stress incontinence, no compensation occurs in the change from supine to standing position; intra-abdominal pressure increases, but urethral closing pressure does not increase, resulting in urinary incontinence.

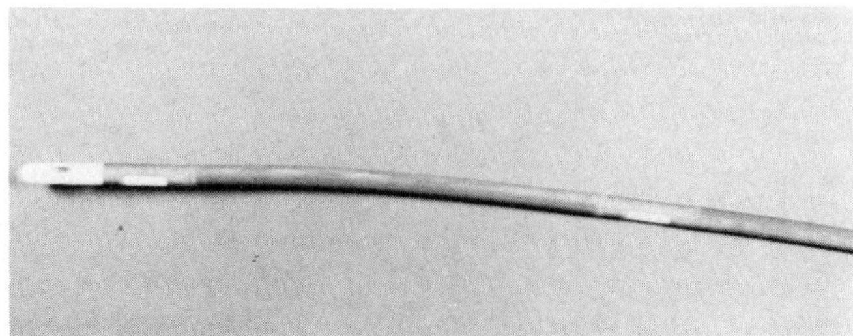

Figure 4–22. Dual-channel microtip transducer with perfusion tip. One centimeter from the proximal end, the first microtip for measuring intravesical pressure is located. Five to 7 cm. from this location, the second microtip is placed for recording of urethral pressure.

OUR OWN METHOD

The microtip catheter (Figure 4–22) is No. 7 French, with two side-facing pressure-sensing areas, each with a surface area of 0.75 mm. (Bruskewitz and Raz, 1979). The most proximal pressure sensor is at the tip of the catheter, and the next is 5 to 7 cm. back from the tip. In performing urethral pressure profiles, the distal sensor records the urethral pressure profile, while the proximal sensor remains in the bladder, allowing simultaneous recording of intravesical and intraurethral pressures. The catheter is manufactured with two silicone in-line strain-gauge pressure transducers designed to sense mechanical pressures and transform them into an electrical signal, which varies in direct proportion to the magnitude of the sensed pressure. The transducer is in turn attached to a transducer control unit and then to an 8-channel strip chart recorder. The unit is calibrated mechanically by submersion in a column of fluid, so that 30 ml. of water is equal to 1 cm. deflection of the recorder needle for the distàl transducer. The catheter is stored in a 500 cc. graduated container filled to a height of 30 cm. with activated dialdehyde solution (Cidex), which is used for the mechanical calibration and sterilization. Electronic calibration is also obtained by a transducer control unit which has an electrically calibrated signal of 100 mm. Hg. In this way, double calibration, electronic and mechanical, can be obtained. The tip of the catheter is covered during storage with a special shield, allowing both sterilization and protection of the sensitive microtips.

The catheter is withdrawn at a continuous rate of 1 mm./second, using a Harvard pump withdrawal system connected to a wire and catheter holder. The strip chart recorder is set at 1 mm./second, providing a direct correlation between the rate of catheter withdrawal and the speed of the strip chart recorder. Reading of the functional length of the urethra is thus simplified.

Urethral pressure profiles are obtained with the bladder both empty and full (filled to 200 ml.), in the supine and standing positions. The patient is asked to cough at each centimeter of catheter withdrawal. Coughing and straining may elicit changes in intravesical pressure, suggesting instability of the bladder and permitting recording of changes in the transmission of intra-abdominal pressure to the bladder and urethra. This information is transferred to the chart recorder, where a third preamplifier simultaneously records the differential pressures between urethra and bladder.

Interpretation of Results

Parameters studied in urethral pressure profile recording are (1) profile length; (2) functional profile length, defined as the distance along the profile curve at which the urethral pressure is above the intravesical pressure; (3) maximum urethral pressure, the difference between the basal pressure and maximal pressure in the profile curve; (4) maximal closing pressure, which is the difference between the maximal pressure and intravesical pressure; and (5) the shape of the curve.

In the young female, the anatomic length of the urethra is about 4 cm. But the average urethral length in patients studied in our unit is 2.8 cm., with a bell-shaped curve. (This is the group with normal continence.) In patients with stress incontinence due to sphincter incompetence (urethral incontinence), we find a shorter functional urethra, about 2 cm. This difference may be due to a characteristic of urinary stress incontinence, the incompetent bladder neck, wide-open and presenting a decreased functional length.

Fifty patients were studied with concomitant perfusion of the bladder and recording of intravesical and intraurethral pressures. Patients with normal continence displayed a functional urethral length of 28 mm. which decreased to 24 mm. after filling; the functional urethral length of the patient with urinary stress incontinence was 20 mm., but with bladder filling, this remained almost unchanged.

What happens to the closing pressure of the urethra? On a supine pressure profile, the normal closing pressure in the young female is 70 to 90 cm. of water. In older patients, who have undergone multiple deliveries and menopausal changes, the closing pressure is between 40 and 60 cm. of water. Patients with stress incontinence due to sphincter incompetence usually have lower closing pressures. Maximal closing pressure averages 32 cm. of water.

Advantages and Disadvantages of Microtip Pressure Recording

The use of a dual channel transducer has improved our understanding of female urethral pathophysiology. We believe the single channel pressure profile recording, unaccompanied by simultaneous recording of bladder pressure, fails to provide sufficient information, except when pressures are high or low. When pressures are extremely high (above 100 cm. of water), patients are usually experiencing inflammatory changes, with increased tonicity in the area of the external sphincter or a tight urethral stricture. If a patient complains of urinary stress incontinence and high urethral pressures are found, sphincteric insufficiency is rare.

A second group of patients in whom single channel recording is useful is that group in whom the urethra shows low maximal pressure (30 cm. of water). These patients generally have intrinsic damage to the urethral mechanism, whether or not pelvic relaxation is present. Damage accompanied by periurethral fibrosis often is a sequel of multiple surgery or irradiation.

With the dual channel microtip transducer, concomitant recording of intravesical and intraurethral pressures allows us to document the gradient of pressure of the urethra over the bladder. Patients with normal continence maintain a positive gradient of pressure with coughing, abdominal straining, or positional change. The intraurethral pressure will remain higher than the intravesical. In patients with urinary stress incontinence due to sphincter insufficiency, the gradient of pressure is decreased, and the intraurethral pressure tends to equal the intravesical pressure, objectively demonstrating sphincteric insufficiency (Figure 4–23).

Postoperative studies using the dual channel microtip transducer have shown that the most important change that occurs is not due to increase in functional length of the urethra, maximum pressure of the urethra, or urethral closing pressure, but rather is the result of a positive gradient of pressure, with adequate transmission of pressure at the time of coughing and straining. The intraurethral pressure remains higher than the intravesical pressure at all times. Anatomic repositioning of the proximal urethra has produced a change in functioning, with closure of the proximal urethra during stress.

In patients with normal continence during coughing and straining, intra-abdominal

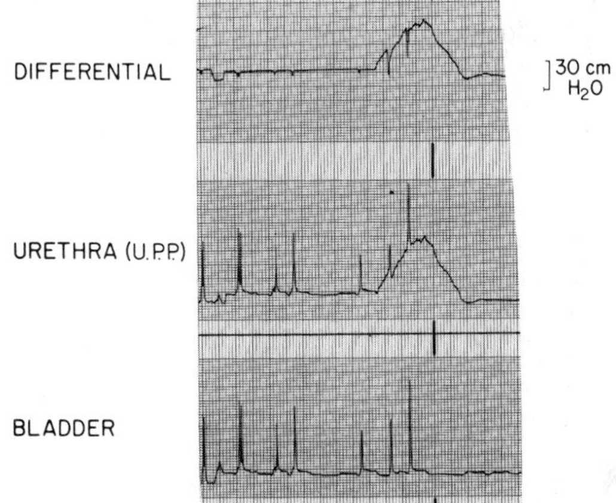

Figure 4–23. Study performed with dual-channel microtip transducer: recording of intravesical and intraurethral pressures and pressure gradient (differential). During profilometry and coughing, the urethra is unable to maintain the closing pressure and a negative pressure gradient occurs. No changes occur in intravesical pressure between coughs. This patient has objective sphincteric incompetence. (Adapted from Bruskewitz, R., and Raz, S.: Urethral pressure profile using microtip catheter in females. Urology *14*:303, 1979.)

pressures are transmitted equally to the proximal urethra above the external sphincter and the bladder, allowing maintenance of a positive gradient of pressures between urethra and bladder. In continent females, the gradient becomes negative distal to the external sphincter with coughing; in patients with severe urethral prolapse without coughing, coughing and straining produce poor transmission of intra-abdominal pressures to the proximal urethra. However, intraurethral pressure will remain higher than intravesical pressure. In patients with pelvic floor relaxation and urinary stress incontinence, coughing or straining produces equalization of intraurethral and intravesical pressures and a negative gradient of pressure (a sharp negative deflection in the differential channel), demonstrating that during coughing or straining the intravesical pressure is equal to the intraurethral pressure. This is when stress occurs. This is a typical and important diagnostic pattern which objectively records urinary stress incontinence due to sphincter insufficiency.

It should be pointed out, however, that both membrane and microtip catheters are sensitive instruments and require close attention to keep them functioning properly. Because the microtip transducer is a delicate, expensive instrument, it is basically a research tool and is not generally available for office practice.

URINARY FLOW

Urinary flow measures the amount of urine voided in a given period of time. This is expressed in milliliters of urine per second. A few principles of fluid dynamics should be understood for the operator to have a full comprehension of urinary flow studies.

The bladder may be compared to a column of fluid and the urethra to a tube from which the urine exits. The first factor which determines urinary flow (ml./second) is the height of the column of water, i.e., the forces of expulsion. If pressure is high, there will be a parallel increase in the flow. There is, accordingly, a direct, proportional relationship between the urinary flow and the pressure exerted by the bladder.

The second factor is the length of the urethra. The longer the urethra, the smaller the flow and the greater the resistance the urine must overcome. Higher resistance, then, will produce a lower flow. Flow, therefore, is in indirect proportion to the length of the urethra.

The third important factor in the determination of urinary flow is the cross section of the urethra. The narrower the urethra, the more restricted the urinary flow, and the wider the cross section of the urethra, the better the flow. These again are relationships of direct proportion: a larger area produces a larger flow. Because the cross section of a circle is twice the radius squared, divided by pi, it is easy to appreciate how a tiny change in an already diminished cross section of the urethra can produce such a severe impact on the urinary flow.

A fourth factor that must be appreciated is that when urine begins to flow, the flow in the bladder neck, in the midurethra, and in the distal urethra is exactly the same. The flow that is maintained along the tube (in this case the urethra) is even. It can be compared to a river in which water is flowing from a reservoir downstream. The amount of water that enters this narrow stream is the same at the beginning or at the end of the stream. The main difference is that there is a very narrow area, where we can observe an increase in the velocity of the water, but if this channel is widened, the velocity of the water will be diminished, and the water will be calm.

This analogy can be applied directly to urinary flow. The flow from the neck of the bladder to the distal urethra is exactly the same all along the length of the urethra. In areas where there is urethral dilatation, the velocity of the urine will be diminished, not

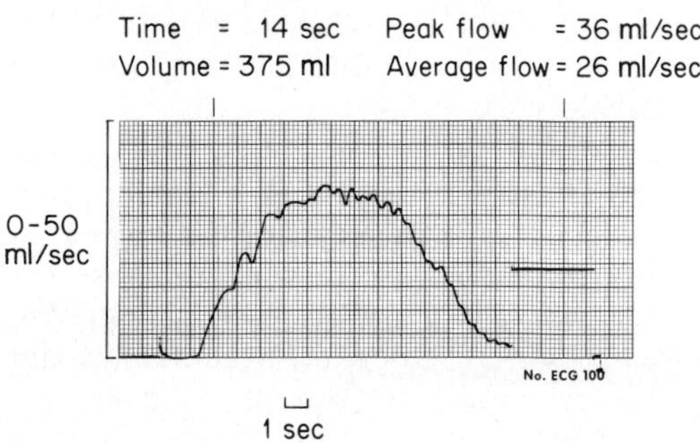

Figure 4–24. Urinary flow rate study in normal patient showing peak flow rate of 36 ml./sec., average flow rate of 26 ml./sec., and volume of 375 ml. voided in 14 sec. This is a normal voiding pattern.

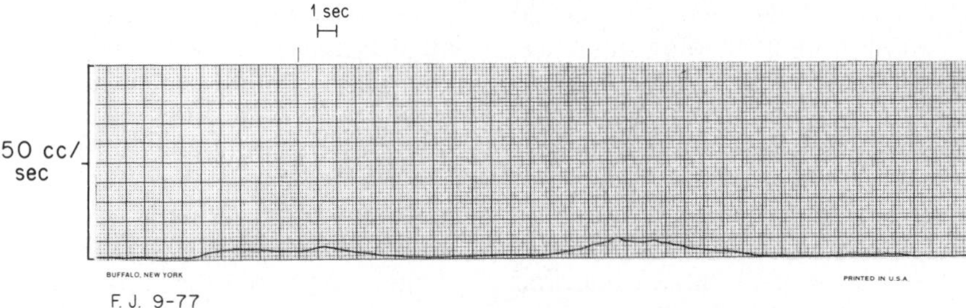

Figure 4–25. Urinary flow rate study in patient with outlet obstruction. Peak flow rate is extremely low and voiding time prolonged. (From Raz, S., and Bradley, W. E.: Neuromuscular dysfunction of the lower urinary tract. *In* Harrison, J. H., et al.: Campbell's Urology. 4th Ed. Philadelphia, W. B. Saunders Co., 1979.)

the flow. But in areas where the urethra is narrow, there will be a sharp increase in velocity to maintain a constant urinary flow.

Urinary flow is not easy to determine, because of the many factors involved. But, in general, flow is a good screening test for voiding dysfunction. Urinary flow depends upon two main factors: the forces of expulsion (intra-abdominal pressures and bladder contraction) and urethral resistance (such as adequate urethral relaxation, funneling of the bladder neck, and so forth).

Normally, the patient will urinate 300 ml., with a peak flow of 20 ml./second and a voiding time of 10 to 15 seconds. The curve is an uninterrupted bell-shaped curve (Figure 4–24).

When the flow curve is examined, several factors must be identified: the time used for voiding (in seconds); the peak flow, i.e., the maximum flow achieved; the average flow (calculated by dividing the voided volume by the time in seconds); and, finally, the volume of urine voided. Each of these factors can change the urinary flow.

As mentioned, the normal curve of flow is an unobstructed, uninterrupted type of stream, which might produce a few spurts of urine, such as we occasionally see with obstruction. Occasionally the peak flow will be high, but if the curve is interrupted, this may be suggestive of an obstructive pattern. Voiding time may be prolonged, also suggesting urinary obstruction (Figure 4–25). Spurts of urine may signify that the patient is voiding by abdominal straining and not by a true bladder contraction.

The amount of urine voided changes the urinary flow drastically. If the volume voided is less than 100 or 150 ml., interpretation will be difficult. When small volumes are voided, the appearance of the curve is obstructive. But if the same patient voids a larger volume, the curve can be entirely normal (Figure 4–26).

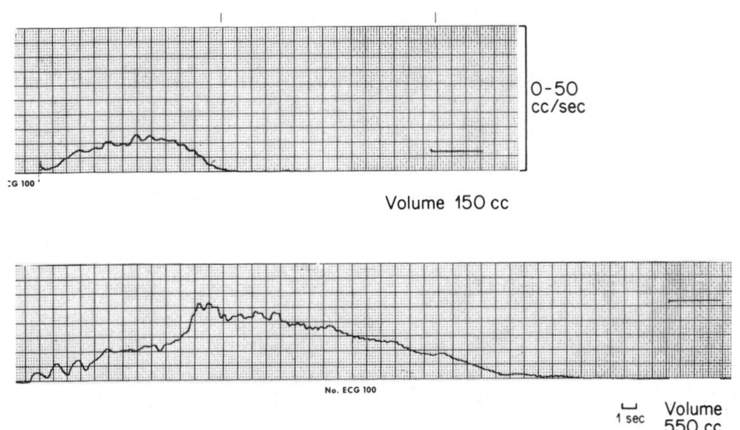

Figure 4–26. Urinary flow rates performed in same patient as in Figure 4–25 but with two different volumes, 150 and 550 ml. The smaller volume (upper graph) shows relatively low peak of only 12 ml./sec., but the greater volume (lower graph) shows peak flow of more than 25 ml./sec., stressing importance of recording voided volume at time of urinary flowmetry.

In general, peak flows of more than 20 ml./second and a normal voiding time suggest a nonobstructive pattern. Peak flows of less than 10 ml./second with a prolonged voiding time, by the same token, suggest obstruction. When the peak flow is between 10 and 20 ml./second, other factors can be considered. A patient with very powerful bladder contractions may have a normal urinary flow, compensating for the obstruction by the high pressures which the bladder can develop. In contrast, in the patient with no obstruction and poor urinary flow a lack of expulsive forces may account for the poor urinary flow.

When the flow is between 10 and 20 ml./second, it is important to determine intravesical pressures. A patient who urinates with high intravesical pressures and poor flow has obstruction. This relationship can be further assessed by studying intravesical pressure at the time of voiding by calculating urethral resistance. We use the simple formula of Resistance $= \frac{P}{F^2}$. This is not meant to reduce the function of urethra to a mathematical formula, but is offered mainly to enable the operator to appreciate obstruction. If the relationship between pressure and flow, as expressed by $R = \frac{P}{F^2}$, is more than 0.4 or 0.5, obstruction is not usually indicated. For example, if a patient voids with intravesical pressures of 40 cm. of water and a peak flow of 20 ml/second, resistance can be calculated thus: $\frac{P}{F^2} = \frac{40}{400} = 0.1$, suggesting obstruction. In the case of another patient, with maximal pressure during voiding of 60 cm. of water and a urinary flow of 10 ml/second, the relationship would be $\frac{60}{100}$, or 0.6, suggesting a pattern of obstruction.

Another important factor which often changes urinary flow is the environment — the lack of privacy that surrounds all of this testing. Much of the time a patient's flow will be affected by the difference in conditions between urinating on the flow chair and urinating in her own home, where her pattern of voiding is likely to be completely different. As much as possible, patients should be able to perform the voiding study in private.

An invasive type of urinary flow recording will also change the whole pattern. If electromyographic needles or recording catheters have been inserted, the urinary flow may be completely different from the flow the patient is able to develop without instrumentation. Thus, a word of caution is in order when urinary flow is performed in conjunction with other urodynamic testing. A noninvasive urinary flow should always be performed for purposes of comparison.

VIDEO-PRESSURE-FLOW STUDIES

Video-pressure-flow studies are a combination of the previously described individual tests, emphasizing voiding and filling cystometry, urinary flow, and fluoroscopic observation of lower urinary tract changes during voiding. Video-pressure-flow studies are an excellent means of documenting the correlation between changes in intravesical pressures and the anatomic findings of individual radiologic studies. The chief drawback of video-pressure-flow studies is the expense of the sophisticated equipment required for the mixing of the radiologic picture with the pressure studies. Consequently, performance of these studies is reserved to selected urodynamic centers.

Materials and Methods

Two catheters are usually inserted into the bladder, a small Foley catheter and a small filling tube. Intra-abdominal pressures are recorded with an intra-abdominal balloon; optionally, electromyographic activity of the pelvic floor may be recorded. Under fluoroscopic observation, intravesical pressures are recorded, and the image is transmitted and mixed by the fluoroscopic video tape image intensifier. The pressure recordings are likewise included in the image, permitting constant monitoring. A microphone can also be introduced on the video tape, so that we can hear the instructions being given to the patient, as well as document the patient's first sensation of urination, voiding sensations, and maximal capacity. All of this provides an excellent physiologic study of the lower urinary tract,

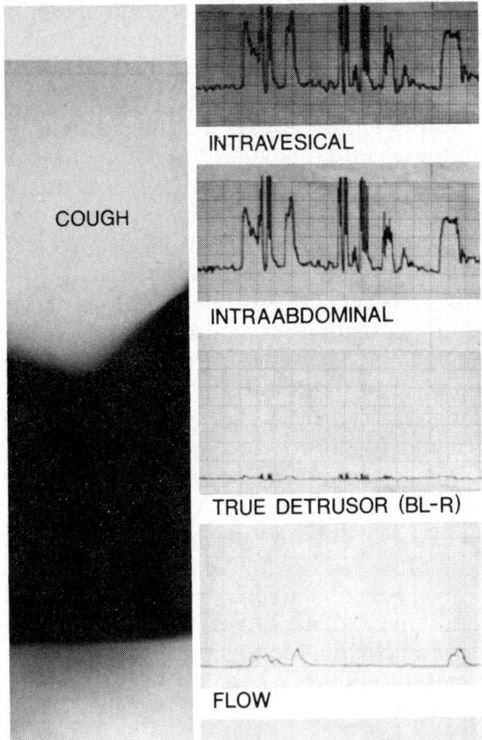

Figure 4–27. Combined true detrusor pressure, urinary flow, and video-imaging. The patient shows increase in intra-abdominal and intravesical pressures during coughing, but no change in true detrusor pressure. Involuntary loss of urine at time of coughing is evidenced by small spikes in flow curve.

combining the best methods for studying lower urinary tract dysfunction.

After filling cystometry with the patient in the supine position, the patient is allowed to stand. We observe the hypermobility of the bladder, the relationship between the urethra and bladder neck, the presence or absence of bladder neck funneling, and the level of continence. When the patient is asked to cough and strain, intravesical, intra-abdominal, and true detrusor pressures are recorded by electronic subtraction. We observe the competence of the bladder neck and the absence or presence of urinary stress incontinence during coughing. If urinary stress incontinence does indeed occur, we must determine if straining causes any change in the true detrusor pressure (Figure 4–27). Urinary stress incontinence due to sphincteric incompetence (urethral incontinence) is defined as involuntary loss of urine occurring during straining without a change in the true detrusor pressure. Patients with bladder incontinence (hyperreflexia or unstable bladder) experience a progressive increase in intravesical pressures and in the true detrusor pressures as well, demonstrating that incontinence has occurred because of changes in the detrusor pressure, rather than because of sphincteric incompetence.

Urinary flow studies are recorded, as well as postvoid residual urine. These studies are easy to review on video tape and can be stored in an efficient fashion, along with diagnostic treatment plans for the patient.

ELECTROMYOGRAPHY

Electromyography is not generally required in a urodynamic assessment. I perform it only when I suspect that a patient is suffering from neurogenic bladder. Sphincter electromyography can be performed by the insertion of needle electrodes or by the use of surface electrodes (Raz and Bradley, 1979). My preference is for needle electrodes, which can be used to explore the muscles of the pelvic floor for evidence of individual denervation potential. Electromyograpy can also be used to test the coughing and straining reflexes of the pelvic floor and patterns of voiding.

RADIOLOGY

Complete evaluation of female urinary incontinence requires a multifaceted approach, of which radiologic assessment is an extremely important part (Shapiro and Raz, in press). Synchronous pressure-flow-cine cystourethrography provides objective data on the anatomy of the female lower urinary tract, which is utilized to aid in therapeutic decision-making. Although this type of approach requires sophisticated equipment that is available only at urodynamic centers, cystography and fluoroscopy should be widely available.

History

Barnes first reported the x-ray use of a chain of beads in 1942 to determine urethral configuration. Ball (1950) showed that the x-ray appearance of a Foley catheter could be used to determine urethral position. Muellner (1949) used fluoroscopy and showed descent of the bladder base on coughing, which caused funneling of the bladder neck as the result of a rise in intra-abdominal pressure. Jeffcoate and Roberts (1952) introduced the concept of the posterior urethrovesical angle (PUV) as a constant anatomic change in the patients with urinary stress incontinence. Hodgkinson, in 1953, using the metallic bead chain technique, found that urethral sphincter dysfunction is characterized by (1) descent of the urethrovesical junction and bladder base on straining without backward rotation of the bladder; (2) conversion of the bladder neck to the most dependent position of the bladder; and (3) funneling of the proximal urerthra. Tanagho (1974) used cystourethrography as the most valuable diagnostic tool in evaluating incontinent female patients, and most physicians still use cystourethrography in their assessment of the problem.

Materials and Methods

Before the study, the patient is asked to empty her bladder; if the patient has a full bladder, she can sit on the flow chair, and a noninvasive urinary flow study can be done before catheter insertion and manipulation take place (Shapiro and Raz, in press). A No. 8 or 10 French Robinson catheter is introduced into the bladder and the postvoid residual measured. The bladder is then filled under low pressure (15 cm. above the pubis) with 30 per cent meglamine diatrizoate (Cystografin). A three-way stopcock can be interposed in the perfusion line and connected to a manometer to record intermittent intravesical pressures during filling. Fluoroscopic observation of the bladder during filling is done with the patient in the supine position. Anteroposterior (AP) and oblique views are obtained, to look for vesicoureteric reflux and observe overall shape. The first sensation of voiding and bladder capacity are then recorded. The perfusion bottle is watched, or the intravesical pressure is recorded through the filling catheter to look for bladder pressures above 15 cm. of water or uninhibited contractions, which will stop the perfusion. The patient is then placed in an upright position on the tilted fluoroscopic table. The femurs are lined up fluoroscopically to give a true lateral view. Relaxing and straining are done in the AP and lateral positions. With the patient in a 30 degree oblique position, the catheter is removed, and the level of continence, or the presence of incontinence, is observed during straining. The position of the bladder neck and urethra with relation to the inferior border of the pubic symphysis is noted. Coughing views are taken to determine if incontinence occurs only during cough or is prolonged after the coughing maneuver stops. The patient then is asked to void with fluoroscopic observation of the outlet. (It is unusual to find a patient with incontinence who cannot void under fluoroscopy.) The patient is asked to stop voiding by contracting her pelvic floor and, after a 5- to 10-second delay, a film is taken to determine if there is closure of the bladder neck. The patient then finishes voiding, and a postvoid film is taken.

Interpretation

The AP film is used mainly to study the mobility and position of the bladder base.

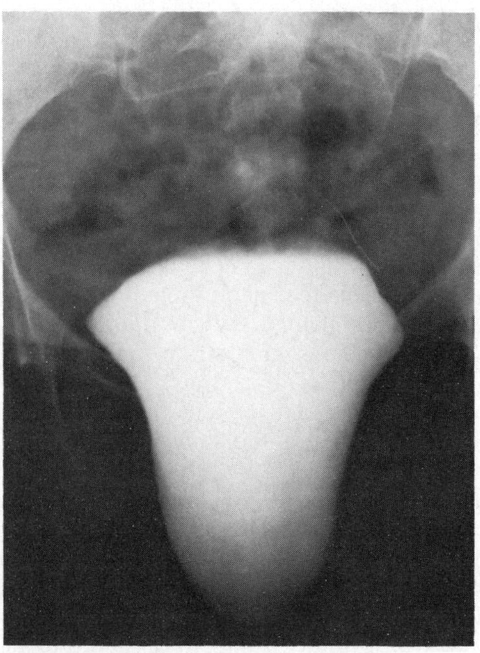

Figure 4–28. Anteroposterior cystogram demonstrates severe cystocele effacing the area of the bladder neck and urethra.

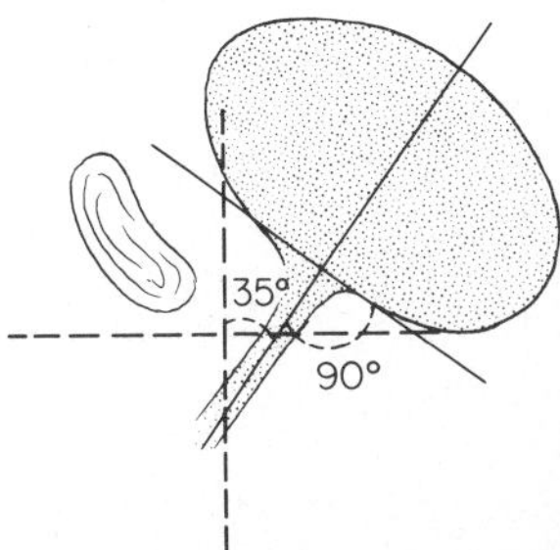

Figure 4–29. Diagram of lateral straining film showing the three elements that must be analyzed during studies: (1) the bladder base, which should not drop below the inferior pubic rami; (2) the relationship between the urethra and trigone (normal urethrotrigonal angle of 90 degrees), signifying a competent, closed bladder neck; (3) the axis of the urethra, which should not normally be greater than 35 or 40 degrees.

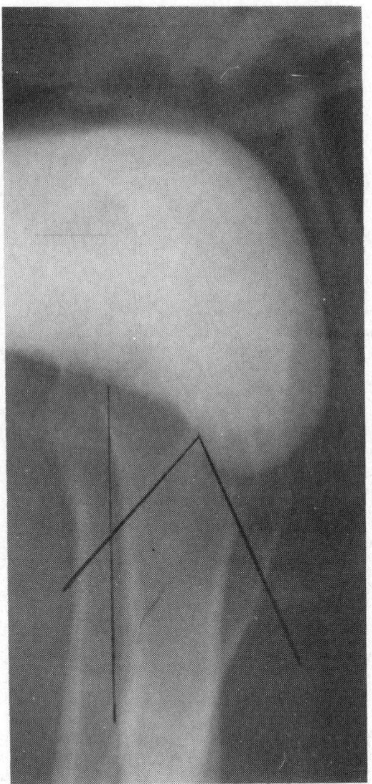

Figure 4–30. Lateral cystography in patient in the standing position during straining demonstrating changes in axis of urethra, urethrotrigonal angle, and relationship of bladder base to pubic symphysis. The urethra is well supported; there is no cystocele or evidence of funneling of the bladder neck.

In adolescents, the bladder is above the pelvis, but with puberty, the base descends to the level of the superior ramus of the pubic symphysis. During abdominal straining, the bladder should descend no farther than the inferior border of the symphysis. A cystocele is indicated by prolapse of the bladder beneath the symphysis on straining films (Figure 4–28). During straining, hypermobility of the bladder can be noted, and in procidentia the entire bladder may be seen under the level of the pubic symphysis. If cystocele is present, the bladder neck and urethra are obscured on the AP films, and their presence can only be appreciated on the lateral films.

True lateral films are the most important studies to assess the anatomic changes of the lower urinary tract. They provide a physical examination of the patient in the straining position, as well as objective evaluations of the position of the bladder neck and urethra and the amount of cystocele. These anatomic aspects are very difficult to evaluate in the supine position; incontinence in the female is a disease of the standing position.

Three elements of the lower urinary tract — the bladder neck, bladder base, and urethra — can prolapse and are best seen on true lateral films (Figures 4–29, 4–30). The most important anatomic abnormality is loss of the posterior urethrotrigonal angle. The normal angle between the urethra and trigone in patients whose level of continence is at the bladder neck is 90 degrees or less. When the angle becomes

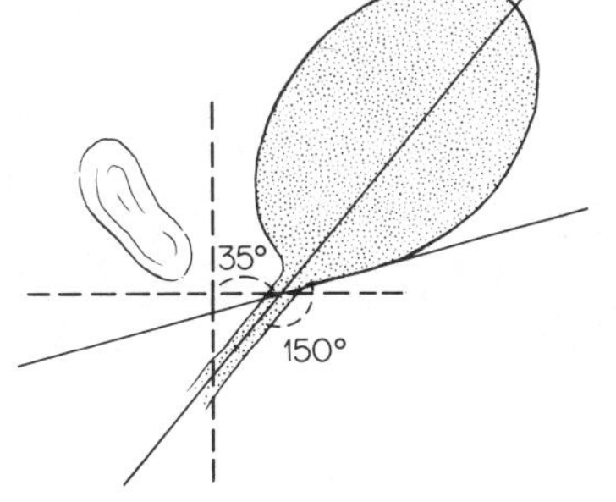

Figure 4–31. Diagram illustrating funneling of the bladder neck. The urethral axis is normal, but the urethrotrigonal angle is increased, and the bladder base is located higher than inferior pubic rami.

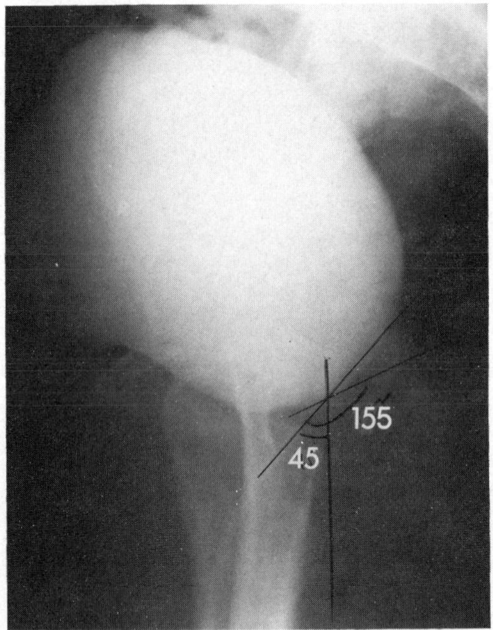

Figure 4–32. Lateral cystography in a patient with a urethral axis of 45 degrees (no urethral prolapse) and no evidence of cystocele, as shown by the location of the bladder base higher than the inferior pubic rami, but with funneling of bladder neck. This patient has multiple sclerosis with a large residual urine volume.

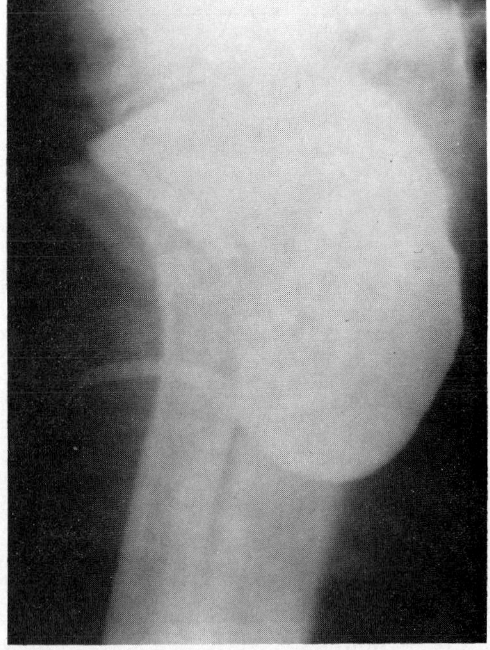

Figure 4–34. True lateral cystogram from a patient with triple anomaly of cystocele, increase in urethral axis (prolapse), and funneling of the bladder neck. These anatomic abnormalities can be seen in patients *without* urinary stress incontinence.

obtuse or disappears (180 degrees), the bladder neck becomes incompetent. Loss of the posterior urethrotrigonal angle is a static radiologic finding and may be seen in patients without sphincteric insufficiency and with normal continence, as well as in patients with incontinence due to neurogenic bladder or poor compliance (Figures 4–31 to 4–34). Ninety-five per cent of patients with true stress incontinence due to sphincteric insufficiency demonstrate bladder neck incompetence. Therefore, if a patient presents with urinary incontinence but a normal urethrotrigonal angle, i.e., competent bladder neck, some other reason for her incontinence, such as hyperreflexia or large residuals, not secondary to anatomic abnormality, may be present.

After removal of the catheter, oblique upright, relaxed and straining films are done under fluoroscopy. Given a competent bladder neck, normal bladder base and urethra, the level of continence is at the bladder neck itself. A horizontal line at the bladder base indicates a competent, closed bladder neck. Bladder neck incompetence at the level of continence is in the area of the midurethra or — very occasionally — in the distal urethra (Figure 4–35).

Documentation of bladder neck incompetence in the standing position is quite important. Findings on the oblique films are

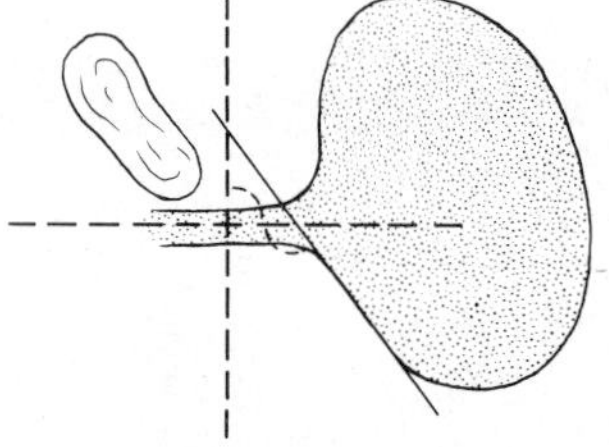

Figure 4–33. Diagram showing the three elements of the lower urinary tract in prolapse: cystocele (bladder lower than the inferior pubic rami); urethral prolapse (increase in urethral axis); and funneling of the bladder neck.

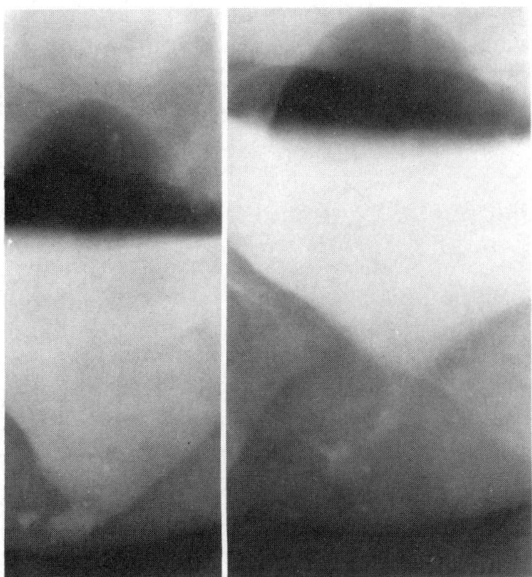

Figure 4–35. Relaxation and straining films after filling in a patient with sphincteric insufficiency show wide-open bladder neck in oblique position and hypermobility of bladder base. Cystocele, funneling of the bladder neck, and objective urinary incontinence during straining are demonstrated.

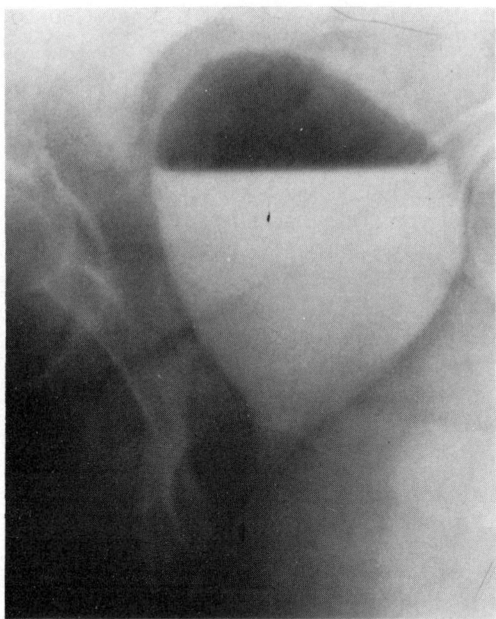

Figure 4–36. Oblique standing cystogram while the patient is coughing. Bladder neck funneling and involuntary loss of urine only at time of coughing are observed.

used to corroborate the findings of the previously discussed true lateral films. Patients with normal posterior urethrotrigonal angles should have a competent bladder neck, with the level of continence at the neck. Patients with a funneled bladder neck on the true lateral film should demonstrate the same findings on the oblique films. To repeat, the patient must have a stable bladder, without uninhibited contractions or changes in the detrusor pressure, for these assumptions to be valid.

It is rare for patients with clinically significant true stress incontinence to be able to maintain continence under fluoroscopy. Coughing films (Figure 4–36) provide objective evidence of urinary incontinence and help to differentiate urgency incontinence from stress incontinence, particularly when a clinical history is ambiguous. Incontinence can be demonstrated by asking the patient to cough before she is catheterized. It is important to time the incontinence in relation to the stress. If there is a delay between coughing and incontinence, or if there is continued incontinence under stress, bladder instability must be suspected. Stress hyperreflexia, or unstable stress incontinence, may result from a cough that causes an uninhibited bladder contraction

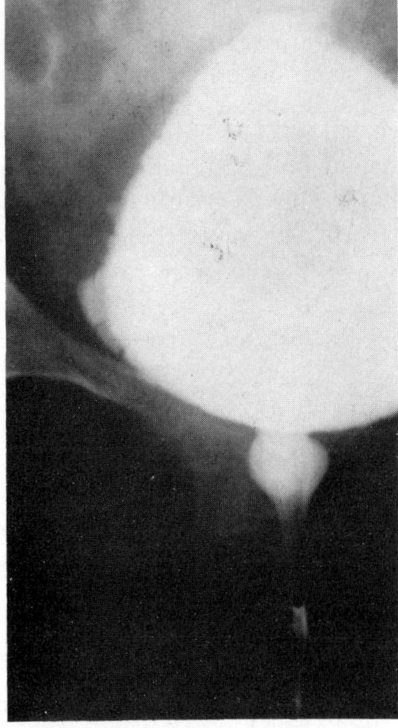

Figure 4–37. Voiding cystogram from a patient with outlet obstruction due to external sphincter dysfunction and neurogenic bladder. The bladder is trabeculated with pseudodiverticula; the urethra is deformed, with severe dilatation of the proximal two thirds and narrowing in the area of the external sphincter.

and sudden relaxation of the pelvic floor, with loss of urine. This is not sphincteric insufficiency, and a patient demonstrating these findings would not benefit from bladder neck suspension.

During voiding under fluoroscopic control, the patient is checked for the presence or absence of abdominal straining and for any abnormalities of the urethral outlet (Figure 4–37). We look for urethral diverticula, outlet obstruction, distal sphincteric dysfunction, vesicoureteral reflux, trabeculation, and diverticula of the bladder. When the patient is asked to stop micturition, she should be able to inhibit voiding, and within 3 to 5 seconds the bladder neck should return to the normal shape, with the level of continence at the bladder neck. In this case a patient with sphincteric insufficiency or hyperreflexia may be able to elevate the base of the bladder, but the bladder neck will remain incompetent. Hyperreflexic patients can actively contract their pelvic floor against a true detrusor contraction, leaving the bladder neck wide open.

On postvoiding films, we have been surprised a number of times to find large residuals of urine in patients complaining of urinary stress incontinence. Patients with severe prolapse may have outlet obstruction because of urethral kinking, which obstructs with abdominal straining or attempted voiding. Patients with acontractile bladders resulting from diabetes or previous surgery may present with stress incontinence due to large postvoid residuals. This problem must be treated, along with the correction of any anatomic abnormalities.

Diagnostic Benefits of Radiologic Evaluation

Radiology may also uncover occult causes of incontinence or voiding dysfunction (Swaiman and Bradley, 1967). For example, a patient referred for stress incontinence was found to have a large urethral diverticulum and urethrovaginal fistula.

Radiologic evaluation is extremely important to the assessment of the lower urinary tract, both pre- and postoperatively, for the problems described above. Cure of urinary stress incontinence resulting from anatomic abnormalities is dependent on relocation of the bladder neck to a new intra-abdominal position in the retropubic space. Failure of surgery is, in most cases, due to inappropriate placement of the bladder neck and urethra (Figure 4–38).

Postoperative radiologic evaluation will provide information on three major aspects: (1) whether the bladder neck is still in a low position (at the inferior border of the symphysis pubis or below). The bladder neck is the most dependent portion of the bladder, so with filling the gravitational forces tend to open and funnel it. (2) Under

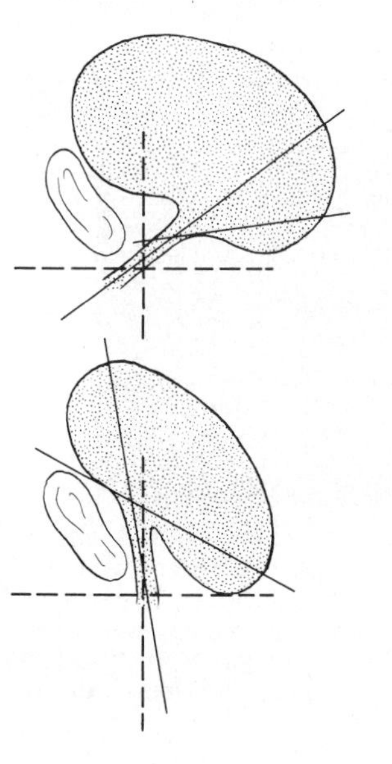

FAILURE

Urethral axis = dropped

Bladder neck = obtuse posterior angle

Bladder floor = normal

SUCCESS

Urethral axis = corrected

Bladder neck = sharp posterior angle

Bladder floor = normal

Figure 4–38. Diagram of results (success and failure) of Marshall-Marchetti operation or any type of bladder neck suspension. The majority of failures occur owing to lack of support and proper positioning of the bladder neck and urethra in a high fixed intra-abdominal position.

fluoroscopy, hypermobility of the bladder base can be seen with straining films. After a good urethropexy, the urethra should be fixed. (3) Lack of correction of the urethral axis can be seen.

Fluoroscopy provides a dynamic method of evaluating female urinary incontinence, using straining and coughing views. Stable incontinence requires that there be involuntary loss of urine, with no change in true detrusor pressure. Using a sequence of films, the incontinent patient can be evaluated objectively to decide if she requires pharmacologic or surgical therapy, self-catherization, or some combination of these.

REFERENCES

Asmussen, M., and Ulmsten, V.: Simultaneous urethral pressure profile measurements with a new technique. Acta Obstet. Gynaecol. Scand. *54*:385, 1975.

Ball, T. L.: Topographic urethrography. Am. J. Obstet. Gynecol. *59*:1243, 1950.

Barnes, A. C.: Roentgenologic study of urethral sphincter strength in the female. J. Urol. *47*:694, 1942.

Blaivas, J.: Cystometry. *In* Raz, S. (Ed.): Female Urology. Philadelphia, W. B. Saunders Co., in press.

Blaivas, J. G., Labib, K. B., Michalik, S., et al.: Cystometric response to propantheline: Clinical implications. J. Urol. *124*:259, 1980.

Bors, E.: A simple sphincterometer. J. Urol. *60*:287, 1948.

Bradley, W. E., Timm, G. W., and Scott, F. B.: Cystometry: III. Cystometers. Urology *5*:843, 1975*a*.

Bradley, W. E., Timm, G. W. and Scott, F. B.: Cystometry: Bladder sensation. Urology *6*:654, 1975*b*.

Bruskewitz, R.: Urethral pressure profile in female lower urinary tract dysfunction. *In* Raz, S. (Ed.): Female Urology. Philadelphia, W. B. Saunders Co., in press.

Bruskewitz, R., and Raz, S.: Urethral pressure profile using microtip catheter in females. Urology *14*:303, 1979.

Dubois, P.: Uber den Druck in der Harnblasse. Arch. Klin. Med. *17*:148, 1876.

Einhorning, G.: Simultaneous recording of intravesical and intraurethral pressure. A study on urethral closure in normal and stress incontinent women. Acta Chir. Scand. (Suppl.) *276*:1, 1961.

Glahn, B. E.: Nueurogenic bladder diagnosed pharmacologically on the basis of denervation supersensitivity. Scand. J. Urol. Nephrol. *4*:13, 1970.

Gleason, D. M., Bottaccini, M. R., and Reilley, R. J.: Comparison of cystometrogram and urethral profiles with gas and water media. Urology *9*:155, 1977.

Glen, E. S., and Rowan, D.: Continuous flow cystometry and urethral pressure profile measurement with monitored intravesical pressure: A diagnostic and prognostic investigation. Urol. Res. *1*:97, 1973.

Harrison, N. W.: The urethral pressure profile. Urol. Res. *4*:95, 1976.

Hodgkinson, C. P.: Relationship of the female urethra and bladder in urinary stress incontinence. Am. J. Obstet. Gynecol. *65*:560, 1953.

Jeffcoate, T. N. A., and Roberts, H.: Observation of stress incontinence of urine. Am. J. Obstet. Gynecol. *64*:721, 1952.

Klevmark, B.: Motility of the urinary bladder in cats during filling at physiologic rates: I. Intra-vesical pressure pattern studies by a new method of cystometry. Acta Physiol. Scand. *90*:565, 1974.

Lapides, J., Friend, C. R., and Ajemian, E. P.: Denervation supersensitivity as a test for neurogenic bladder. Surg. Gynecol. Obstet. *114*:141, 1962.

Lewis, L. G.: A new clinical recording cystometer. J. Urol. *41*:638, 1939.

McGuire, E. J., Lytton, B., Pepe, V., et al.: Stress urinary incontinence. Obstet. Gynecol. *47*:255, 1976.

Melzer, M.: The Urecholine test. J. Urol. *108*:729, 1972.

Merrill, D. C., Bradley, W. E., and Markland, C.: Air cystometry: I. Technique and definition of terms. J. Urol. *106*:678, 1971.

Merrill, D. C., and Rotta, J.: A clinical evaluation of detrusor denervation supersensitivity during air cystometry. J. Urol. *3*:27, 1974.

Muellner, S. R.: Etiology of stress incontinence. Surg. Gynecol. Obstet. *88*:237, 1949.

Raz, S., and Bradley, W. E.: Neuromuscular dysfunction of the lower urinary tract. *In* Harrison, J. H., Gittes, R. F., Perlmutter, A. D., et al. (Eds.): Campbell's Urology. 4th Ed. Vol. 2. Philadelphia, W. B. Saunders Co., 1979, pp. 1215–1270.

Robertson, J. R.: Gas cystometrogram with urethral pressure profile. Obstet. Gynecol. *44*:72, 1974.

Ruch, T. C.: Central control of the bladder. *In* Field, J. (Ed.): Handbook of Physiology. Vol. II, Sec. 1. Washington, D.C., American Physiology Society, 1960.

Shapiro, R. A., and Raz, S.: Clinical applications of the radiologic evaluation of female incontinence. *In* Raz, S. (Ed.): Female Urology. Philadelphia, W. B. Saunders Co., in press.

Summers, J. L., Ford, L. M., Keitzer, W. A., et al.: Fatal air embolism following air cystometrogram. Urology *4*:95, 1974.

Swaiman, K. F., and Bradley, W. E.: Quantitation of collagen in the wall of the human urinary bladder. J. Appl. Physiol. *22*:122, 1967.

Tanagho, E. A.: Simplified cystography in stress urinary incontinence. Br. J. Urol. *46*:295, 1974.

Tanagho, E. A., Miller, E. R., Meyers, F. E., et al.: Observations on the dynamics of the bladder neck. Br. J. Urol. *38*:72, 1966.

Togure, A. G., Bee, D. E., Whorton, E. B., et al.: Parameters of gas urethral pressure profiles: Part I. J. Urol. *122*:195, 1979.

Turner-Warwick, R., and Brown, N. D. G.: A urodynamic evaluation of urinary incontinence in the female and its treatment. Urol. Clin. North Am. *6*:203, 1979.

Wein, A. J., Malloy, T. R., Hanno, P. M., et al.: The reproducibility and significance of carbon dioxide urethral pressure profilometry. J. Urol. *122*:651, 1979.

Zinner, N. R., Sterling, A. M., and Ritter, R. C.: Role of inner urethral softness in urinary incontinence. Urology *16*:115, 1980.

5

THE UROLOGIC EXAMINATION

BERNARD FALLON, M.D.
DAVID A. CULP, M.D.

Radiographic and instrumental examinations are the primary diagnostic tools of the urologist; however, history and physical examinations provide the basic opinion upon which further investigations are founded.

HISTORY-TAKING

Voiding and Other Common Symptoms

Complaints of frequency, burning on urination, dysuria, or nocturia are among the most common presented to any physician. Details of duration, severity, and precipitating factors should be obtained. A childhood history of urinary tract infections and enuresis should be sought. Bubble baths have been incriminated as one cause of such symptoms, particularly in children. The relationship of symptoms to sexual intercourse may be significant. Associated complaints of cloudy, foul-smelling urine indicate strongly a urinary tract infection.

These symptoms may be related to upper or lower urinary tract infection. Fever suggests upper tract involvement, although in children cystitis may be associated with low-grade fever. A pelvic mass encroaching upon the bladder, reducing the functional bladder volume, is also compatible with such symptoms, as are bladder tumors, either primary or secondary, or previous radiation therapy of the pelvis.

Hematuria

Hematuria demands investigation to determine the etiology and location of the lesion producing the bleeding. In the younger patient, with or without voiding symptoms, it may be a signal of infection, but parenchymal renal disease must also be considered, especially glomerulonephritis. Bloody urine is also a cardinal symptom of urinary tract neoplasia or of genital neoplasia invading the urinary tract. Persistent hematuria in the child or young adult should be investigated further, although malignancy is rare in this group. In the older patient, diagnostic studies should be early and very complete.

Pain

Urinary tract pain reflects, to some extent, the site of disease. As with all pain, the location, radiation, and precipitating and relieving factors should be noted. The type and severity of pain may point directly to the diagnosis. The colic of acute ureteral obstruction by stone, clot, or ligature is very different from the constant dull ache of chronic obstruction, whether by tumor, stricture, fibrosis, or other long-term pathologic lesions. The pain associated with infection in or obstruction of the upper tract is usually located in the costovertebral angle or in the flank. It may radiate to the lower quadrants or to the genitalia and along the inner thigh. With time the pain may decrease as the disease progresses, producing chronic obstruction.

Bladder pain may be located in the low back or suprapubic or perineal area. While often of a constant, low-grade nature, unchanged by voiding, it may be sharp and severe with relief obtained after voiding, such as in interstitial cystitis with Hunner's ulcer. Frequently there is no pain associated with bladder disease.

Urethral pain is described by patients as an ache, discomfort, burning, or stinging, usually associated with the act of voiding. Unfortunately for these patients, they may be obliged to void more frequently than usual.

Dyspareunia in the female may be associated with urethral or bladder disease as well as vaginal or deep pelvic lesions.

Incontinence

Urinary incontinence (see Section 3) is associated with many conditions, and frequently the physician can make a provisional diagnosis during the initial conversation with the patient (see Chapter 23). Most important, one should ascertain whether the patient has ever been truly continent. If not, congenital anomalies such as ectopia vesicae (exstrophy), epispadias, ectopic ureteral orifice, or a neurogenic bladder may be responsible. Is there continuous dribbling (characteristic of urinary retention), overflow, or total failure of the bladder to act as a reservoir? Is it merely occasional escape of urine in small or large quantities which might indicate stress or urge incontinence? What factors precipitate leakage — straining, sensation of full bladder, coughing? How many pregnancies has the patient had?

PHYSICAL EXAMINATION

As for other body regions, physical examination should be performed systematically.

External Genitalia and Perineum

We are not concerned primarily with the male in this presentation, but states of intersexuality must be considered. Examination of the labia may reveal fusion or other abnormalities. The size of the phallus is significant. Size and location of the urethral meatus must be noted. In some circumstances, minor variations from normal should arouse suspicion of virilization. Failure of anterior urethral wall fusion (epispadias) will be readily apparent. Unlike exstrophy (failure of anterior bladder wall fusion), epispadias is not associated with fertility or gynecologic problems (Stanton, 1974).

Urethral prolapse and caruncle can be differentiated by the circummeatal, rosette-like herniation of mucosa in the former and the dorsal midline nodule of tissue in the latter (Klaus and Stein, 1973). Both commonly present with bleeding that may be thought to be of vaginal origin. Skene's glands can be expressed vaginally while retracting the urethral meatus to observe the character of the expressed material. Persistent hymen can be a factor in urinary tract infection and in postvoiding urinary dribbling.

On vaginal examination a urethrovaginal or vesicovaginal fistula should be suspected when a persistent drainage of fluid is encountered (see Chapter 21). Urethral diverticulum presents as a swelling in the anterior midline that may be soft to palpation, particularly if it contains pus or urine, or hard when it contains a stone. An ectopic ureteral orifice can occasionally be identified in the vagina or vestibule. A lower ureteral stone, especially if large, may be palpated in the lateral vaginal fornix.

The Bladder

The distended bladder is an easily located, rounded, midline suprapubic mass that may be tender to palpation and dull to percussion. However, the mass can be positively identified as the bladder only by catheterization followed by palpation to determine that the mass has disappeared after the bladder is emptied.

Palpation after voiding may help in assessing residual urine or a poorly emptying diverticulum when a soft, ill-defined fluid mass is noted in the suprapubic region or on bimanual examination. Observation of cystocele and a positive Marshall-Bonney stress test are important in the diagnosis of stress incontinence. The ability to stop the urine leakage with the application of paraurethral support indicates the likelihood of a favorable surgical result.

Bimanual palpation of the bladder will sometimes identify an intravesical stone or the intramural or paravesical induration, mass, or fixation associated with a pelvic neoplasm.

The Ureters

Attempts to palpate the ureters are usually unsuccessful. Only in the presence of induration associated with dilatation, such as in tuberculosis, or when there is deficient volume of abdominal musculature, as in the prune-belly syndrome with hydroureteronephrosis, is it possible to palpate the ureter.

The Kidneys

Located deep in the upper abdomen and protected by the ribs, the kidneys are difficult to palpate, although the lower pole may be felt in a thin person, particularly on the right side, where the kidney lies somewhat lower. The knees should be flexed and supported to enhance abdominal muscle relaxation. A large renal mass may be observed as a rounded, upper quadrant swelling. The best method of palpation uses the fingers of one hand in the costovertebral angle and the fingers of the other hand pressing abdominally. There should be movement with respiration and the mass should be ballotable. On the left, differentiation from the spleen is possible by noting the rounded, medial border which lacks a notch, the downward direction of enlargement, and the band of colonic resonance lying anterior to the kidney. Also, the examining fingers can be inserted between the ribs and a renal mass, not between the ribs and spleen. An ectopic kidney may be palpable as a pelvic or abdominal mass.

Examination of the back is important. Scoliosis may be due to renal inflammation on the concave side of the spine. A gentle tap in the costovertebral angle elicits tenderness, and there may often be a bulge with erythema or edema in the presence of a perinephric abscess.

Auscultation of the renal artery is performed anteriorly 1 inch above and 1 inch lateral to the umbilicus. Frequently, however, auscultation at the costovertebral angle is preferable, since this is closer to the renal artery and there is no interference from intestinal peristalsis.

Adrenal Glands

Except in the case of a large carcinoma, it is impossible to palpate the adrenal glands. However, accompanying systemic signs of adrenal pathologic change are easily noted. Blood pressure should be checked to rule out the possibility of pheochromocytoma. Hirsutism, abnormal fat distribution and skin color, and other signs of endocrine problems accompany adrenal disease.

RADIOLOGIC EXAMINATION

Excretory Urography

The mainstay of urologic evaluation is excretory urography. In the routine study, the initial exposure is a plain film of the abdomen, followed by other films made at 5, 10, and 15 minute intervals after the intravenous injection of contrast medium. Pre- and postvoid bladder films complete the series.

Alterations in the routine study should be tailored to demonstrate anticipated abnormalities in renal function or urinary transport in individual situations. In the evaluation of hypertensive patients, films are taken at 20 seconds, 40 seconds, and 1 minute following the injection of the contrast medium to observe the earliest arrival of contrast medium in the nephrogenic filling of the parenchyma. A difference in the size and density of the renal substance on these early films suggests a delay in delivery of contrast material associated with lesions such as renal artery stenosis.

The most common alteration made in excretory urographic technique is done to elucidate the site of partial or complete ureteral obstruction. Up to as long as 24 hours after the injection, delayed films should be made in an attempt to visualize the collecting system. During some portion of the examination the patient should be in the upright or prone position to permit gravity filling of the ureter when peristalsis is diminished or absent. Thus, information can be gained as to whether the obstruction is intrinsic or extrinsic, its severity, its location, and possibly its duration, since chronic obstruction tends to cause a greater dilatation of the collecting system, perhaps with renal cortical loss.

In the presence of poor excretion, due to obstruction or intrinsic renal disease, better visualization of the kidneys and collecting system may be obtained with infusion urography and nephrotomography, in which 250 ml. or more of the contrast medium is rapidly infused. Mild dilatation of the collecting system and ureters may occur with infusion studies because of the osmotic diuretic effect. Also, if urinary specific gravity is to be checked, it should be measured prior to excretory urography, since it will be spuriously high after this procedure owing to the large content of high molecular weight contrast medium.

Ideally, prior to performance of excretory urography, the patient should be dehydrated and the bowel cleansed to enhance the concentration and visualization of contrast medium in the collecting system. However, patient preparation is not mandatory. Adequate films may be obtained without any preparation. In deciding whether the patient should be prepared for the examination, the purpose of obtaining this study should be considered. If the finest detail is required, it may be wiser to delay the examination until the patient has been properly prepared. Performance of excretory urography is not contraindicated in multiple myeloma, as is commonly thought, since the incidence of acute renal failure following pyelography is essentially no different in this than in other diseases producing chronic renal parenchymal manifestations. To help avoid problems, the patient should be well hydrated prior to the study, and the load of contrast medium should be kept as low as is compatible with a good study.

A history of previous reaction to the contrast medium is the only true contraindication to the performance of this diagnostic examination. However, it should be added that most such episodes are only minor reactions to the intravenous injection, and in many cases a second study can be done later without reaction. Skin and conjunctival testing prior to the excretory urogram is valueless; the best precaution is to have corticosteroids, Benadryl, epinephrine and a resuscitation cart available should problems arise.

Retrograde Pyelography

In the event that excretory studies cannot be employed, or if they fail to visualize the urinary tract, the upper tract may be well outlined by means of retrograde injection of contrast medium via a ureteral catheter at the time of cystoscopy. This study provides finer detail and has the advantage of obtaining renal pelvic urine for microscopic study, culture, or cytology. In addition, a catheter may be left indwelling as an aid to ureteral identification during an operative procedure. Some object to this practice because it creates a false sense of security since, in the presence of pathologic lesions, it is sometimes difficult to palpate the catheter within the ureter. Furthermore, it leaves a foreign body in the urinary tract that often acts as a source of infection.

Retrograde ureteropyelograms are particularly useful for confirming or ruling out urinary tract obstruction in the anuric patient, as well as in the evaluation of the patient with ureteral perforation or fistula (Figure 5–1). An occlusive ureterogram is preferred to passing a catheter to the renal pelvis since it is more likely to identify a ureteral leak.

Cystography

Leakage of contrast medium from the retrograde-filled bladder provides invaluable information about vesical fistulas. Oblique films help to localize the position of the fistulous opening. Postevacuation films are needed often to confirm intraperitoneal or extraperitoneal extravasation. Bladder diverticula, vesicoureteral reflux, and external pressure defects on the bladder can be seen. Voiding cystourethrograms provide the added dimension of a dynamic study and more often demonstrate reflux than does a static film. Residual pockets of contrast medium behind the symphysis pubis are indicative of a urethral diverticulum.

Retrograde Urethrography

An injection study of the male urethra is an easily performed examination that may give extremely valuable information. The short length of the female urethra, however, makes this a difficult investigation to

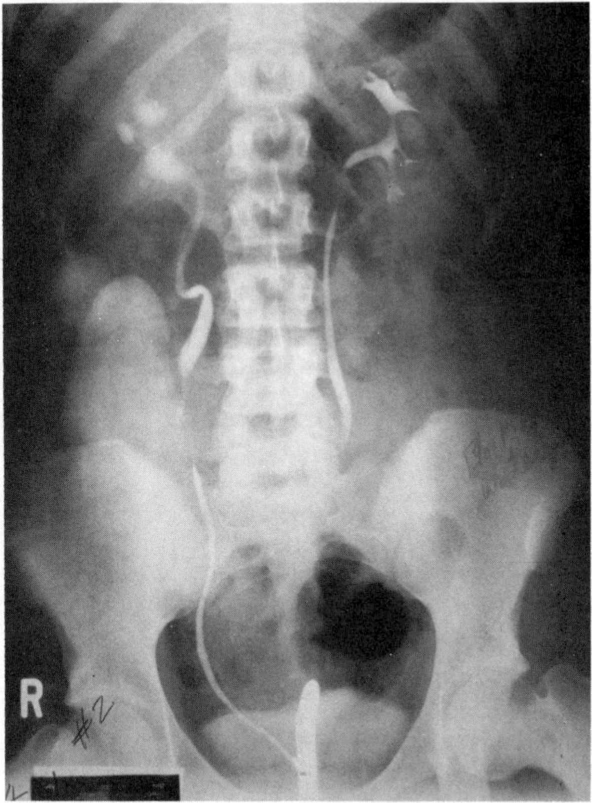

Figure 5–1. Retrograde pyelogram demonstrates right midureteral perforation with extravasation of contrast medium into flank urinoma. Moderate right hydronephrosis is also evident.

perform. This problem may be overcome through the use of a double balloon catheter, with placement of one balloon proximally at the bladder neck and the other in an adjustable position at the external urinary meatus. Contrast medium can enter and fill the urethra through a hole in the side of the catheter between the two balloons. Urethral length can be determined and diverticula outlined (Figure 5–2). Urethrovaginal fistulas may also be located by this method.

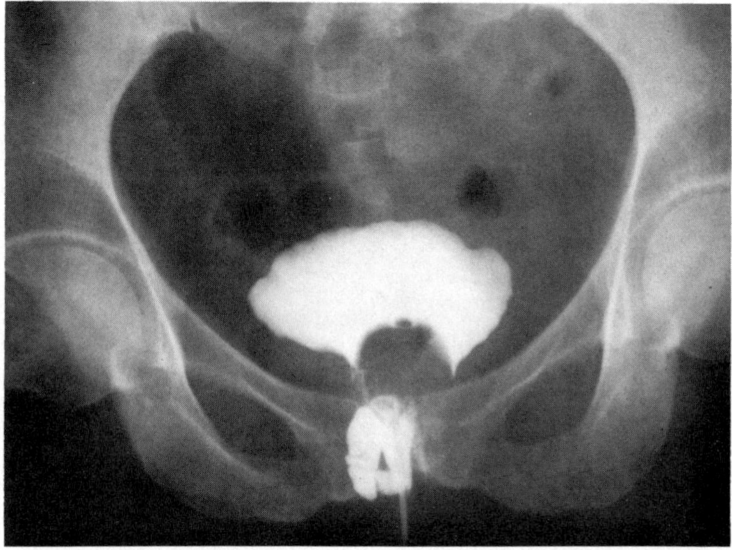

Figure 5–2. Retrograde urethrogram performed with double balloon catheter demonstrates urethra with diverticulum extending off to the right side. Some contrast medium has escaped into the bladder.

Loopography

In patients who have undergone urinary diversion by ileal or colonic conduit, follow-up visualization of the upper tracts can be achieved by retrograde filling of the conduit with contrast medium. Most conduits are constructed *without* antireflux techniques so that the ureters and renal pelves will usually be well visualized by retrograde filling. Lack of filling or dilatation with delay in drainage may indicate fibrotic or malignant stenosis. Such changes noted within a short period of surgery usually indicate postoperative fibrosis at the anastomosis of ureter with bowel; after a longer interval, they are more likely to represent recurrent malignancy. The loopogram should be combined with an excretory urogram to obtain the fullest information.

Nephrostography (Antegrade pyelography)

Temporary renal drainage can be obtained in the woman whose ureter is obstructed (often related to a ureterovaginal fistula) by the insertion of a nephrostomy tube. This may involve either a straight catheter or a loop catheter placed at surgery, or a percutaneous nephrostomy catheter. Renal and ureteral status and management can be assessed periodically by measurement of the intrapelvic pressure, residual renal pelvic urine, and radiographic appearance and function of the pelvis and ureter by instillation of contrast medium through the nephrostomy catheter (Figure 5–3). The need for removal or retention of the nephrostomy tube or for further surgical procedures can be thus determined.

Angiography

The major use of angiography in urinary tract disease is the assessment of renal circulation (Figure 5–4) and renal or adrenal mass lesions. Renal artery stenosis, sometimes associated with hypertension, can be demonstrated. Differentiation of cystic and solid masses is facilitated. Adrenal tumors such as pheochromocytomas may be locat-

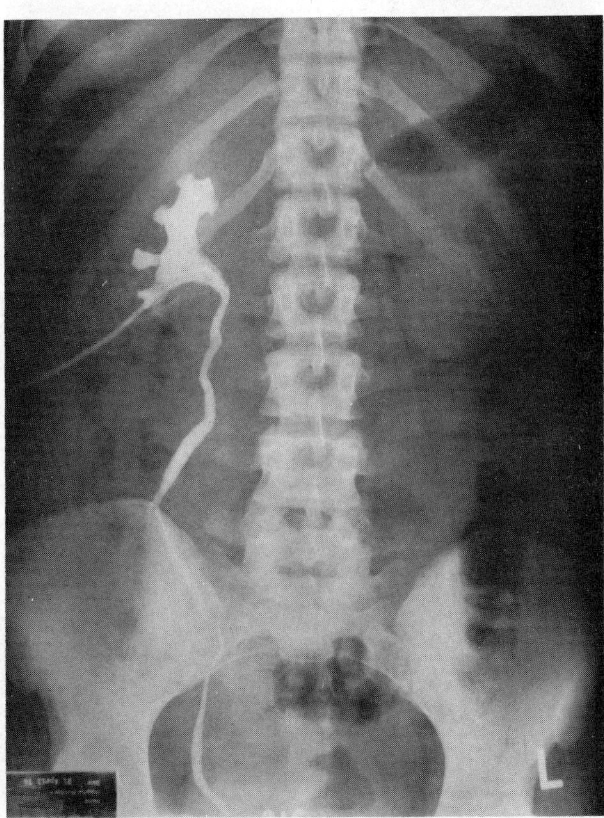

Figure 5–3. Same patient as in Figure 5–1. Nephrostogram 6 weeks following loop nephrostomy drainage of kidney demonstrates healing of perforation with no extravasation. Nephrostomy tube was removed following this study.

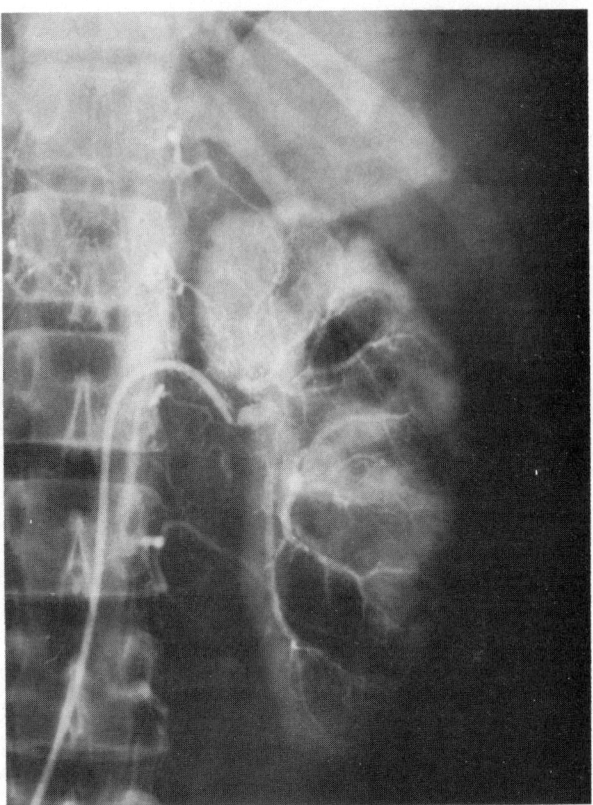

Figure 5–4. Selective left renal angiogram demonstrates enlarged kidney with excellent cortical perfusion. This indicates a good prognosis for recovery of function in this kidney, which was obstructed during a radical hysterectomy 6 weeks earlier.

ed and outlined. In the pelvis, arteriography is less useful. For the urologist, its main benefit is in the assessment of bladder wall lesions. Selective catheterization of vesical arteries may outline a bladder tumor, and the extent of neovascularity may assist in assessing bladder muscle invasion.

Radionuclide Scans

Although lacking the detail of the excretory urogram, radioisotope renograms are an excellent mode of studying renal function in the patient allergic to contrast medium. They are useful in pregnancy (Rudolph and Wax, 1967) because of the low radiation dosage. Adverse reaction to the various isotopes is virtually unknown. Scanning techniques may be adapted for the evaluation of comparative function of two kidneys, possible obstruction, vesicoureteral reflux, and residual urine. The gallium scan may be of value in localizing an obscure abdominal or pelvic abscess or neoplasm, although its use does demand a delay of several days in diagnosis and treatment.

Computed Tomography (CT)

Computed tomography has assumed major importance in assessment of normal and abnormal tissues in the abdomen and pelvis (Kellett et al., 1980). With regard to the urinary tract, visualization of kidneys, ureters, and bladder is greatly enhanced by the use of contrast medium. The position and contour of the urinary organs can be well seen, and any extrinsic tissue mass can frequently be localized if it is greater than 1 cm. in diameter. Enlarged pelvic and retroperitoneal lymph nodes are demonstrated, although a tissue diagnosis is still necessary before therapeutic decisions can be made. A biopsy procedure can be planned with the aid of the CT scan. Bladder wall thickness can be assessed, and, in certain cases of malignant pelvic disease, an abnormality of this parameter may raise the question of direct bladder wall invasion. While x-rays may demonstrate a pressure defect in the

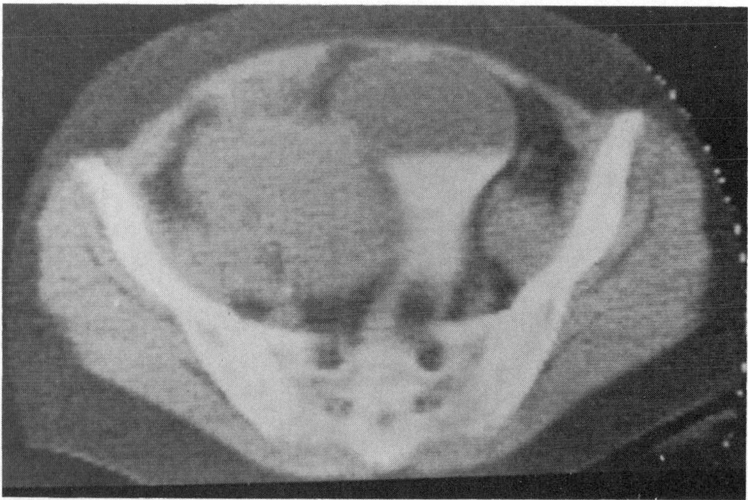

Figure 5–5. CT Scan of pelvis demonstrates large left pelvic mass, which is solid in nature and compressing the bladder toward the right side. Also noted is a smaller mass of metastatic lymph nodes along the right pelvic wall. (From Brown, R. C., and Go, R. T.: Diagnostic radiographic techniques in gynecologic oncology. *In* Sciarra, J. J. (Ed.): Gynecology and Obstetrics, Vol. 4, Harper and Row, Hagerstown, Maryland, 1980.)

bladder outline, CT scan (Figure 5–5) will often accurately localize the mass, define its size, and determine if it is solid or fluid-filled.

Ultrasonography

The increasing use of CT scanning has caused a decline in the use of ultrasound in evaluation of pelvic and abdominal lesions affecting the urinary tract. Ultrasound is not as definitive in delineating or characterizing a mass, particularly if it is less than 3 cm. in diameter. Overlying bony shadows in the pelvis make the interpretation of mass density difficult, so that study results are often ambiguous. The major advantages of ultrasonography are ease and rapidity of performance and lower cost. The proper place of ultrasound quite likely is in the initial assessment of a problem discovered on radiologic and clinical examination. When the situation remains unclear, CT scanning may elicit more information.

ENDOSCOPIC EXAMINATION

Prior to the introduction of a cystoscope, the urethra should be calibrated, assessing the caliber of the external meatus, distal urethral (submeatal) ring, and the bladder neck. In the adult female, a urethral caliber of less than No. 22 French is abnormal, and it may be that a small urethral caliber is of some significance in the etiology of urinary tract infection. Dilatation with bougies or other instruments can be performed as a therapeutic measure and to facilitate passage of a cystoscope. After inserting the cystoscope, residual urine should be measured and the bladder interior examined and evaluated with a variety of lenses, particularly the right angle and Foroblique telescopes. With current technology, visualization of the entire bladder interior is very satisfactory. The character of the bladder mucosa is seen along with the location, number, and appearance of the ureteral orifices, the presence of tumor, stones, or inflammatory process, invasion by tumors from neighboring organs, and edema resulting from malignant infiltration of bladder muscle without mucosal invasion. Pressure defects from extrinsic masses can be noted and some idea of bladder capacity and reflexes obtained. Almost always, the lithotomy position is adequate, but on occasion, to visualize the anterior bladder wall or bladder neck adequately, the knee-chest position may be used.

Urethroscopy should be performed and may aid in localizing an ectopic ureteral orifice or a urethral diverticulum. Intravaginal pressure on the diverticulum will help to define its orifice by expressing the contents or widening the opening in the urethra. Catheterization of the diverticulum aids identification during surgical repair. In attempts to locate an ectopic ureteral orifice, methylene blue or another vital dye should be administered intravenously at some time sufficiently prior to the examination to permit excretion from the kidney. Since most renal segments draining through an ectopically placed orifice do not function well, there may be considerable delay in the appearance of the dye.

Coincident with cystoscopy, bladder washings can be obtained for cytologic examination of the sediment. Lubricant greatly reduces the ease of performance and reliability of this test and therefore should be used sparingly. Biopsy of a suspicious bladder lesion can be obtained. The cup biopsy forceps is adequate for mucosal specimens, but when deeper tissues are desired, the biopsy is best secured with the resectoscope. Fistula margins should be biopsied.

Ureteral catheters may be passed for a variety of diagnostic or therapeutic maneuvers, and radiologic equipment should be attached to the cystoscopic table for maximal benefits during this investigation.

Vaginoscopy should also be performed, particularly when a fistula is suspected. Intravenous or intravesical dyes are useful in helping to localize the vaginal orifice of fistulous tracts.

Papanicolaou Smears

At the time of pelvic or cystoscopic examination, the urologist should perform a Papanicolaou (Pap) smear examination on adult female patients who are not under the regular care of a gynecologist. Occult cervical carcinoma occasionally will be discovered.

Anesthesia

Although local anesthesia or no anesthesia is adequate for most female cystoscopic examinations, one must consider the indications for performing these procedures. When investigating a case of primary or recurrent malignancy in any pelvic organ, cystoscopic examination under general or spinal anesthesia provides an opportunity to secure adequate biopsies and perform complete bimanual examination. The various maneuvers necessary for proper evaluation of a fistula following surgery or irradiation should not be compromised by pain or distress to the patient, which would abbreviate the procedure. Thus, in many circumstances, the examination can be performed more leisurely and safely, and valuable additional information gained, when adequate anesthesia is employed.

LABORATORY EVALUATION

In any preoperative or pre–radiation therapy patient, various blood and urinary studies must be obtained. These are particularly important in patients with the complications of malignant disease or previous unsuccessful therapy. Of particular interest in evaluating renal function is the creatinine clearance test, which unfortunately is frequently not performed. An accurate evaluation of renal function is essential prior to any major operative procedure, and the blood urea nitrogen or serum creatinine values simply do not provide sufficient information.

Examination of urinary sediments and urine culture techniques are discussed in Chapters 24 and 28.

SOME APPLICATIONS OF THE UROLOGIC EXAMINATION

Carcinoma of the Cervix

The most common radiographic change is hydronephrosis secondary to lower ureteral obstruction. Radiographic appearance ranges from ureteral tapering to complete nonvisualization of the lowermost portion of the ureter, with varying degrees of hydronephrosis, or even nonvisualization of the involved upper urinary tract (Figure 5–6). Ureteral course may be altered by an extrinsic tumor mass. Upper ureteral involvement is rarely seen, mainly because there are no continuous lymphatics along the ureter (Miller and Spear, 1973). Symp-

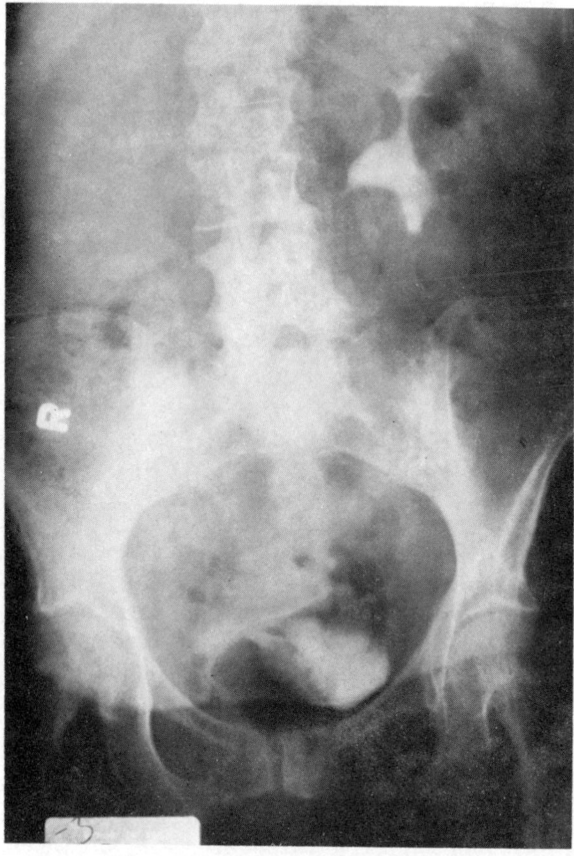

Figure 5–6. Three-hour delayed film of excretory urogram in a patient with carcinoma of the cervix. Minimal function of an enlarged right kidney is noted. The right bladder base is deformed by infiltrating tumor.

toms are nonspecific and consist principally of backache, chills, and fever.

Cystoscopy is helpful in staging cervical tumors. The earliest indication of bladder muscle wall invasion is mucosal edema. Actual tumor invasion into the bladder wall can be diagnosed only by biopsy.

Following radiation therapy for carcinoma of the cervix, asymptomatic ureteral stricture or recurrent carcinoma may arise, so periodic excretory urography should be performed (Figure 5–7). Symptoms of radiation cystitis such as frequency, dysuria, and hematuria may demand cystoscopy. A careful bladder biopsy is necessary to rule out recurrent tumor.

Fistulas

Urinary fistula formation is one of the dreaded complications of gynecologic surgery for benign or malignant conditions. Repeat surgery for recurrent disease is associated with an increased incidence of fistula formation. Likewise, radiation therapy frequently predisposes to fistula formation. Other recognized predisposing factors are arteriosclerosis, hypertension, diabetes mellitus, obesity, and pelvic inflammatory disease (Van Nagell et al., 1974).

Urethrovaginal Fistula

Symptoms vary according to the location. In the proximal urethra, stress incontinence is most likely, while in the distal two thirds of the urethra, the main complaint is postvoid dribbling due to leakage of urine collected in the vagina during voiding (Gray, 1968). These fistulas are relatively easily located by vaginal examination, urethroscopy, and vaginoscopy. They are usually found along the midline of the anterior vaginal wall. As with all fistulas, if there is a history of malignant disease, a biopsy should be taken from the margins.

Vesicovaginal Fistula

Vesicovaginal fistula (see also Chapter 21) may be more difficult to locate. If there

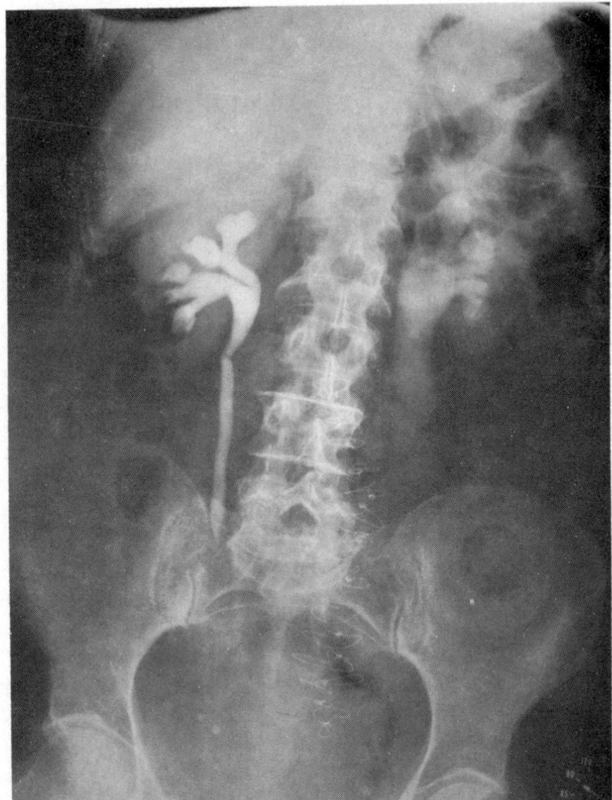

Figure 5–7. Excretory urogram demonstrates bilateral partial ureteral obstruction from recurrent carcinoma of the cervix.

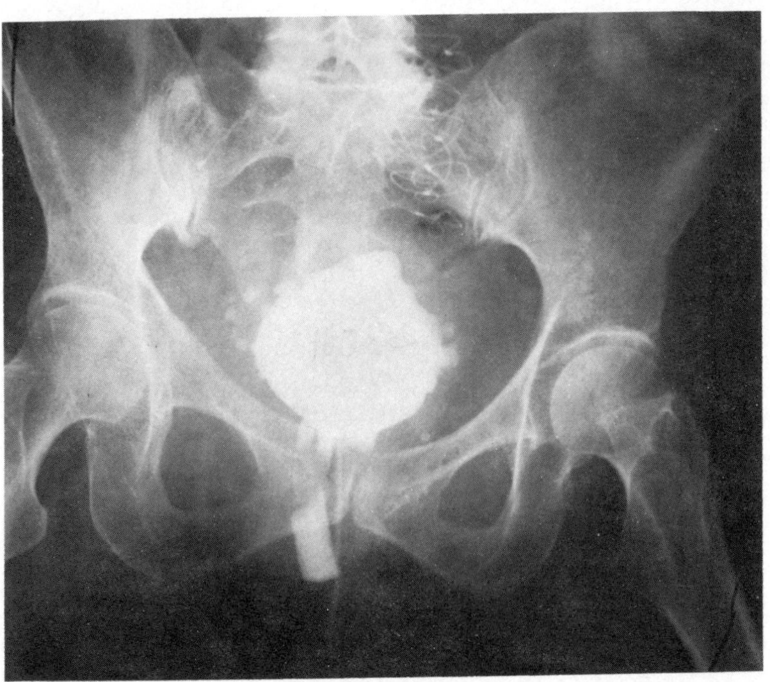

Figure 5–8. Cystogram demonstrates a vesicovaginal fistula. Contrast medium injected through a Foley catheter into the bladder stains a vaginal tampon.

is fluid leakage, the first step is to confirm that it is from the urinary tract, by administration of indigo carmine or another vital dye intravenously. The drainage will be stained with the dye material if it is urine. Analysis of the fluid for urea, creatinine, and protein content will help to distinguish it from lymph. Location of the fistula in the bladder can be confirmed by the intravesical instillation of a dye and radiographic media, or sterile milk, to avoid staining surrounding tissue (Figure 5–8). If a vaginal tampon becomes discolored, the fistula is a vesicovaginal fistula, provided vesicoureteral reflux is not present.

Cystoscopy should be performed to determine the exact location of the fistula. Careful examination is required to ensure that there are not multiple fistulous areas. In those cases where neoplasm is a possible etiologic factor, biopsy of the margin should be performed.

If the fistula is small, it may be difficult to locate amid the inflammatory reactive tissue. Occasionally, it is helpful to fill the bladder with air and perform vaginoscopy in the knee-chest position with water in the vagina. Air bubbles may be seen to exit from the fistulous tract (O'Conor and Nanninga, 1975). To facilitate vaginoscopy, an extra hole can be cut in the side of a Foley catheter and the tip of the catheter also cut off. A Foroblique lens can then be inserted through the side hole along the lumen of the catheter and out through its tip. When the catheter balloon is inflated, water can be retained in the vagina, permitting better visualization of the distended vagina (Figure 5–9) (Diaz-Ball and Moore, 1969).

Ureterovaginal Fistula

Urinary incontinence with a coexistent normal voiding pattern will be present when a ureterovaginal fistula exists. Intravesical and intravenous injection of methylene blue aids in the diagnosis.

An excretory urogram usually reveals an abnormal ureter (Figure 5–10). In this respect ureterovaginal fistula differs from the vesicovaginal type, in which the ureter is generally normal unless the vesical damage involves the ureteral orifice. The affected ureter is usually dilated in the early phase by edema and in the later phase by fibrosis (Weyrauch and Rous, 1966). A collection of extravasated urine may be seen on the plain film as a pelvic ground-glass density, or in the excretory phase as a dilute area of contrast medium outside the confines of the urinary tract. The location of the fistula may be visualized on a blocking ureterogram as an area of extravasation or an

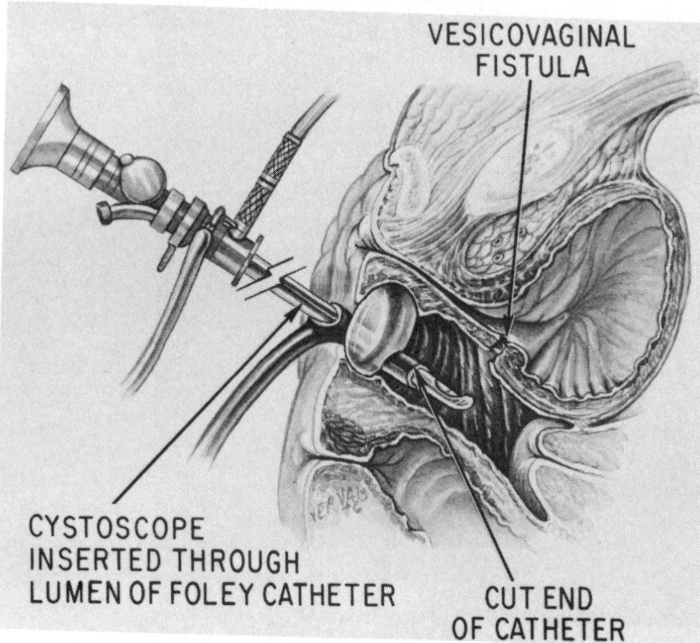

Figure 5–9. Cystoscope is inserted through a hole cut in the side of a Foley catheter and projects through the cut end of the catheter. When the balloon is inflated, the vagina can be distended with water, permitting better visualization of its interior. A vesicovaginal fistula is illustrated.

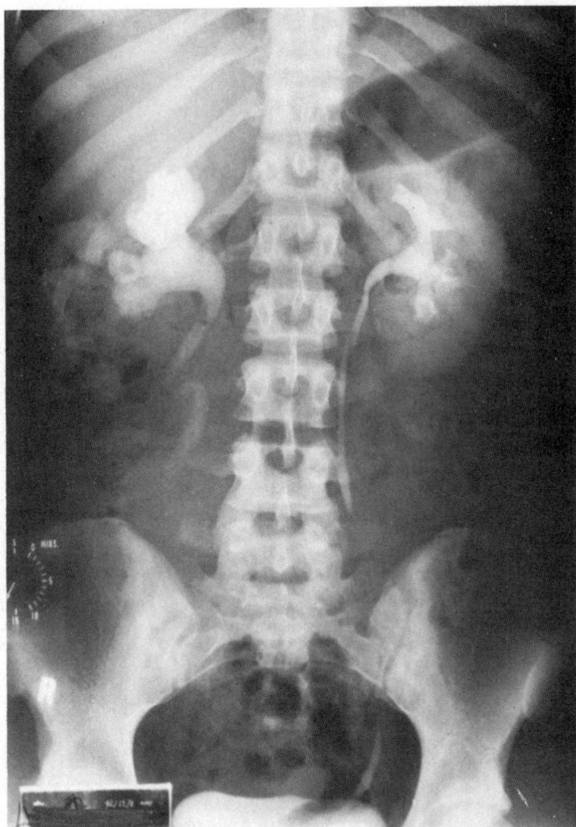

Figure 5–10. Excretory urogram demonstrates moderate hydronephrosis associated with ureteral fistula. The lower half of the ureter is not visualized. Delayed films identified the site of ureteral injury and resultant ureterovaginal fistula.

abrupt termination of the column of contrast medium in the pelvic area without extravasation. When this occurs, the passage of a ureteral catheter is blocked by the distal ureteral obstruction.

Vesicouterine Fistula

The principal etiologic factor in vesicouterine fistula has been obstetric trauma, although therapeutic abortions are now a common cause. A vesicouterine fistula may exist unrecognized for several weeks. Symptoms include cyclic hematuria, urinary infection, and urinary leakage from the vagina. Cystoscopy, cystography, and hysterography pinpoint the location of the fistula.

Ureteral Transection and Obstruction

"The venial sin is to injure the ureter; the mortal sin is not to recognize it" (Higgins, 1967). Routine intravenous injection of indigo carmine or methylene blue toward the end of a pelvic procedure will help to detect transection, although it is not a substitute for adequate caution and surgical exposure.

Presentation of symptoms of ureteral injury may be early, with urinary leakage from the wound, a palpable mass, pelvic or flank tenderness, fever, elevated white blood cell count, and mild elevation of blood urea nitrogen from reabsorption of extravasated urine (Glenn, 1962). A urinalysis usually shows microscopic hematuria. Other laboratory tests are of virtually no help. Immediate anuria results from bilateral ligation.

The most frequent changes on excretory urography are hydronephrosis, extravasation, and nonvisualization of the affected side. Retrograde ureteropyelography confirms the diagnosis (Figure 5–11).

Bilateral partial ureteral obstruction may initially be associated with an excellent

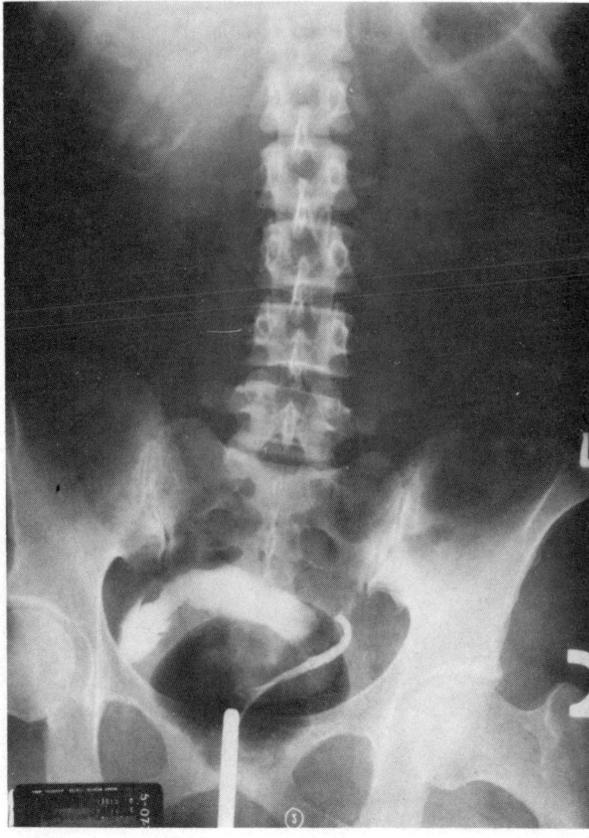

Figure 5–11. Retrograde study demonstrates complete obstruction of left ureter. The distal site of obstruction makes ureteroneocystostomy feasible and preferable to ureteroureterostomy.

urinary output, but gradually anuria develops as edema completes the obstruction.

Delayed presentation of ureteral injury should be suspected when the patient develops backache, urinary tract infection, unremitting fever, or prolonged paralytic ileus (Spence and Boone, 1961).

Other Gynecologic Malignancies

Neither ovarian nor endometrial carcinoma often involves the urinary tract. Excretory urography and cystography are advised to detect changes in ureteral or bladder anatomy from extrinsic compression (Figure 5–12). Urethral or bladder invasion in vulvovaginal carcinoma is easily diagnosed by inspection, palpation, endoscopy, and biopsy.

Incontinence

The functions of the bladder are to store urine and expel it when necessary and appropriate. Incontinence results when the bladder is unable to provide these two functions. Incontinence may be classified as overflow, urge, stress, or true. The diagnosis is established by a combination of history, physical examination, and radiologic (Figure 5–13), endoscopic, and urodynamic examinations. Cinefluorography is an excellent method of investigation (Lund et al., 1957) but exposes the patient to a high radiation dosage; in addition, facilities for this procedure are not generally available.

The various types of incontinence and the neurogenic bladder are discussed in Chapters 3 and 23.

Intersexuality

The morphologic criteria for the assignment of sex are classified in the following categories: (1) chromosomal or genetic, (2) gonadal or histologic, (3) appearance of the external genitalia, (4) the phenotype, (5) the sex of rearing, and (6) the gender role

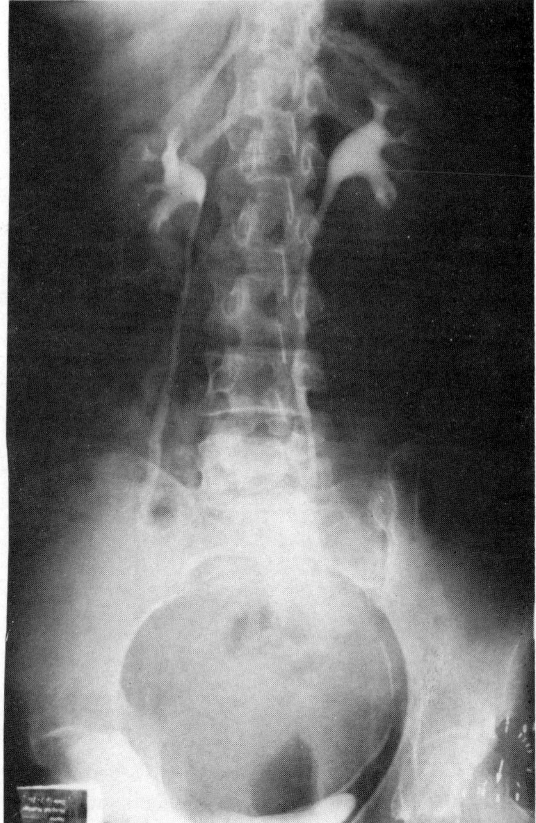

Figure 5–12. Excretory urogram of patient with carcinoma of the ovary. Bilateral ureteral displacement in the pelvis from the ovarian mass is demonstrated.

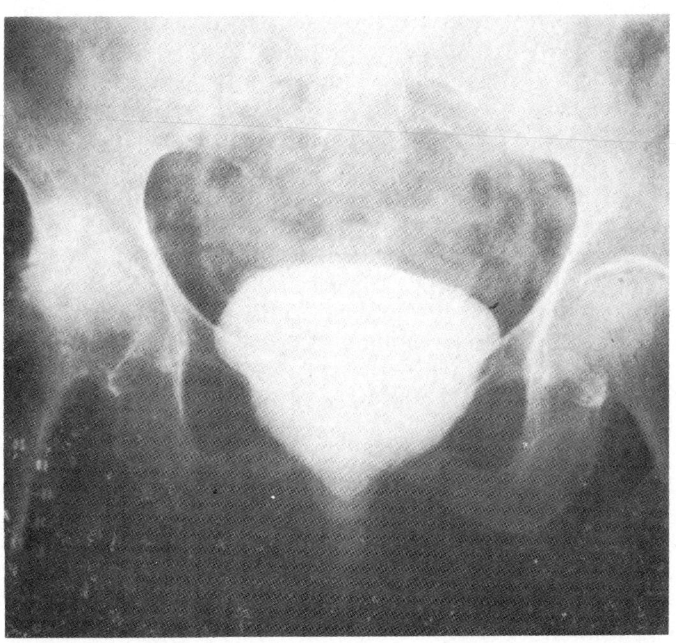

Figure 5–13. Cystogram portion of excretory urogram demonstrates a cystocele. The cystocele deformity can be exaggerated by having the patient strain or stand upright while the film is exposed.

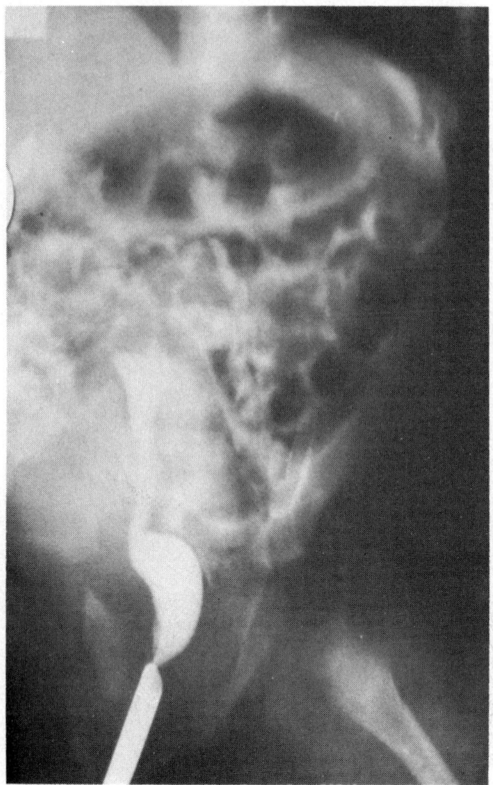

Figure 5–14. Genitography: vagina and uterine cavity demonstrated in a patient with adrenogenital syndrome. The injection was made via a cystoscope in the urogenital sinus.

(Bunge, 1962). Intersexuality occurs when there are contradictions in the morphologic criteria of sex. It is a multidisciplinary problem in which gynecologic, endocrinologic, and urologic evaluation is essential.

The obstetrician will be the first physician to see a child with adrenogenital syndrome. Careful genital examination following delivery reveals the ambiguous genitalia, which should prompt further investigation. Family history, occurrence of problems in siblings, and measurements of serum electrolytes, urinary 17-ketosteroids, and pregnanetriol are all helpful in establishing the diagnosis. Endoscopy and genitography (Figure 5–14) elucidate the status of the internal organs. Cytologic evaluation of a buccal smear is a simple test for the evaluation of genetic sex of the individual (Moore and Barr, 1955). In some cases, chromosomal studies must be performed.

In any patient with an intersex problem, all evident gonadal structures should be palpated carefully. In true intersex, when both ovarian and testicular tissues are present, the ovotestis possesses firm and soft areas, the former more likely ovarian and the latter more likely testicular (Van Niekerk, 1974). Although its early effects are strong, leading to inhibition of ipsilateral müllerian structures and masculinization of the external genitalia, the testicular tissue hyalinizes at puberty or shortly thereafter (Jones et al., 1965). The ovarian tissue remains functional throughout life.

An inguinal hernia in a female may be associated with testicular feminization syndrome. Abnormal chromatin studies are indicative of the latter, but exploration with biopsy of the gonad is conclusive proof of the diagnosis. The syndrome is due to absence or deficiency of 5-alpha-reductase, which converts testosterone to dihydrotestosterone (Northcutt et al., 1969) or of the binding globulin responsible for androgen transport to its nuclear site of action (Allen, 1976).

Infertility

Ten to 15 per cent of marriages are infertile. Of these, 40 per cent may be related to male factors. Evaluation is begun only after at least one year of failure to conceive in the absence of birth control measures. Because of the ease of performance, investigation of the male partner should be undertaken first. Semen analysis is an index of the male fertility potential. Normal parameters are liquefaction within 30 minutes, a volume of 2 to 5 ml., a sperm count of at least 20 million per ml., abnormal forms less than 30 per cent, and viability of 70 per cent (Bunge, 1965). The semen sample should be obtained by masturbation or withdrawal techniques. The postcoital Sims-Huhner cervical smear alone is not satisfactory (Cohen, 1975).

The absence of fructose from the semen suggests congenital absence or disease of the seminal vesicles and vasa deferentia (Bunge and Moon, 1968). Patency of the ductus can be ascertained by endoscopic catheterization and injection of contrast medium into the ejaculatory ducts or vasography performed through a scrotal exposure.

Before embarking upon an extensive, long-term therapeutic regimen, testicular biopsy should be performed in men with aspermia or low counts to determine whether the abnormality is reversible.

Sperm-agglutinating antibodies have been reported in the sera of some infertile men with normal semen analysis (Alexander, 1977). The significance of such antibodies has not yet been elucidated. However, the wives of such patients have conceived by artificial insemination of donor semen. Sperm-immobilizing antibodies and seminal plasma precipitants may also be involved in infertility problems. Spermatogenic suppression with testosterone permits the antibody titer to fall and later successful impregnation to occur. The female of the partnership may also be sensitized, and when antisperm antibodies are found in the wife's serum, a condom should be used during each contact for one year, in an attempt to desensitize her by removing the antigen.

In some infertile marriages, a psychologic factor in either partner is indicated by the occasional conception following adoption.

REFERENCES

Alexander, N. J.: Sperm antibodies and infertility. *In* Cockett, A. T. K., and Urry, R. L. (Eds.): Male Infertility. New York, Grune & Stratton, 1977, pp. 123–144.

Allen, T. D.: Disorders of sexual differentiation. Urology *7*(Suppl.1):1, 1976.

Bunge, R. G.: Sex determination. J. Iowa Med. Soc. *52*:715, 1962.

Bunge, R. G.: Male inferility. J. Iowa Med. Soc. *55*:125, 1965.

Bunge, R. G., and Moon, K. H.: Observations on the biochemistry of human semen. Fertil. Steril. *19*:186, 1968.

Cohen, M. R.: Evaluation of the infertile couple. *In* Gold, J. J. (Ed.): Gynecologic Endocrinology. Hagerstown, Md., Harper & Row, 1976.

Diaz-Ball, F. L., and Moore, C. A.: A diagnostic aid for vesicovaginal fistula. J. Urol. *102*:424, 1969.

Glenn, J. F.: External ureteral trauma. Trauma *4*:47, 1962.

Gray, L. A.: Urethrovaginal fistulas. Am. J. Obstet. Gynecol. *101*:28, 1968.

Higgins, C. C.: Ureteral injuries during surgery. J.A.M.A. *199*:118, 1967.

Jones, H. W., Ferguson-Smith, M. A., and Heller, R. H.: Pathologic and cytogenetic findings in true hermaphroditism. Obstet. Gynecol. *25*:435, 1965.

Kellett, M. J., Oliver, R. T. D., Husband, J. E., and Fry, I. K.: Computed tomography as an adjunct to bimanual examination for staging bladder tumors. Br. J. Urol. *52*:101, 1980.

Klaus, H., and Stein, R. T.: Urethral prolapse in young girls. Pediatrics *52*:645, 1973.

Lund, C. J., Benjamin, J. A., Tristan, T. A., et al.: Cinefluorographic studies of the bladder and urethra in women. Am. J. Obstet. Gynecol. *74*:896, 1957.

Miller, W. A., and Spear, J. L.: Periureteral and ureteral metastases from carcinoma of the cervix. Radiology *107*:533, 1973.

Moore, K. L., and Barr, M. L.: Smears from the oral mucosa in the detection of chromosomal sex. Lancet *2*:57, 1955.

Northcutt, R. C., Island, D. P., and Liddle, G. W.: An explanation for the target organ unresponsiveness to testosterone in the testicular feminization syndrome. J. Clin. Endocrinol. Metab. *29*:422, 1969.

O'Conor, V. J., and Nanninga, J. B.: *In* Whitehead, E. Douglas (Ed.): Current Operative Urology. Hagerstown, Md., Harper & Row, 1975, p. 792.

Rudolph, J. H., and Wax, S. H.: The ^{131}I renogram in pregnancy. II. Normal pregnancy. Obstet. Gynecol. *30*:386, 1967.

Spence, H. M., and Boone, T.: Surgical injuries to the ureter. J.A.M.A. *176*:1070, 1961.

Stanton, S. G.: Gynecologic complications of epispadias and bladder exstrophy. Am. J. Obstet. Gynecol. *119*:748, 1974.

Van Nagell, J. R., Jr., Parker, J. C., Jr., Maruyama, Y., et al.: Bladder or rectal injury following radiation therapy for cervical cancer. Am. J. Obstet. Gynecol. *119*:727, 1974.

Van Niekerk, W. A.: Intersexuality. Clinics in Obstet. Gynaecol. *1*:553, 1974.

Weyrauch, H. M., and Rous, S. N.: Transvaginal-transvesical approach for surgical repair of vesicovaginal fistula. Surg. Gynecol. Obstet. *123*:12105, 1966.

6

OFFICE URETHROSCOPY

THOMAS A. McCARTHY, M.D.
DONALD R. OSTERGARD, M.D.

INTRODUCTION

Endoscopic evaluation of the female urethra was introduced and described more than 15 years ago by Robertson (1966, 1980). Recently, female urethroscopy has emerged as a recognized diagnostic tool in the clinical evaluation of the incontinent patient. As a result, gynecologic urology is now an important clinical discipline.

HISTORY

Early in the nineteenth century Bozzini developed the first endoscope, which was designed for visualization of the bladder. A candle was used to provide light to see the various structures inside the bladder. His efforts were not well received and Bozzini was ostracized from the medical community. His instrument met a similar fate.

Late in the nineteenth century, Howard Kelly (1908) of Johns Hopkins Hospital developed a simple cystoscope used in conjunction with a head mirror. With patients in the knee-chest position, the insertion of this simple tubular instrument caused air to enter and distend the bladder. Using this technique, Kelly was the first to perform ureteral catheterization under direct visualization. Since Kelly was the director of the first modern gynecologic residency training program, gynecologists were classically trained as genitourinary surgeons.

At about the time Kelly was developing his air cystoscope, Nitze in Austria developed a new indirect water cystoscope. Urologists adopted this endoscope and its developmental offshoots as invaluable tools for evaluation of the bladder. This endoscope incorporated a 30 degree lens, allowing the physician to visualize the majority of the bladder wall, which is impossible with a direct 0 degree lens. With the addition of a 70 degree lens, virtually the entire bladder can be inspected.

A problem emerged, however, in regard to the female urethra. Although the indirect endoscopes are excellent for viewing the bladder, they are poor substitutes for a direct 0 degree viewing system for the female urethra. The 30 degree endoscope does not give an adequate view of the urethra. As a result, the female urethra has long been overlooked as a source of significant pathology.

Robertson was the first to develop an endoscope designed primarily for use in the female urethra (1973). He made two major changes from the standard cystoscope. First, the lens system is a direct 0 degree view. This affords more complete visualization of the urethra, especially the distal and posterior aspects, where much of the pathologic detail is found. Second, Robertson pioneered the use of endoscopes with optics designed to employ carbon dioxide. There are several advantages to carbon dioxide as the distending medium. The technique is less cumbersome and more rapid than the water system, which is a major advantage in the office setting. Additionally, the gas system gives a clearer view of the pertinent structures than does the water system.

Others have attempted to improve various aspects of the original Robertson urethroscope. Judd revised the inlet valve system, allowing for more expeditious filling and drainage of the bladder. Changes in the lens and optical aspects of the system to improve lighting and resolution have also been made. The basic characteristics, though, of a 0 degree viewing lens and a gas filling medium remain unchanged and are the critical aspects of the technique.

CLINICAL DEVELOPMENTS

Initially designed as an instrument to view the bladder base, trigone, and urethra, the urethroscope is playing an expanded role in the evaluation of lower urinary tract symptoms (Figure 6–1). In women with urinary incontinence, an important aspect of evaluation is to rule out inappropriately timed bladder contractions as the etiology of urine loss (unstable bladder). With the addition of a pressure/volume recorder to the gas supply of the urethroscope, a simple cystometer is available to evaluate bladder stability during the endoscopic procedure (Figs. 6–2 and 6–3). Another aspect of the evaluation of the incontinent patient is obtained through a measurement of the resistance capability of the urethra. Using opening pressure measurements as described later in this chapter, a crude measurement of urethral function is made (Fig. 6–4). In conjunction with other findings, this may help to define the etiology of a patient's urinary incontinence.

EQUIPMENT

Since many female urethroscopes and filling systems are available and the variety of equipment may confuse the practitioner, the following is a rough guide to the requirements and characteristics for a basic system.

Urethroscope. As described above, this should have a 0 degree lens system with a

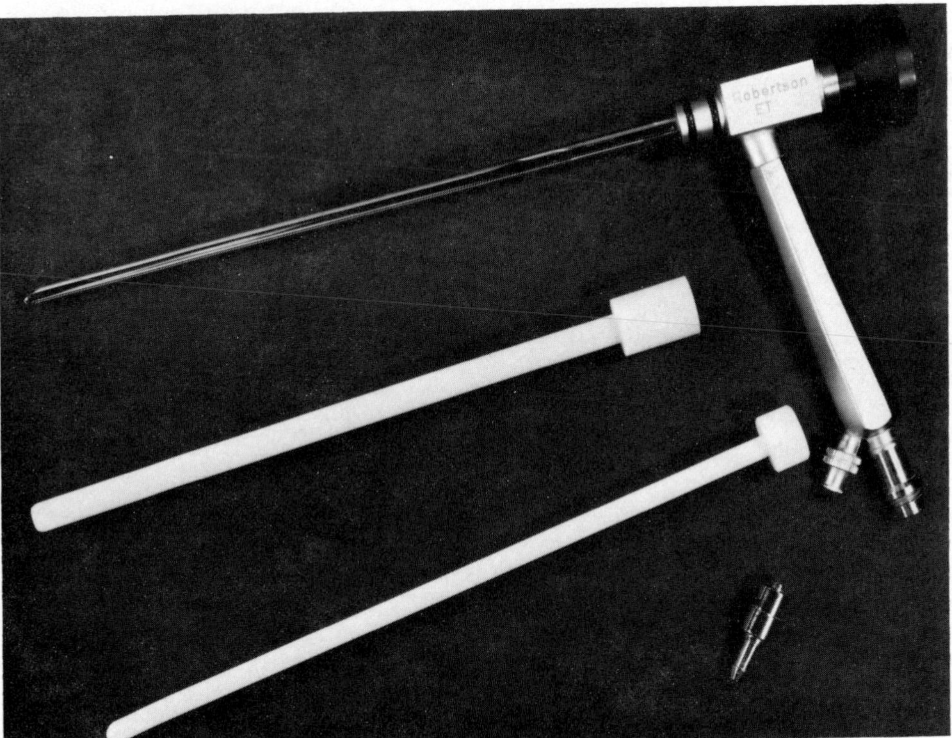

Figure 6–1. The Robertson Female Urethroscope, sheath and obturator. (Endotek Corporation, Santa Barbara, CA.)

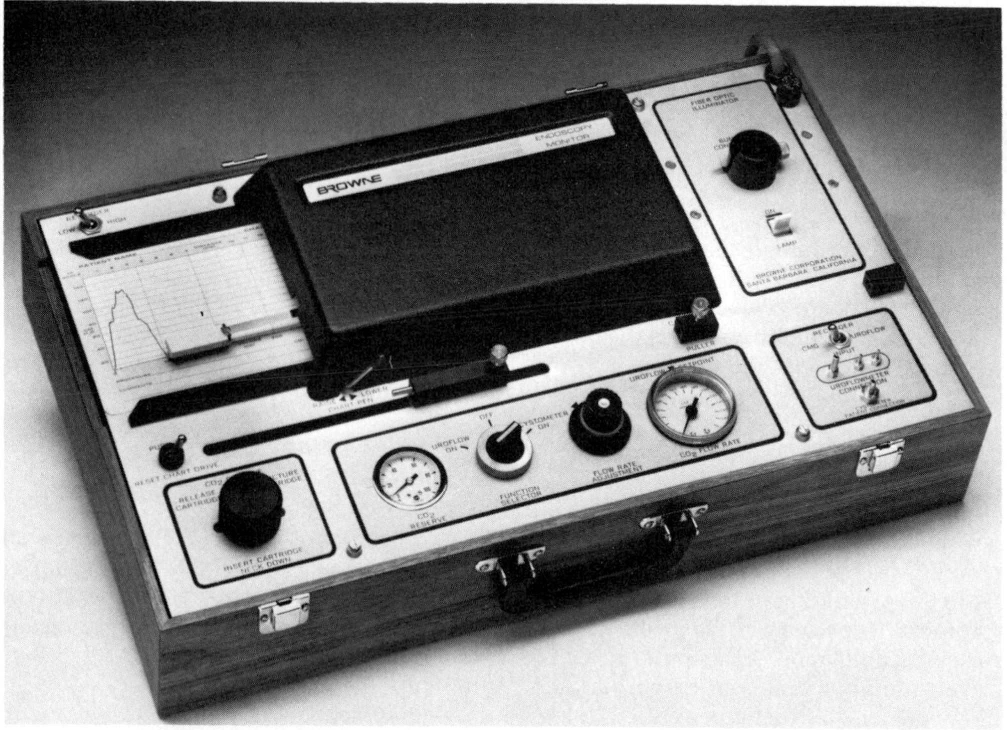

Figure 6–2. The Browne Endoscopy Monitor. A single channel CO_2 infusion instrument providing a graph of CO_2 pressure and volume and a fiberoptic light source. (Browne Corporation, Santa Barbara, CA.)

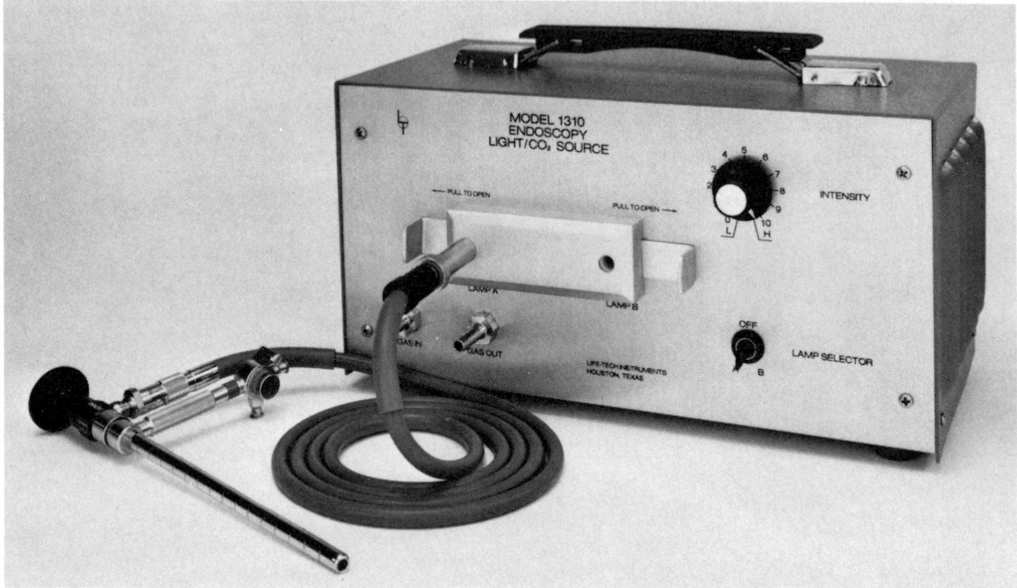

Figure 6–3. The Life-Tech Endoscopy Monitor, with a CO_2 pressure recording chart and a fiberoptic light. (Life-Tech Instruments, Houston, TX. © 1981, Chisholm, Rich & Assoc.)

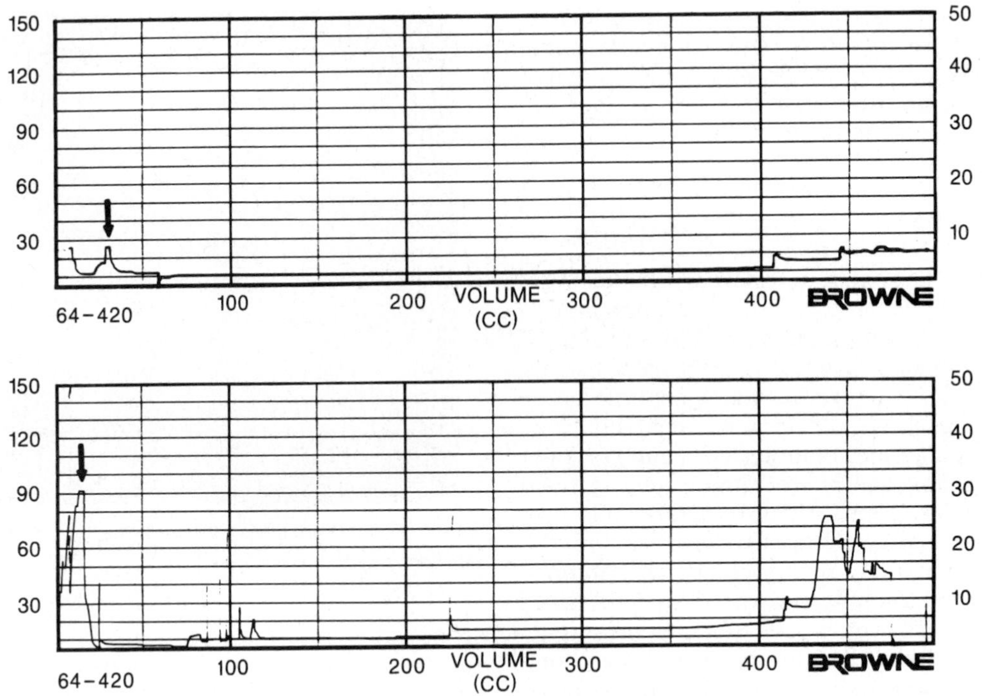

Figure 6–4. Urethral opening pressures. *Upper graph,* A patient with stress incontinence. Note low pressure of 26 cm H_2O (arrow). *Lower graph,* A normal patient. Note normal pressure of 90 cm H_2O (arrow).

CO_2 source for filling (Figure 6–1). Virtually all urethroscopes are constructed in this manner. The only real variables in urethroscopic instruments are: (1) optical quality, (2) viewing area, (3) light transmission, (4) convenience of the filling and drainage valve mechanisms, (5) the "feel" of the instrument in your hands, and (6) cost. Each instrument has its own strengths and relative disadvantages. The particular needs of the physician should dictate the choice of instrument.

CO_2 Cystometer. The cystometer, or pressure/volume recording instrument, is an integral part of the urethroscopic system (Figures 6–2 and 6–3). Unlike the urethroscope, there are many varieties of recorders available, each having different characteristics and capabilities. The basic instrument is a simple cystometer. Realistically this is all that is needed in the evaluation of most patients. This produces a graphic display of pressure/volume relationships at all times during gas flow through the instrument. This, then, may be used to measure and record urethral opening pressure and to perform cystometry either through the urethroscope or through a catheter. Ideally the recorder could be turned off when not needed for pressure recording while gas flow continues for inspection of the lower urinary tract.

Certainly much more sophisticated equipment is available in this area. There are recorders capable of performing CO_2 urethral pressure profiles, electronic uroflowmetry, and electromyographic (EMG) recording. The need for these tests in the majority of patients is minimal. There are easier and less expensive methods of performing office uroflowmetry. If complex urodynamic analysis is required, it is best carried out in an established laboratory in which these tests are routinely performed. In essence, the simpler the equipment, the better the results of office urethroscopy or cystometry.

URETHROSCOPIC TECHNIQUE

Preparation of the Patient

With the patient resting comfortably in the lithotomy position, the nurse prepares the patient by cleansing the urethral meatus and adjacent vulva with povidone-iodine solution. Psychologic support is given to the patient through a thorough explanation of the anticipated procedure.

Anesthesia

Any anesthetic technique, whether topical or by local injection, has the potential to interfere with the subsequent urethroscopic examination. Topical anesthesia is usually given by the introduction of a cotton-tipped applicator soaked in 4 per cent lidocaine hydrochloride solution (Xylocaine) or 2 per cent lidocaine hydrochloride jelly injected into the urethra. Unfortunately, this produces erythema in the sensitive urethral epithelium and may give the false impression of an inflammatory reaction. Since almost all women can tolerate the procedure without anesthesia, it is the author's recommendation that no local anesthetic be given.

Introduction of the Urethroscope

With the CO_2 flowing at a rate of 120 cc./minute, the tip of the urethroscope is gently introduced through the urethral meatus with the CO_2 serving as an obturator. It is essential that the physician observe the urethral mucosa during the initial introduction of the urethroscope, since instrumentation will produce erythema of the mucosa and confuse subsequent interpretation. Observation of the pressure increase during the initial insertion of the urethroscope provides an indication of opening pressure. Opening pressure is usually low with genuine stress incontinence (< 30 cm. of H_2O) and high in other patients (> 50 cm. of H_2O) (Figure 6–4). Since there is a great deal of overlap between the opening pressures in patients with stress incontinence and in those with incontinence on another basis, this measurement cannot be relied upon, by itself, as a diagnostic aid. Opening pressure is one piece of information that will contribute to the establishment of an accurate diagnosis.

Not infrequently, the first indication of meatal stenosis is encountered as the physician attempts, but fails, to insert the urethroscope through the external urethral meatus. At this point, calibration of the meatus will inform the endoscopist as to whether or not urethral dilatation will be required to complete the procedure. In the event that dilatation is required, subsequent erythema in the urethra must be interpreted in light of the trauma caused by the dilatation.

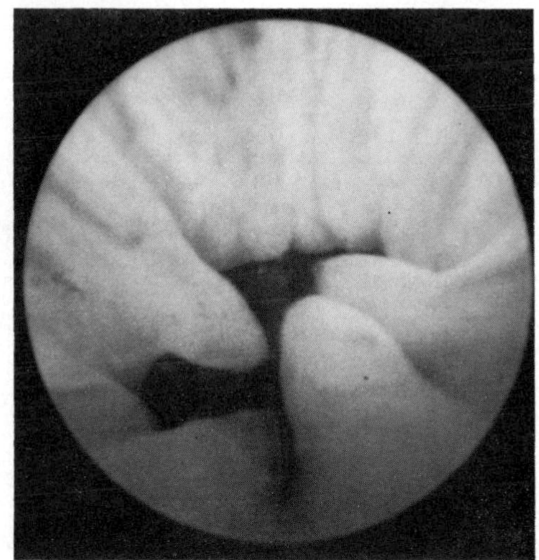

Figure 6–5. Inflammatory fronds at the urethrovesical junction.

As the tip of the urethroscope slowly traverses the length of the urethra, the CO_2 will partially distend the urethral lumen. The physician carefully inspects the urethral lumen for evidence of inflammation, exudate from posterior periurethral glands, polyps, condyloma, diverticular orifices, and the very rare ectopic ureter or primary carcinoma (Figure 6–5). When the bladder itself is visualized, the flow of CO_2 is stopped, and at this point the urethrovesical junction and the trigone are inspected for the presence of inflammatory polyps, granularity, shagginess, exudate, and other pathologic findings. If the CO_2 is allowed to continue flowing, polyps may be missed as a result of their being compressed by the CO_2 against the epithelium. Similarly, trigonal pathology may be missed for the same reason. The presence of urine at the urethrovesical junction and on the trigone allows these polyps to float freely and thus become visible.

The bladder is then emptied of all urine.

If only a few minutes have passed since voiding, this may be recorded as the patient's residual urine. The trigone is then reinspected and each ureteral orifice is visualized and its function verified by the observation of urine exiting from its lumen.

Dynamic Assessment of the Function of the Urethrovesical Junction

With the CO_2 flow still turned off, the urethroscope is withdrawn until the entire circumference of the urethrovesical junction is visible (Figure 6-6). The lumen should occupy about 80 per cent of the total area visualized through the urethroscope. The patient is then asked to "hold urine" or to "squeeze her rectum"—i.e., to contract her pelvic floor (Figure 6-7)—to perform a Valsalva maneuver, and finally to cough. The junction is observed for closure, opening, or absence of change. The response of the urethrovesical junction to each of these commands is recorded as well as an estimate of the descent of the urethrovesical junction with the Valsalva maneuver and on coughing. During Valsalva maneuver and coughing, the tip of the urethroscope must move coincidentally with the downward descent of the urethrovesical junction if an accurate assessment of its response to this stress is to be made. Generally, asking the patient to perform the Valsalva maneuver slowly or to cough initially with minimal force facilitates this observation.

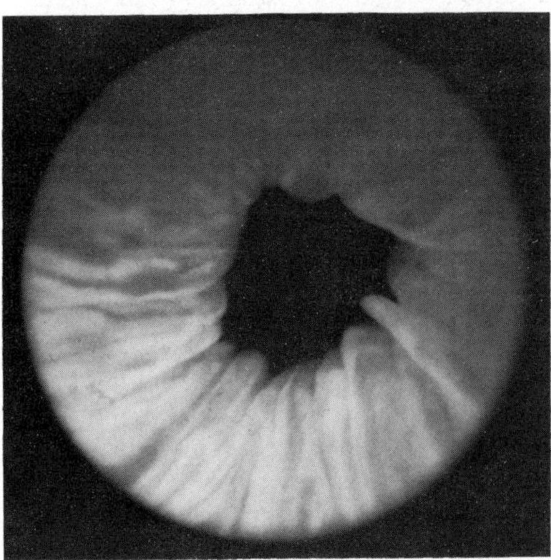

Figure 6-6. The urethrovesical junction of a normal patient.

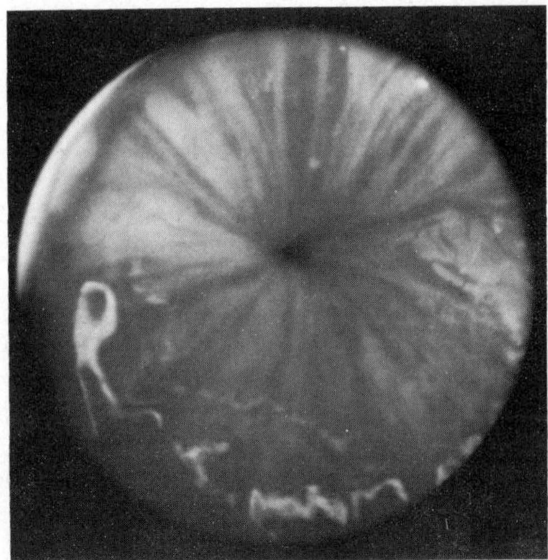

Figure 6-7. The urethrovesical junction of a normal patient in response to a command to hold the urine.

Carbon Dioxide Cystometry

The next step is to obtain a CO_2 cystometrogram through the urethroscope. Using a flow rate of 120 cc./minute, the bladder is progressively filled with CO_2. First sensation, fullness, and maximal volume are all recorded, and the urethrovesical junction is continuously observed during filling. When fullness occurs, the dynamic response of the urethrovesical junction to "hold," Valsalva maneuver, and cough is again assessed.

During cystometrography, any pressure increase is suspected of resulting from a detrusor contraction. However, Valsalva maneuver by the patient must be distinguished from true intrinsic detrusor activity. Without simultaneous intrarectal pressure recordings, the surest way to make this distinction is to observe the patient's breathing. Since the patient cannot breathe and perform the Valsalva maneuver at the same time, this will usually provide evidence of the true etiology of the observed pressure increase. If the pressure increase is not due to Valsalva maneuver, the patient must be asked to try to inhibit this intrinsic detrusor activity in order to determine her control over this spontaneous activity of her bladder.

At the point of absolute maximal fullness, and with the CO_2 still running, the patient is then asked to void while the physician observes the response of the urethra and the urethrovesical junction to this command. Generally, the entire urethra can be visualized during voiding, and the CO_2 will escape around the urethroscope. Again, the patient's ability to control this voluntary vesical activity is observed by asking the patient to stop voiding. If the patient cannot void, the CO_2 should be evacuated through the urethroscope.

Withdrawal of the Urethroscope

After completion of vesical evacuation, the CO_2 flow is again turned on and the urethroscope is gradually withdrawn. Distention of the urethra during withdrawal is accomplished by digital transvaginal compression of the urethra at the urethrovesical junction. This is particularly helpful in visualizing diverticular orifices and ectopic ureters. Again, the physician observes the entire urethra for polyps, fronds, and exudate as the instrument is completely withdrawn. The search for periurethral gland exudate and the more copious diverticular contents is facilitated by gentle urethral massage.

Interpretation: Static Urethroscopic Findings

The normal urethral mucosa has a pale pink to bright red appearance, which may become very pale in the hypoestrogenic woman. There are no specific findings in the urethral epithelium to substantiate or refute the diagnosis of chronic urethritis. However, the combined presence of reddened mucosa, inflammatory polyps, tenderness, and, classically, exudate from the periurethral glands suggests urethritis.

Since asymptomatic women may demonstrate exudate from the posterior periurethral glands, the presence of exudate probably adds little to the diagnosis of chronic urethritis. Large quantities of exudate suggest an origin from a larger contiguous cavity or from several cavities, which may indicate the presence of a single or multiple urethral diverticula. This indicates the need for a diligent search for diverticular orifices. The presence of clear fluid in the urethra suggests the possibility of an ectopic ureter. This should be visible through the urethroscope. However, in questionable cases an intravenous pyelogram will confirm its presence. At the urethrovesical junction, inflammatory polyps are commonly present; their pathologic significance is really not known (Fig. 6–5). Larger polyps are suspected of being neoplastic and should be excised. The trigone commonly has a granular appearance, which is more likely to be due to localized aggregations of lymphoid tissue. Its exact significance continues to be questioned. The shaggy appearance of the trigone, especially when combined with exudate, indicates a chronic inflammatory reaction and deserves the diagnosis of trigonitis.

The normal functioning of the ureters is easily observed through the urethroscope as they intermittently discharge urine. Occasionally, ureteroceles and ureteral tumors may be seen, requiring further evaluation by a qualified urologist.

Interpretation: Dynamic Urethroscopic Findings

When the normal patient is requested to "hold urine" or to "squeeze the rectum," the urethrovesical junction should respond with immediate and complete closure over the end of the urethroscope (Fig. 6–7). Occasionally a normal patient will have a minimal response to the command of "hold urine" but a definitive response to the "squeeze the rectum" command owing to her inability to contract the pelvic floor with the "hold urine" request. Some patients will actually perform the Valsalva maneuver instead of contracting the pelvic floor in response to either command.

The patient with an unstable bladder will frequently respond to these commands in an identical fashion to the normal patient. The patient with genuine stress incontinence, however, responds to "hold urine" and "squeeze the rectum" with a sluggish and usually incomplete closure of the urethrovesical junction.

Absence of any voluntary activity in response to the commands of "hold urine" or "squeeze the rectum" may indicate the presence of a rigid, fibrotic, scarred urethra subsequent to periurethral surgical procedures. This urethral drainpipe represents an end stage of incontinence due to multiple surgical procedures. Further urodynamic studies are necessary to fully evaluate these patients.

When the normal patient performs a Valsalva maneuver or coughs, the urethrovesical junction should promptly close without any significant mobility during these stresses. However, since normally continent patients may also have a mobile urethrovesical junction, this response is variable. Patients with vesical instability respond similarly, except that some may have a detrusor contraction stimulated by these stresses. When the patient with genuine stress incontinence performs Valsalva maneuvers or coughs, the junction's diameter usually remains the same or opens further. This usually occurs with a coincidental marked descent of the urethrovesical junction.

Interpretation: CO_2 Cystometry

Several aspects of CO_2 cystometry have already been discussed. These include the need to distinguish pressure increases as a result of Valsalva maneuvers from those due to intrinsic vesical activity. Since the latter may indicate vesical instability, the distinction is crucial. This distinction is not always possible, and, therefore, it represents one of the limitations of CO_2 cystometry. Normal women should experience a first sensation with a volume of 50 to 100 cc. CO_2, fullness at about 300 cc., and a maximal volume of 350 cc. Unfortunately, CO_2 is a very irritating substance, with direct effects on the vesical mucosa and also with effects secondary to its combination with water to form carbonic acid. Additionally, the spherical nature of the bladder when filled with CO_2 is decidedly nonphysiologic. All of these are irritative factors, which tend to markedly lower the volumes of first sensation and fullness, even in the normal patient. Reflex stimulation may be so marked that uninhibited vesical contractions occur, which give the false impression of vesical instability. These false positives may occur as frequently as in 50 per cent of cases, and, therefore, water cystometry is indicated to validate the existence of an unstable bladder (Chapter 3).

As the physician observes the urethrovesical junction during filling with CO_2 in the normal patient, a gradual and definite closure occurs as filling progresses. The patient with genuine stress incontinence, however, shows a lesser degree of closure, which is rarely complete. This is due to the altered anatomic relationships found in these patients and the inefficient functioning of the urethrovesical junction under these circumstances.

When a patient has a detrusor contraction of either voluntary or involuntary origin, the patient's ability to stop it must be determined. During the contraction, the urethrovesical junction opens widely, and the urethra may be viewed from one end to the other. At the peak of voiding, there is usually a widening of the urethra in its middle third. The greatest usefulness of CO_2 cystometry through the urethroscope is its use as a screening technique, provided that the observations fall into the normal range. However, when there are indications of an unstable bladder, water cystometry is required to validate the diagnosis.

ROLE OF OFFICE URETHROCYSTOMETRY AND URETHROSCOPY

The urethroscope and the CO_2 cystometer play a useful role in the evaluation of women with various lower urinary tract complaints (Robertson, 1980). In particular, women having urinary incontinence of any type should have an endoscopic evaluation and a screening cystometrogram. The value lies in increasing the ability to choose correct therapy in individual cases. Clearly, patients having urethral diverticula as the cause of their urinary incontinence will not improve with surgery designed to correct genuine stress incontinence. Without urethroscopy, diverticula are commonly overlooked and patients are subjected to incorrect treatment. Similarly, patients having recurrent lower tract infections or irritative symptoms without cultivable infection (urethral syndrome) should undergo endoscopic evaluation. Evidence of urethral pathology, whether urethritis, trigonitis, diverticulum, or tumor, will clearly be missed in most cases without this type of investigation.

For too long, women have been mislabeled as neurotic because the physician only studied the bladder. It is now evident that the female urethra is a source of common pathology and must not be overlooked. With proper instruments and adequate training in their use, there is a definite improvement in our ability to care for women with lower urinary tract complaints.

REFERENCES

Kelly, H. A.: Medical Gynecology. New York, Appleton, 1908.

Robertson, J. R.: Office Cystoscopy: Substituting the culdoscope for the Kelly cystoscope. Obstet. Gynecol. *28*:219, 1966.

Robertson, J. R.: Gynecologic urethroscopy. Am. J. Obstet. Gynecol. *115*:986, 1973.

Robertson, J. R.: Dynamic Urethroscopy. *In* Ostergard, D. R. (Ed.): Basic and Advanced Gynecologic Urology, Theory and Practice. Baltimore, Williams & Wilkins, 1980.

7

CLINICAL ASPECTS OF GENITAL AND URINARY TRACT ANOMALIES

FREDERICK KEITH CHAPLER, M.D.

The close temporal and anatomic relationship established during the embryologic development of the urogenital system results in an increased percentage of anomalies in one tract when the other is involved. This concept provides the clinician with the rationale for investigating the urinary system when defects are present in the genital system. It is important to identify urinary tract anomalies because these patients are generally more prone to renal disease. Renal disease may result from infection as a consequence of malrotation or malposition, or it may be idiopathic.

Two groups of patients present at high risk for concomitant congenital anomalies involving the reproductive and urinary tracts: One group has primary amenorrhea; the other has secondary infertility or reproductive difficulty as the presenting complaint. Of course, many congenital anomalies of the reproductive tract go undetected. Only the patient who presents with problems, or whose physician is alert and aware of the subtle signs of the anomalies, will have the proper investigative procedures. Reproductive tract anomalies may be discovered during pelvic examination, at surgical exposure, or by hysterosalpingography. The urinary tract is usually investigated by excretory urography or intravenous pyelography. (Despite some theoretical differences, the two terms have been used interchangeably — see Witten et al., 1977.) Retrograde pyelography, urethroscopy, cystoscopy, or more sophisticated techniques can be utilized in selected patients (Buchsbaum and Chapler, 1976) (Chapter 5).

PRIMARY AMENORRHEA

Primary amenorrhea can be divided into three subclasses according to etiology: (1) congenital anomalies of the genital tract, (2) hypoestrogenism, and (3) discrepancy between the gonad and phenotype (Figure 7–1). Urinary tract anomalies can accompany all three conditions.

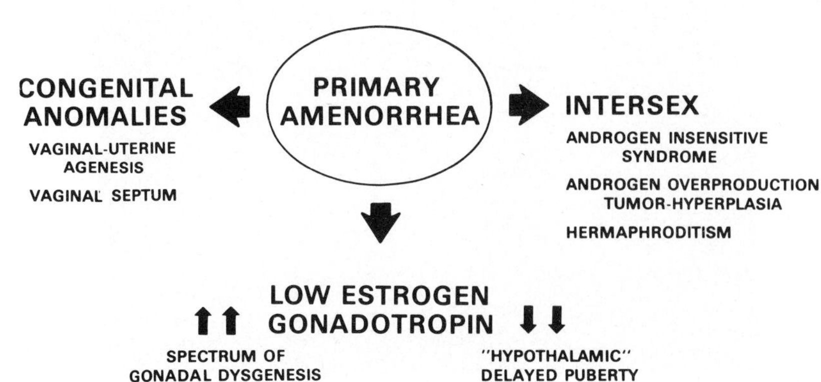

Figure 7–1. Primary amenorrhea.

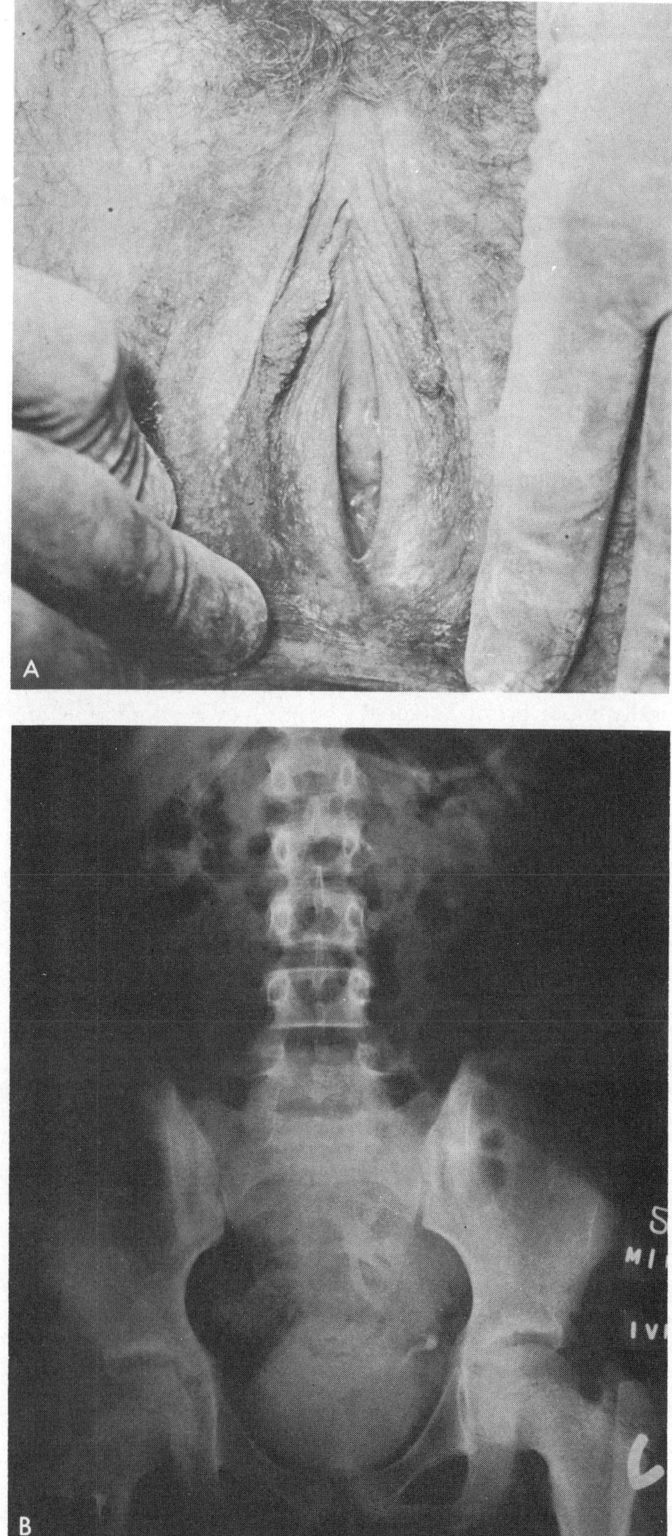

Figure 7–2. Vaginal agenesis. *A,* External genitalia. *B,* Excretory urogram illustrating pelvic kidney in patient with vaginal agenesis.

Congenital Anomalies of the Genital Tract

Vaginal Agenesis

Despite its rather infrequent incidence — 1:4000 in the general population (Capraro and Gallego, 1976), vaginal agenesis is the most common anomaly in this group. Twenty per cent of primary amenorrhea patients present with congenital malformations of the genital tract (Ross and Vande Wiele, 1981). Two types of patients have been identified. One is phenotypically female and has scant or absent pubic and axillary hair, an XY karyogram, intra-abdominal testicles, and a male hormone profile. He represents an end-organ failure to androgen hormone. Although his condition is commonly called testicular feminization, there is an increasing trend to refer to it as an androgen-insensitive syndrome. An intracellular deficit of dihydrotestosterone (DHT) cytosol or nuclear receptor protein, or both, seems to be the basis for this lack of tissue responsiveness to androgens (Bardin, 1973; Chan and O'Malley, 1976). Since androgen is necessary for normal male external genitalia differentiation, this patient has typical female external genitalia. Müllerian development is inhibited because the testicles elaborate the müllerian inhibiting substance. Consequently, these patients have no uterus or vagina, and they present with amenorrhea with absence of müllerian structures. Urinary tract anomalies are rare, but have been reported, in these patients (Swanson and Chapler, 1978).

The second, more common type with an absent vagina presents with normal pubic hair (Figure 7–2*A*), an XX karyogram, normal ovaries, and a normal female hormone profile. A high incidence of renal anomalies, ranging from 25 to 50 per cent, is associated with congenital absence of the vagina in the otherwise normal female patient (Chawla et al., 1966; Cali and Pratt, 1968; Leduc et al., 1968; Grover et al., 1970; Griffin et al., 1976).

Pelvic Kidney. Particular attention has been paid to the frequent (7 to 15 per cent) finding of a pelvic kidney in patients with an absent vagina (Fore et al., 1975). This is striking when one considers that the incidence of pelvic kidneys in the general population is 1:20,000 (Sokolski, 1960). The ectopic kidney may present as a pelvic mass of unknown etiology. A preoperative intravenous pyelogram is mandatory in all patients undergoing vaginal reconstruction. In the most common type of vaginoplasty, a modified McIndoe procedure, a space is dissected between the urethra and the rectum to the peritoneum to accommodate the mold with the skin graft. Accurate localization of the kidney and ureter is essential so that injury to these structures may be avoided (Wharton, 1947). Figure 7–2*B* shows a pelvic kidney on a preoperative pyelogram of a patient scheduled to have a vaginal reconstructive procedure.

TABLE 7–1. RENAL ANOMALIES ASSOCIATED WITH VAGINAL AGENESIS

Ectopic pelvic kidney
Solitary kidney
Malrotation
Duplication of pelves

The explanation for the pelvic kidney and absent vagina lies in the wolffian duct's close anatomic relation to and its influence on müllerian duct development. Ectopic pelvic kidneys and absence of müllerian structures represent an arrest in medial deviation during migration. This results from a teratogenic influence on the wolffian duct between the sixth and ninth weeks of intrauterine development (Gruenwald, 1941; Goldstein et al., 1973; Fore et al., 1975). Other urinary tract anomalies associated with vaginal agenesis are shown in Table 7–1.

The need for complete urologic study of patients with congenital absence of the vagina is apparent. All patients should have intravenous pyelograms and, if indicated, cystoscopy and retrograde ureteral pyelography.

Transverse Vaginal Septum

Failure of canalization of the vaginal plate, or lack of union of the two vaginal primordia, the urogenital sinus and the müllerian derivatives, may result in a transverse vaginal septum that occludes outflow of menstrual blood (Deppisch, 1972). This anomaly is difficult to correct but is fortunately rare. If the transverse septum is complete, the patient presents with primary

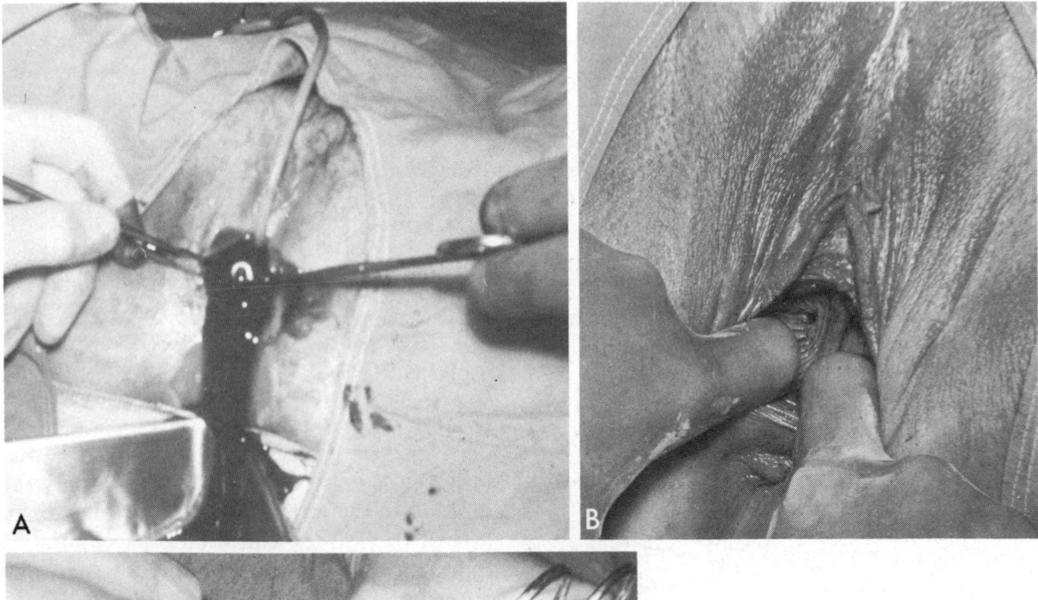

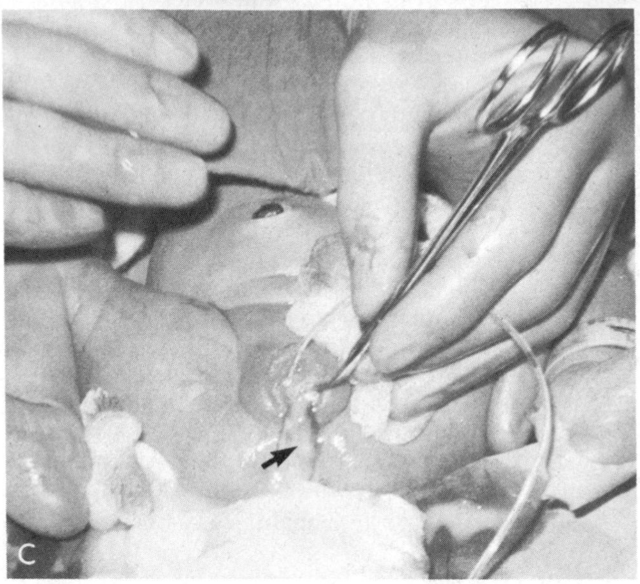

Figure 7–3. Examples of vaginal septa. *A*, Draining hematometrocolpos following incision of transverse vaginal septum. *B*, Longitudinal vaginal septum. *C*, Infant with hydrometrocolpos. Mucoid material can be seen on perineum (arrow).

amenorrhea, abdominal pain, and a palpable pelvic mass. The symptoms result from the accumulation of menstrual blood, hematometra, and hematocolpos. Incision of the septum relieves the obstruction (Figure 7–3*A*), but total excision of the septum is necessary to prevent recurrence. Thin septae, which are located low in the vaginal tract, can be mistaken for an intact hymen.

Treatment for relief of hematometra or hematocolpos resulting from an intact hymen and from a transverse septum is the same. The incidence of urinary tract anomalies accompanying these disorders, however, is quite different: Urinary tract anomalies are common in patients with transverse septum and very unusual in patients with intact hymen. The presence of a longitudinal vaginal septum (Figure 7–3*B*) also increases the likelihood of concomitant renal anomalies (Bowman and Scott, 1954).

Occasionally a low transverse septum results in a hydrometrocolpos (Figure 7–3*C*). Instead of blood, the uterus and vagina are filled with a mucous secretion, the exact cause of which is uncertain. There is an increased incidence of associated urogenital anomalies with this condition (Smith and

Goodwin, 1971). Reed and Griscom (1973) reviewed 26 patients, 12 of whom had intravenous pyelography. Eight of the 12 infants had unilateral renal agenesis. Uterine malformation was also noted. Four patients with imperforate hymen had no other abnormalities. These observations demonstrate the advisability of obtaining intravenous pyelograms in patients with transverse vaginal septum or longitudinal vaginal septum, and in infants with hydrometrocolpos.

Labial Adhesions

Although labial adhesions are not a congenital malformation, they are included here because they frequently indicate a "possible absent vagina" or present as ambiguous genitalia requiring further investigation. Urinary tract infection is common in these patients because the free flow of urine is obstructed by the adhesions. Primary urinary tract infections can also predispose to the formation of adhesions, secondary to denudation of the immature labial epithelium. Topical application of an estrogen cream, twice daily for 6 weeks, will usually correct the problem. In a report of 50 patients with adhesions of the labia minora, attention was brought to the unexpected finding of four anomalies of the urinary tract (Capraro and Greenberg, 1972). These included malrotations and a hypoplastic kidney. This deserves consideration, since most physicians do not routinely obtain intravenous pyelograms in patients with labial adhesions. Certainly, any patient with posttreatment recurrent urinary tract symptoms should have excretory urography.

Gonadal Dysgenesis (Hypoestrogenism)

Elevated gonadotropin levels, a sex chromatin–negative buccal smear, hypoestrogenism, and assorted somatic abnormalities characterize the classic XO female with abnormal ovarian development (Figure 7–4*A*). A spectrum of gonadal dysgenesis occurs, with accompanying variation of the classic findings. Mosaics may be sex-chromatin positive, and karyograms will be abnormal. Some patients have minimal somatic findings. Nevertheless, those presenting with primary amenorrhea, hypoestrogenism, and hypergonadotrophism most likely fit somewhere into the gonadal dysgenesis group. In addition to the usual endocrine-related laboratory tests and chromosomal studies, the patient with XO gonadal dysgenesis should have excretory urography. Over 50 per cent of the classic Turner's syndrome patients have abnormalities of the urinary tract (Hung and Lo Presti, 1965; Reveno and Palubinskas, 1966; Matthies et al., 1971). The most common anomalies have been horseshoe kidneys (Figure 7–4*B*), malrotations, unilateral agenesis, and bifid pelves. The incidence of horseshoe kidney in the general population is 1:500, but is closer to 1:5 in Turner's syndrome patients (Jeune et al., 1962). Malrotation problems are the most common abnormality reported.

Almost all patients with urinary tract anomalies have some associated somatic problems, but there does not seem to be a consistent relationship between specific abnormalities and renal problems (Haddad and Wilkins, 1959). Therefore, the presence or absence of any particular stigma of gonadal dysgenesis cannot be used to predict the presence of a urinary tract anomaly. The presence of a horseshoe kidney in a patient with XY gonadal dysgenesis has been reported (Swanson and Chapler, 1978). Two cases of renal failure in association with XY gonadal dysgenesis have also been reported (Harkins et al., 1980). This observed association of XY gonadal dysgenesis and renal problems should stimulate thorough investigation of the urinary tract in these patients.

Matthies and co-workers (1971) believe a failure of normal "migratory or position specification phenomena during embryonic development" accounts for this association of abnormal gonadal and renal development. Such failure could be due to a shortage of necessary chemical substance, theoretically present in normal germ cells but lacking in aneuploid germ cells. This hypothesis awaits final proof, but it would satisfactorily explain the findings in Turner's syndrome patients and help to answer the question of why mosaics with XX/XO and pure gonadal dysgenesis pa-

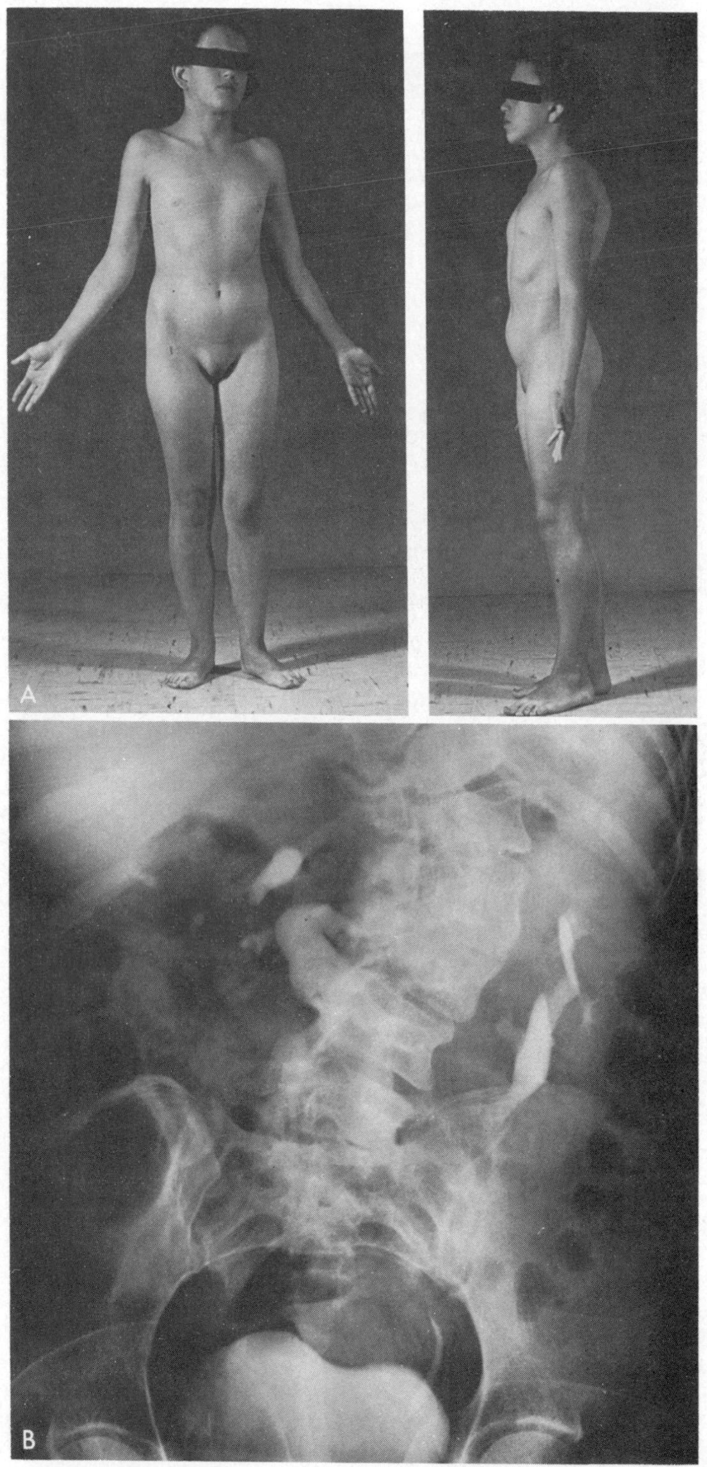

Figure 7–4. Turner's syndrome. *A*, Classic somatic stigmata: webbed neck, wide carrying angle and short stature. *B*, Excretory urogram showing horseshoe kidney in patient with XO gonadal dysgenesis.

tients do not have a higher incidence of renal anomalies.

All patients with XO and XY gonadal dysgenesis should have an intravenous pyelogram. If an anomaly is found, close observation is warranted because of predisposition to renal disease.

Intersex

Hyperandrogenism during genital tract development can result in masculinization of the external genitalia in otherwise normal-appearing females. If the source of the androgens is a hyperplastic adrenal gland, resulting from a compensatory hypersecretion of ACTH due to a 21-hydroxylase enzymatic deficiency with compromised cortisol production, the condition is termed the adrenogenital syndrome (Root et al., 1971). This is the most common cause of ambiguous genitalia the gynecologist encounters (Summitt, 1972; Park et al., 1975).

Varying degrees of androgenization of the urogenital sinus derivatives exist, including clitoral hypertrophy, labial fusion, and a persistent urogenital sinus. Timing and amount of androgen exposure determine the extent of involvement. As a rule, the earlier and the greater the exposure, the more severe the anomaly. Figure 7–5 shows a classic example of early exposure as evidenced by the fused labia, clitoral hypertrophy, and persistent urogenital sinus. Panendoscopy or radiographic visualization of the urogenital sinus, or a combination of these techniques, is often used to document the presence of the vagina and location of the urethra. Intersexuality resulting from this congenital adrenal hyperplasia is always associated with a vagina whose communication with the urogenital sinus is posterior and does not enter the urethra (Jones and Scott, 1971). This has practical importance to the surgeon correcting the anomaly, for the vagina can usually be exteriorized without fear of damaging the urethra. An apparent association of upper urinary tract anomalies and the adrenogenital syndrome has been reported (McMillan et al., 1976). Two of 10 patients had a partial duplication of the collecting system and one patient had unilateral renal agenesis.

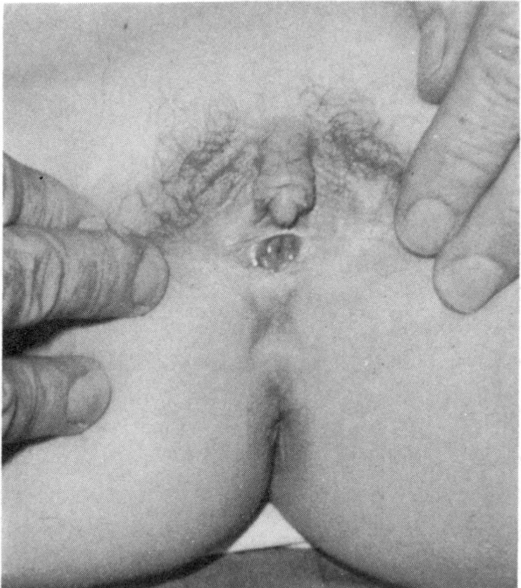

Figure 7–5. Clitoral hypertrophy, labial fusion and urogenital sinus in adrenogenital syndrome.

Other urogenital sinus anomalies associated with intersexuality should be approached and evaluated on an individual basis to determine the correct arrangement of the lower urogenital tract. Because of the many possible anatomic variations, panendoscopy and genitography are both helpful.

SECONDARY INFERTILITY AND REPRODUCTIVE PROBLEMS

Even though this grouping is quite arbitrary, it seems that most patients who have abnormalities of uterine development are first seen in relation to infertility or reproductive problems. The majority of patients with uterine anomalies do not have difficulty conceiving, but close to 30 per cent have difficulty in carrying a pregnancy to term (Gray and Skandalakis, 1972).

Uterine Malformation

Thirty per cent of women with uterine malformation have a demonstrable urinary tract anomaly. Conversely, women with urinary tract anomalies have a high percentage of müllerian duct anomalies. For example, Semmens (1962) reported that 37 per cent of his patients with major uterine anomalies had unilateral renal agenesis, while Collins (1932) reported that 90 per cent of his female patients with unilateral renal agenesis had accompanying uterine anomalies. This coexistence of anomalies results from the close embryologic development of the two systems. This has long been recognized and given due emphasis (Phelan et al., 1953). However, with an incidence of uterine anomalies of 1:600, the individual clinician may encounter such patients only rarely, and the possibility of accompanying urinary tract abnormalities may be overlooked. Therefore, the importance of routine intravenous pyelography in all with genital tract anomalies cannot be overemphasized (Polishuk and Ron, 1974).

Many classifications of uterine malformations are available (Jarcho, 1946; Jones and Baramki, 1975), covering all approaches from embryologic to "functional" (Semmens, 1962). Each has its individual usefulness depending on the needs of the clinician or investigator. From a practical standpoint, the most common anomalies are the didelphic uterus, the bicornuate uterus (unicollis or bicollis), and the septate uterus (complete or partial) (Figure 7–6). Each has definite anatomic characteristics, unique configuration on hysterogram, and different clinical implications. For instance, early abortion is associated with a septate uterus, third-trimester fundal notching is seen in a bicornuate uterus, and septal dystocia may be present in a didelphic uterus. The hysterosalpingogram reveals two cervices and two uterine horns in a didelphic uterus (Figure 7–7*A*), a wide angle between the two horns in a bicornuate uterus (Figure 7–7*B*), a narrow angle in a septate uterus (Figure 7–7*C*), and a fundal concavity of more than 1 cm. but less than 1.5 cm. in an arcuate uterus (Figure 7–7*D*) (Siegler, 1974).

If surgical correction is indicated, the preferred procedures are the Strassman for the didelphic or bicornuate uterus, and the Jones or Thomkins for the troublesome septate uterus. Didelphic and bicornuate uteri have two distinct palpable horns; the septate uterus is smooth across the fundus. A longitudinal vaginal septum is most often seen in a didelphic uterus. Two cervices are always present in a didelphic uterus, occasionally in a bicornuate (bicollis) uterus, and infrequently in a septate (total) uterus. Obviously, there is great overlapping of these observations, and gynecologists who perform metroplasties are frequently sur-

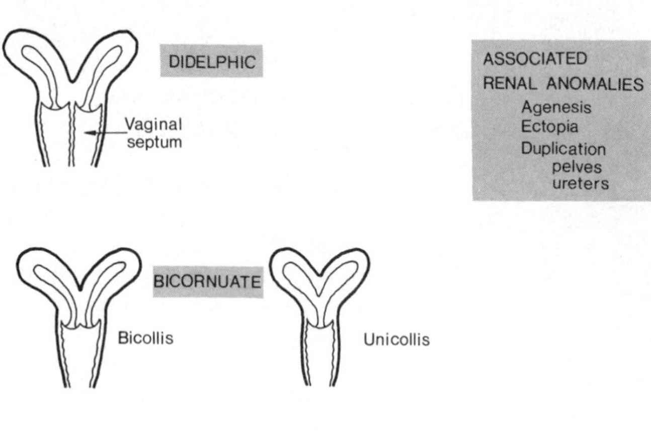

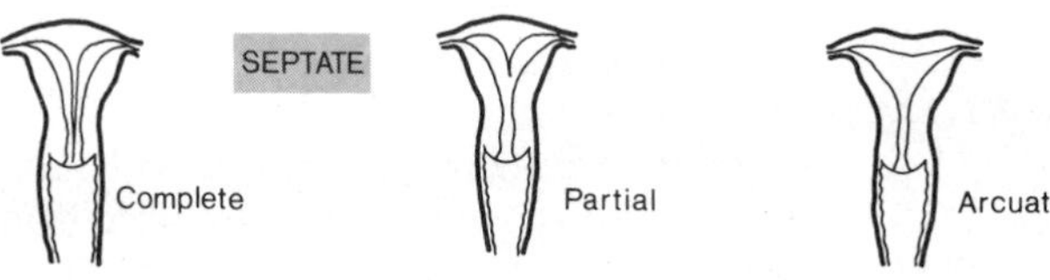

Figure 7–6. Common uterine malformations and associated urinary tract anomalies.

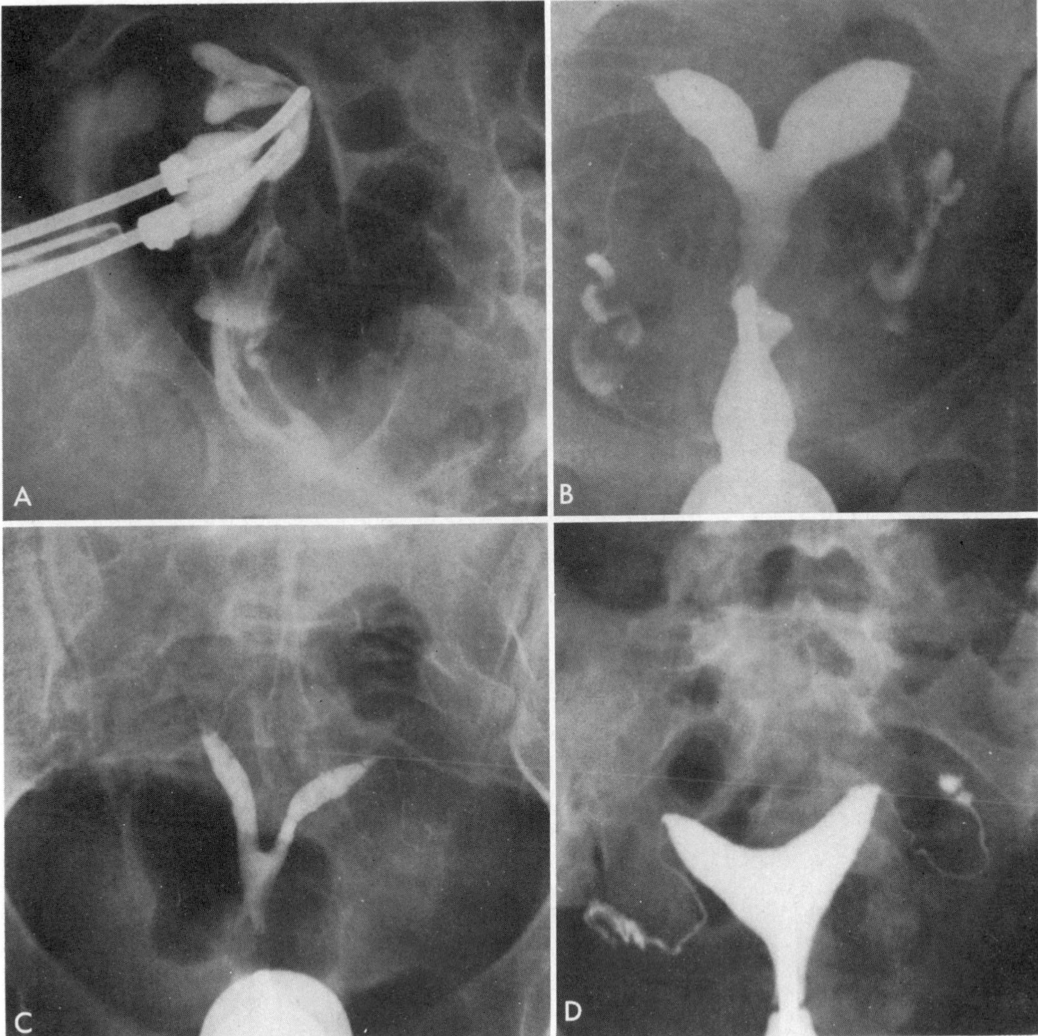

Figure 7–7. Hysterosalpingograms illustrating the common uterine malformations: *A,* Didelphic. *B,* Bicornuate. *C,* Septate. *D,* Arcuate.

prised by the actual uterine anomaly presented at the time of surgery, despite all preoperative evaluations.

Abnormalities of the urinary tract can be found in conjunction with all three uterine malformations. Certain conditions warrant special mention because of the extremely high degree of correlation. Obstructive malformations almost always have an accompanying renal agenesis on the obstructed side. This mechanism of a mesonephric duct abnormality resulting in both renal and uterine anomalies is found in the so-called ACI rat, thus providing an animal model for further studies of this problem (Marshall, 1978). Wiersma and co-workers (1976) recently reviewed the problem of uterus bicornis bicollis with a partial vaginal septum with resultant hematometra and hematocolpos on the obstructed side. This is also referred to as a double uterus with obstructed hemivagina and ipsilateral renal agenesis (Rock and Jones, 1980). This malformation complex has been referred to by a urologist as type II unilateral renal agenesis, and represents faulty differentiation of the mesonephric duct and ureteral bud and an abnormal laterally placed müllerian duct that forms the blind pouch (Magee et al., 1979). Figure 7–8*A* shows a hemihysterectomy specimen from such a patient. Her tube and ovary had previously been removed from

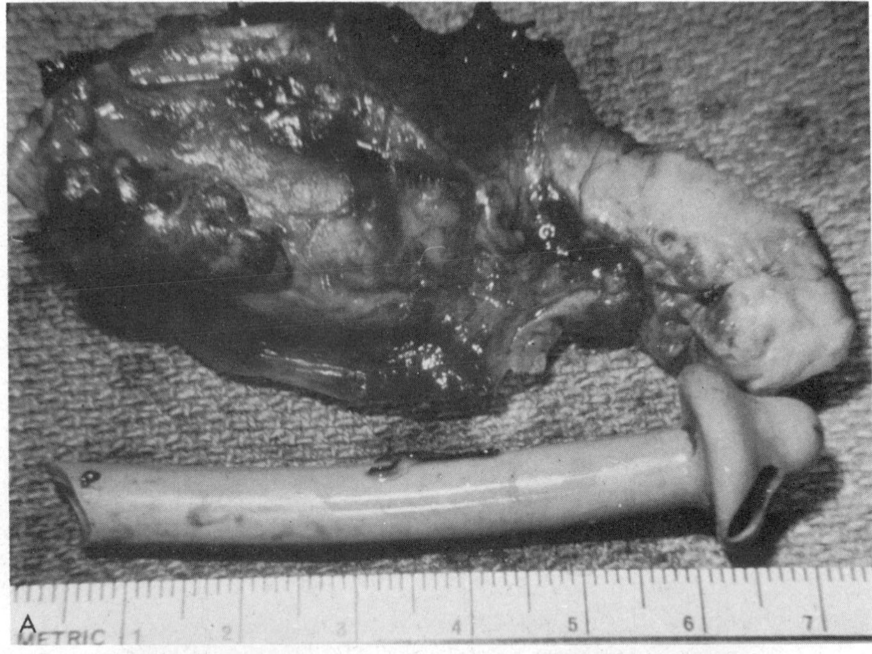

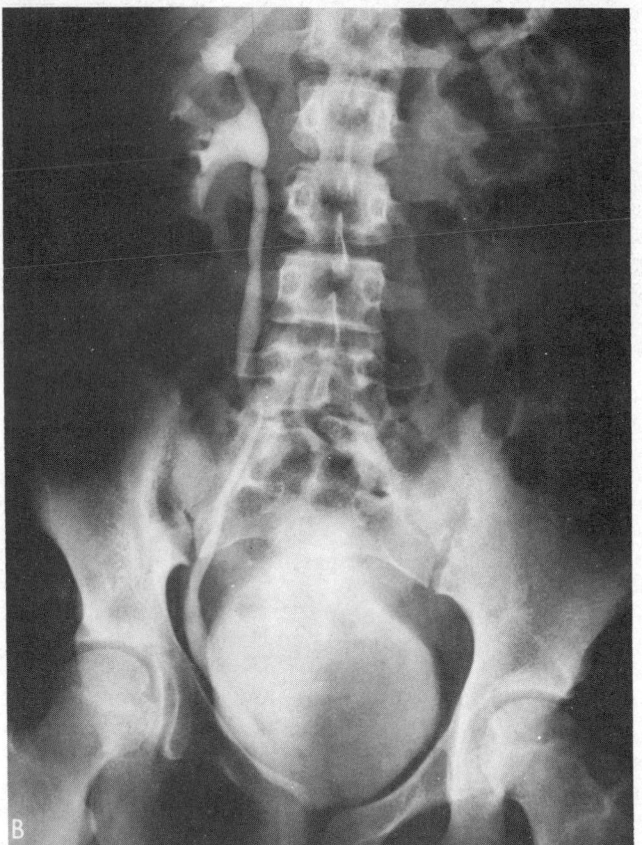

Figure 7–8. *A,* Excised uterine horn with "lost" catheter previously used to drain the obstructed hemivagina. *B,* Ipsilateral renal agenesis in same patient.

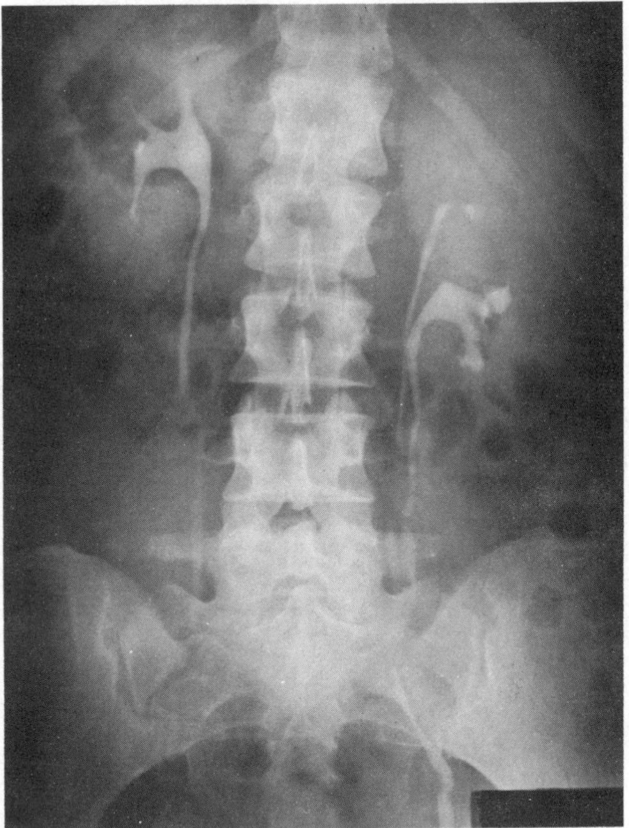

Figure 7–9. Intravenous pyelogram illustrating duplication of ureters in patient with müllerian malfusion (bicornuate uterus).

the obstructed side, with the remaining uterine horn and hemivagina being drained by the catheter shown in the picture. The catheter was lost, and after a year of continual vaginal drainage, "found" at time of surgery in the previously unrecognized obstructed hemivagina. The patient's intravenous pyelogram (Figure 7–8*B*) shows the expected renal agenesis on the side that had müllerian ductal obstruction. Other examples of asymmetrical development of the müllerian ducts, such as the communicating uteri (Toaff, 1974), also have associated major urologic defects. Other urinary tract anomalies seen with uterine malformation are pelvic kidney, horseshoe kidney, and duplication of the renal pelvis and ureter (Woolf and Allen, 1953) (Figure 7–9).

Although the majority of uterine anomalies probably go undetected, since most of these patients are able to achieve a pregnancy, there are certain signals that serve to alert the clinician to the possibility of a müllerian malformation. These have been summarized by Semmens (1975), and the principal ones are listed in Table 7–2. Discriminatory selection of patients with one or more of these symptoms or findings will identify those who should be candidates for a hysterogram, hysteroscopy, and in some cases, laparoscopy. If an anomaly is found, an intravenous pyelogram is indicated.

TABLE 7–2. SIGNS AND SYMPTOMS SUGGESTING MÜLLERIAN MALDEVELOPMENT

Recurrent abortions
Premature deliveries
Abnormal presentations
Abnormal uterine contour
Vaginal septum
Asymmetrical cervical placement
History of trapped placenta
Transverse lie
Postpartum bleeding
Recurrent pyelitis in pregnancy
Dysmenorrhea
Dyspareunia
Pelvic mass

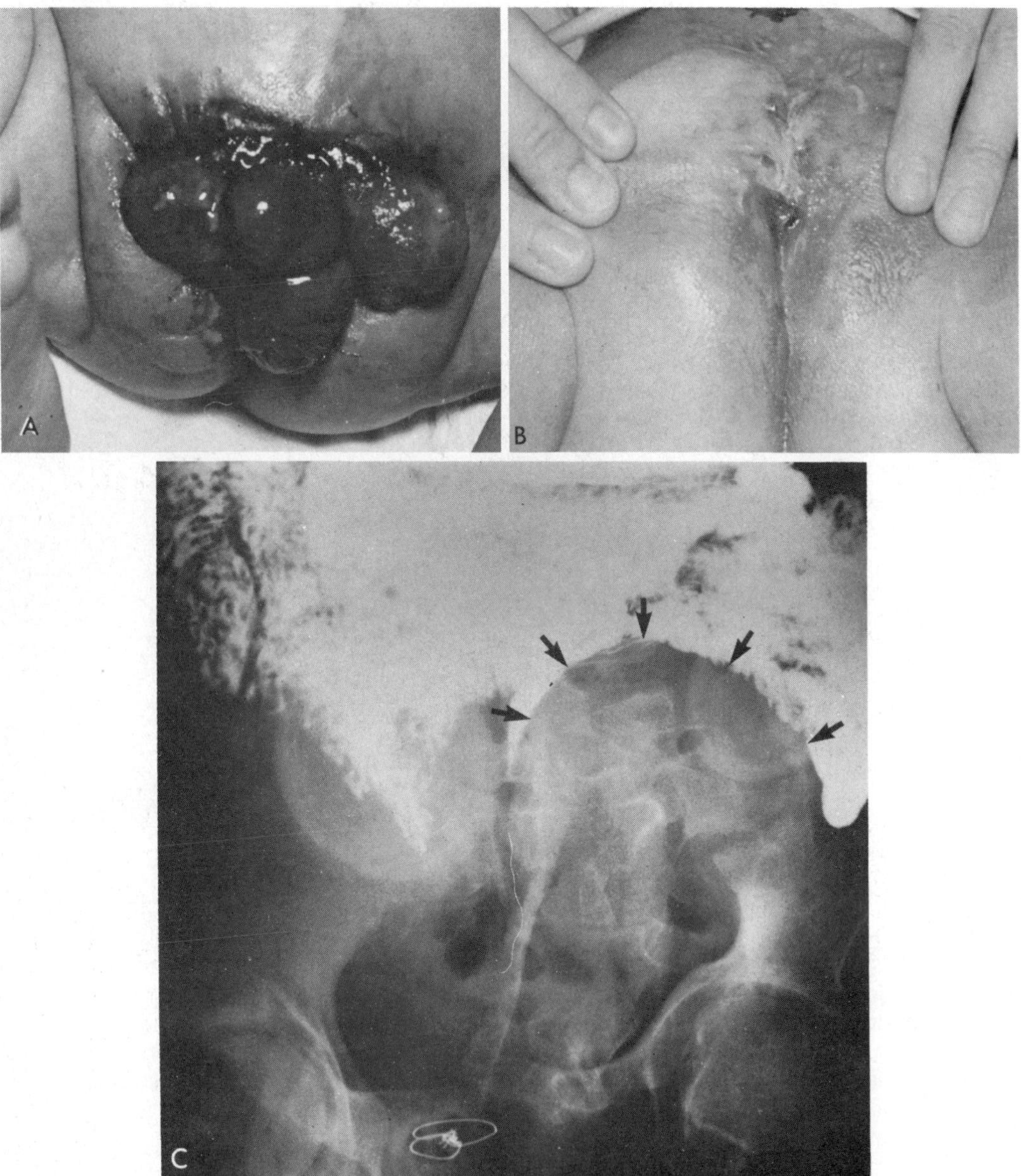

Figure 7–10. *A*, Infant with congenital bladder exstrophy. *B*, Same patient, age 14. Note vaginal agenesis. *C*, Same patient, age 16, with hematometra outlined in small bowel series radiograph.

DES-Exposed Women

Structural abnormalities of the uterus have been reported in women exposed to diethylstilbestrol (DES) in utero. Abnormal hysterosalpingograms were noted in over 60 per cent of such women. The most common findings were: a T-shaped uterus, intrauterine constrictions, and a small cavity. Patients with demonstrated abnormalities had a high pregnancy wastage, including premature delivery, spontaneous abortion, and ectopic pregnancies (Kaufman et al., 1980*a*). Surprisingly there does not seem to be any increase in upper urinary tract anomalies. There was no statistical difference in the numbers of abnormal intravenous pyelograms in women exposed to DES, with or without abnormal hysterosalpingograms and a control group (Kaufman et al., 1980*b*). This suggests that the effects of stilbestrol were confined to the müllerian system.

Miscellaneous Conditions

Exstrophy of the Bladder

This rare condition is frequently associated with genital tract anomalies. Absence of the vagina and müllerian malfusion problems have been reported (Jones, 1973). Figure 7–10*A* shows a patient with bladder exstrophy shortly after birth. A "double uterus" was noted at the time of one of her

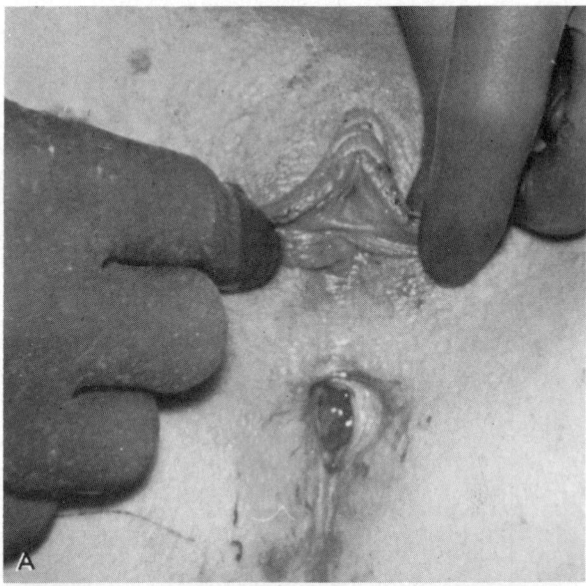

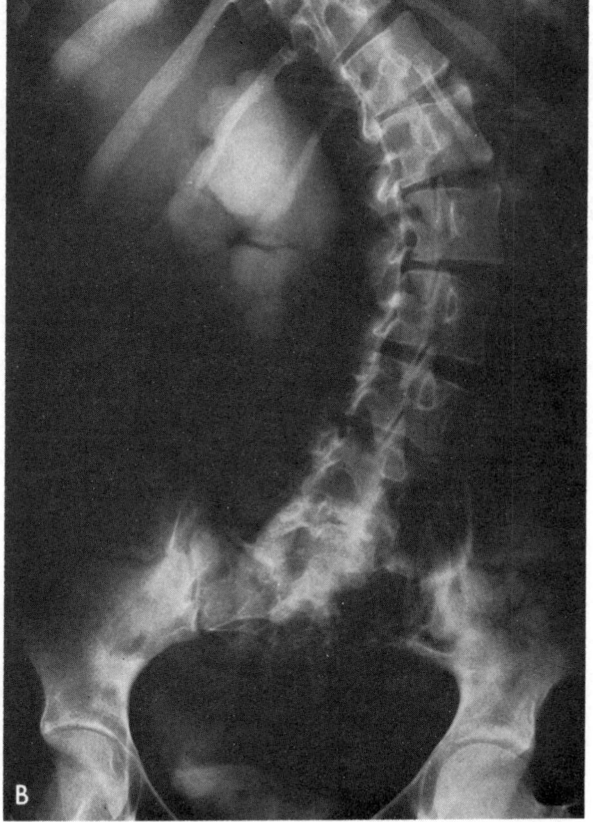

Figure 7–11. *A,* Vaginal agenesis in patient with multiple anomalies, including uterine malformation and anal atresia (note "pull through" repair site). *B,* Excretory urogram illustrating congenital hydronephrosis secondary to congenital bladder neck obstruction.

several reparative surgical procedures. Later, absence of the vagina was noted (Figure 7–10*B*). The patient then presented at age 16 years with a painful pelvic mass as outlined in Figure 7–10*C*. This represented a large hematometra, which was surgically removed. Her external genitalia and vaginal anomaly will be corrected in the future.

Anal Atresia

This more common defect, also called imperforate anus, has a similarly high degree of associated reproductive and urinary tract anomalies (Stephens, 1968; Gray and Skandalakis, 1972). Figure 7–11*A* shows the external genitalia of a patient prior to her vaginoplasty. She had been noted to have a bicornuate uterus, and the horns were removed separately during two of her many previous surgical procedures. Her congenital hydronephrosis as seen in the intravenous pyelogram (Figure 7–11*B*) was the result of congenital bladder neck obstruction. This patient also had several coexisting anomalies of the gastrointestinal tract. Six months following her vaginoplasty, she was married and is currently doing well.

REFERENCES

Bardin, C.: Androgen metabolism and mechanism of action in male pseudohermaphroditism. II. Recent Progr. Hormone Res. *29*:65, 1973.

Bowman, J., and Scott, R.: Transverse vaginal septum. Obstet. Gynecol. *3*:441, 1954.

Buchsbaum, H., and Chapler, F.: Gynecology. *In* Liechty, R., and Soper, R. (Eds.): Synopsis of Surgery. St. Louis, The C. V. Mosby Co., 1976.

Cali, R., and Pratt, J.: Congenital absence of the vagina. Am. J. Obstet. Gynecol. *100*:752, 1968.

Capraro, V., and Greenberg, H.: Adhesions of the labia minora. Obstet. Gynecol. *39*:65, 1972.

Capraro, V., and Gallego, M.: Vaginal agenesis. Am. J. Obstet. Gynecol. *124*:98, 1976.

Chan, L., and O'Malley, B.: Mechanism of action of the sex steroid hormones. N. Engl. J. Med. *294*:1430, 1976.

Chawla, S., Bery, K., and Indra, K.: Abnormalities of the urinary tract and skeleton associated with congenital absence of vagina. Br. Med. J. *2*:1398, 1966.

Collins, D. C.: Congenital unilateral renal agenesis. Ann. Surg. *95*:715, 1932.

Deppisch, L.: Transverse vaginal septum. Obstet. Gynecol. *39*:193, 1972.

Fore, S., Hammon, C., Parker, R., and Anderson, E.: Urologic and genital anomalies in patients with congenital absence of the vagina. Obstet. Gynecol. *46*:411, 1975.

Goldstein, A., Ackerman, E., Woodruff, R., and Poyas, J.: Vaginal and cervical communication with mesonephric duct remnants: Relationship to unilateral renal agenesis. Am. J. Obstet. Gynecol. *116*:101, 1973.

Gray, S., and Skandalakis, J.: Embryology for Surgeons, Philadelphia, W. B. Saunders Co., 1972.

Griffin, J., Edwards, C., Madden, J., Harrod, M., and Wilson, J.: Congenital absence of the vagina. Ann. Intern. Med. *85*:224, 1976.

Grover, S., Solanki, B., and Banerjee, M.: A clinicopathologic study of müllerian duct aplasia with special reference to cytogenetic studies. Am. J. Obstet. Gynecol. *107*:133, 1970.

Gruenwald, P.: Relation of the growing müllerian duct to the wolffian duct and its importance for the genesis of malformation. Anat. Rec. *81*:1, 1941.

Haddad, H., and Wilkins, L.: Congenital anomalies associated with gonadal aplasia—review of 55 cases. Pediatrics *23*:885, 1959.

Harkins, P., Haning, R., Jr., and Shapiro, S.: Renal failure with XY gonadal dysgenesis: report of the second case. Obstet. Gynecol. *56*:751, 1980.

Hung, W., and Lo Presti, J.: Urinary tract abnormalities in gonadal dysgenesis. Am. J. Roentgenol. *95*:439, 1965.

Jarcho, J.: Malformations of the uterus. Am. J. Surg. *71*:106, 1946.

Jeune, M., Bertrand, J., Deffrenne, R., and Forget, M.: Frequence des anomalies renales dans le syndrome de Turner chez l'enfant. Pediatrie *17*:897, 1962.

Jones, H., Jr., and Scott, W.: Hermaphroditism. Genital Anomalies and Related Endocrine Disorders. 2nd Ed. Baltimore, The Williams & Wilkins Co., 1971.

Jones, H., Jr.: An anomaly of the external genitalia in female patients with exstrophy of the bladder. Am. J. Obstet. Gynecol. *117*:748, 1973.

Jones, H., Jr., and Baramki, T.: Congenital anomalies. *In* Behrman, S., and Kistner, R. (Eds.): Progress in Infertility. 2nd Ed. Boston, Little, Brown and Co., 1975.

Kaufman, R., Adam, E., Binder, G., and Gerthoffer, E.: Upper genital tract changes and pregnancy outcome in offspring exposed in utero to diethylstilbestrol. Am. J. Obstet. Gynecol. *137*:299, 1980*a*.

Kaufman, R., Adam, E., Grey, M., and Gerthoffer, E.: Urinary tract changes associated with exposure in utero to diethylstilbestrol. Obstet. Gynecol. *56*:330, 1980*b*.

Leduc, B., Van Campenhout, J., and Simard, R.: Congenital absence of the vagina. Am. J. Obstet. Gynecol. *100*:512, 1968.

Magee, M., Lucey, D., and Fried, F.: A new embryologic classification for uro-gynecologic malformations: the syndromes of mesonephric duct induced müllerian deformities. J. Urol. *121*:265, 1979.

Marshall, F., and Beisel, D.: The association of uterine and renal anomalies. Obstet. Gynecol. *51*:559, 1978.

Matthies, F., MacDiarmid, W., Rallison, M., and Tyler, F.: Renal anomalies in Turner's syndrome. Clin. Pediatr. *10*:561, 1971.

McMillan, D., McArthur, G., Williams, J., and Birdsell, D.: Upper urinary tract anomalies in children with adrenogenital syndrome. J. Pediatr. *89*:953, 1976.

Park, I., Aimakhu, V., and Jones, H., Jr.: An etiologic and pathogenetic classification of male hermaphroditism. Am. J. Obstet. Gynecol. *123*:505, 1975.

Phelan, J., Counseller, V., and Green, L.: Deformities of the urinary tract with congenital absence of the vagina. Surg. Gynecol. Obstet. *97*:1–3, 1953.

Polishuk, W., and Ron, M.: Familial bicornuate and double uterus. Am. J. Obstet. Gynecol. *119*:982, 1974.

Reed, M., and Griscom, N.: Hydrometrocolpos in infancy. Am. J. Roentgenol. *118*:1, 1973.

Reveno, J., and Palubinskas, A.: Congenital renal anomalies in gonadal dysgenesis. Radiology *86*:49, 1966.

Rock, J., and Jones, H.: The double uterus associated with an obstructed hemivagina and ipsilateral renal agenesis. Am. J. Obstet. Gynecol. *138*:339, 1980.

Root, A., Bongiovanni, A., and Eberlein, W.: The adrenogenital syndrome. *In* Cristy, N. (Ed.): The Human Adrenal Cortex. New York, Harper & Row, Publishers, Inc., 1971.

Ross, G., and Vande Wiele, R.: The ovaries. *In* Williams, R. (Ed.): Textbook of Endocrinology. 6th Ed. Philadelphia, W. B. Saunders Co., 1981.

Semmens, J.: Congenital anomalies of female genital tract. Functional classification based on review of 56 personal cases and 500 reported cases. Obstet. Gynecol. *19*:328, 1962.

Semmens, J.: Congenital defects of the reproductive tract: clinical implications. Contemp. Ob/Gyn. *5*:95, 1975.

Siegler, A.: Hysterosalpingography. 2nd Ed. New York, Medcom Press, 1974.

Smith, R., and Goodwin, W.: Congenital hydrocolpos and associated urogenital malformations. J. Urol. *105*:683, 1971.

Sokolski, E.: Pregnancy complicated by solitary pelvic kidney. Obstet. Gynecol. *16*:365, 1960.

Stephens, F.: The female anus, perineum and vestibule: embryogenesis and deformities. Aust. N.Z. J. Obstet. Gynaecol. *8*:55, 1968.

Summitt, R.: Differential diagnosis of genital ambiguity in the newborn. Clin. Obstet. Gynecol. *15*:112, 1972.

Swanson, J., and Chapler, F.: Renal anomalies in the "XY female." Obstet. Gynecol. *51*:237, 1978.

Toaff, R.: A major genital malformation — communicating uteri. Obstet. Gynecol. *43*:221, 1974.

Wharton, L.: Congenital malformations associated with developmental defects of the female reproductive organs. Am. J. Obstet. Gynecol. *53*:37, 1947.

Wiersma, A., Peterson, L., and Justema, E.: Uterine anomalies associated with unilateral renal agenesis. Obstet. Gynecol. *47*:654, 1976.

Witten, D., Utz, D., and Myers, G.: Emmett's Clinical Urography. 4th Ed. Philadelphia, W. B. Saunders Co., 1977.

Woolf, R. B., and Allen, W. M.: Concomitant malformations. The frequent simultaneous occurrence of congenital malformations of the reproductive and urinary tract. Obstet. Gynecol. *2*:236, 1953.

SECTION

2

CLINICAL GYNECOLOGY

8

OFFICE AND SURGICAL GYNECOLOGY

H. J. BUCHSBAUM, M.D.

The physician in gynecologic practice commonly encounters conditions that cause functional and anatomic changes in the urinary tract. Drugs and operative procedures used in the management of these conditions can further compromise or even injure the urinary tract. The changing nature of gynecologic and obstetric practice has added new problems to the old. Erosion into the bladder by porcelain pessaries is no longer seen; problems related to methods of contraception and abortion are now taking on increasing importance.

OUTPATIENT GYNECOLOGY

Coitus-Related Injury

A rare type of urinary tract trauma that the gynecologist may encounter is injury related to coitus. Injuries severe enough to damage the bladder can occur in forcible rape and in women experiencing first coitus at a young age. Foda (1959) found two instances of "defloration in recently married women" among 220 cases of urinary fistulae.

Disorders Related to the Use of Contraceptives

The most effective and widely used methods of contraception, the oral contraceptive and intrauterine device, have been introduced into clinical practice in the last 20 years. Both have a demonstrated effect on the urinary tract.

Oral Contraceptive

There are approximately 50 million women presently taking hormone drugs for contraception. The metabolic effects of these drugs have been recognized and widely reported. Less clear is the effect these drugs have on the urinary tract. Koide and Lyle (1975), in an extensive review of the literature, were able to identify the more common effects of this group of drugs. Ureteral dilatation, like that of pregnancy, is found in a greater number of patients taking oral contraceptives than in control subjects. The proximal two thirds of the ureter dilates; the distal ureter is normal in caliber. The mechanism causing this dilatation is not well understood. It is probably the effect of hormones, since the changes regress after discontinuation of the drugs. In a study evaluating the side effects of oral contraceptives in over 16,000 women, Ramcharan and associates (1980) found a higher incidence of urinary tract infections and bacteriuria in users than in controls.

Estrogen-containing oral contraceptives have been implicated in the recently described "loin pain/hematuria syndrome." The patients complain of severe, recurrent, unilateral or bilateral kidney pain and tenderness, often accompanied by hematuria.

The symptom complex is similar to pyelonephritis, but the urine is invariably sterile and excretory urograms are normal, as are blood studies. The only abnormality is in the peripheral intrarenal vessels demonstrated on renal angiography (Burden et al., 1979). The entity developed in 5 of 9 patients within 2 months of starting an estrogen-containing oral contraceptive.

Intrauterine Device (IUD)

The second most common form of contraception is the IUD, with approximately 15 million in use. Considerable modifications in design have been introduced since the first commercially available devices came on the market. The most common serious complication of this method of contraception is perforation of the uterus. Perforation is rare (1 per 1000) and usually occurs at the time of insertion. The site of perforation is the fundus or the anterior uterine wall in the retroflexed and retroverted uterus. The device usually enters the peritoneal cavity; less commonly it becomes lodged in the broad ligament.

We cared for a 37-year-old para 2-0-3-2 with frequency, urgency, dysuria, and lower abdominal pain. The patient had had an IUD (Copper 7) inserted two years earlier and developed symptoms of recurrent bladder infection. An excretory urogram revealed normal upper tracts. A scout film (Figure 8–1*A*) showed two densities in the true pelvis: one consistent with a bladder calculus, the other a small discrete foreign body. Cystoscopic examination confirmed the presence of the stone. A suprapubic cystolithotomy was attempted, but the stone was formed around the IUD, which had perforated the uterus and bladder wall. A hysterectomy was then performed, with closure of the bladder defect. One week following surgery the patient developed total urinary incontinence, and a vesicovaginal fistula was demonstrated on intravenous pyelography (Figure 8–1*B*). The fistula was successfully repaired 4 months later, using an omental interposition technique.

Perforation of the uterus and bladder by a Lippes Loop, 7 years after insertion, has also been reported (Saronwala et al., 1974).

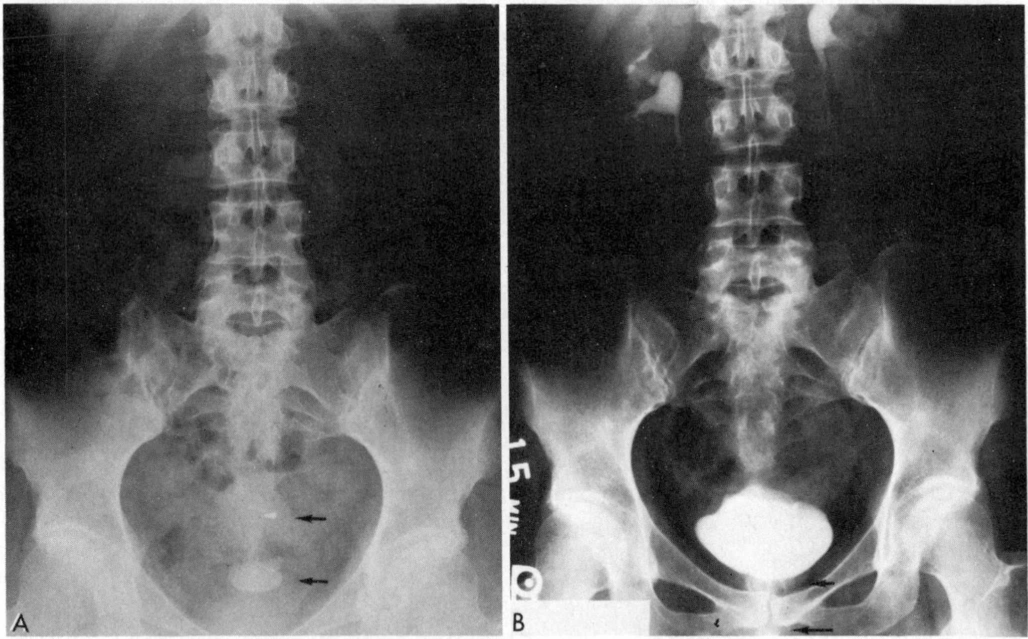

Figure 8–1. Patient with IUD perforating bladder.

A, Scout film of abdomen showing two foreign bodies in pelvis. Lower arrow identifies density consistent with calculus; upper arrow points to a more discrete foreign body.

B, Intravenous pyelogram following hysterectomy and cystolithotomy. The IUD had perforated uterine and bladder walls and was embedded in the bladder stone. Contrast material (arrows) is seen in vagina, demonstrating vesicovaginal fistula. Defect was subsequently closed surgically.

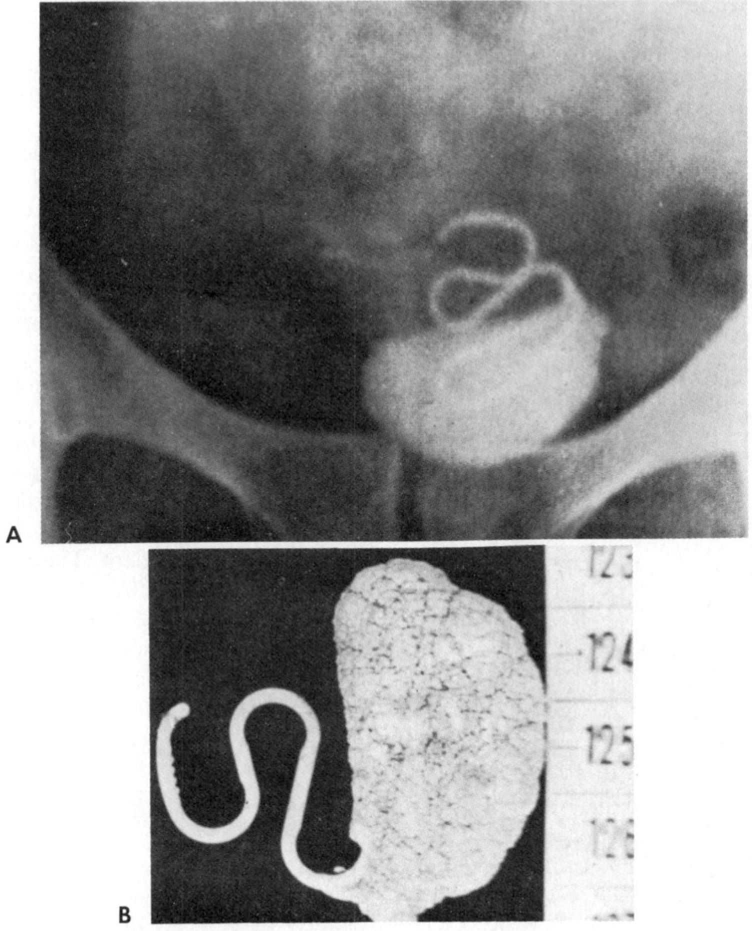

Figure 8–2. *A,* Detail from anteroposterior film of pelvis in patient 7 years after insertion of a Lippes Loop. *B,* IUD removed from bladder, incorporated into stone. (From Saronwala, K. C., Singh, R., and Dass, H.: Obstet. Gynecol. *44*:424, 1974, with permission of Harper & Row, Publishers.)

The patient experienced severe bladder symptoms, and a scout film of the pelvis revealed a foreign body and the IUD (Figure 8–2*A*). The Lippes Loop was retrieved from the urinary bladder, where it was partially incorporated into a 4 × 2 cm. calculus (Figure 8–2*B*). In addition to the cases already mentioned, bladder perforations have been reported with the Dalcon Shield (Neutz et al., 1978) and the Copper T (Avello et al., 1977).

Injury During Pregnancy Termination

Concern about unwanted pregnancy is as old as recorded history, and references to instrumentation of the pregnant uterus to induce abortion can be found in ancient literature. Attempts at inducing abortion have always carried two major risks: (1) infection and (2) perforation, with associated injury to other viscera. Since the legalization of abortion in this country, demand for such procedures has been constantly increasing; over 1 million pregnancy terminations are performed annually. With the increased demand for these services, other methods of emptying the uterus have been developed. Some of these procedures are done in outpatient facilities. Menstrual extraction, suction aspiration, and dilatation and sharp curettage have all been used in early pregnancy. The risks of perforation are directly related to the size of the uterus and the method of termination, and inversely related to the experience of the physician.

Uterine Perforation

Perforation of the uterus with sound or dilator occurs in approximately 0.5 per cent of diagnostic dilatations with curettage. Risks of perforation and urinary tract injury in menstrual extraction using a flexible cannula are extremely low. With vacuum and sharp curettage the need for dilatation of the cervix and sounding of the uterus greatly increases the risk of perforation. Dilators and sounds account for well over one half of uterine perforations in pregnancy termination. The most common site of perforation is the anterior uterine wall through the isthmus, particularly in the retroverted and retroflexed uterus (Beric et al., 1973).

Bladder Perforation

Both vacuum aspiration (Rouse et al., 1971) and sharp curettage (Sood, 1971) in the performance of pregnancy termination have resulted in bladder perforation. Bladder perforation through the anterior uterine wall injures the posterior aspect of the bladder, generally above the trigone. If the bladder has not been emptied, urine will be discharged through the external cervical os. If bladder perforation is suspected, 100 to 200 ml. of methylene blue–colored saline should be instilled into the bladder and a tampon placed in the vagina. If a defect is demonstrated or suspected, cystoscopic examination must be performed to rule out injury to the trigone. Management of these injuries should be individualized (Chap. 9).

Ureteral Injury

While the bladder is at greatest risk among urinary structures in pregnancy termination, ureteral injury has also been reported. Ureteral injury outside the bladder is most likely to occur with sharp curettage. The site of ureteral injury is usually at the pelvic brim where the ureter is relatively immobile, overlying bone (Beneventi and Twinem, 1950; Beyer, 1959; Gordon, 1973; Barton et al., 1978).

Dimopoulos and colleagues (1977) reported a patient who sustained avulsion of an entire ureter during suction curettage at 3 months' gestation. The cannula perforated the cervix and bladder before injuring the ureter. Nephrectomy and repair of the bladder were then performed.

GYNECOLOGIC SURGERY

More urinary tract injuries occur in the performance of gynecologic surgery than in any other type of surgery. The problems encountered in radical pelvic surgery for malignancy are discussed in Chapter 9; the anatomic and physiologic alterations of the urinary tract resulting from common malignant and inflammatory gynecologic conditions are described in Chapter 26. Symmonds (1976) estimates that 75 per cent of urinary fistulas result from surgery on the female genitalia; 80 to 90 per cent of these are ureterovaginal, and three quarters of all fistulas follow total abdominal hysterectomy. The reported incidence of injuries to the urinary tract in gynecologic surgery (exclusive of radical procedures) varies from 0.2 to 2.5 per cent. The most common site of injury is the bladder; the most serious is injury to the ureter. Unrecognized bladder injury generally results in the formation of a vesicovaginal fistula; unrecognized ureteral injury in fistula or obstruction.

Laparoscopic Procedures

Since its introduction into clinical practice, the fiberoptic laparoscope has been widely applied in gynecology. It has replaced the culdoscope as a diagnostic tool and now finds its greatest application in tubal sterilization.

Bladder Perforation

In placement of the insufflation (Veerhis) needle and the trocar, the bladder may be perforated. It is estimated that 2 per cent of laparoscopic complications involve the bladder (Phillips et al., 1974). The risk of bladder injury can be reduced if the bladder is emptied immediately before the procedure. If the bladder is entered with the needle, prolonged bladder drainage with an indwelling catheter is all that is needed. If the injury is larger, as with a trocar, the defect should be repaired in two layers with 2-0 chromic catgut.

Ureteral Thermal Injury

A less frequent but more serious complication is ureteral thermal injury. Two cases of ureteral burn during tubal cauterization have been reported (Stengel et al., 1974; Irvin et al., 1975), and one following diagnostic laporoscopy (Schapira et al., 1978). The ureteral fistulas communicated with the peritoneal cavity, and all three patients developed "urinary ascites." Another ureteral thermal injury was reported by Cheng (1976) during fulguration of endometriotic implants on the uterosacral ligaments. Repair of such injuries is difficult since the vascular injury may be quite extensive, requiring resection of the ureter. When the site of the burn is at the pelvic brim, transureteroureterostomy is an appropriate method of management (see Chapter 9).

Abdominal Surgery

The avoidance of urinary tract injury begins with a knowledge of the surgical anatomy and the recognition that disorders of the genital tract can cause displacement and distortion of the ureters and bladder. While we do not believe in the *routine* use of preoperative urograms or cystoscopic examinations, these studies can prove helpful in cases where significant urinary tract changes can be anticipated because of the patient's history or findings on physical examination. At such times urograms not only can alert the surgeon to ureteral displacement but also will document the presence of genitourinary anomalies, e.g., double ureter or pelvic kidney. If preoperative urography is not performed, the pelvic surgeon must palpate both kidneys prior to removing a retroperitoneal pelvic tumor. Few surgical errors are more tragic and avoidable than removing a solitary pelvic kidney.

Ureteral Catheters. Controversy exists about the value of ureteral catheters in pelvic surgery. Their routine use is to be condemned. We believe that they have very limited application in gynecologic surgery. The placement of ureteral catheters requires an additional operative procedure, traumatizes the urothelium, and carries the risk of perforation. In pelvic inflammatory disease and endometriosis, the tissue surrounding the ureter is often so indurated that the ureteral catheter cannot be palpated through the thickened tissue, giving the surgeon a false sense of security. Under such conditions the ureter should be identified at the pelvic brim and traced caudad to the site of disease to ensure its safety. The surest protection for the ureter is the knowledge of pelvic anatomy.

Bladder Injury

Bladder Catheterization. All patients undergoing pelvic celiotomy should have bladder catheterization under sterile conditions immediately before the surgery. For all but the simplest procedures, an indwelling catheter assures decompression of the bladder throughout the surgery. The distended bladder fills the pelvis, obstructs the surgeon's field of vision, and is more susceptible to injury.

Entering the Peritoneal Cavity. Bladder injuries occurred in 1.9 per cent of 819 total abdominal hysterectomies reported by Graber and associates (1964). The bladder can be injured at the very beginning of the procedure upon entering the peritoneal cavity. Regardless of the skin incision (vertical or transverse), the peritoneum should be opened vertically. To avoid bladder injury, the peritoneal cavity is best entered near the umbilicus, and the peritoneum incised toward the pelvis. It is important for the surgeon to remember that the bladder is an *extraperitoneal* structure. If the peritoneum is opened carefully, injury to the bladder can be avoided.

Mobilization of the Bladder. In total abdominal hysterectomy the bladder must be mobilized inferiorly to ensure its safety and that of the ureters, and to allow removal of the uterus. The vesicouterine fold of the visceral peritoneum is best entered laterally after the round ligaments have been divided and ligated. The peritoneum over the cervix is elevated with tissue forceps and a curved incision directed to that point. Too often the bladder incision is made too high on the corpus of the uterus. This causes bleeding, which obscures the field, exposing the bladder to possible injury. When the peritoneum can be tented by elevating it with tissue forceps, one can be assured that the incision will be atraumatic. The edge of the inferior bladder flap can then be grasped with forceps and the bladder dissected off the cervix and vagina. The areolar tissue allows the plane to be developed easily, preferably with a gauze-wrapped finger or with a dental roll dissector. The bladder

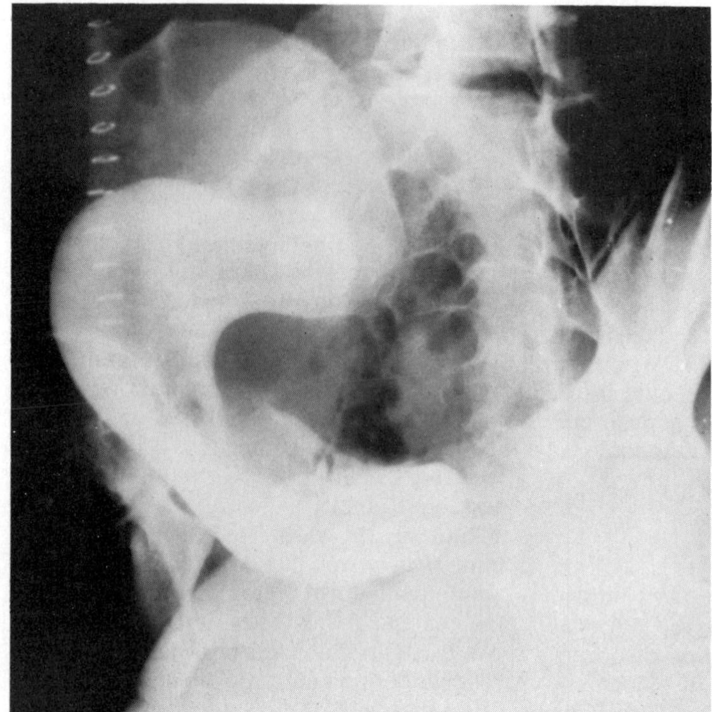

Figure 8–3. Retrograde cystogram (oblique view) 6 days following total abdominal hysterectomy. Note surgical clips on left. Postoperatively the patient developed tachycardia and hypotension without evidence of external bleeding. Cystogram shows distortion of bladder by large pelvic hematoma.

must be mobilized enough to allow access to the vagina.

In patients with previous surgery (e.g., low segment transverse cesarean section) the tissue planes are obliterated. In such cases dissection is best performed with scissors, with the tip directed against the cervix.

If the bladder is inadvertently entered, the defect should be marked with a suture and repair delayed until the bladder dissection is completed. The bladder is closed in two layers, utilizing 2-0 chromic catgut suture.

Other Surgical Precautions. The bladder is again at risk after the uterus has been removed in total hysterectomy. In closing the vaginal vault, a suture can incorporate the bladder wall. This suture through the vaginal mucosa and bladder mucosa is likely to result in the formation of a vesicovaginal fistula. Finally, the bladder can be injured in the reperitonealization. Care must be taken to avoid piercing the bladder with sutures placed in the lower edge of the peritoneum.

Bladder Fistula. Unrecognized bladder injury can result in a vesicoperitoneal communication, with urinary ascites and bacterial or chemical peritonitis, or in the formation of an extraperitoneal urinoma. The site of the fistula is usually high in the posterior aspect of the bladder, behind the trigone. Surgical injury rarely involves the trigone.

In Graber and O'Rourke's series (1964), 11 bladder injuries in 819 total abdominal hysterectomies were recognized and repaired primarily. Only one vesicovaginal fistula developed in this group, while five other patients in whom bladder injury was not appreciated developed vesicovaginal fistulas.

Bladder Hemorrhage. An intraoperative bladder injury severe enough to cause frank hemorrhage is rare. If bleeding is noted following surgery, gravity retrograde cystography using at least 250 ml. of iodinated contrast material should be performed to rule out urinary extravasation. If bladder perforation can be excluded, the bleeding can usually be managed by resting the bladder via a urethral catheter for a period of 5 to 7 days and by maintaining high urinary output.

In the rare situation not amenable to urethral catheter drainage and bladder rest, control of bleeding can be effected by transurethral fulguration. When this occurs, the clinician should suspect intrinsic bladder disease. The author has not personally seen or noted any reports of bladder hemorrhage related to gynecologic surgical injury severe enough to require hypogastric artery ligation, instillation of intravesical formalin, or supravesical diversion. Bladder hemorrhage of such magnitude suggests severe underlying disease, such as primary or secondary bladder malignancy, radiation cystitis, or disseminated intravascular coagulation.

Postoperative pelvic bleeding with hematoma formation can cause marked distortion of the bladder (Figure 8–3). Significant cystographic findings are most commonly found after radical hysterectomy, but bladder compression by hematoma can follow any pelvic procedure that is accompanied by bleeding. There is no evidence to suggest that bladder function is compromised after resolution of the hematoma.

Ureteral Injury

Ureteral injury carries more dire consequences than does intraoperative bladder trauma. Few controlled studies are available to assess the frequency of this injury in gynecologic surgery. St. Martin and associates (1953) obtained pre- and postoperative intravenous pyelograms on 332 women undergoing gynecologic surgery, excluding radical procedures. They found ureteral alterations in eight cases (2.4 per cent); of these, five were minor, with temporary hydronephrosis, and all cleared spontaneously by the fifth postoperative week. Solomons and co-workers (1960) conducted a similar study in 200 women undergoing hysterectomy for benign conditions. After total abdominal hysterectomy, there were changes suggestive of intraoperative damage to the ureter on the pyelogram in three of 171 patients (1.8 per cent).

Location of Injury. In the performance of total abdominal hysterectomy, adnexectomy, or both, there are five points at which the ureter can be injured:

1. *Infundibulopelvic ligament*. The proximity of the ureter to this vascular pedicle is shown in Figure 8–4. Under normal circumstances the ovary can be elevated and the

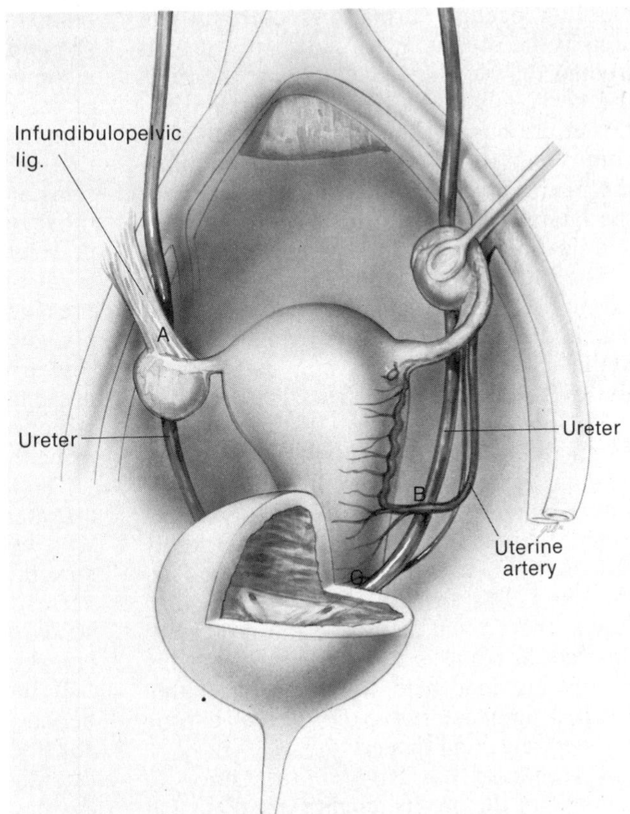

Figure 8–4. Anatomic relationships between genital and urinary structures in the female pelvis. Sites of common ureteral injury in the performance of gynecologic surgery: infundibulopelvic ligament (A), uterine artery (B), cardinal ligament and vaginal angle (C).

ligament stretched, allowing it to move away from the ureter. In pelvic inflammatory disease and endometriosis, the anatomy is distorted and the tissue is indurated, so that great care must be taken to avoid ureteral injury in clamping the infundibulopelvic ligament. The operator can avoid injury to the ureter in this situation by opening the peritoneum over the lateral wall between the round and infundibulopelvic ligaments and identifying the ureter. This is easily done by finger dissection. The ureter is on the medial leaf of the peritoneum and can be found coursing into the pelvis just medial to the bifurcation of the common iliac artery. With the ureter under direct vision, the infundibulopelvic ligament can be safely clamped, divided, and ligated.

In Higgins' series (1967) of 59 ureteral injuries following gynecologic surgery, 5 (8.5 per cent) occurred during salpingo-oophorectomy for ovarian cysts.

2. *Uterine artery.* The ureter is approximately 2 to 2.5 cm. from the lateral margin of the cervix where the uterine artery crosses anteriorly (see Figure 8–4). If bleeding occurs during dissection in the area of the uterine artery, attempts at controlling the bleeding by clamping lateral to the cervix place the ureter at great risk. Direct pressure with a sponge stick usually controls the bleeding long enough to allow the operator to open the peritoneum over the lateral pelvic wall, identify the ureter, and ligate the hypogastric artery.

The use of hemostatic preparations such as microfibrillar collagen to control bleeding should be avoided in the vicinity of the ureter. These substances may cause fibrosis severe enough to obstruct the ureter.

3. *Cardinal ligaments.* When total abdominal hysterectomy is performed, the cardinal ligaments are serially clamped and suture-ligated. In intrafascial hysterectomy, the risk to the ureter is markedly reduced. When the clamps are placed inside the collar formed by the pubocervical fascia, there is no danger to the ureters. If this fascial plane is not developed and the clamps are inadvertently reversed so that the tips point laterally, the ureters can be grasped, cut, and ligated.

4. *Angle of the vagina.* Just prior to removal of the uterus, clamps are placed at the vaginal angles to control bleeding and stabilize the vault. If the bladder has not been adequately mobilized with the ureters displaced laterally, they are in jeopardy at this point as they course anteriorly and medially (see Figure 8–4).

5. *Reperitonealization.* After the specimen has been removed, during closure of the pelvic peritoneum, a careless suture on the medial leaf of the peritoneum can incorporate the ureter, puncture it, or kink it.

TABLE 8–1. MECHANISMS OF URETERAL INJURY

1. Ligation
2. Transection
3. Excision
4. Crushing
5. Puncture
6. Kinking
7. Ischemia and necrosis

Mechanism of Injury. The ureter can be injured by one or more of seven mechanisms listed in Table 8–1. Ischemia and necrosis occur almost exclusively following radical pelvic surgery. Crushing with subsequent fibrosis, kinking, or ligation causes a compensatory hypertrophy and dilatation of the proximal ureter, with hydroureteronephrosis and diminished renal function on that side. This may produce classic symptoms or be completely silent, particularly in the face of a normally functioning contralateral kidney. Likewise, measurements of renal function may be normal even in the presence of a completely ligated ureter with a normal functioning contralateral kidney. The urinary sediment may be normal in the presence of complete or near complete obstruction of the ureter, since little or no urine from that side enters the bladder.

The finding of urinary extravasation from a ureteral fistula will usually be correlated with pyelographic evidence of ureteral obstruction and hydroureteronephrosis. Conversely, the finding of partial ureteral obstruction should alert the physician to possible fistula formation.

If the patient develops urinary incontinence postoperatively, the surgeon should consider ureterovaginal fistula in the differential diagnosis. A systematic approach to the evaluation of postoperative fistula will establish the diagnosis. If suspicion of ureteral injury exists, the surgeon should obtain postoperative intravenous pyelograms, or have retrograde studies performed, or both. Procrastination could result in loss of the kidney. Complete loss of kidney function in the absence of any signs or symptoms can occur within 2 months of complete ureteral ligation.

Clinical Findings

If ureteral injury is suspected intraoperatively, the intravenous administration of 5 ml. of indigo carmine in the presence of reasonable kidney function can help to identify the site of injury. The extravasation of blue urine directs the surgeon's attention to the site of injury. If ureteral ligation is suspected intraoperatively, the ureter should be identified proximal to the suspected site and 1 ml. of sterile methylene blue injected through a fine needle into the lumen of the ureter. If the urine in the collection system does not take on a blue coloration it is fair to assume that the ureter is completely blocked.

The symptoms of ureteral injury depend on whether ureteral obstruction alone or ureteral perforation with extravasation or fistula formation is present. The typical symptom complex of ureteral obstruction consists of unilateral dull to severe flank pain, fever, chills, malaise, and reflex ileus.

Diagnostic Aids. An excretory urogram will show impaired visualization of an enlarged hydronephrotic kidney, and delayed films will identify the point of ureteral obstruction. However, if the obstruction has been present for a long time, the kidney may never show more than a nephrogram. The intravenous study is limited in that it may not visualize the compromised side; however, it will demonstrate a normal contralateral kidney. An abdominal ultrasound study can help in confirming the clinical impression of an enlarged kidney with hydroureteronephrosis (Leopold and Asher, 1975). The ultrasound is particularly useful in patients who are sensitive to iodinated intravenous contrast material.

If these studies do not yield conclusive results, cystoscopy with ipsilateral retrograde pyeloureterography should be performed. This study should commence with a bulb ureterogram to identify the normal distal ureter as well as the point of obstruction. If contrast material does flow across the point of obstruction into the dilated system, the passage of a ureteral catheter is warranted in an attempt to overcome the obstruction and drain the hydroureteronephrosis. This is usually not possible because the obstruction, compounded by the tissue reaction, makes the passage of a ureteral catheter quite difficult. Untreated acute ureteral obstruction and hydronephrosis will rarely result in hypertension.

In ureteral injury, the patient may complain primarily of fever, chills, flank pain, and later note drainage of urine either through the vagina, to the skin, or across the rectal sphincter. Ureterovaginal fistulas appear most commonly 3 to 7 days following surgery. If the fistulous tract has not reached the surface, there may be only pain and tenderness around the point of urinary extravasation. An excretory urogram will show ipsilateral mild to moderate hydroureteronephrosis, and the fistulous tract or urinoma cavity may be outlined with contrast material. Again, cystoscopy and ipsilateral ureteropyelography can identify the point of injury and the fistulous tract. An attempt should be made to pass a ureteral catheter to bridge the gap, although this is usually unsuccessful.

A concomitant vesicovaginal fistula should be ruled out by the performance of a retrograde cystogram. An ampule of indigo carmine should be added to the contrast material and a vaginal tampon inserted. If the bladder is intact, the cystogram will be normal and there will be no dye staining the tampon. On the other hand, if the test is repeated with intravenously administered indigo carmine, the tampon will be stained blue in the presence of a ureterovaginal fistula and sufficient kidney function on the side of injury.

Other aids in the diagnosis of urinary fistula include (1) injection of a skin tract (fistulogram) to document a ureterocutaneous connection and (2) oral administration of charcoal or carmine red. When a communication exists between the ureter and the gastrointestinal tract, these materials can be identified in the urine (Glenn, 1962).

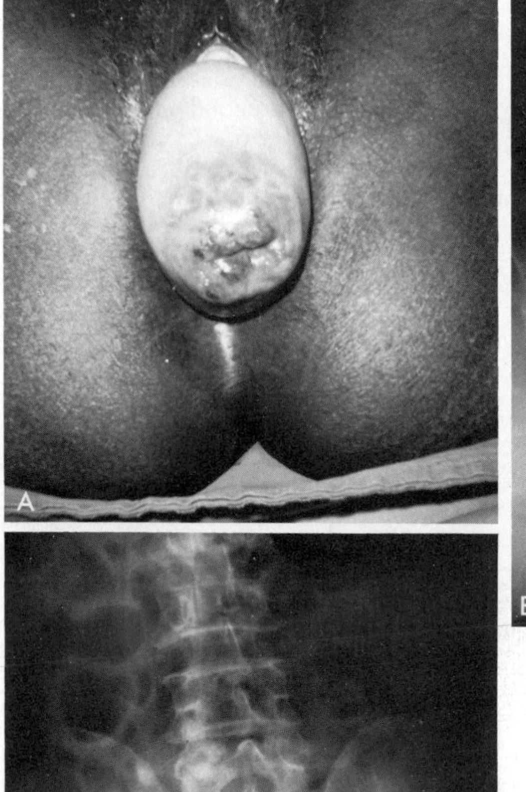

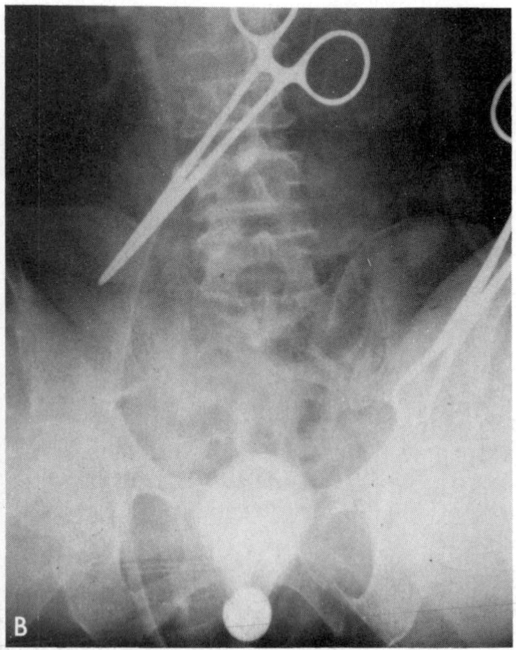

Figure 8–5. *A,* Patient with third degree uterine prolapse. Uterine cervix and corpus are projecting through the introitus. *B,* Retrograde cystogram taken on the operating table prior to surgical procedure. Note extrapelvic location of trigone, identified by Foley catheter bulb. *C,* Postoperative cystogram, with elevation of bladder following vaginal hysterectomy and anterior colporrhaphy. Patient was continent of urine.

Vaginal Hysterectomy

Of the many vaginal operations devised for the treatment of uterine prolapse, only vaginal hysterectomy continues to be widely used. The Manchester (Donald or Fothergill) operation is used in selected cases, whereas the others have largely been abandoned. The indications for vaginal hysterectomy have been expanded so that it is now performed for carcinoma in situ of the uterine cervix, dysfunctional uterine bleeding, and endometrial carcinoma, and in a few clinics for abortion and sterilization (Laufe and Kreutner, 1971; van Nagell and Roddick, 1971). In some clinics, vaginal hysterectomy and colporrhaphy represent half of the gynecologic surgical procedures performed. In vaginal as in abdominal hysterectomy, the bladder must be mobilized before the uterus can be removed. It is in the course of this dissection that the bladder and ureters are placed in jeopardy. Careful technique and good exposure will reduce the incidence of urinary tract injuries.

An effective technique for repair of large anterior defects in patients with third degree uterine prolapse (Figure 8–5) is use of concentric sutures of 2–0 polyglycolic acid.

After the first suture is placed and tied, the defect is greatly reduced. A second such suture is generally all that is needed to close the defect, although a third suture can be used if necessary.

Surgical Precautions

With a tenaculum on the cervix, traction is exerted to bring the uterus down the vaginal canal. The mucosa on the portio is incised circumferentially below the bladder. Care must be taken to incise the mucosa only, lest the wrong plane be developed. The mucosa is grasped and elevated and bluntly dissected until the bladder attachment to the cervix, the vesicouterine fascia, is identified. This is best cut in the midline using Metzenbaum scissors, with the tips directed against the cervix (Figure 8–6*A*). The areolar tissue next encountered is easily dissected with a gauze-wrapped finger, pushing the bladder off the anterior aspect of the cervix and lower portion of the corpus (Figure 8–6*B*). The vesicouterine fold of the peritoneum is next encountered as a smooth structure. This should be grasped with a tissue forceps and incised. After the peritoneum has been entered, the incision is enlarged and a narrow ribbon retractor placed anteriorly to displace the bladder (Figure 8–6*C*).

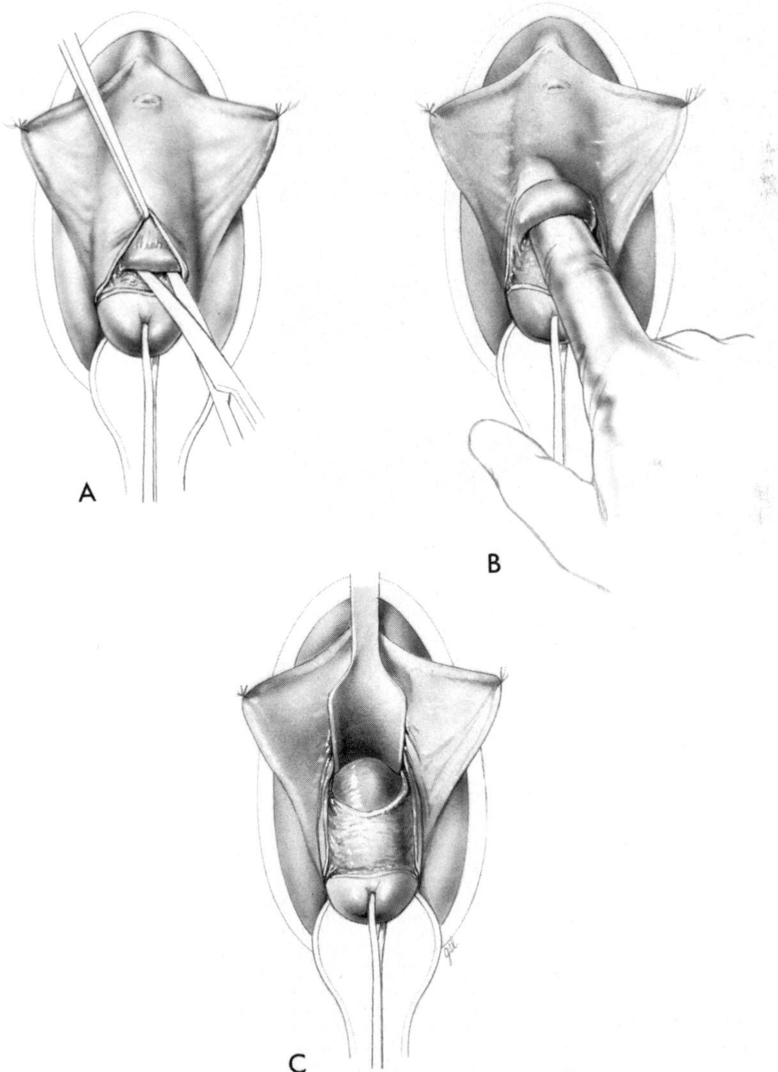

Figure 8–6. Technique of mobilizing bladder and displacing ureters in vaginal hysterectomy. See text for description.

If difficulty is encountered in this dissection, the operator should not persist. The overly cautious surgeon may, as Gray (1963) suggests, ". . . dissect through the wall of the uterus into the endometrial cavity while trying to avoid injury to the interior of the bladder." The reward for persistence is increased bleeding, which obscures the surgical field and adds to the surgeon's frustration.

If there is difficulty in entering the peritoneum anteriorly, it is safest to abandon these attempts and enter the peritoneum posteriorly, through the cul-de-sac. The index finger can be brought anteriorly over the fundus to guide the operator. It is also possible to deliver the fundus of the uterus, after the pedicles have been clamped, through the cul-de-sac opening and incise the vesicouterine fold of the visceral peritoneum, as in abdominal hysterectomy, albeit upside down.

Considering the proximity of the bladder and uterus, the restricted field, and limited exposure, it is surprising how rarely the bladder and ureters are injured in the performance of vaginal hysterectomy. Bladder injury appears to be more common in pa-

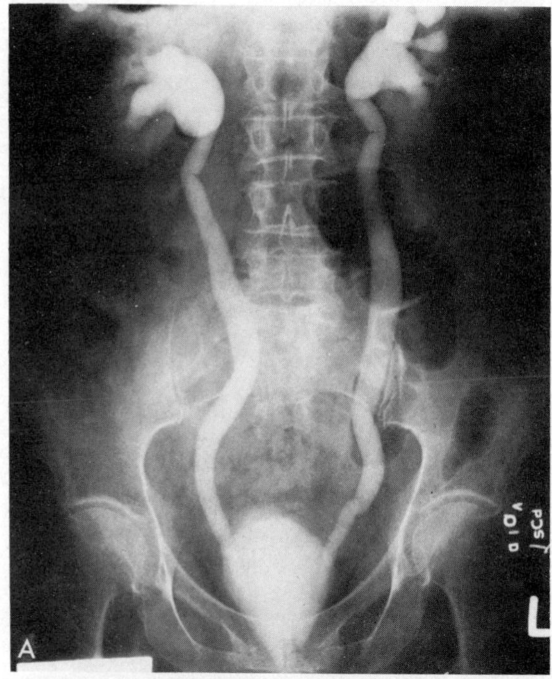

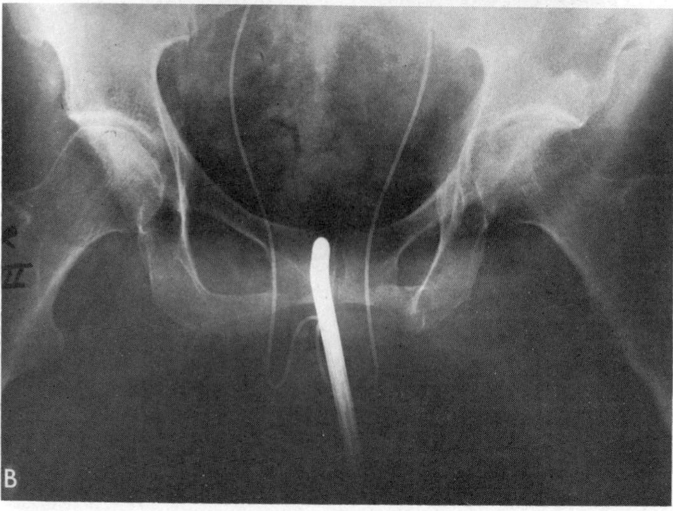

Figure 8–7. Patient with uterine prolapse.

A, Preoperative intravenous pyelogram demonstrating bilateral hydroureteronephrosis. Note the bladder neck below symphysis.

B, Ureteral catheters demonstrating caudal displacement. Trigone is well below symphysis.

Illustration continued on opposite page

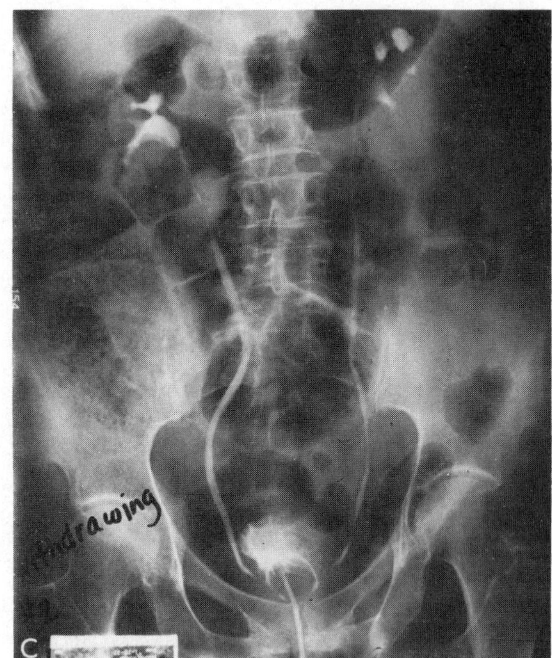

Figure 8–7. *Continued.* *C,* Postoperative retrograde ureterograms at the time of withdrawal of ureteral catheters. Note location of bladder base and caliber of ureters 4 days following vaginal hysterectomy and anterior colporrhaphy.

tients with pelvic inflammatory disease (Copenhaver, 1962), but previous pelvic surgery, including cesarean section, does not increase the frequency of inadvertent cystotomy (Coulam and Pratt, 1973). Hager and Ledermair (1979) reported on 132 women who had had vaginal hysterectomy, for a variety of indications, following at least one prior gynecologic procedure. Twelve patients had had two, and two had had three, prior pelvic operations. Although three bladder injuries occurred, all were repaired primarily and no fistulae resulted. This outcome compared favorably to a control group of over 3000 vaginal hysterectomies.

Bladder Perforation

If the bladder is entered, the injury should be repaired utilizing two layers of 2-0 chromic catgut, lest the defect be enlarged. The site of injury is generally the posterior wall of the bladder above the trigone. The trigone is at greater risk of injury in vaginal than in abdominal hysterectomy, since the dissection is begun at a more caudal point. If the bladder injury permits, it is wise to examine the interior of the bladder before beginning the repair to determine the proximity of the defect to the trigone.

Incidence. The reported incidence of bladder injury in vaginal hysterectomy varies from 0.2 per cent to 1.6 per cent (Copenhaver, 1962; Gray, 1963; Rubin, 1966; Porges, 1970; Pratt, 1976; Burmucic, 1975). Tasche (1968) reported bladder injury in four of 1700 consecutive vaginal hysterectomies, with only one vesicovaginal fistula. If the bladder injury is recognized and repaired, there are usually no sequelae. In Copenhaver's (1962) series of 1000 vaginal hysterectomies, there were 11 cystotomies recognized and repaired. Of the two vesicovaginal fistulas that developed in this series, only one occurred in the 11 cases recognized and repaired.

Ureteral Injury

Although the bladder is of greatest concern in vaginal hysterectomy and anterior colporrhaphy, ureteral injury can also occur.

Ureteral Compression in Uterine Prolapse. The role that uterine prolapse, the most frequent indication for this surgery, plays in ureteral injury is interesting to speculate about. Froriep, as early as 1824, and Virchow, in 1847, called attention to the upper urinary tract changes accompanying complete prolapse of the uterus. Significant hydroureter and hydronephrosis were present in 15 of the 23 cadavers with uterine prolapse examined by Halban and Tandler (Lieberthal and Frankenthal, 1941). The changes are bilateral in about half of these cases; when unilateral obstruction is present, neither side predominates. The degree of upper tract changes is probably related to the age of the patient and the severity and duration of prolapse (Figure 8-7,*A,B*).

The mechanism and exact site of this ureteral obstruction are not clear. Some investigators (Brettauer and Rubin, 1923; Wallingford, 1939) have thought that the obstruction is caused by the uterine arteries, which, when the uterus descends, cause the ureters to form a sling. Others have believed that it is the broad and cardinal ligaments that cause extrinsic pressure on the ureters (Lieberthal and Frankenthal, 1941; Chapman, 1975). Hadar and Meiraz (1980), among others, believe that the ureteral compression is at the urogenital diaphragm. In one study (Elkin et al., 1974) of 19 patients (18 with uterine procedentia and one with prolapse of the vaginal vault), all had some degree of upper tract changes. In 16 of 18 (89 per cent), the changes were bilateral. Pelvic arteriography in two patients showed that the site of ureteral obstruction was well below the level of the uterine arteries; the dilatation in these patients reached the bladder. The authors suggest, therefore, that the obstruction may be in the intramural portion of the ureter.

Gregoir and colleagues (1976) agree that the ureteral obstruction is at the vesical junction. Based on studies on 14 patients, they believe that the dilatation and stasis develop in two stages, each having a different mechanism. In the first stage, the prolapse of the uterus leads to stretching of the terminal ureter, with narrowing and reduction of caliber. This narrowing inhibits peristalsis and the flow of urine, resulting in a proximal dilatation. With prolonged prolapse, there is rotation of the ureters, with obstruction at the intramural portion.

Regardless of its etiology, the ureteral compression can lead to pyoureter and fatal uremia. Treatment of the uterine prolapse corrects the ureteral obstruction, with rapid return to normal (Figure 8-7, *C*). In performing vaginal hysterectomy for complete uterine prolapse, the surgeon must be aware that the ureters may be dilated and displaced medially. The anterior peritoneal incision should be wide enough to accommodate a large retractor, and the pedicles must be clamped close to the uterus.

Nonpuerperal uterine eversion is a rare entity, usually found with benign or malignant smooth muscle tumors. In a recent report, a patient presented with acute urinary retention and bilateral hydronephrosis (Pride and Shaffer, 1977). The fundus could not be reposited to relieve the obstruction; the condition was surgically corrected by hysterectomy.

Surgical Trauma. Although the risk to the ureter is low in vaginal hysterectomy, Copenhaver (1962) reported two known ureteral injuries in 1000 cases (0.2 per cent). Ureteral abnormalities were found in five of 27 *symptomatic* patients studied with intravenous pyelograms following vaginal hysterectomy (van Nagell and Roddick, 1972). In one, the obstruction was "surgical," while in the other four the obstruction was by extrinsic masses. These were the symptomatic patients among the 617 who had undergone vaginal hysterectomy. Burmucic (1975) reported one operative ligation of a ureter and two postoperative ureterovaginal fistulas among 2309 vaginal hysterectomies. Since ureteral obstruction can be "silent" and renal function lost without clinical signs or symptoms, the true incidence of ureteral damage in vaginal hysterectomy is still unknown.

The most common type of injury the ureter sustains in vaginal hysterectomy is crushing and ligation near the bladder. Harrow (1954) reported a case of bilateral ureteral obstruction following anterior colporrhaphy, and cites three other cases.

If ureteral injury is suspected, retrograde ureteral catheters should be passed with the patient still anesthetized. If this is unsuccessful, immediate correction should be undertaken. It is best to approach the site of obstruction via an extraperitoneal abdominal incision. Reimplantation via ureteroneocystotomy is the most appropriate method of repair.

Urethrovaginal Fistula

Gray (1968) has reported another urinary complication of vaginal hysterectomy and anterior colporrhaphy: urethrovaginal fistula. He encountered this problem in 10 of 950 patients who had vaginal hysterectomy and anterior colporrhaphy. We have found such defects to be extremely rare. If the patient is symptomatic, the fistula should be repaired by a layered closure over an indwelling urethral catheter.

REFERENCES

Avello, E. J., Torga, L. G., Villanueva, J. L., et al.: Perforacion uterina y migracion vesical de un dispositivo intrauterino. Observacion casuistica. Acta Ginecol. *30*:79, 1977.

Barton, J. J., Grier, E. A., and Mutchnik, D. L.: Uretero-uterine fistula as a complication of elective abortion. Obstet. Gynecol. *52*(Suppl.):81s, 1978.

Beneventi, F. A., and Twinem, F. P.: Transection of the ureter following uterine instrumentation. J. Urol. *63*:224, 1950.

Beric, B., Kupresanin, M., and Kapor-Stanulovic, N.: Accidents and sequelae of medical abortions. Am. J. Obstet. Gynecol. *116*:813, 1973.

Beyer, E.: Ureterabriss bei krimineller Abtreibung. Munch. Med. Wsch. 101:358, 1959.

Brettauer, J., and Rubin, I. C.: Hydroureter and hydronephrosis; frequent secondary changes in cases of prolapse of the uterus and bladder. Am. J. Obstet. Gynecol. *6*:696, 1923.

Burden, R. P., Etherington, M. D., Dathan, J. R., et al.: The loin-pain/hematuria syndrome. Lancet *1*:897, 1979.

Burmucic, R.: Die vaginale Uterusexstirpation au der Univ. Frauenklinik Graz im der Zeit von 1955 bis 1970. Geburtsh. Frauenheilkd. *35*:767, 1975.

Chapman, R. H.: Ureteric obstruction due to uterine prolapse. Br. J. Urol. *47*:531, 1975.

Cheng, Y. S.: Ureteral injury resulting from laparoscopic fulguration of endometriotic implant. Am. J. Obstet. Gynecol. *126*:1045, 1976.

Copenhaver, E. H.: Vaginal hysterectomy. An analysis of indications and complications among 1,000 operations. Am. J. Obstet. Gynecol. *84*:123, 1962.

Coulam, C. B., and Pratt, J. H.: Vaginal hysterectomy: Is previous pelvic operation a contraindication? Am. J. Obstet. Gynecol. *116*:252, 1973.

Dimoupoulos, C.,, Giannopoulos, A., Pantasopoulos, D., et al.: Avulsion of the ureter from both ends as a complication of interruption of pregnancy with vacuum aspirator. J. Urol. *118*:108, 1977.

Elkin, M., Goldman, S. M., and Meng, C.-H.: Ureteral obstruction in patients with uterine prolapse. Radiology *110*:289, 1974.

Foda, M. S.: Evaluation of methods of treatment of urinary fistulas in women: report of 220 cases. J. Obstet. Gynaecol. Br. Emp. *66*:372, 1959.

Glenn, J. F.: External ureteral trauma. Trauma *4*:45, 1962.

Gordon, M.: First trimester abortion. *In* Osofsky, H. J., and Osofsky, J. D.: The Abortion Experience. Hagerstown, Harper & Row, 1973.

Graber, E. A., O'Rourke, J. J., and McElrath, T.: Iatrogenic bladder injury during hysterectomy. Obstet. Gynecol. *23*:267, 1964.

Gray, L. A.: Vaginal Hysterectomy. 2nd Ed. Springfield, Ill., Charles C Thomas, 1963, p. 144.

Gray, L. A.: Urethrovaginal fistulas. Am. J. Obstet. Gynecol. *101*:28, 1968.

Gregoir, W., Schulman, C. C., and Chantrie, M.: Ureteric obstruction associated with uterine prolapse. Eur. Urol. *2*:29, 1976.

Hadar, H., and Meiraz, D.: Total uterine prolapse causing hydroureteronephrosis. Surg. Gynecol. Obstet. *150*:711, 1980.

Hager, H., and Ledermair, O.: Die vaginale Uterusexstirpation nach vorausgegangeneu gynakologischen oder geburtshilflichen Laparotomien. Geburtsh. Frauenheilkd. *39*:98, 1979.

Harrow, B. R.: Renal function after complete bilateral ureteral obstruction following colporrhaphy. Am. J. Surg. *87*:842, 1954.

Higgins, C. C.: Ureteral injuries during surgery. J.A.M.A., *199*:82, 1967.

Irvin, T. T., Goligher, J. C., and Scott, J. S.: Injury to the ureter during laparoscopic tubal sterilization. Arch. Surg. *110*:1501, 1975.

Koide, S. S., and Lyle, K. C.: Unusual signs and symptoms associated with oral contraceptive medication. J. Reprod. Med. *15*:214, 1975.

Laufe, L. E., and Kreutner, A. K.: Vaginal hysterectomy: A modality for therapeutic abortion and sterilization. Am. J. Obstet. Gynecol. *110*:1096, 1971.

Leopold, G. R., and Asher, W. M.: Fundamentals of Abdominal and Pelvic Ultrasonography. Philadelphia, W. B. Saunders Co., 1975.

Lieberthal, F., and Frankenthal, L.: The mechanism of ureteral obstruction in prolapse of the uterus. Surg. Gynecol. Obstet. *73*:828, 1941.

Neutz, E., Silber, A., and Meredino, V. J.: Dalkon shield perforation of the uterus and urinary bladder with calculus formation: case report. Am. J. Obstet. Gynecol. *130*:848, 1978.
Phillips, J., Keith, D., and Keith, L.: Gynecological laparoscopy 1973: The state of the art. *In* Phillips, J. M., and Keith, L.: Gynecological Laparoscopy: Principles and Techniques. New York, Stratton Intercontinental Medical Book Corp., 1974.
Porges, R. F.: Vaginal hysterectomy at Bellevue Hospital. Obstet. Gynecol. *35*:300, 1970.
Pratt, J. H.: Common complications of vaginal hysterectomy: thoughts regarding their prevention and management. Clin. Obstet. Gynecol. *19*:645, 1976.
Pride, G. L., and Shaffer, R. L.: Nonpuerperal uterine inversion. Report of an unusual case. Obstet. Gynecol. *49*:361, 1977.
Ramcharan, S., Pellegrin, F. A., Ray, R. M., et al.: The Walnut Creek contraceptive drug study. J. Reprod. Med. *25*:358, 1980.
Rouse, S. N., Major, F., and Gordon, M.: Rupture of the bladder secondary to uterine vacuum curettage: A case report and review of the literature. J. Urol. *106*:685, 1971.
Rubin, A.: Complications of vaginal operations for pelvic floor relaxation. Am. J. Obstet. Gynecol. *95*:972, 1966.
Saronwala, K. C., Singh, R., and Dass, H.: Lippes Loop perforation of the uterus and urinary bladder with stone formation. Obstet. Gynecol. *44*:424, 1974.
Schapira, M., Dizereus, H., Essinger, A., et al.: Urinary ascites after gynaecological laparoscopy. Lancet *1*:871, 1978.
Solomons, E., Levin, E. J., Bauman, J., et al.: A pyelographic study of ureteric injuries sustained during hysterectomy for benign conditions. Surg. Gynecol. Obstet. *111*:41, 1960.
Sood, S. V.: Some operative and postoperative hazards of legal termination of pregnancy. Br. Med. J. *4*:270, 1971.
St. Martin, E. C., Trichel, B. E., Campbell, J. H., et al.: Ureteral injuries in gynecologic surgery. J. Urol. *70*:51, 1953.
Stengel, J. N., Felderman, E. S., and Zamora, D.: Ureteral injury: complication of laparoscopic sterilization. Urology *4*:341, 1974.
Symmonds, R. E.: Ureteral injuries associated with gynecologic surgery: prevention and management. Clin. Obstet. Gynecol. *19*:623, 1976.
Tasche, L. W.: 1700 vaginal hysterectomies in general practice. Minn. Med. *51*:1705, 1968.
van Nagell, J.R ., Jr., and Roddick, J. W., Jr.: Vaginal hysterectomy as a sterilization procedure. Am. J. Obstet. Gynecol. *111*:703, 1971.
van Nagell, J. R., Jr., and Roddick, J. W., Jr.: Vaginal hysterectomy, the ureter and excretory urography. Obstet. Gynecol. *39*:784, 1972.
Wallingford, A. J.: The changes of the urinary tract associated with prolapse of the uterus. Am. J. Obstet. Gynecol. *38*:489, 1939.

9

MANAGEMENT OF URINARY TRACT INJURIES

J. D. SCHMIDT, M.D.

This chapter will focus mainly on injuries to the ureter. Because of local tissue and renal function changes developing as the interval between injury and clinical recognition increases, ureteral injuries are better discussed according to their time of discovery. The recognition and repair of injuries to the bladder and urethra (whether due to gynecologic or obstetric surgery) are also covered in Chapters 8 and 31.

MANAGEMENT OF URETERAL INJURY

Injuries Discovered at Surgery or Early Postoperatively

The management of ureteral injuries discovered during gynecologic surgery differs from that of injuries detected later. Correction and repair initially can often spare the patient lengthy operative procedures and insure renal function (Hoch et al., 1975). Treatment of ureteral injuries by immediate repair is successful in approximately 80 to 90 per cent of cases (Béland, 1977). In a recent report (Mendez and McGinty, 1978), good results were achieved in only 67 per cent of patients whose ureteral injuries were recognized and thus managed late. The same authors reported 100 per cent good results in their group of patients whose ureteral injuries were recognized and treated early.

Ureteroureterostomy

If the area of ureteral injury is localized (e.g., ligation), the injured segment of ureter should be excised rather than the ligature simply removed. The proximal and distal ends of the normal ureter can be identified and spatulated, and a ureteroureterostomy performed using interrupted 4–0 sutures for watertight closure. Drainage is extraperitoneal. Two centimeters or more of injured ureter can be excised and repaired in this fashion.

Ureteroneocystostomy

When injury occurs in the distal ureter, as is often the case following gynecologic surgery, a ureteroureterostomy may not be technically feasible. The method of choice in these cases is ureteral reimplantation into the urinary bladder (ureteroneocystostomy) (Schmidt, 1979). The diseased ureter can be excised or simply bypassed by ligation, and the proximal ureter implanted into the bladder.

Technical considerations in ureteroneocystostomy include the choice of ureterovesical anastomosis, i.e., either refluxing or antirefluxing. In general, the antireflux submucosal tunnel technique should be utilized; this is technically easy in a normal-sized ureter. A ratio of 2:1 or 3:1 (submucosa tunnel length to the width of the ureter) should be used. The anastomosis between the spatulated ureter and the bladder mucosa should be made with 4–0 chromic catgut sutures.

In cases where the ureter cannot reach the bladder without tension, the bladder can be mobilized toward the ureter and the adjacent bladder wall sutured to the iliopsoas muscle ("psoas hitch") (Ehrlich et al., 1978) (Figure 9–1). Another alternative in the presence of a normal or large capacity bladder is the Boari-Ockerblad technique, which raises a flap or pedicle of anterior bladder wall (Ockerblad, 1947). The bladder tube is generally long enough to reach the ureter; the ureter can be anastomosed directly to this tube, either in a refluxing or antireflux manner. Such ureteral anastomoses are usually stented with a No. 5 or No. 8 French polyethylene feeding tube for a period of 5 to 7 days. The urinary bladder is closed with absorbable suture material and is drained with either a urethral or suprapubic catheter; the ureterovesical anastomosis is drained extraperitoneally.

Transureteroureterostomy

Transureteroureterostomy effectively bypasses the injured area and is suitable when the ureter proximal to the area of injury cannot readily reach the urinary bladder (Smith, 1969). The anastomosis of one side of the urinary tract to its contralateral mate is not new, but until recently has not been widely used. Its advantages include the avoidance of use of segments of intestine to assist in the diversion (Schmidt et al., 1972).

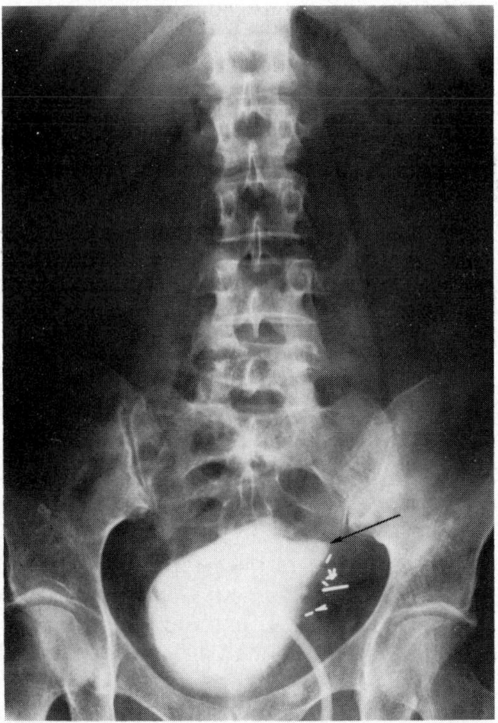

Figure 9–1. Cystogram following anti-refluxing left ureteral reimplantation and "psoas hitch" maneuver as definitive repair of posthysterectomy left ureteral obstruction. No ureteral reflux is seen. Arrow indicates bladder sutured to psoas muscle.

The simplest form of transureteroureterostomy involves the mobilization of one ureter at or above the level of the sacral promontory in a retroperitoneal tunnel, where it is anastomosed end-to-side to the contralateral ureter (Figure 9–2). A watertight anastomosis, using continuous or interrupted 4–0 chromic catgut suture material, is constructed with extraperitoneal drainage. Ureteral stenting is optional. The recipient ureter is mobilized only enough to allow exposure of a surface for the anastomosis. The distal segment of the recipient ureter continues to the urinary bladder. This type of ureteroureterostomy is best accomplished when one or both ureters are somewhat dilated and have an increased blood supply. It is particularly suitable for treatment of unilateral obstruction, fistula or reflux when the opposite ureterovesical junction is normal.

Although complications at transureteroureterostomy are uncommon, Ehrlich and Skinner (1975) have reported five cases requiring further surgery. Poor blood supply and anastomotic tension were responsible for the failures. On occasion, a dilated distal recipient ureter may be of sufficient length and have adequate blood supply to be brought to the skin of the abdomen or flank as a cutaneous ureterostomy (see Figure 9–2). An important technical consideration is the excision of a full-thickness core of abdominal wall to prevent skin or fascial obstruction (baffle effect) by abdominal wall musculature. The ureters can be stented via the skin ureterostomy. This technique can be used only when there is sufficient terminal ureter on either side to bring to the skin level. If the patient has had pelvic irradiation, the dangers of using ischemic ureter with attendant poor healing are magnified. In addition, neither ureter may be sufficiently dilated for safe stomal formation at the skin level. Lastly the late complications of stomal stenosis will result in bilateral ureteral obstruction and renal failure.

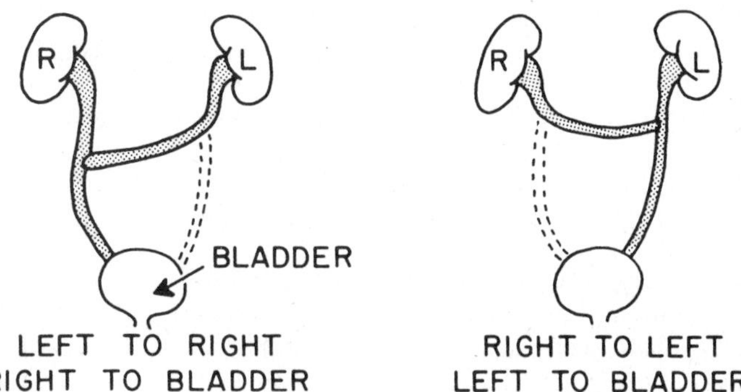

Figure 9–2. Variations of transureteroureterostomy.

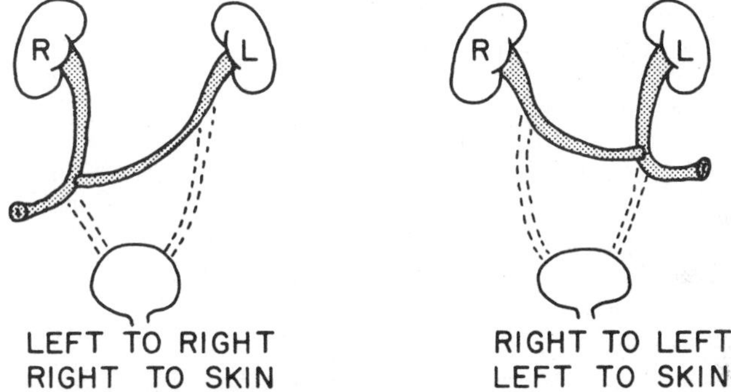

If a fistula is present in the recipient ureter, treatment with an indwelling catheter may be sufficient for closure of the fistula, as shown in the following case.

E. H., a 57-year-old woman, developed a left ureterovaginal fistula and right ureteral perforation several days following radical hysterectomy for cervical cancer. Postoperatively she was treated by bilateral ureteral catheters, but the urinary extravasation persisted after 10 days. The patient was re-operated, and a left-to-right transureteroureterostomy was performed, along with drainage of the right ureteral injury and continued ureteral stenting for 14 days. Recovery was then uneventful.

Delayed Treatment of Ureteral Injury

Nephrostomy and Diversion

Immediate drainage of the obstructed kidney should be performed when recognition of ureteral injury and obstruction has been delayed. Nephrostomy can be carried out by one of several methods.

Standard Tube Nephrostomy. Standard tube nephrostomy is best performed on a kidney obstructed to a moderate or marked degree. A flank extraperitoneal exposure is made and the dilated proximal ureter or renal pelvis entered sharply. Using a curved instrument directed into the intrarenal collecting system and out the parenchyma over a midline or inferior calyx, a large caliber 4-wing Malecot or Foley retention catheter is drawn into the kidney. The opening in the ureter or pelvis is left open or loosely sutured and the wound drained.

In the case of a kidney with marked obstruction and considerable thinning of the parenchyma over the distended calyces, dissection of the pelvis or ureter may be eliminated and a stab incision made directly into the dilated inferior or middle calyx via the parenchyma. The drainage tube is inserted into the collecting system and brought out through either the incision or a stab wound, and the flank wound is closed in layers with drainage.

Silastic Loop or Circle Nephrostomy. For patients who require long-term or permanent nephrostomy drainage, a loop nephrostomy is most appropriate (Hawtrey et al., 1974). In this procedure a length of

Silastic tubing (No. 12, 16, or 22 French) with precut holes for urinary drainage is brought through two portions of the upper urinary tract and then out the flank. Modifications include (1) both entry and exit points through the renal parenchyma, (2) entry through the renal parenchyma and exit out an opening in the renal pelvis or ureter, and (3) entry through the renal parenchyma and exit through the ureteral lumen to the skin as an intubated cutaneous ureterostomy. Such tubes are commercially available and have the advantage of being nonreactive and easy to change without the need for x-ray or fluoroscopic control. Accidental displacement or extrusion from the urinary tract is rare with such a tube.

Percutaneous Nephrostomy. The percutaneous insertion of a small Teflon catheter under fluoroscopic control into the dilated collecting system can produce immediate and effective urinary drainage (Ho et al., 1980). With the help of a urologist or radiologist skilled in this technique, a No. 5 French catheter is inserted across the renal parenchyma under local anesthesia. The effects of ureteral obstruction can then be allowed to resolve. Definitive reparative surgery of the ureteral injury can be scheduled when the patient is in optimal condition. The percutaneous nephrostomy tube, like the other nephrostomy tubes, can be left in place following the definitive ureteral repair as a "safety valve." The tube can be removed later when the repair has healed and ureteral transport is normal (Figures 9–3*A* and *B*).

An exciting aspect of percutaneous nephrostomy is the extension of the technique to the antegrade insertion of ureteral stents (Lang et al., 1979). Because of extra side holes, a ureteral stent so inserted drains the affected urinary tract and may even be passed through and beyond the area of injury. The stent can remain externalized and attached to straight drainage or be converted to an internalized drainage system using the double-J (double pigtail)

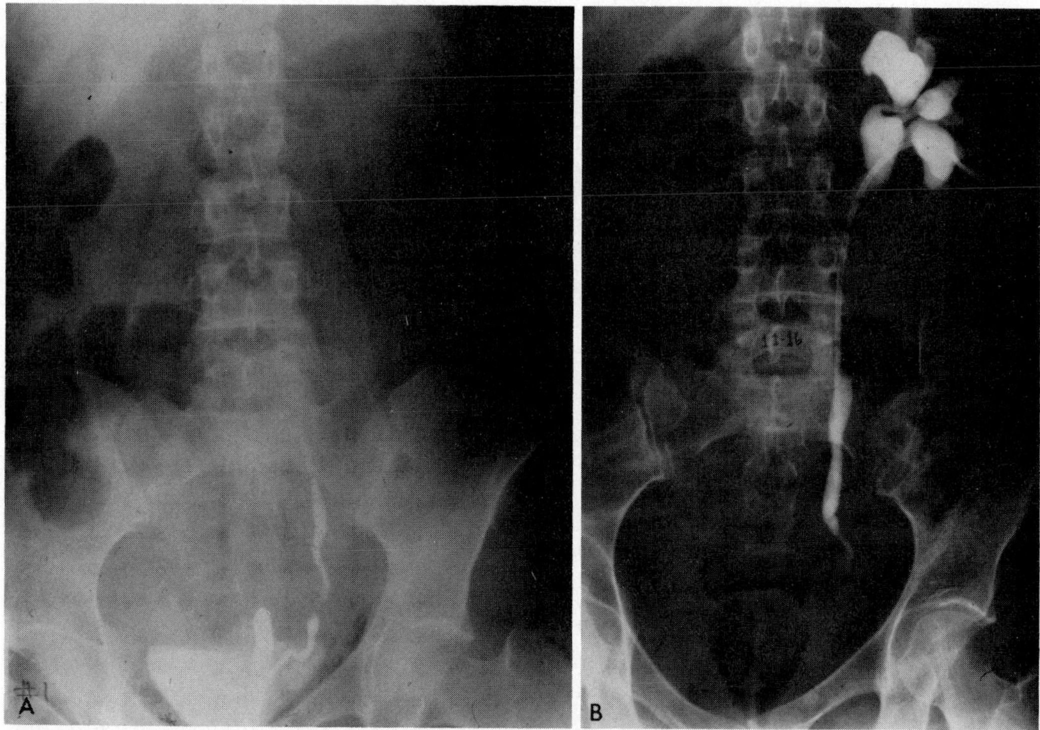

Figure 9–3. *A*, Left retrograde ureterogram reveals significant distal ureteral narrowing in this 35-year-old woman who developed left flank pain and fever following hysterectomy and left salpingo-oophorectomy for endometriosis.

B, Left percutaneous nephrostomy catheter is passed into dilated proximal ureter; antegrade contrast injection demonstrates site of postoperative obstruction.

stent (Camacho et al., 1979; Ho et al., 1980). When this maneuver is completed, the proximal end of the stent is in the renal pelvis and the distal end is in the urinary bladder (Figure 9–4). Definitive repair of the injury can be planned electively when renal function returns to normal and the patient has recovered from the initial procedure.

Bilateral Nephrostomies. Bilateral nephrostomies require the patient to wear two drainage tubes and their attached systems, and are generally undesirable. Any of the already mentioned nephrostomy procedures can be combined with transureteroureterostomy or transpyelopyelostomy. In these situations, a retroperitoneal anastomosis of the two dilated collecting systems avoids manipulation of the bowel and obviates the need for more than one external appliance or drainage tube. Also, at the time of nephrostomy, the proximal ureter can be intentionally ligated should there be a distal fistula present that would otherwise persist and drain urine.

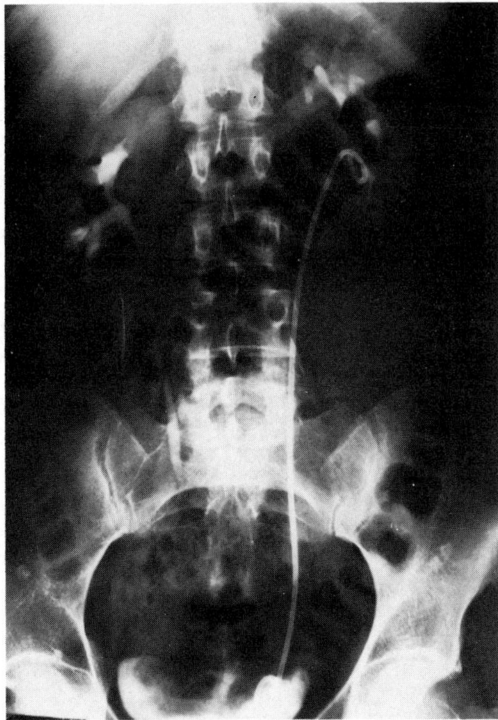

Figure 9–4. Percutaneous nephrostomy catheter in same patient as in Figure 9–3 has been exchanged percutaneously for internalized double-J (double pigtail) ureteral stent. Excretory urogram reveals resolution of left hydronephrosis.

Definitive Repair

The second stage in the management of late-recognized ureteral injury can take place weeks to months following preliminary nephrostomy and diversion. The options available for repair are identical to those mentioned, including resection of the injured area with ureteroureterostomy, ureteral reimplantation into the urinary bladder, and transureteroureterostomy. Ureteral stents may be used as an option since the previously placed nephrostomy catheter will act as a safety valve following the repair. In fact, the presence of the nephrostomy tube is helpful in monitoring the response of the patient to the repair.

For example, an antegrade pyelogram or nephrostogram can be obtained at some convenient time following the primary repair to demonstrate ureteral transport and the presence or absence of persistent urinary leakage. If the antegrade study shows good transport across the repaired ureter without extravasation, the next step is simply clamping the nephrostomy tube for one or more days. The patient is observed for signs of recurrent ureteral obstruction such as fever, chills, and flank pain. Should this happen, the nephrostomy tube is reopened and allowed to drain. If the patient does well, the nephrostomy tube can safely be removed, and in the absence of distal obstruction, the nephrostomy tract should seal within 24 to 48 hours.

Use of Intestinal Segments. Another method of bypassing an injured ureteral segment is the use of an isolated loop of small bowel (Goodwin et al., 1959; Irvin et al., 1975; Morales et al., 1959; Perry et al., 1975). As in the performance of the standard ileal conduit operation (Chapter 11), a segment of terminal ileum of suitable length is isolated and sutured proximally to the renal pelvis or proximal ureter and distally to the distal ureter or to the bladder. The disadvantages of an ileovesical anastomosis are (1) free reflux of urine, which may reach the kidney, causing subsequent damage and infection, (2) potential urine absorption across the small bowel mucosa with resultant renal damage (Krupp et al., 1970) and (3) excessive ileal mucus secretion.

Bilateral Ureteral Injury

If a well-hydrated, normotensive patient is anuric postoperatively, the patency of the urethral-bladder catheter must first be checked. Wesolowski (1969) found 25 cases of bilateral ureteral injury reported in the literature between 1949 and 1969. The majority of cases followed radical hysterectomy for cervical carcinoma, but this complication also occurred in six patients undergoing hysterectomy for benign disease.

The early management of bilateral ureteral injury may combine the placement of at least one nephrostomy tube with repair of ureteral injury, using either ureteroureterostomy, ureteral reimplantations, or transureteroureterostomy. One side may be bypassed using the transureteroureterostomy, with the contralateral injury repaired by ureteral reimplantation and stenting. Nephrostomy drainage can be added as a "safety valve." Should the bilateral ureteral injuries be severe and the urinary bladder be of small capacity or otherwise diseased, primary supravesical diversion, such as creation of an ileal conduit, with or without preliminary or concomitant nephrostomy drainage, is the procedure of choice.

Autotransplantation

Current techniques for kidney perfusion make autotransplantation a suitable alternative in repair of high ureteral injuries. In this procedure the kidney is removed after careful dissection of the renal pedicle to keep the ureteral blood supply intact. The kidney is positioned in the ipsilateral or opposite iliac fossa, with the renal artery sutured to the hypogastric artery, the renal vein sutured to the external iliac vein, and the ureter reimplanted into the urinary bladder. However, the technique should not be employed in poor-risk patients with good function of the contralateral kidney or if standard methods of repair of the injury are possible (Stewart et al., 1976).

Nephrectomy

Removal of the ipsilateral kidney obviously results in cure of a ureteral obstruction or fistula. In the older, debilitated patient, nephrectomy may be the most prudent method of treatment. It should otherwise be reserved for those situations in which prior procedures to conserve renal function and urinary transport have failed. Of historical note is the fact that the first planned nephrectomy was performed for a ureterovaginal fistula.

Ureteral Catheters

Ureteral catheters have a place in the management of patients with ureteral injuries and obstruction. A ureteral catheter can be passed retrograde through the area of injury to drain the obstructed proximal segment. This allows renal function to return to normal, drains the area of infection, and buys time to allow definitive surgical repair. Ureteral catheters can be left in place for 1 to 2 weeks, allowing some injuries to heal spontaneously.

For the poor-risk patient, the passage of a ureteral catheter may be the first step in successive dilatations of the ureter, allowing later passage of one of the newer ureteral stents. Either the Gibbons Silastic ureteral stent (Gibbons et al., 1976) or the double-J (double pigtail) ureteral stent can be left in place for several weeks to months (Figure 9–5). These relatively nonreactive foreign bodies drain the obstructed kidney and allow for spontaneous healing in the area of injury. These ureteral stents can easily be removed and, if necessary, reinserted cystoscopically. Their insertion does not preclude definitive surgical management of any continuing obstruction. Of technical interest, these ureteral stents can also be inserted at surgery via the open bladder or upper urinary tract.

Pyelostomy

Standard tube pyelostomy is a fast and simple technique, requiring only the insertion of a large-caliber Foley catheter through the dilated renal pelvis into the kidney, where it is sutured in place (Ihse et al., 1975). However, the speed and simplicity of this procedure are more than offset by its temporary nature; such a tube usually becomes dislodged fairly readily and cannot easily be replaced. This form of upper

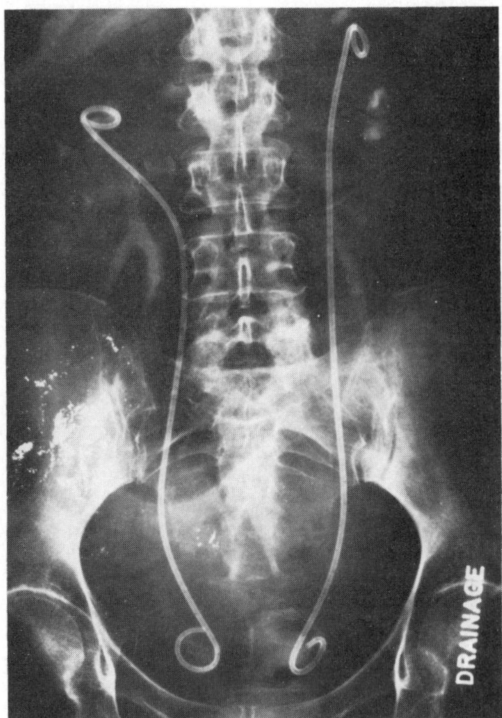

Figure 9–5. Postdrainage film of retrograde cystogram demonstrates bilateral double-J (double pigtail) ureteral stents in good position. Stents were inserted cystoscopically in a 57-year-old woman who developed bilateral ureteral obstruction following radical hysterectomy. Reflux up the stents explains presence of contrast medium in the kidneys. Residual barium from a prior study is also present.

tract diversion should be considered only a "safety valve" procedure at best.

Ureterostomy

End cutaneous ureterostomy is one of the simplest and quickest forms of supravesical urinary diversion, particularly in a patient with only a single functioning kidney (Straffon et al., 1969). This method, in which the ureter is brought directly to the skin, is the procedure of choice when the involved ureter is markedly dilated with an increased blood supply due to chronic obstruction. The dissection of such a ureter should be kept well away from the adventitia, which contains all of the nutrient vessels necessary to keep the ureter viable. This procedure should not be performed if the ureter has been irradiated or if the ureter is fairly normal in caliber. The ideal dilated, well-vascularized ureter may require temporary intubation but usually functions well thereafter with only an external appliance.

Ureterostomy In Situ

A less common temporary diversion for the obstructed ureter is the technique of ureterostomy in situ. An extraperitoneal (often muscle-splitting) approach to the dilated proximal ureter is made. The ureter is opened sufficiently to allow passage of a catheter into the renal pelvis. This catheter exits the loosely closed ureterostomy and then is brought through the abdominal wall via a separate stab incision. The catheter used must be of a caliber large enough to drain well and of a length sufficient to be attached to a bedside drainage receptacle. Since ureterostomy in situ catheters cannot be changed easily, they are best utilized either in the terminally ill patient or when definitive repair can be performed at a reasonably early date.

MANAGEMENT OF BLADDER INJURY

Most injuries to the urinary bladder will be recognized intraoperatively and thus be repaired immediately. Principles of repair include (1) debridement of any injured tissue, (2) bladder wall closure utilizing absorbable suture material, and (3) adequate bladder drainage. The latter aspect can be effected by either an indwelling Foley urethral catheter or a suprapubic cystostomy brought out via a separate stab wound in the bladder and abdominal walls.

Small bladder perforations can be closed by an inner layer of interrupted 2–0 or 0 chromic suture reinforced by an outer layer of continuous suture. The mucosa itself need not be included in the closure. Not only will this avoid the formation of bladder calculi, but mucosal regeneration is rapid, provided that the musculature has been carefully reapproximated.

For larger bladder injuries, I prefer a purse-string type of closure. A single 0 chromic continuous suture is placed in the bladder muscle (avoiding mucosa) surrounding the perforation. The defect is closed simply by tightening and then tying the purse-string. Several Lembert-type sutures of 0 or 2–0 chromic gut are used to reinforce the area. Extraperitoneal drainage is provided for at least 5 days.

Bladder drainage should be maintained for at least 5 days, and up to 10 to 14 days in the case of larger injuries. A gravity cystogram should be performed to demonstrate normal bladder integrity before a trial of voiding.

If the intramural ureter or ureteral orifice is injured, as well as the bladder wall, ureteral reimplantation is required.

SUMMARY

The management of urinary tract injuries following gynecologic surgery begins with a systematic evaluation to establish site of injury. Treatment depends on time elapsed since injury, status of the urinary tract, and the patient's general condition. Ureteral injuries may require immediate upper tract diversion. Definitive repair can be delayed until acute reactions have subsided and the patient is in optimal condition.

REFERENCES

Béland, G.: Early treatment of ureteral injuries found after gynecological surgery. J. Urol. *118*:25, 1977.

Camacho, M. F., Pereiras, P., Carrion, K., et al.: Double-ended pigtail ureteral stent: useful modification to single-end ureteral stent. Urology *13*:516, 1979.

Ehrlich, R. M., Melman, A., and Skinner, D. G.: The use of vesicopsoas hitch in urologic surgery. J. Urol. *119*:322, 1978.

Ehrlich, R. M., and Skinner, D. G.: Complications of transureteroureterostomy. J. Urol. *113*:467, 1975.

Gibbons, R. P., Correa, R. J., Jr., Cummings, K. B., et al.: Experience with indwelling ureteral stent catheters. J. Urol. *115*:22, 1976.

Goodwin, W. E., Winter, C. C., and Turner, R. D.: Replacement of the ureter by small intestine: clinical application and results of the ileal ureter. J. Urol. *81*:406, 1959.

Hawtrey, C. E., Boatman, D. L., Brown, R. G., et al.: Clinical experience with loop nephrostomy for urinary diversion. J. Urol. *112*:36, 1974.

Ho, P. C., Talner, L. B., Parsons, C. L., et al.: Percutaneous nephrostomy: experience in 107 kidneys. Urology *16*:532, 1980.

Hoch, W. H., Kursh, E. D., and Persky, L.: Early aggressive management of intraoperative ureteral injuries. J. Urol. *114*:530, 1975.

Ihse, I., Arness, O. B., and Jonsson, G.: Surgical injuries of the ureter. A review of 42 cases. Scand. J. Urol. Nephrol. *9*:39, 1975.

Irvin, T. T., Goligher, J. C., and Scott, J. S.: Injury to the ureter during laparoscopic tubal sterilization. Arch. Surg. *110*:1501, 1975.

Krupp, P., Hoffman, M., and Roeling, W.: Terminal ileum as ureteral substitute. Obstet. Gynecol. *35*:416, 1970.

Lang, E. K., Lanasa, J. A., Garrett, J., et al.: The management of urinary fistulas and strictures with percutaneous ureteral stent catheters. J. Urol. *122*:736, 1979.

Mendez, R., and McGinty, D. M.: The management of ureteral injuries. J. Urol. *119*:192, 1978.

Morales, P., Askari, S., and Hotchkiss, R. S.: Ileal replacement of the ureter. J. Urol. *82*:304, 1959.

Ockerblad, N. F.: Reimplantation of the ureter into the bladder by a flap method. J. Urol. *57*:845, 1947.

Perry, C. P., Massey, F. M., Moore, T. N., et al.: Treatment of irradiation injury to the ureter by ileal substitution. Obstet. Gynecol. *46*:517, 1975.

Schmidt, E.: Ureterocystoneostomy using the Politano-Leadbetter procedure in adults. Helv. Chir. Acta *46*:373, 1979.

Schmidt, J. D., Flocks, R. H., and Arduino, L.: Transureteroureterostomy in the management of distal ureteral disease. J. Urol. *108*:240, 1972.

Smith, I.: Trans-uretero-ureterostomy. Br. J. Urol. *41*:14, 1969.

Stewart, B. H., Hewitt, C. B., and Banowsky, L. H. W.: Management of extensively destroyed ureter: special reference to renal autotransplantation. J. Urol. *115*:257, 1976.

Straffon, R. A., Kyle, K., and Corvalan, J.: Techniques of cutaneous ureterostomy and results in 51 patients. Trans. Am. Assoc. Genitourin. Surg. *61*:130, 1969.

Wesolowski, S.: Bilateral ureteral injuries in gynaecology. Br. J. Urol. *41*:666, 1969.

10

THE URINARY TRACT AND RADICAL HYSTERECTOMY

H. J. BUCHSBAUM, M.D.

There is a natural tendency to limit the dissection to avoid ureteral damage. This is in error, for the most important complication following a radical pelvic dissection is recurrence.

L. Parsons (1975)

The lower ureters and bladder are at considerable risk from carcinoma of the cervix. At its primary site, in its local spread, and in the regional lymph nodes, cervical carcinoma can involve the lower urinary tract. It is not surprising, therefore, that these structures are also placed at risk in radical hysterectomy, the appropriate surgical treatment for early invasive cervical cancer.

HISTORICAL REVIEW

Freund first performed an abdominal hysterectomy for cervical carcinoma in 1878. He did not isolate or dissect the ureters. Later, Clark identified the ureters during the operative procedure in order to remove more of the paracervical tissue. Wertheim in 1898 first reported the extensive dissection of both ureters to facilitate the wide removal of paracervical and parametrial tissue. Clark later suggested resection of the distal ureters (with ureteroneocystotomy) to reduce the incidence of fistulas and to achieve a wider lateral margin of resection.

Radiation therapy was applied to the treatment of cervical carcinoma in the early years of the twentieth century. Rapid improvements in x-ray equipment, the clinical use of radium, and uniformity of dosimetry far outstripped advances in the surgical areas, so that by the late 1920s radiation therapy had practically replaced surgery in the treatment of cervical cancer. A few surgeons such as Taussig, Bonney, and Meigs continued to perform radical abdominal hysterectomy and to perfect the procedure. Their fistula rate was little changed from that of Wertheim.

The urologic problems that face the surgeon today performing radical pelvic dissection differ only slightly from those that faced the pioneer surgeons. Surgery is now performed in earlier stages of cervical carcinoma, generally limited to patients with Stage Ib and IIa lesions. Radical hysterectomy requires considerable dissection of the ureters to allow removal of all the connective tissue between the cervix and lateral pelvic wall; mobilization of the bladder is also necessary to allow removal of the upper vagina to ensure an adequate margin of resection. Radical hysterectomy, therefore, places the ureters and bladder at considerable risk.

The past two decades have seen renewed interest in the surgical treatment of cervical carcinoma. Specifically, surgeons have addressed themselves to the urinary tract problems that follow radical hysterectomy. While intraoperative injury of the urinary tract is rare, urinary problems continue to be the most significant complications following radical hysterectomy. These postoperative complications include ureteral fistulas and stricture, vesicovaginal fistulas, and bladder dysfunction.

PREOPERATIVE EVALUATION

The prevention of urinary tract problems begins with the preoperative evaluation. All patients undergoing radical hysterectomy should have urographic and cystoscopic studies performed as part of a tumor survey. These studies can identify anomalies and pathologic processes that can affect the lower urinary tract. Wertheim (1912), without benefit of pyelography, found double ureters in 4 of 500 surgical cases. Parsons (1970) estimated that 1 in 25 patients who have preoperative pyelography will have a double ureter.

Preoperative intravenous pyelography is a routine part of the staging survey for patients with cervical carcinoma. In 80 consecutive patients undergoing radical hysterectomy, we found renal and ureteral anomalies in six (7.5 per cent). The anomalies ranged from double ureters in two patients to surgically less important findings such as bifid renal pelvis and fetal lobulation of the kidney in the others.

The preoperative placement of ureteral catheters in patients scheduled for radical hysterectomy has been advocated by some authors. We have never used ureteral catheters, and along with most surgeons who perform radical pelvic operations, we condemn their use. Catheters traumatize the urothelium, distort the anatomy, and by tenting the ureter may make it more susceptible to injury. The ureter is rarely injured during surgical dissection, and a knowledge of its location and course through the pelvis is a far better guarantee of its safety than are indwelling ureteral catheters. Ureteral dissection accompanying radical hysterectomy should not be performed by the occasional surgeon. The experienced surgeon, familiar with the route of the ureter, has no need for the potentially dangerous catheters.

INTRAOPERATIVE MANAGEMENT

Prevention of Ureteral Fistula

The ureter is the only vital structure between the lateral aspect of the cervix and the lateral pelvic wall. Cervical carcinoma spreads along the tissue planes laterally. The ureteral or parametrial lymph node, when present, is the first of the regional lymph nodes involved. In order to remove the paracervical tissue and ensure an adequate margin of resection, the ureters must be mobilized to some degree. Wertheim as early as 1912 identified the operative and postoperative conditions that contribute to fistula formation: trauma and infection.

The early pelvic surgeons dealing with cervical carcinoma recognized the risk of postoperative urinary tract complications, particularly ureterovaginal fistulas. Reviewing the experience at Kelly's clinic for the years 1889 to 1902, Sampson (1902) reported that 19 of 32 ureteral injuries occurred in patients undergoing surgical treatment of cervical carcinoma. The reported fistula rate in the last 75 years has varied from under 1 per cent to as high as 30 per cent. Recent series of 92 (Underwood et al., 1979) and 130 (Sall et al., 1979) radical hysterectomies reported no ureteral fistulas.

The experience of the surgeon is perhaps the most important factor related to the development of postoperative urinary tract fistulas. A number of other factors have been identified which contribute to fistula formation. Brunschwig and Frick (1956), Calame and Nelson (1967), and Mack (1969) found the fistula rate directly related to the stage of disease. The fistula rate was doubled when cervical carcinoma extended beyond the cervix from approximately 10 per cent in Stage I to 20 per cent in Stage II.

Most authorities believe that prior radiation therapy, with its compromise of small blood vessels, increases the incidence of fistulas (Mack, 1969; Mickal et al., 1972; Lang et al., 1973; Green, 1975; Mikuta et al., 1977; Underwood et al., 1979; Benedet et al., 1980). Talbert and co-workers (1965) reported that radiation therapy prior to surgery had no influence on fistula formation. Webb and Symmonds (1979) examined the influence of radiation therapy on the development of ureteral fistula following 610 radical hysterectomies performed for a variety of genital malignancies. Nearly one quarter of the patients (23.6 per cent) had some prior radiation therapy. The overall ureteral fistula rate was 2.5 per cent — 6.4 per cent in patients with radiation therapy, and only 1.4 per cent in the nonirradiated group.

The role of preoperative radiation therapy in the development of ureteral fistula is dependent on a variety of features, including the type of radiation therapy and the intraoperative and postoperative management of the ureter. The presence of pelvic inflammatory disease, endometriosis, bowel diverticulosis, recent conization, or prior supracervical hysterectomy makes ureteral dissection more hazardous and is associated with an increased fistula rate. A less obvious factor, the patient's socioeconomic status, which may reflect her nutritional and immunologic state, may play a role in fistula formation.

URETERAL BLOOD SUPPLY

During mobilization and dissection of the ureter, its external nutrient vessels are compromised. The distal one third of the ureter receives a variable number of branches from the hypogastric artery and its branches. The superior and inferior vesical, the superior and inferior gluteal, the uterine, and the obturator arteries all contribute nutrient vessels to the ureter. It has been estimated that the vesical arteries provide almost half of the total number of vessels to the ureter (McCormack and Anson, 1950). Varverikos (1952) found that, in one third of women, the sole blood supply to the ureter within the pelvis came from branches from the uterine artery as it crosses the ureter. The ureteral vessels from the hypogastric artery and its branches seldom divide before they reach the ureter. When they reach the ureter, they bifurcate and send branches superiorly and inferiorly. The small branches form a plexus on the ureter, lie in close association with the adventitia, and run parallel to the long axis of the ureter. Compromise of this vascular plexus of the ureter in the course of dissection leads to ischemia and ultimately necrosis.

Sampson in 1904 and more recently Masterson (1957) have shown experimentally that the external vessels to the lower ureter can be ligated without compromising the integrity of the ureter, so long as the adventitial plexus is undisturbed. Circular denudation should be avoided in the course of dissection. It is our practice to mobilize the ureter with sharp and blunt dissection, leaving it attached by a "mesentery" to the posterior and later lateral leaf of the peritoneum. The ureter is never handled with instruments or retracted with drains or umbilical tape. Absorbable sutures should be used on pedicles that lie in proximity to the ureters, and mass ligatures near the ureter should be avoided since they may obstruct or kink it.

SURGICAL TECHNIQUES

Specific intraoperative maneuvers have been described in order to reduce the incidence of ureteral fistula and obstruction. Burch and co-workers (1965) suggested ligating the uterine artery medial to the ureter, as is done during the radical vaginal operation. This maneuver maintains the uterine artery branches to the ureter. Utilizing this technique Burch and associates (1965) have reported a significant reduction in the number of fistulas (Table 10–1).

Novak (1956) does not divide the uterine artery until the dissection is nearly complete. This allows the small branches from the uterine artery to the ureter to be maintained in spite of the surgical manipulation. At the completion of the procedure Novak places the ureter, from the level of the common iliac artery caudad, in the peritoneal cavity. He feels this diminishes kinking and obstruction of flow. Furthermore, the ureter is left in a cleaner environment. Utilizing this technique Novak (1969) has been able to reduce the number of fistulas in patients operated on in his clinic (see

TABLE 10–1. FISTULA RATE RELATED TO CHANGE IN INTRAOPERATIVE MANAGEMENT OF THE URETERS

Author	Years of Study	Number of Cases	Fistula Rate (Per Cent)
Burch et al. (1965)	1957	56	8.8
	1965	144	1.4
Novak (1969)	1920–1946	372	9.4
	1947–1953	246	11.4
	1954–1968	1,306	2.1
Green (1975)	1962–1966	286	5.6
	1966–1975	225	0.9

Table 10–1). Others (Werner and Sederl, 1975; Lash, 1973) suspend the ureter from the lateral pelvic wall and use a pedicle of omentum to cover the exposed ureter. Bonney (1935), Meigs (1954), and Symmonds and Pratt (1961) simply extraperitonealize the ureters, closing the pelvic peritoneum.

Ureteral Suspension

After the surgical dissection is complete and the uterus and paracervical tissues removed, the ureter dips into the hollow of the pelvis (Figure 10–1). There it lies in a pool of blood, lymph, and exudate in direct communication with the contaminated vagina. Green (1966) described a technique for suspending the ureter from the superior vesical artery (anterior division of the hypogastric artery) by fine chromic catgut sutures. Several sutures of 5–0 chromic catgut are passed through the ureteral adventitia and the wall of the vessel between the ureterovesical junction and the origin of the superior vesical artery (Figure 10–2). This maneuver allows the ureter to assume a more gently curving course similar to its normal one. This more normal anatomic position favors the return of physiologic function, keeps the ureter out of the hollow of the pelvis where exudate and lymph collect, and allows for earlier and better application of the ureter to the pelvic sidewall, where it can obtain additional blood supply. Unfortunately, the superior vesical artery may have to be excised during the procedure, or it may be injured, necessitating ligation. Utilizing this technique Green has been able to dramatically reduce fistula formation (see Table 10–1). Macasaet and

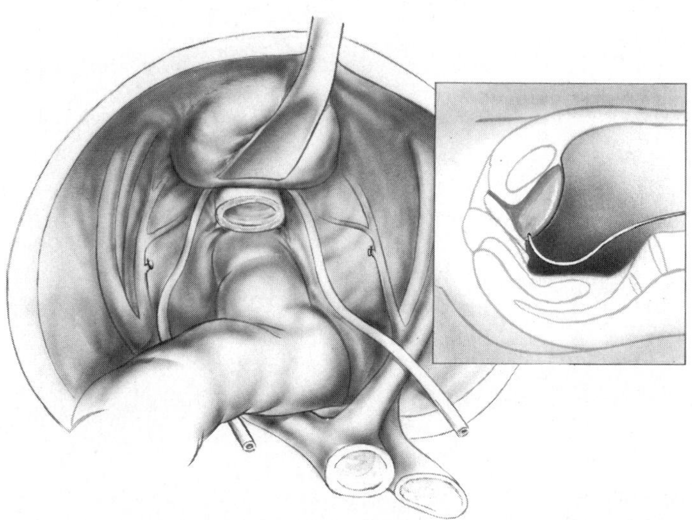

Figure 10–1. Appearance of pelvis after completion of radical hysterectomy and pelvic lymphadenectomy. Note ureters dip into hollow of pelvis. Inset: Sagittal section showing position of ureter.

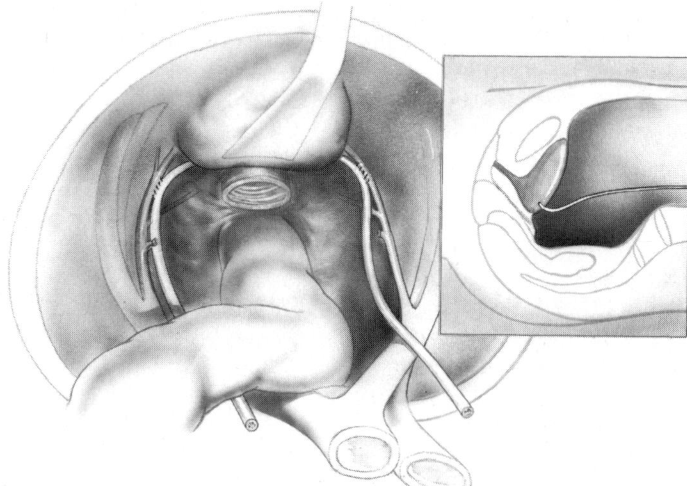

Figure 10–2. Ureteral suspension (Green) from anterior branch of hypogastric artery after completion of surgery. Inset: Sagittal section showing elevation of ureter achieved by this technique.

co-workers (1976) report great success in reducing the incidence of ureteral fistulas with this method.

Ohkawa Technique

In 1971 we became aware of a surgical technique devised by Dr. Ohkawa of the Nippon Medical School (1970). Following completion of the procedure, the ureters are placed in a peritoneal envelope. The rationale behind this technique is as follows: The ureters are elevated and removed from the potentially infected retroperitoneal space and can develop a new blood supply from the peritoneum. Ohkawa (1970) reported ureteral fistulas in 1.1 per cent of 375 patients undergoing radical hysterectomy in which the ureter was managed in this fashion. One drawback to this method of developing a peritoneal envelope for the ureters is that it is time-consuming, adding as much as 45 minutes to the operative procedure. In addition, there may not be enough peritoneum to complete the envelope on both sides.

Present Series

We used Green's method of ureteral suspension, the Ohkawa technique, and simple retroperitoneal placement in the intraoperative management of the ureter in 80 consecutive radical hysterectomies. The majority of the procedures were performed by post-residency gynecologic oncology fellows under the supervision of the author. In 1970 and 1971 the Green technique was used, from late 1971 to 1975 the Ohkawa technique was utilized, and most recently the ureters have simply been placed in the retroperitoneal space.

The histology and stage of cervical neoplasia in these 80 patients are described in Table 10–2. The patients have been followed from 3 to 11 years and three were lost to follow-up. Three patients died of persistent or recurrent disease at 8, 9, and 12 months following surgery. One patient died in an auto accident 2½ years after surgery without evidence of recurrence, after having had a normal postoperative intravenous pyelogram at 3 months.

Ureteral fistulas developed in 3.7 per cent or three of the 80 patients. As will be seen later the incidence of fistula formation varies greatly with the surgical management of the ureter. In assessing results of ureteral management in this series, we will

TABLE 10–2. INDICATIONS FOR RADICAL HYSTERECTOMY

		Number of Patients
Cervical carcinoma		79
Stage Ib	76	
Stage IIa	3	
Sarcoma botryoides		1
Total		80

be examining each ureter and kidney as a separate unit, since in some patients the right and left ureters were managed differently. In two patients, the type of management could not be ascertained from the operative note, leaving 156 units for evaluation.

Ureteral Suspension (Green). Nine patients had bilateral suspension of the ureters from the superior vesical artery and four had unilateral suspension for a total of 22 units. There were *no* fistulas and *no* cases of ureteral obstruction in these 22 units.

Reperitonealization. As noted earlier, the ureters are left in the extraperitoneal space, and the pelvic peritoneum is closed with a continuous chromic catgut suture. The retroperitoneal space is drained with suction catheters. This method of management was used on a total of 39 units, bilaterally in 16 patients and unilaterally in seven. *No* patient in this group developed a fistula or an obstruction.

Ohkawa Technique. Forty-four patients had bilateral Ohkawa peritoneal envelopes developed, while seven had the procedure performed on one side for a total of 95 units. Three ureteral fistulas developed in the 95 units managed with the Ohkawa technique. All were ureterocutaneous fistulas and developed in patients who had retroperitoneal sump drains brought out through the abdominal wall. Seven ureters became blocked postoperatively; five required surgical intervention (see later discussion).

POSTOPERATIVE MANAGEMENT

Changes or modifications in surgical technique do not take place in a vacuum, and it is often impossible to assign proportional credit to innovations. The lowered fistula rate resulting from modifications in the intraoperative management of the ureter occurred during a time that saw the introduction of prophylactic antibiotics, prolonged bladder drainage, and suction drainage of the retroperitoneal space. Green (1975), for instance, was able to reduce urinary fistulas following radical hysterectomy from 11 to 5.6 per cent by prolonged postoperative bladder drainage. With the intraoperative suspension of the ureters he was able to further reduce the fistula rate from 5.6 to 0.9 per cent.

A modification of the prolonged bladder catheterization has been the use of suprapubic bladder drainage. The advantages over the urethral catheter are patient comfort, lowered incidence of cystitis, and convenience in measuring residual urines. We routinely use an 18 French Silastic Foley catheter introduced into the bladder under direct vision at the completion of the procedure. The bladder is distended with approximately 200 ml. of saline, the Foley catheter being introduced through a stab wound and affixed to the bladder wall with a purse-string suture of 2–0 chromic catgut. The catheter is brought out extraperitoneally and affixed to the abdominal wall. The catheter is attached to straight drainage and later to a leg bag and left in place for 3 to 6 weeks. During this time the patient is placed on a urinary antimicrobial regimen. The catheter is removed in the outpatient clinic after a residual urine volume of under 50 ml. is demonstrated. In 85 patients managed in this fashion three problems were encountered: two catheters fell out (and were replaced by a urethral catheter), and one patient experienced leakage around the catheter, which necessitated its removal and replacement with a urethral catheter.

Van Nagell and Schiwietz (1976) used suprapubic bladder drainage in 109 patients for an average of 47 days and reported that these patients had a urinary fistula rate half that of patients who had urethral catheters (5 per cent versus 11 per cent).

Wertheim (1912) suggested that the retroperitoneal space be drained following radical hysterectomy. He noted that after the operation is completed, the ureter ". . . finds itself in a puddle of liquid swarming with products of putrefaction which reacts unfavorably upon the ureter's nutrition." Symmonds and Pratt (1961) nearly 50 years later reported great success with suction catheters placed in the retroperitoneal space and brought out through the abdominal wall. The benefits are removal of exudate, reduction of lymphocysts, and the more rapid adherence of the peritoneum and the ureter to the lateral pelvic wall.

We have found this a useful technique

and utilize it in all patients. The Jackson-Pratt drains have proved to be very effective. Several hundred milliliters of fluid is removed in the first three postoperative days. The hematocrit level for the fluid on the first day is generally 6 to 8 volume per cent and on the second day 3 per cent. The fluid usually becomes clear by the third day, suggesting that its source is not bleeding but lymph and reactive exudate. The drains are attached to a constant wall suction at moderate pressure (80 to 120 mm. Hg). The catheters are generally removed on the fourth postoperative day when the volume of drainage has decreased to less than 25 ml. in 24 hours.

Ureteral Fistula

Incidence

Although fistulas represent the more common and clinically more striking postoperative ureteral complication, ureteral stricture is the more threatening. In Green's series (1966), among 12.5 per cent ureteral complications, 8.5 per cent were fistulas and 4.0 per cent strictures. Similar complications were reported by Talbert and co-workers (1965): 8 per cent of 112 patients developed ureteral fistulas following radical hysterectomy, while 4.5 per cent developed ureteral strictures. Urinary tract fistulas generally develop between the first and third weeks following surgery.

Symptoms

Flank or side pain and fever accompany the developing ureterovaginal fistula in the majority of patients, whereas both may be absent with the developing vesicovaginal fistula. All three of our patients who developed ureteral fistulas had right flank or lower quadrant pain and fever. On the tenth, tenth, and eleventh postoperative days, respectively, the temperature returned to normal and the patient noted leakage of urine.

Diagnosis

If a fistula is suspected in the postoperative period, systematic evaluation will generally establish the diagnosis. Vesicovaginal fistulas can be distinguished from ureterovaginal fistulas by the instillation of 200 to 300 ml. of methylene blue–colored saline into the bladder after the placement of a tampon in the vagina. The patient is asked to stand, after which the tampon is removed and examined for color. Blue color on the tampon suggests the presence of a vesicovaginal fistula.

In the absence of leakage from the bladder, a fresh tampon is placed in the vagina and 10 ml. of indigo carmine is administered intravenously. After about 30 minutes, the tampon is again removed and examined for color. The presence of blue color suggests a ureterovaginal fistula, but does not identify side or site. Neither can a combination of vesicovaginal and ureterovaginal fistulas be distinguished by these simple tests.

Intravenous pyelograms can be of help in determining the side of the ureterovaginal fistula. When extravasation is seen on intravenous pyelogram the side and site of the fistula can be established (Figure 10–3). A direct method for establishing the side of the fistula is to observe the ureteral orifices through a cystoscope after the intravenous administration of indigo carmine. The spurt of dye from the orifice suggests that the ureter is intact on that side.

The most definitive way of establishing the side and site of fistulas is during surgery, when both ureters have been isolated above the pelvis. With a Foley catheter in the bladder and a tampon in the vagina, methylene blue is injected into one ureter. If the dye is noted in the bladder (via the Foley catheter) but not on the tampon, it is likely that the ureter is intact. If the dye fails to show in the bladder and instead stains the tampon, the fistula can be assumed to be on the side given the dye.

Treatment

In our series, all three fistulas developed in patients in whom the ureters were managed by the Ohkawa technique. None closed spontaneously. Two patients had right-to-left transureteroureterostomy (Figure 10–4) with satisfactory outcome. The third patient had an early recurrence of cancer and died.

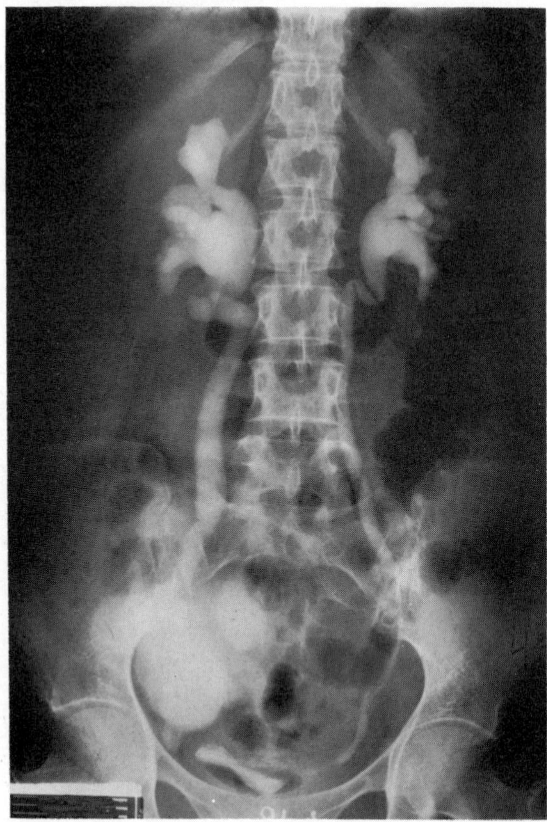

Figure 10–3. Intravenous pyelogram 10 days after radical hysterectomy in patient with ureteral fistula. Extravasation of contrast material from the right ureter is seen.

When a ureteral fistula is close to the bladder, ureteroneocystotomy is the most appropriate corrective procedure; if higher, a bladder flap can be used. If the fistula is above the pelvic brim, a transureteroureterostomy (see Figure 10–4) or the interposition of a portion of ileum can be used in the surgical correction. End-to-end anastomoses are generally unsatisfactory and should be avoided (see Chapter 9).

Ureteral Stricture

The leakage of urine directs the physician's attention to a ureteral fistula; a blocked ureter may be asymptomatic and lead to loss of renal function. The one kidney lost in our series of 80 radical hysterectomies resulted from the asymptomatic blockage of a ureter (autonephrectomy). When pain and fever are present and there is no evidence of urinary leakage, ureteral stricture should be suspected. It is essential that intravenous or retrograde pyelography or both be performed as early as possible. Talbert and co-workers (1965) and Mattsson (1975) have called attention to the significance of early changes on intravenous pyelography. Unilateral early dilatation suggests probable ureteral compromise. If there has been considerable delay in establishing the presence of ureteral stricture and the kidney does not visualize on intravenous pyelography, a renogram should be obtained to determine viability of the kidney. Although opinions vary on the length of time that it takes for an obstructed kidney to lose function, most urologists feel that irreversible changes occur after 2 months.

There were seven cases of ureteral stricture in our series of 80 patients. Two were transitory, regressing without treatment; two patients required temporary nephrostomy; and one patient with obstruction 2 to 3 cm. from the ureterovesical junction had a ureteroneocystotomy after the obstruction failed to clear with nephrostomy drainage. In one patient ureteral stricture was

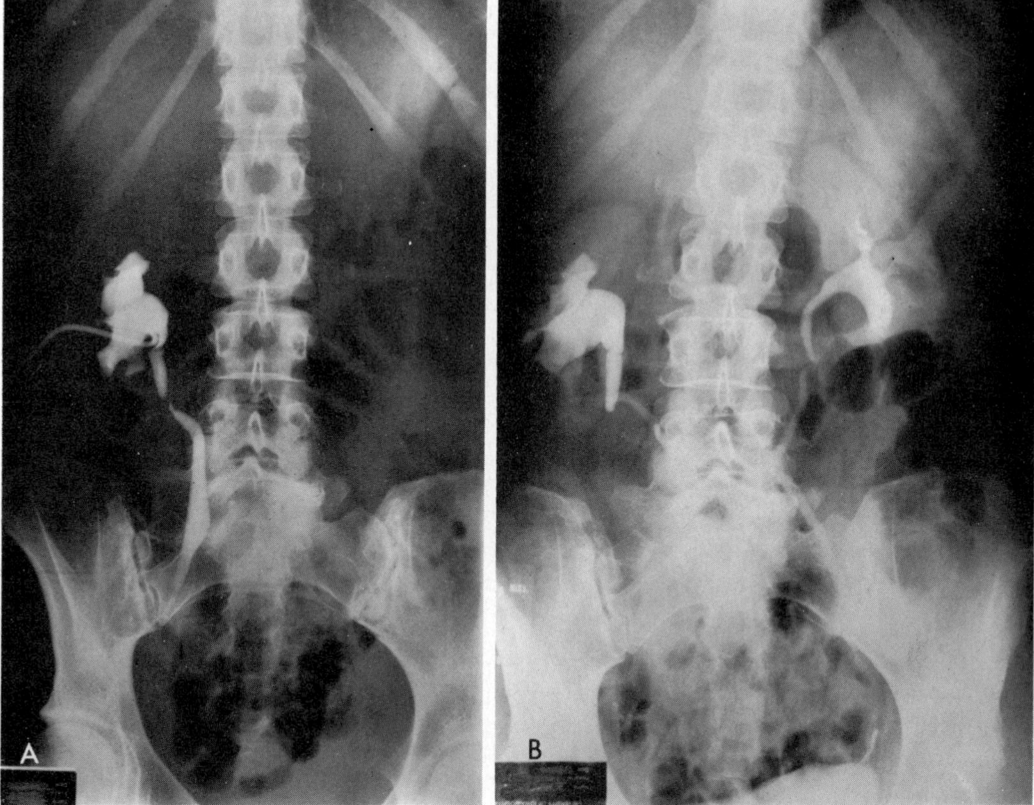

Figure 10–4. Correction of postoperative ureteral stricture.

A, Antegrade pyelogram following radical hysterectomy and right nephrostomy, showing ureteral obstruction at level of common iliac vessels. This patient had both ureters placed in peritoneal envelopes (Ohkawa), and the obstruction is at site where ureter enters envelope.

B, Intravenous pyelogram after right-to-left transureteroureterostomy to relieve right ureteral obstruction.

caused by a lymphocyst (Figure 10–5). The obstruction cleared after the lymphocyst was surgically drained. Renal function was lost in one patient 6 months after surgery and a nephrectomy was performed.

The importance of early intervention by nephrostomy cannot be overemphasized. In a number of patients, the obstruction will clear without further treatment after a period of diversion. After diversion (generally by loop nephrostomy), the patient should be evaluated with urography at 3 months and again at 6 months. If the obstruction persists at 6 months, appropriate surgery can then safely be carried out.

A rare complication of ureteral fistula is the formation of urinoma (Everett, 1957). A ureteral fistula that communicates with the peritoneum, either primarily or following stricture, results in urine leaking into the peritoneal cavity. The abdomen becomes protuberant, distended by urine. We have seen one such patient, with approximately 3000 ml. of urine contained in a pseudocyst formed by the omentum anteriorly and the parietal peritoneum posteriorly.

Vesicovaginal Fistula

Vesicovaginal fistulas are far less frequent following radical hysterectomy than are ureteral fistulas. Green and colleagues (1962) reported 14 vesicovaginal fistulas (2.2 per cent) in 623 patients, compared to an 8.5 per cent ureterovaginal fistula rate. In most series the ureterovaginal fistula rate is 2 to 4 times that of vesicovaginal fistulas (Talbert et al., 1965: Green, 1966; Mikuta et al., 1977; Sall et al., 1979; Benedet et al., 1980). Calame and Nelson (1967) found no vesicovaginal fistulas in 209 patients under-

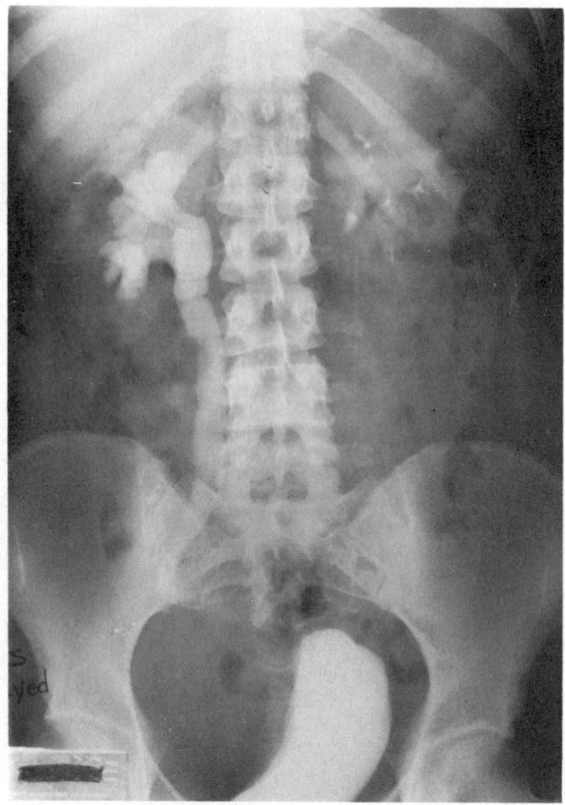

Figure 10–5. Delayed film after intravenous pyelogram in patient with postoperative pelvic lymphocyst. Obstruction of ureter and indentation of bladder by lymphocyst can be seen on the right.

going radical hysterectomy but reported a 13.4 per cent incidence of ureterovaginal fistulas. The low incidence of vesicovaginal fistulas relates to the better blood supply of the bladder. The vesical branches are generally retained.

Two vesicovaginal fistulas developed in our series. One occurred in a patient whose bladder was injured during surgery and the defect repaired. Bladder drainage was maintained for 2 weeks. Approximately 5 weeks after discharge from the hospital the patient noted leakage of urine from the vagina. The second patient developed a spontaneous vesicovaginal fistula several weeks following surgery. Both patients were maintained on long-term continuous bladder drainage, but neither fistula healed spontaneously. Both were surgically repaired, one 4 and the other 13 months postoperatively.

Postoperative Intravenous Pyelogram

Intravenous pyelograms (IVP) should be part of the routine postoperative evaluation of patients treated with radical hysterectomy. In asymptomatic patients, the first study should be performed within 4 weeks of surgery and repeated at 3 and 6 months. In this fashion, the physician is able to identify postoperative ureteral obstruction early enough to prevent loss of the kidney.

The IVP in a patient following radical hysterectomy and lymphadenectomy must be interpreted in light of the recent surgery. Between 20 and 30 per cent of patients will show significant alterations (Green, 1962; Mattsson, 1975) on IVP: the nephrogram phase is accentuated and the pyelogram phase delayed. The most striking alteration is dilatation of the upper tract. There is dilatation of the pelvicalyceal system and the upper two thirds of the ureter. The distal one third of the ureter may be normal or narrowed (Figure 10–6) (Hanafec et al., 1958). The dilatation of the upper tract and the narrowed appearance of the lower portion of the ureter are found regardless of the intraoperative management of the ureter. Mallik (1960) originally believed that these changes start or at least appear on pyelog-

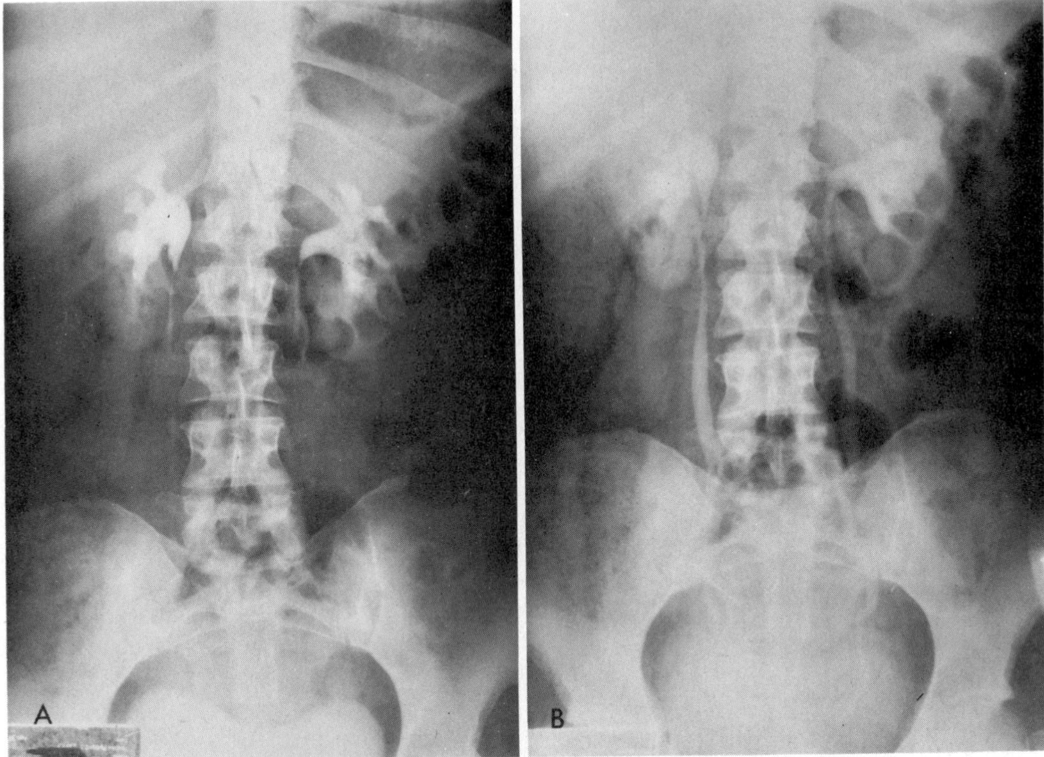

Figure 10–6. Early upper urinary tract alterations following radical hysterectomy.
A, Preoperative study.
B, Pyelogram taken 2 weeks after radical hysterectomy and pelvic lymphadenectomy, demonstrating bilateral and symmetrical upper tract dilatation. The lower third of both ureters is narrowed.

raphy late in the third or early in the fourth week following surgery. Talbert and associates (1965) found these changes as early as 24 hours following surgery. Our experience supports Talbert's findings in that these typical changes may appear within the first week. Mallik (1960) suggested that hydronephrosis developing before the third week was an ominous sign indicative of ureteral fistula or ureteral stricture. This has not been our experience. We have seen the typical bilateral upper tract dilatation in many patients in whom these changes have later reverted to normal. In most patients these changes regress so that by the end of 1 year the intravenous pyelogram shows a return to the preoperative condition (Figure 10–7).

It is not known for certain what causes these upper tract changes, but they probably result from a combination of factors. Compromise of the ureteral blood supply, denervation as a result of dissection, periureteral adhesions, and edema of the ureteral wall probably contribute. It is difficult to determine whether the lower ureter retains its normal caliber while the upper tract is dilated or whether the lower tract is narrowed with the subsequent dilatation of the upper tract. Since these changes occur so commonly, regardless of method of ureteral management, it appears best to consider them a functional abnormality, as suggested by Green (1975).

Mattsson (1976) ascribes great prognostic significance to abnormal findings on postoperative pyelograms. In 61 of 168 patients, pyelograms were interpreted as abnormal at 3 to 12 weeks post radical hysterectomy. Twenty-eight later reverted to normal, 13 remained unchanged, and 6 worsened. Fifteen of 61 patients (25 per cent) with abnormal pyelograms, and only 16 of 107 (15 per cent) with normal IVPs, later died of cancer.

Bladder Dysfunction

Sensory and micturition problems following radical hysterectomy have received

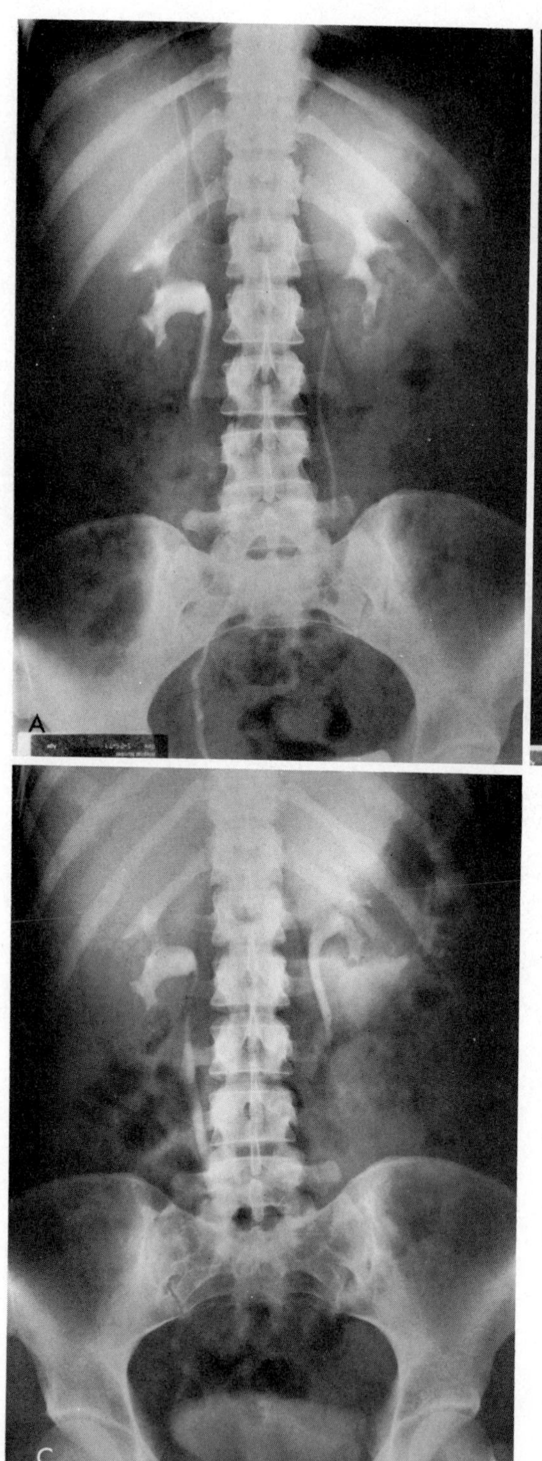

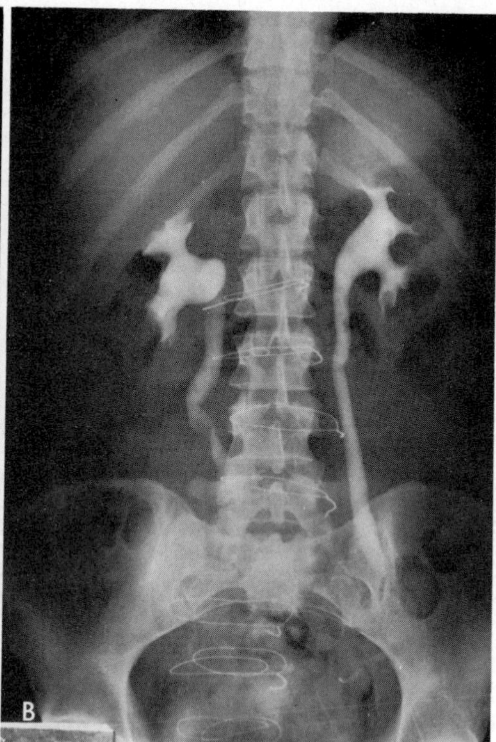

Figure 10–7. Regression of upper urinary tract changes following radical hysterectomy.

A, Intravenous pyelogram prior to surgery.

B, Upper tract changes 5 weeks following surgery. Bilateral mild hydroureter and hydronephrosis are seen.

C, Intravenous pyelogram 2 years after surgery, showing return of caliber of ureters to preoperative state.

TABLE 10–3. BLADDER DYSFUNCTION FOLLOWING RADICAL HYSTERECTOMY (17 OF 80 PATIENTS)

Symptom	Number of Patients
Sensory loss	7
Urgency	4
Difficulty initiating stream	3
Strain to empty bladder	3
Stress incontinence	3
Spasm	1
	21*

*Some patients had more than one symptom.

far less attention in the medical literature than have postoperative urinary fistulas. Bladder dysfunction is far more common, its etiology less well understood, and its management more vexing.

Incidence

The incidence of postoperative bladder dysfunction has been reported to be as high as 50 per cent (Lewington, 1956; Fraser, 1966; Low et al., 1981). Seventeen of 80 patients (21 per cent in our series) had a total of 21 bladder problems (Table 10–3). Although most bladder problems are transitory, with normal function returning by 6 months, when symptoms persist beyond 6 months they may become permanent. One patient with persistent sensory loss developed an atonic bladder in spite of prolonged bladder drainage. Similarly, a patient with stress incontinence persisting beyond 1 year had a failed surgical repair and continues to be bothered by involuntary loss of urine.

Pathophysiology

Patients experience both sensory and functional disorders following radical hysterectomy and pelvic lymphadenectomy. The bladder dysfunction presents in a variety of ways: sensory loss, a lessened perception of bladder distention, lowered capacity, inability to empty the bladder, and, less commonly, urinary stress incontinence. The pathophysiology of these changes is still not completely understood.

The sympathetic fibers innervating the bladder arise from the para-aortic sympathetic chain at the T11 to L12 level. These synapse in the superior mesenteric ganglion and course into the pelvis over the promontory and sacrum. They enter the pelvis via the hypogastric nerve, synapse in the pelvic plexus, and reach the bladder through the fixed bladder base. In the pelvic plexus, the fibers synapse with parasympathetic fibers from S2, S3, and S4, which traverse the pelvis via the pelvic nerve and enter the pelvic plexus from either side of the rectum. The postganglionic fibers may be exclusively sympathetic, exclusively parasympathetic, or mixed.

The autonomic fibers innervating the bladder can be disrupted at several stages during radical hysterectomy: (1) during dissection of the presacral or superior gluteal nodes, (2) during paravaginal dissection and mobilization of the bladder, and (3) during resection of the cardinal ligament.

It has been known for some time that a hypertonic bladder dysfunction follows radical hysterectomy and is manifested by a diminished capacity, elevated resting pressure, and increased residual urine volume (Fraser, 1966; Glahn, 1970; Barclay and Roman-Lopez, 1975). Most earlier investigators attributed the hypertonic condition to a parasympathetic dominance and ascribed little significance to the role of the sympathetic innervation.

Seski and co-workers (1977) confirmed the findings of previous investigators regarding bladder capacity, intravesical pressure, and residual urine volume, but carried their investigations a step further. By administering a parasympatholytic drug, they were unable to reduce the postoperative hypertonia, suggesting that it was not a result of parasympathetic dominance. They further found no bladder neck dysfunction as measured by electromyography of the sphincter. While they acknowledge that some degree of neural injury takes place, they believed that the major factor contributing to the postoperative hypertonic bladder is an increase in the myogenic tone of the detrusor itself, and that this is only a transitory condition.

Studies by Forney (1980) and by Low and associates (1981) have suggested a different etiology. Forney, at Southwestern Medical School, studied 22 patients (11 with complete cardinal ligament resection and 11 with less radical resection, which spared the distal and inferior 1 to 2 cm of cardinal ligament) with preoperative and serial postoperative CO_2 cystourethroscopy, as well as urethral and bladder pressure measurements.

The mean time following radical hysterectomy before a patient could void with a residual of less than 50 ml. was 51 days in the complete resection group, and only 20 days in the incomplete group ($P<0.01$). Sensory loss was equally diminished in both groups; the mean volume required to elicit the sensation of fullness was 160 ml. in the complete resection group and 140 ml. in the incomplete resection group. Postoperatively, all 11 patients with complete cardinal resection, and only 4 of 11 with the lesser procedure, had hypertonic cystometry. Five patients (4 patients in the complete resection group), who previously were asymptomatic, developed urinary stress incontinence postoperatively. In 1 of 2 patients with preexisting incontinence, the problem became worse; in the other, it was symptomatically unchanged.

These findings by Forney documented a correlation between the extent of surgery— i.e., resection of cardinal ligament—and postoperative bladder function.

Low and colleagues (1981) performed preoperative and postoperative cystometry with simultaneous recording of bladder and urethral pressures in 20 patients undergoing radical hysterectomy for cervical carcinoma. Preoperatively, there was a modest rise of 10 cm. of water in the bladder after filling with 500 ml. of water. The more significant postoperative rise is seen in Figure 10–8.

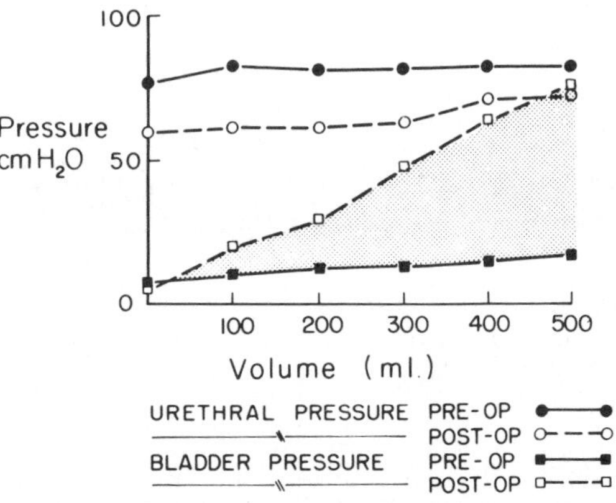

Figure 10–8. Preoperative and postoperative bladder and urethral pressures. Bladder and urethral pressures during continuous infusion of 500 ml. of water into the bladder. Note appreciable post–radical hysterectomy rise in vesical pressure and the diminution in urethral pressure. (From Low, J. A., Mauger, C. M., and Carmichael, J. A.: The effect of Wertheim hysterectomy upon bladder and urethral function. Am. J. Obstet. Gynecol. *139*:826, 1981.)

Also shown is a decline of 29 per cent in mean urethral pressure following surgery. A preoperative and postoperative urethral pressure profile with the patient at rest is shown in Figure 10–9. The mean maximum preoperative urethral pressure was 90 cm. of water at a point 2.0 cm. proximal to the urethral meatus. Postoperatively, the maximum urethral pressure had fallen to 64 cm. of water at a point 1.5 cm. from the meatus.

Both Forney (1980) and Low and colleagues (1981) reviewed the literature on bladder innervation and concluded that

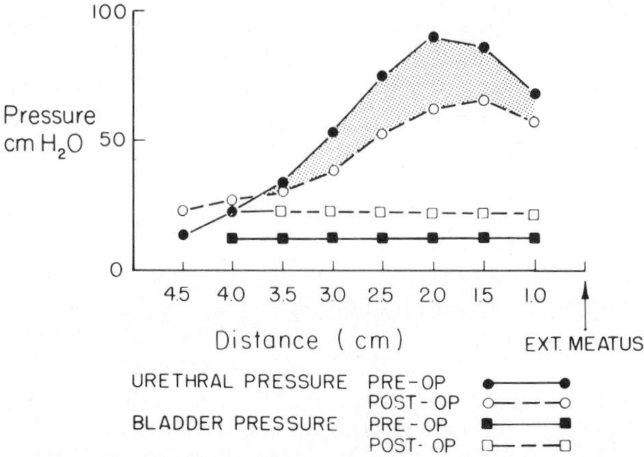

Figure 10–9. Preoperative and postoperative urethral pressure profile. Note post–radical hysterectomy diminution in urethral maximal pressure. Preoperatively, the maximum urethral pressure was 90 cm. of water at 2.0 cm. above the external urethral meatus. Postoperatively, the maximum urethral pressure was 64 cm. of water at a point 1.5 cm. from the external urethral meatus. (From Low, J. A., Mauger, C. M., and Carmichael, J. A.: The effect of Wertheim hysterectomy upon bladder and urethral function. Am. J. Obstet. Gynecol. *139*:826, 1981.)

sympathetic loss plays a major role in the postoperative bladder changes. The postganglionic sympathetic nerves terminate in both alpha- and beta-adrenergic receptors, with the former localized in the urethra and bladder neck and the latter diffusely scattered throughout the detrusor muscle. Under normal circumstances, stimulation of the beta fibers causes inhibition of the detrusor, thereby lowering intravesical pressure and giving the bladder its compliance. Compromise of beta-adrenergic function will thereby increase intravesical pressure.

Furthermore, there is a suggestion that sympathetic alpha-adrenergic stimulation may have an inhibitory effect on parasympathetic transmission to the detrusor muscle. This may explain the incidence of the detrusor dyssynergia that Low and colleagues (1981) found in their post–radical hysterectomy studies. Finally, loss of alpha-adrenergic stimulation of the smooth muscle in the urethra and bladder neck may contribute to the fall in urethral pressure, resulting in the higher incidence of urinary stress incontinence following radical hysterectomy.

Considerably more work needs to be done before the mechanisms operational in postoperative bladder dysfunction are completely understood. Forney's study (1980) suggests a method of moderating the adverse effects of the surgery on bladder function: sparing the distal and inferior 1 to 2 cm. of cardinal ligament.

Hypotonic Phase. Overdistention of the bladder in the early postoperative period can lead to a hypotonic bladder. Since there is some degree of sensory loss postoperatively, with patients often perceiving a full bladder by substitute sensations (e.g., pressure in pelvis, discomfort, or fullness of abdomen), it is essential that the bladder not be allowed to overdistend. Furthermore, compromise of detrusor function requires that patients utilize ancillary muscles in emptying the bladder. They are not likely to use the abdominal muscles while the ventral incision is still healing because this would cause considerable pain.

POSTOPERATIVE BLADDER DRAINAGE. For reasons already given, prolonged postoperative bladder drainage has been used since the report of Green and colleagues (1962). By using continuous bladder drainage via an indwelling catheter the patient is spared the need to restrict fluid, frequent voiding, and possible need for catheterization. We now use an indwelling suprapubic catheter placed in the bladder at the completion of the operation. It offers convenience, patient comfort and acceptance, and an acceptably low incidence of bladder infection.

Postoperative Urinary Tract Infection (UTI)

The high frequency with which patients develop UTI following radical hysterectomy is now becoming evident. Sall and colleagues (1979) reported that 37 per cent of their patients had postoperative UTI; Webb and Symmonds (1979) reported 15.4 per cent.

A number of preoperative and postoperative factors contribute to this high incidence of UTI. Most patients will have had cystoscopic examination prior to the operative procedure, many close enough to the day of surgery to not have had adequate antimicrobial prophylaxis. Furthermore, all patients will have an indwelling catheter postoperatively.

Mattsson (1976) treated 19 of 168 patients (11.3 per cent) who had bacteriuria on admission prior to radical hysterectomy. Postoperatively, nearly 53 per cent of all patients were found to have significant bacteremia; 14.9 per cent of these had had normal and 37.7 per cent abnormal postoperative excretory urograms.

These findings would suggest that patients should be screened preoperatively, and those found to have bacteriuria treated. The patients should be evaluated frequently during the postoperative period for bacteriuria and, if such is found, specific antimicrobial therapy instituted.

REFERENCES

Barclay, D. L., and Roman-Lopez, J. J.: Bladder dysfunction after Shauta hysterectomy. One year follow-up. Am. J. Obstet. Gynecol. *123*:519, 1975.

Benedet, J. L., Turko, M., Boyes, D. A., et al.: Radical hysterectomy in the treatment of cervical cancer. Am. J. Obstet. Gynecol. *137*:254, 1980.

Bonney, V.: The treatment of carcinoma of the cervix by Wertheim's operation. Am. J. Obstet. Gynecol. *30*:815, 1935.

Brunschwig, A., and Frick, H. C., III: I. Urinary tract fistulas following radical surgical treatment of carcinoma of the cervix. Am. J. Obstet. Gynecol. *72*:479, 1956.

Burch, J. C., Chalfant, R. L., and Johnson, J. W.: Technique for prevention of ureterovaginal fistula following radical abdominal hysterectomy. Ann. Surg. *161*:832, 1965.

Calame, R. J., and Nelson, J. H., Jr.: Ureterovaginal fistula as a complication of radical pelvic surgery. Arch. Surg. *94*:876, 1967.

Everett, H. S.: Ureteroperitoneal fistula with urinary ascites. J. Urol. *78*:585, 1957.

Forney, J. P.: The effect of radical hysterectomy on bladder physiology. Am. J. Obstet. Gynecol. *138*:374, 1980.

Fraser, A. C.: The late effects of Wertheim hysterectomy on the urinary tract. J. Obstet. Gynaecol. Br. Commonw. *73*:1002, 1966.

Glahn, E.: The neurogenic factor in vesical dysfunction following radical hysterectomy for carcinoma of the cervix. Scand. J. Urol. Nephrol. *4*:107, 1970.

Green, T. H., Jr.: Ureteral suspension for prevention of ureteral complications following radical Wertheim hysterectomy. Obstet. Gynecol. *28*:1, 1966.

Green, T. H., Jr.: Ureteral suspension — an operative technique for the prevention of ureteral complications following radical Wertheim hysterectomy. *In* Taylor, M. L., and Green, T. H., Jr. (eds.): Progress in Gynecology. Vol. VI. New York, Grune & Stratton, 1975.

Green, T. H., Jr., Meigs, J. V., Ulfelder, H., et al.: Urologic complications of radical Wertheim hysterectomy. Incidence, etiology, management and prevention. Obstet. Gynecol. *20*:293, 1962.

Hanafec, W., Ottoman, R. E., and Wilk, S. P.: Roentgen diagnosis of urinary complications following radical hysterectomy and pelvic lymph node dissection. Radiology *70*:46, 1958.

Lang, E. K., Wood, M., Brown, R., et al.: Complications in urinary tract related to treatment of carcinoma of the cervix. South. Med. J. *66*:228, 1973.

Lash, A. F.: Ureteral protection in radical abdominal and vaginal hysterectomy as surgical treatment of cervical carcinoma. Int. Surg. *58*:352, 1973.

Lewington, W.: Disturbances of micturition following Wertheim hysterectomy. J. Obstet. Gynaecol. Brit. Emp. *63*:861, 1956.

Low, J. A., Mauger, G. M., and Carmichael, J. A.: The effect of Wertheim hysterectomy upon bladder and urethral function. Am. J. Obstet. Gynecol. *139*:826, 1981.

Macasaet, M. A., Lu, T., and Nelson, J. H., Jr.: Ureterovaginal fistula as a complication of radical pelvic surgery. Am. J. Obstet. Gynecol. *124*:757, 1976.

Mack, W. S.: Urological complications of pelvic surgery. Br. J. Urol. *41*:641, 1969.

Mallik, M. K. B.: A study of the ureters following Wertheim hysterectomy. J. Obstet. Gynaecol. Br. Commonw. *67*:556, 1960.

Masterson, J. G.: An experimental study of ureteral injuries in radical pelvic surgery. Am. J. Obstet. Gynecol. *73*:359, 1957.

Mattsson, T.: Complications of treatment and metastatic spread of cervical carcinoma with special regard to roentgenological studies. Acta Obstet. Gynecol. Scand. *58*(Suppl):1, 1976.

Mattsson, T.: Frequency and management of urological and some other complications following radical surgery for carcinoma of the cervix uteri, stages I and II. Acta Obstet. Gynecol. Scand. *54*:271, 1975.

McCormack, L. J., and Anson, B. J.: Arterial supply of the ureter. Q. Bull. Northwest. Univ. Med. School *24*:292, 1950.

Meigs, J. V.: Surgical Treatment of Cancer of the Cervix. New York, Grune & Stratton, 1954.

Mickal, A., Torres, J. E., and Schlosser, J. V.: Complications of therapy for carcinoma of the cervix. Am. J. Obstet. Gynecol. *112*:556, 1972.

Mikuta, J. J., Giuntoli, R. L., Rubin, E. L., et al.: The problem radical hysterectomy. Am. J. Obstet. Gynecol. *128*:119, 1977.

Novak, F.: Procedure for the reduction of the number of ureterovaginal fistulas after Wertheim's operation. Am. J. Obstet. Gynecol. *72*:506, 1956.

Novak, F.: The prevention of ureterovaginal fistulas after the Wertheim operation. Int. J. Obstet. Gynecol. *7*:301, 1969.

Ohkawa, K.: Ureteral management in radical pelvic surgery with special reference to the peritoneal flap. New York, Sixth World Congress of Gynecology and Obstetrics, April 11, 1970.

Parsons, L.: Urologic complications following gynecological surgery. *In* Sturgis, S. H., and Taymor, M. L. (eds.): Progress in Gynecology. Vol. V. New York, Grune & Stratton, 1970.

Perez, C. A., Camel, M., Kao, M. S., et al.: Randomized study of preoperative radiation and surgery or irradiation alone in the treatment of stage I_B and II_A carcinoma of the uterine cervix: Preliminary analysis of failures and complications. Cancer *45*:2758, 1980.

Roberts, J. M., and Homesley, H. D.: Observations on bladder function following radical hysterectomy using carbon dioxide cystometry. Surg. Gynecol. Obstet. *147*:558, 1978.

Sall, S., Pineda, A. A., Canalog, A., et al.: Surgical treatment of stages I_B and II_A invasive carcinoma of the cervix by radical abdominal hysterectomy. Am. J. Obstet. Gynecol. *135*:442, 1979.

Sampson, J. A.: Ligation and clamping the ureter as complications of surgical operations. Am. Med. *4*:693, 1902.

Sampson, J. A.: Complications arising from freeing the ureters in the more radical operations for carcinoma cervicis uteri, with special reference to postoperative ureteral necrosis. Bull. Johns Hopkins Hosp. *15*:123, 1904.

Seski, J. C., Diokno, A. C., and Anderson, D. G.: Bladder dysfunction after radical hysterectomy. Am. J. Obstet. Gynecol. *128*:643, 1977.

Symmonds, R. E., and Pratt, J. H.: Prevention of fistulas and lymphocysts in radical hysterectomy. Obstet. Gynecol. *17*:57, 1961.

Talbert, L. M., Palumbo, L., Shingleton, H., et al.: Urologic complications of radical hysterectomy for carcinoma of the cervix. South. Med. J. *58*:11, 1965.

Underwood, P. B., Jr., Wilson, W. C., Kreutner, A., et al.: Radical hysterectomy: A critical review of twenty-two years' experience. Am. J. Obstet. Gynecol. *134*:889, 1979.

van Nagell, J. R., and Schiwietz, D. P.: Surgical adjuvants in radical hysterectomy and pelvic lymphadenectomy. Surg. Gynecol. Obstet. *143*:735, 1976.

Varverikos, E. D.: Variability of vascular supply to the ureter. Am. J. Obstet. Gynecol. *63*:774, 1952.

Webb, M. J., and Symmonds, R. E.: Wertheim hysterectomy: A reappraisal. Obstet. Gynecol. *54*:140, 1979.

Werner, P., and Sederl, J.: The technique of Wertheim's radical operation. *In* Meigs, J. (ed.): Surgical Treatment of Cancer of the Cervix. New York, Grune & Stratton, 1975, p. 197.

Wertheim, E.: The extended abdominal operation for carcinoma uteri (based on 500 operative cases). Am. J. Obstet. Dis. Women Child. *66*:169, 1912.

11

URINARY DIVERSION IN PELVIC EXENTERATION

J. D. SCHMIDT, M.D.
H. J. BUCHSBAUM, M.D.

The role of pelvic exenteration is now firmly established in the treatment of pelvic malignancies. It has been used in the treatment of bowel and urinary bladder cancer and in soft tissue sarcomas, but has found its widest application in the management of primary and recurrent female genital malignancies. Operative morbidity and mortality have been greatly reduced, and the five-year survival rate has improved. These results have contributed to a wider acceptance and application of pelvic exenteration in the treatment of pelvic neoplasms.

Many factors have led to the improved outcome, including selection of patients, improved surgical techniques and better-trained pelvic surgeons. Improved anesthesia, new antibiotics, and availability of blood and blood products have also made significant contributions. A better understanding of postoperative fluid requirements, resulting from wider use of central venous pressure monitoring and urinary osmolality, has contributed to a lowered operative mortality.

One of the most important factors contributing to long-term survival following pelvic exenteration has been the improvement in methods of urinary diversion. All authors agree on its importance in improving short- and long-term survival. Brunschwig and Daniel (1960) noted that ". . . among these patients who die after years, complications of the urinary tract are the leading causes of death."

PRINCIPLES OF URINARY DIVERSION

The *ideal* method of urinary diversion accompanying pelvic exenteration should include all of the following: (1) unobstructed drainage of urine from the kidney(s), (2) continent storage of urine, (3) separation of fecal and urinary streams, (4) minimal reabsorption of urine and electrolytes, (5) absence of reflux, (6) patient acceptance, (7) maintenance of normal renal function, and (8) simplicity of technique.

Urinary diversions are grouped into supravesical and vesical categories. Since, in the performance of exenterative procedures, the urinary bladder and the urethra are removed, vesical forms of diversion will not be discussed.

Supravesical methods of urinary diversion applicable to total and anterior pelvic exenteration include:

1. Direct diversion
   a. Nephrostomy (open surgical or percutaneous)
   b. Cutaneous ureterostomy
2. Indirect diversion via intestine
   a. Intact bowel — ureterosigmoidostomy or wet colostomy

b. Rectal pouch
c. Isolated segment of bowel — ileal, sigmoid or transverse colon conduit.

Direct Supravesical Diversion

Nephrostomy and cutaneous ureterostomy have not found wide application in exenterative surgery. Conventional nephrostomy diversion leaves the patient with two tubes that require changing and continual care. Stricture at the fascia, stomal problems and the lack of satisfactory appliances militate against cutaneous ureterostomies. Scott (1965) suggested that the care of two cutaneous ureterostomies ". . . is more than twice as difficult as the care of one. . . . " Furthermore, patients with total pelvic exenteration will also have a colostomy stoma to contend with.

The technique of transureteroureterostomy allows the two ureters to join in a common stem, which in turn may be brought to the skin as an end cutaneous ureterostomy or to a bowel segment or even intact bowel. Transureteroureterostomy was used in 32 patients reported at the University of Iowa (Schmidt et al., 1972). Of these, 18 had a malignancy, including 9 with gynecologic tumors: carcinoma of the cervix with ureteral stricture, vesicovaginal or ureterovaginal fistula (7) and endometrial cancer (2).

Seven complications occurred in the entire series: stomal stenosis, i.e., with end cutaneous ureterostomy (3), urinary extravasation of more than two weeks' duration (2), bowel obstruction (1), and one instance of calculous pyelonephritis requiring nephrectomy and occurring 21 years after right-to-left transureteroureterostomy and left ureterosigmoidostomy.

Intestinal Diversion

Use of the Intact Bowel

In the earlier experience with pelvic exenteration, the most common method of urinary diversion was implantation of the ureters into the intact bowel: Ureterosigmoidostomy in anterior exenteration, and wet colostomy in total exenteration. Brunschwig and Daniel (1960), twelve years after the original description of exenteration, reported the methods of urinary diversion in 587 patients who had pelvic exenteration (Table 11–1).

A total of 71.4 per cent of patients had ureters implanted into the intact bowel without separation of fecal and urinary streams. The ease and speed of ureterocolonic anastomosis made this a very desirable method. Furthermore, patients with total exenteration had a single stoma (i.e., colostomy), and patients with anterior exenteration had none.

TABLE 11–1. TYPES OF URINARY DIVERSION IN 587 PATIENTS UNDERGOING PELVIC EXENTERATION*

	Total Exenteration	Anterior Exenteration	Total Number of Patients
Wet colostomy	245		(387) 245
Ureterosigmoidostomy		142	142
Cutaneous ureterostomy	55	15	70
Ileal conduit	32	38	70
Proximal bowel	25	10	35
Rectal bladder		11	11
Other	3	11	14
Total	360	227	587

*From Brunschwig and Daniels, 1960.

Postoperative Problems. Two major problems were subsequently identified in patients diverted by either ureterosigmoidostomy or wet colostomy where the ureters were implanted into the intact bowel: (1) electrolyte and acid-base problems and (2) ascending infections. Both phenomena severely compromise renal function.

Douglas and Sweeney (1957) reported 23 pelvic exenterations in which urinary diversion was either by ureteral implantation into the sigmoid colon or by cutaneous ureterostomies. Seventy-eight per cent of the patients developed urinary tract infections, 74 per cent developed bilateral hydronephrosis, 13 per cent had unilateral hydronephrosis, and 3 per cent required revisions of ureterostomies.

Symmonds and co-workers (1968), reporting on the large experience at the Mayo Clinic, found 60 urinary complications in 57 patients with ureterosigmoidostomy or wet colostomy. One third of the patients had electrolyte problems, 13 of 57 (23 per cent) had severe pyelitis or renal calculi, and a similar number had loss of renal function. Symmonds (1968) reported that approximately one half of deaths during the first two months following anterior exenteration were related to the method of urinary diversion by ureterosigmoidostomy.

ELECTROLYTE AND ACID-BASE PROBLEMS. Ferris and Odel (1950) first identified the electrolyte problems in patients with ureterocolonic implants. The unidirectional absorption across the bowel mucosa of chloride ion from urine allowed to pool in the bowel lumen resulted in hyperchloremic acidosis. Some degree of renal impairment as a result of concomitant or previous obstruction or of pyelonephritis compounds the problem. Selective chloride absorption was later studied by Irvine and colleagues (1960). Seventy-five per cent of patients with ureterocolonic anastomoses developed hyperchloremic acidosis; half showed clinical signs and symptoms.

ASCENDING INFECTION. Preoperative antibiotic and mechanical preparation cannot completely and effectively sterilize the colon. In the intact intestine the ureters are exposed to potentially dangerous coliform bacteria. Before long, an ascending infection develops that damages the kidney and impairs effective transport of urine along the collecting system. Progressive parenchymal destruction takes place, compromising renal function.

Rectal Pouch

A modification of ureteral implantation into the intact bowel was the formation of a rectal pouch, first described by Mauclaire in 1895 (Smith and Hinman, 1955). In this technique, applicable in anterior exenteration, an end sigmoid colostomy is performed, the proximal end of the rectum is closed, and both ureters are implanted into the "rectal bladder."

The capacity of reservoir ranges from 175 to 300 ml. Paull and Hodges (1955) showed that residual pressures were low in this reservoir. An isolated segment of this type can more easily be sterilized, and the likelihood of ascending infection is reduced. Unresolved remains the question of whether it is better to have rectal control of the fecal stream with a continuous urine output via a conduit or questionable rectal control of urine and a colostomy.

The concept of rectal sphincter continence appears reasonable. Unfortunately, the extensive pelvic dissection present, often in older patients, many of whom had had prior radiation therapy, compromised rectal sphincter function. These patients were continent for formed stool but could not retain urine.

With this procedure, there is no appliance to control leakage of urine, and life for these patients can become quite oppressive. Jensen and Symmonds (1965) evaluated the rectal pouch in 14 patients undergoing anterior pelvic exenteration. Eleven patients had prior radiation therapy. Ten of the patients were satisfied with this method of urinary diversion, whereas four were not. In the former group, three were totally continent; seven others were continent during the day but had some degree of urinary incontinence at night.

All but one patient in this series showed some degree of metabolic acidosis; four had hyperchloremia, and hyperkalemia was noted in over half the patients. Jensen and Symmonds (1965) concluded that the results with the rectal bladder were disappointing, particularly in the patients previously irradiated.

The Isolated Bowel Segment

From collected series, it became evident that separation of fecal and urinary streams was necessary. Twelve years after the first report of pelvic exenteration, Brunschwig and Daniel (1960) expressed a preference for conduit diversion. By 1970 Brunschwig, reflecting on a 20-year experience with pelvic exenteration, suggested that the colon conduit was far superior to ureteral implantation into the intact bowel. In 925 cases reported by 1970, the use of urinary diversion by conduit had increased to 30 per cent. That separation of the fecal and urinary streams could significantly improve prognosis was also noted by others studying the long-term effects of ureterosigmoidostomy (McConnell and Stewart, 1975; Symmonds et al., 1968). In order to separate the fecal from the urinary stream, an isolated segment of bowel taken out of continuity, with its blood supply maintained by mesentery, is used as a conduit.

The isolated intestinal segment is not meant to act as a reservoir but rather as a channel or "conduit" for conveying the urine to the outside and into an external collecting device. The advantages of this type of urinary diversion are: (1) the fecal and urinary streams are separated, thereby reducing the likelihood of ascending infection; and (2) the urine is not allowed to pool in the lumen of the bowel, thereby reducing absorption of electrolytes and resultant metabolic acidosis.

Ileal Conduit. The first report of clinical application of conduit diversion was by Bricker (1950). He used an isolated segment of ileum for the conduit. Earlier animal work had been reported by two Austrian surgeons, but the method had not been applied in the human. Shortly after Bricker's original reports, ileal conduit diversion was enthusiastically accepted by surgeons doing pelvic exenterations.

In an early report from the M.D. Anderson Hospital, Rutledge and Burns (1965) utilized three types of urinary diversion: ileal conduit, sigmoid conduit, and rectal pouch. Seventy-four patients had diversion by ileal conduit, 16 by sigmoid conduit and 7 by rectal pouch. The urinary complications were the most common postoperative problems. Twenty-six patients (35 per cent) developed urinary problems, including fistulas, malfunction, obstruction, and infection. Swan and Rutledge (1974) later reported the M.D. Anderson Hospital experience in 189 cases of pelvic exenteration with conduit diversion. Of these patients, 159 had ileal conduit diversion; 30 had diversion by sigmoid conduit.

Experience with the ileal conduit for urinary diversion has been reported by many authors. The operative mortality rates for patients with cancer have ranged from 6.2 to 14.1 per cent (Harbach et al., 1971; Ellis et al., 1971; Schmidt et al., 1973); perioperative deaths occurred from anastomotic leakage and urosepsis, acute renal failure, and gastrointestinal bleeding. Late complications in the group treated for cancer included bowel obstruction, ureteroileal obstruction, pyelonephritis, renal calculi, and stomal problems.

The highest morbidity and mortality rates have been reported in those patients with prior pelvic irradiation (Harbach et al., 1971; Ellis et al., 1971; Schmidt et al., 1973). The many problems related to ileal conduit diversion in general have been detailed by Schmidt and co-worker (1973). In a review of urinary diversions for gynecologic surgery, Leadbetter (1975) preferred the ureterosigmoidostomy alone or with a proximal colostomy for anterior exenteration and a wet colostomy or ileal conduit for total pelvic exenteration. The effects of prior radiotherapy were not mentioned.

The histologic changes in ileal conduits have been reported by Goldstein and associates (1967). Progressive villous atrophy starting at one week and complete by two years following surgery was noted in 22 patients, most of whom had received pelvic irradiation prior to diversion. Dreschner and colleagues (1973), studying multiple biopsies from an ileal conduit constructed nine months earlier, found a spectrum of atrophic changes from mild to severe. This finding suggests that the villous atrophy occurs as a patchy phenomenon.

Wrigley and co-authors (1976) reported 32 patients treated by pelvic exenteration

(17 anterior and 15 total) for gynecologic malignancy. Urinary diversion was by the standard ileal conduit. Eight patients (25 per cent) sustained ten major complications, including eight urinary fistulas and two fistulas from the ileoileal anastomosis. The authors believed that radiation therapy (used preoperatively in most of their patients) caused sufficient local tissue damage to contribute to the high morbidity rate. They recommended that the distal ileum not be used as a urinary conduit in patients who had received radiotherapy to the pelvis. The interposition of healthy tissue between the urinary conduit and the pelvis was suggested as a means of further reducing complications in total exenteration.

Sigmoid Conduit. Although the ileal conduit appeared to meet the criteria for a satisfactory method of urinary diversion, several problems were encountered by surgeons using this method for diversion in pelvic exenteration. The ileum is generally in the field of maximum irradiation when a pelvic neoplasm is treated (Figures 11–1 and 11–2). The problems encountered when the ileum is used for urinary diversion in irradiated patients are those related to healing of the ileoileal anastomosis and implantation of irradiated ureters into a heavily irradiated segment of small bowel. The radiation damage to the small bowel, sigmoid colon, and rectum has been detailed. Ptacek (1975) reported on 14 women in a three-year period requiring surgery for bowel damage related to radiation therapy for carcinoma of the cervix. Three of the patients died of further bowel complications. An alternative to ileum for conduit construction is sigmoid colon.

Parsons and Taylor (1955) reported a significant decrease in mortality in patients with diversion by a sigmoid conduit, compared to patients with ureterosigmoidostomies. There were five deaths in 27 patients with sigmoid conduits (19 per cent mortality), compared to 11 deaths in 29 patients undergoing ureterosigmoidostomy (38 per cent mortality).

Schmitz and co-workers (1960) described the use of sigmoid conduits in four patients undergoing pelvic exenteration and commented favorably on its use. More detailed evaluation of the sigmoid conduit appears

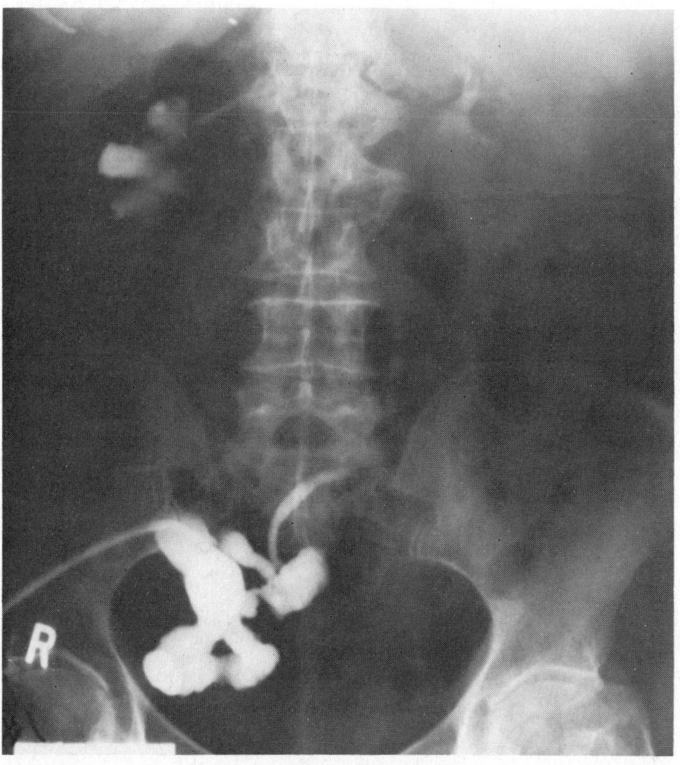

Figure 11–1. "Loopogram" showing severe radiation damage to the segment of ileum used for ileal conduit. This 63-year-old woman developed a vesicovaginal fistula subsequent to pelvic radiotherapy for cervical cancer. The ileal segment is irregular with inflamed mucosa. Bilateral reflux is seen.

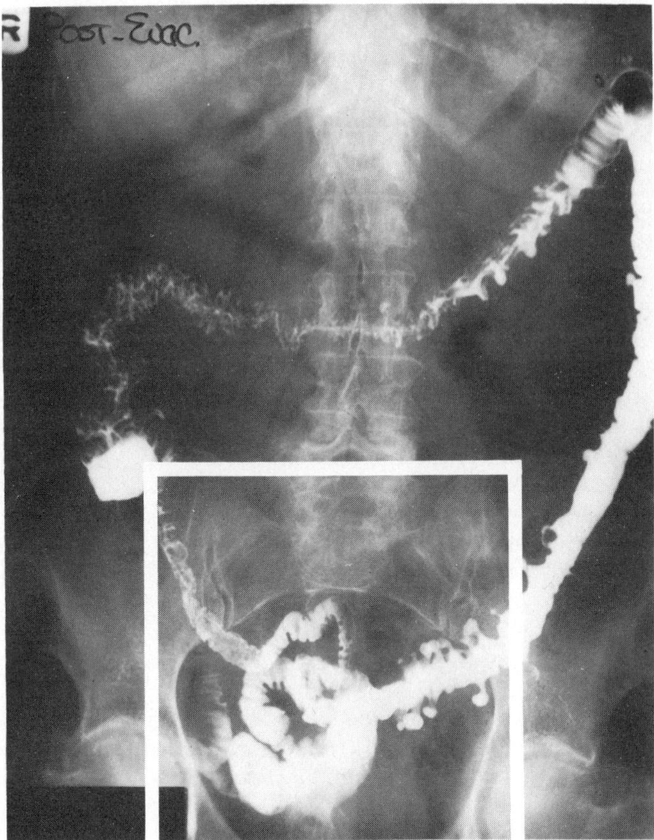

Figure 11–2. Postevacuation barium enema radiograph with field of pelvic irradiation for carcinoma of cervix outlined. Terminal ileum is within field. Note sigmoid diverticula also in field.

in reports by Kaplan and associates (1967) and by Symmonds and Gibbs (1970). Kaplan and co-workers found the residual urine in sigmoid conduits to range from 7 to 36 ml., with an emptying time of 25 to 30 minutes. The contractile pattern of the isolated sigmoid segment appeared to be mass contractions every 1 to 1½ minutes, lasting 20 to 30 sec., and reaching a pressure of 20 to 60 mm Hg.

An isolated segment of sigmoid can be effectively sterilized, thus reducing the likelihood of ascending infection. The lumen is large, allowing for adequate stomal formation. Of perhaps greater importance is the fact that a bowel anastomosis is avoided. Symmonds and Gibbs (1970), reporting on their experience with 26 sigmoid urinary conduits, thought that this offered a very satisfactory alternative to the ileal conduit. Most of their patients had had pelvic irradiation for gynecologic malignancy and were treated by total exenteration. Six patients developed hyperchloremia but none had acidosis. They recommend the ileal conduit for anterior exenteration and the sigmoid colon conduit for total exenteration. Morley and co-workers (1971) utilized sigmoid conduits in 19 of 23 women (82 per cent) undergoing anterior pelvic exenteration.

Symmonds and Jones (1975) reported on their experience with 42 sigmoid conduits in patients with pelvic exenterations. Thirteen patients developed stomal complications, five pyelonephritis, and 17 hyperchloremic acidosis. Three patients were noted to have urinary stones following surgery, one of whom had a prior stone. These authors concluded that the sigmoid conduit preserved a normal urinary tract in 12 of 34 patients studied, improved the function of previously abnormal urinary tracts in nine and failed to improve the function of abnormal urinary tracts in four patients. In nine patients there was some degree of renal deterioration following sigmoid conduit diversion.

Altwein and Hohenfellner (1975) reported the use of the sigmoid colon conduit for urinary diversion in 42 patients. The number of patients treated for malignancy or who had prior irradiation was not stated; the operative mortality was only 2 per cent (one of 42 patients).

Transverse Colon Conduit. The use of the transverse colon conduit seems ideally suited for patients undergoing pelvic exenteration following irradiation for genital malignancy. Because of a short mesentery, the transverse colon is held out of the pelvis and thus out of the field of radiation (see Figure 11–2). Its large diameter reduces the likelihood of stenosis at the site of bowel anastomosis or at the fascial or skin level. Its mobility allows stomal placement in either the right or left upper or lower quadrant. As a conduit, this bowel segment functions very satisfactorily. The transverse colon is also less likely to be the site of intrinsic disease, e.g., diverticula, than is the sigmoid colon. In this procedure the ureters can be transected well above the field of pelvic irradiation. In anterior exenteration the fecal stream can be reconstituted by a colocolic anastomosis.

The transverse colon conduit was first described by Nelson (1969). Seventeen women had urinary diversion by transverse colon conduit either as part of pelvic exenteration or for urinary tract complications following pelvic irradiation. No patient died as a result of the urinary diversion. Nelson chose the transverse colon as an alternative "to isolate an un-irradiated intestinal segment at a point high enough so that the ureter can be transected above the pelvic brim and still be long enough to perform ureterointestinal anastomoses." He later reported on over 70 women with transverse colon conduit; only three (4 per cent) developed ureterocolic strictures and hydronephrosis (Nelson, 1975).

Our earlier experience with eight patients (four having cervical carcinoma) with transverse colon conduit was reported by Schmidt and colleagues (1975). In three patients the conduit was constructed as part of an exenteration operation; the fourth woman required urinary diversion following radiation therapy for cervical cancer. Two of the eight paitents developed ureterocolic urinary leakage, presumably due to the use of irradiated ureters. Of three patients with normal preoperative excretory urograms, two remained normal. All five patients with hydronephrosis on preoperative urography showed improvement on postoperative studies.

A later report on the transverse colon conduit was based on 22 patients (Schmidt et al., 1976); included were 11 patients with cervical cancer. Indications for diversion were: radiation cystitis (7), vesicovaginal fistula (7), pelvic exenteration in previously irradiated patients (6), and ureteral obstruction (2). The operative mortality rate was 4 per cent (one death); six patients required additional surgery for complications. Preoperatively normal upper urinary tracts remained normal in six of seven patients. Of 15 patients with preoperative hydronephrosis, 10 were improved, one was stable, and one became worse after diversion; three patients were not available for urographic follow-up. Stomal problems were minimal, and renal function plus electrolyte pattern remained normal or stable. The transverse colon conduit was considered the preferred method of urinary diversion in such irradiated patients. The authors felt that the procedure should be used more extensively to prevent the problems associated with the use of damaged tissues, rather than only as a "salvage" technique.

Morales and Golimbu (1975) reported on 46 patients with diversion by colon conduit, 39 by transverse colon and seven by sigmoid colon. Over one half of their patients had a malignancy, but the number previously treated with pelvic irradiation was not stated. These authors preferred a two-layer, non-refluxing ureterocolonic anastomosis.

The authors' personal experience using transverse colon conduits in pelvic exenteration and other situations of extensive prior pelvic irradiation now totals over 40 patients. We now prefer to use this form of supravesical urinary diversion as part of a planned primary treatment, if possible, rather than as a "bail-out" procedure for complications of prior therapy. There seems to be no difference in upper urinary tract function and anatomy compared with the use of the ileal conduit segment, although experience with the latter technique has been longer and greater.

TABLE 11–2. FACTORS FOR CONSIDERATION IN CHOICES OF URINARY DIVERSION IN PATIENTS WITH MALIGNANCY

1. Curative vs. palliative approach
2. Single vs. staged procedures
3. Status of upper urinary tracts
4. Status of renal and hepatic function
5. Psychologic make-up of patient
6. Status of anal and urinary sphincters
7. Site of primary tumor; need for cystectomy
8. Presence of fistula
9. Multidisciplinary management
10. Effects of radiotherapy

SURGICAL CONSIDERATIONS

The purpose of any technique for urinary diversion is to alter the manner by which the urinary tract empties outside the body. The method of diversion must be tailored to the specific patient problem at hand. The various areas to be evaluated prior to diversion are listed in Table 11–2.

An understanding of some of the technical details of diversion, along with the advantages and disadvantages of each method, will aid in the selection of optional diversion procedures for patients undergoing pelvic exenterations. Each of the techniques of urinary diversion mentioned in this chapter and in Chapter 10 has a place in the management of obstetric and other gynecologic problems.

Use of Isolated Intestinal Segments

Ileal Conduit (Ureteroileocutaneous Anastomoses)

The standard form of supravesical urinary diversion using a segment of intestine is the ileal conduit or ileal bladder. In a typical operation the ureters are transected at or just above the level of the sacral promontory, are spatulated as needed, and then are sutured in a refluxing, end-to-side manner to the antimesenteric portion of an isolated segment of terminal ileum (Figures 11–3 through 11–5). This segment of terminal ileum (10 to 25 cm. in length), previously selected and isolated from the intestinal tract with its mesenteric blood supply intact, is used for the conduit. Intestinal continuity is reestablished with a single layer of nonabsorbable sutures for the ileoileostomy.

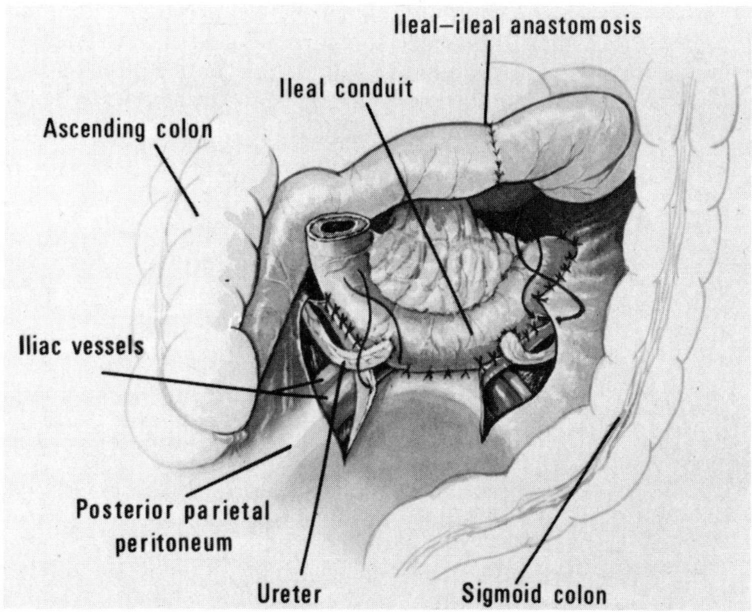

Figure 11–3. Retroperitonealization of ureteroileal anastomoses using adjacent flaps of posterior parietal peritoneum. (From Schmidt, J. D., et al.: Complications, results and problems of ileal conduit diversions. J. Urol. *109*:210–216, 1973. Copyright © The Williams & Wilkins Co., Baltimore. Reproduced by permission.)

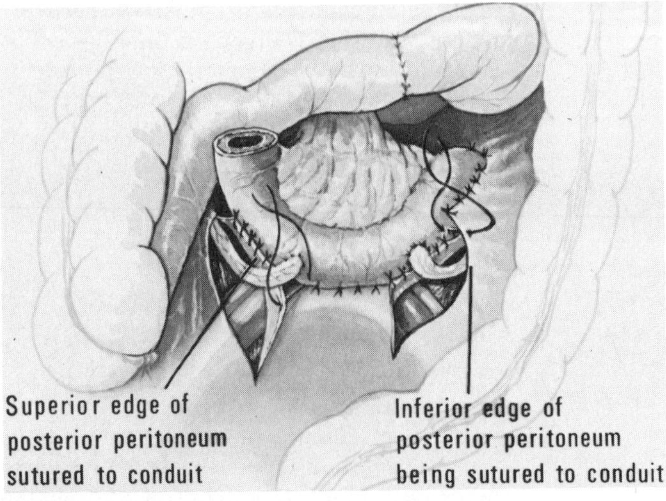

Figure 11–4. Close-up of retroperitonealization procedure. (From Schmidt, J. D., et al.: Complications, results and problems of ileal conduit diversions. J. Urol. *109:* 210–216, 1973. Copyright © The Williams & Wilkins Co., Baltimore. Reproduced by permission.)

The proximal or blind end of the isolated ileal segment is closed in one layer with the distal or stomal end brought through a full-thickness defect in the right lower quadrant or right lateral abdomen (Figures 11–6 and 11–7). Suitable stomal and appliance sites are selected prior to surgery. The ureteroileal anastomoses are made with a single layer of interrupted absorbable sutures; some authors recommend a second reinforcing layer of nonabsorbable sutures. The anastomoses are usually made separately. One variation includes a conjoint ureteral anastomosis; in another variation, the left ureter is anastomosed to the blind or proximal end of the ileal segment. The ureteroileal anastomoses can be stented or left unstented.

There has been more experience with the ileal conduit type of urointestinal diversion in exenteration than with any other form. The use of the ileum affords a segment of intestine that is generally sterile and is easy to prepare mechanically prior to surgery. Unless previously irradiated or otherwise compromised, the ileoileostomy heals per primam. The ileal segment functions as a conduit rather than as a reservoir. Thus, urinary absorption with resultant hyperchloremic acidosis is not generally a problem unless there is preexisting renal insufficiency or chronic pyelonephritis with cal-

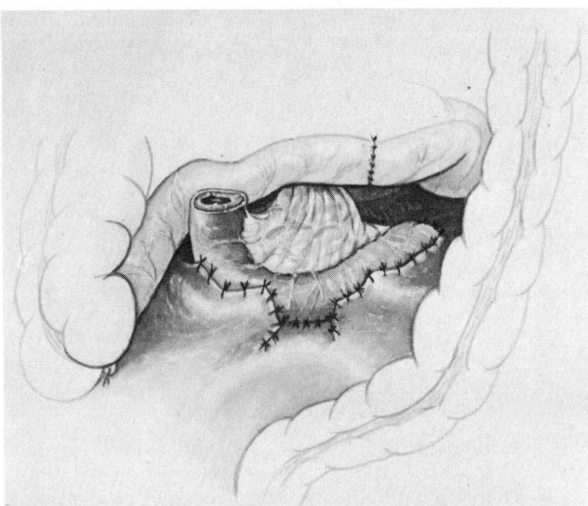

Figure 11–5. Completion of retroperitonealization of ureteroileal anastomoses. (From Schmidt, J. D., et al.: Complications, results and problems of ileal conduit diversions. J. Urol. *109*:210–216, 1973. Copyright © The Williams & Wilkins Co., Baltimore. Reproduced by permission.)

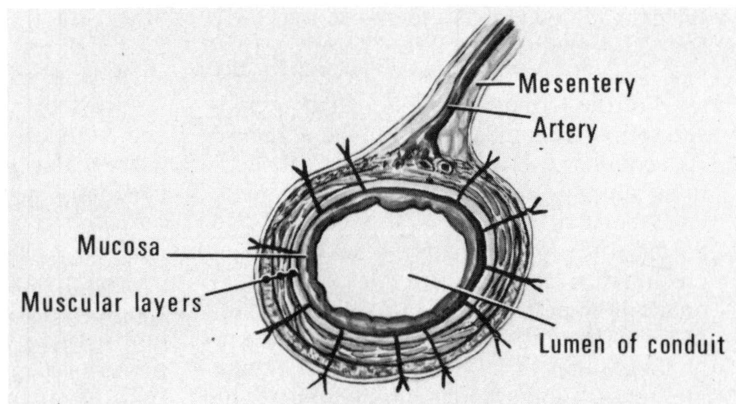

Figure 11–6. Coronal section of ileal conduit demonstrates placement of fascial sutures with reference to mesentery. (From Schmidt, J. D., et al.: Complications, results and problems of ileal conduit diversions. J. Urol. *109*:210–216, 1973. Copyright © The Williams & Wilkins Co., Baltimore. Reproduced by permission.)

culi. On the other hand, if the patient has had extensive pelvic irradiation, the segment of ileum to be used is very likely already injured by radiotherapy; its use may result in poor healing of the ileoileostomy or the ureteroileal anastomoses; or both. Subsequent problems include bowel obstruction, urinary fistula and extravasation, and pelvic abscess. In such instances a far better choice for diversion is the use of the transverse colon conduit, discussed later (Schmidt et al., 1975, 1976).

High Ileal or Pyeloileal Conduit

Variations of the ileal conduit include the *high ileal conduit* and the *pyeloileal conduit*. With the high ileal conduit, the anastomoses between the ureters and the segment of ileum take place in the proximal one third of the ureter rather than at the level of the sacral promontory. This higher location for the anastomoses is particularly useful if there is any question about the functional integrity of the ureters in cases of long-standing obstruction.

The pyeloileal conduit utilizes an end-to-side or side-to-side anastomosis directly between the renal pelvis and the segment of ileum. This is an alternative technique for use in patients with markedly dilated renal pelves where anastomoses can be performed from the anterior aspect transperitoneally. Should there be any question about the functional or mechanical integrity of the ureter, the pyeloileal conduit is indicated. The ureter below the ureteropelvic junction should be either resected or transected and ligated.

An important technical consideration for the performance of either the high ileal or the pyeloileal conduit is that the reconsti-

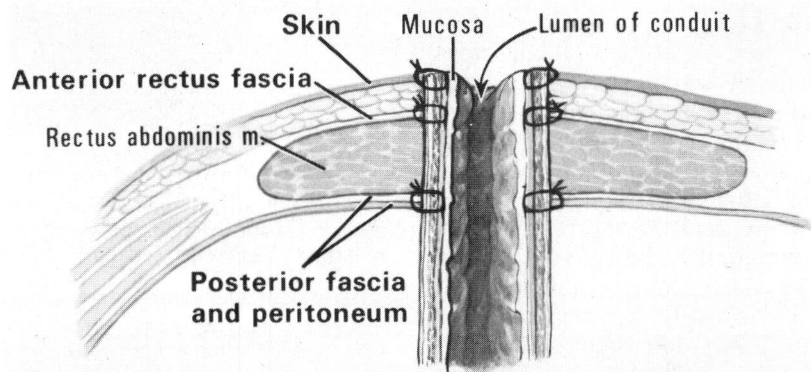

Figure 11–7. Cross section of ileal conduit traversing full-thickness abdominal wall defect. Note three-layer fixation; as an alternative, the peritoneum and anterior fascia can be combined as one layer. (From Schmidt, J. D., et al.: Complications, results and problems of ileal conduit diversions. J. Urol. *109*:210–216, 1973. Copyright © The Williams & Wilkins Co., Baltimore. Reproduced by permission.)

tuted small bowel must be placed inferiorly and the segment superiorly. A retroperitoneal tunnel for the conduit is made at the level of the kidneys. This is exactly opposite to the technique used for the standard ileal conduit, in which the ileum is reconstituted superiorly and anteriorly and the isolated segment is dropped inferiorly and posteriorly. Also, since in the pyeloileal conduit the bowel segment must reach from one kidney pelvis across to the other kidney pelvis and then to the skin, a sufficiently long segment of ileum with adequate mesentery and blood supply must be planned well in advance of the anastomoses.

Jejunal Conduit

The use of an isolated segment of jejunum, sutured either to the ureters or directly to dilated renal pelves, has been used alternatively in patients in whom for technical reasons (e.g., adhesions or irradiation) the ileum was not available. But in the presence of pelvic irradiation, the jejunum may also have suffered damage and would be best left alone, with the transverse colon conduit procedure substituted. Another major disadvantage of a jejunal conduit is the excessive absorption of urine and electrolytes with resultant severe metabolic changes. These include hypochloremic acidosis with hyponatremia, hyperkalemia, and azotemia (Morales and Whitehead, 1973).

Colonic Conduits

Transverse Colon Conduit. The transverse colon conduit is the optimal supravesical urinary diversion in exenteration for a patient who has had pelvic radiation therapy. Although the transverse colon can be ptotic or redundant, its mobility precludes its receiving the dose of irradiation usually received by the small bowel, rectosigmoid and distal ureters. The hepatic and splenic flexures are always out of the standard radiation therapy field for genital cancer (see Figure 11–2). Its redundant feature allows sufficient mobilization for anastomosis to the proximal ureters well above the field of irradiation or, if necessary, to dilated renal pelves directly. Preoperative preparation includes good mechanical cleansing of the colon as well as administration over 24 hours of a non-absorbable antibiotic such as neomycin or kanamycin sulfate.

After the pelvic exenteration has been completed, ureters that appear well vascularized and well above the field of pelvic irradiation are identified and mobilized sufficiently to bring them to the midline if necessary. The greater omentum is dissected sharply off the anterior surface of the transverse colon for a distance sufficiently long to allow the segment to reach from the posterior parietal peritoneum to either the right or left upper quadrant. If necessary, the hepatic or splenic flexure of the colon may be brought down. Care is exercised not to interfere with the blood supply via the middle colic artery in the transverse mesocolon (Figure 11–8). After a suitable length (10 to 15 cm.) has been selected, the

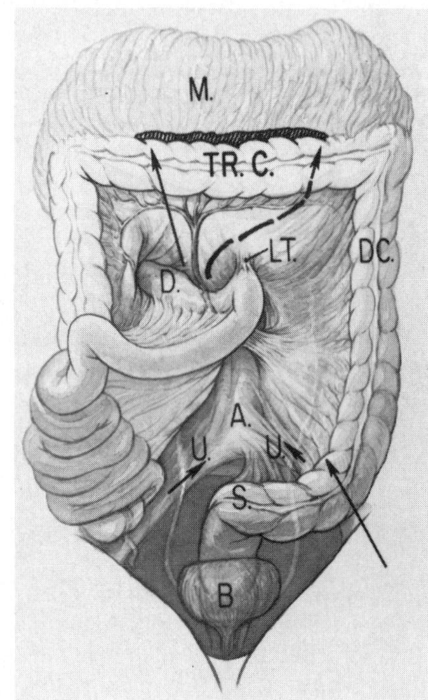

Figure 11–8. Technique of transverse colon conduit diversion: selection of segment. *M.*, Greater omentum; *TR.C.*, transverse colon; *D.*, duodenum; *LT.*, ligament of Treitz; *DC.*, descending colon; *A.*, aorta; *U.*, ureter; *S.*, sigmoid colon; *B.*, bladder. Arrows indicate positions of incisions in colon and mesocolon. Dotted arrow indicates longer mesocolic incision to increase conduit mobility. (From Schmidt, J.D., et al.: Transverse colon conduit: a preferred method of urinary diversion for radiation-treated pelvic malignancies. J. Urol. *113*:308–313, 1975. Copyright © The Williams & Wilkins Co., Baltimore. Reproduced by permission.)

transverse colon and its mesentery are divided. Mesenteric transillumination is often helpful to visualize the blood supply.

Since the colon empties by mass action and not by peristalsis, either proximal or distal end can be chosen for the stoma and the opposite end for the "blind" portion. In a typical operation, the blind end is closed with continuous 4–0 chromic gut for the mucosal-submucosal layer and with interrupted 3–0 silk for the seromuscular layer. This end is attached to the posterior parietal peritoneum near the midline with interrupted 3–0 silk sutures. Bowel continuity is reestablished by a two-layer colocolostomy, which should be free of tension (Fig. 11–9). The previously mobilized ureters are brought through a retroperitoneal tunnel to a point adjacent to the sutured blind end of the transverse colon segment, spatulated as needed and then anastomosed end-to-side to the colon near that end of the segment (Fig. 11–10). Usually a single layer of interrupted 3–0 or 4–0 chromic gut is sufficient.

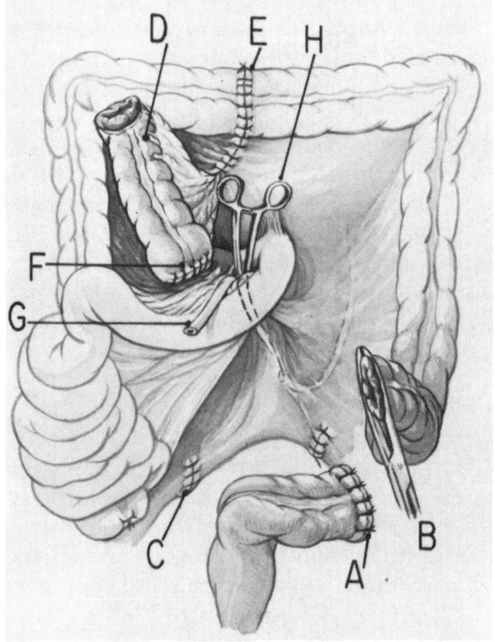

Figure 11–9. Technique of transverse colon conduit diversions. *E,* Colonic continuity restored. *D* and *F,* Isolated segment. *G* and *H,* Ureters dissected. *A* and *B,* Sigmoid resection and colostomy are optional for total exenteration. *C,* Peritoneal closure. (From Schmidt, J.D., et al.: Transverse colon conduit: a preferred method of urinary diversion for radiation-treated pelvic malignancies. J. Urol. *113*:308–313, 1975. Copyright © The Williams & Wilkins Co., Baltimore. Reproduced by permission.)

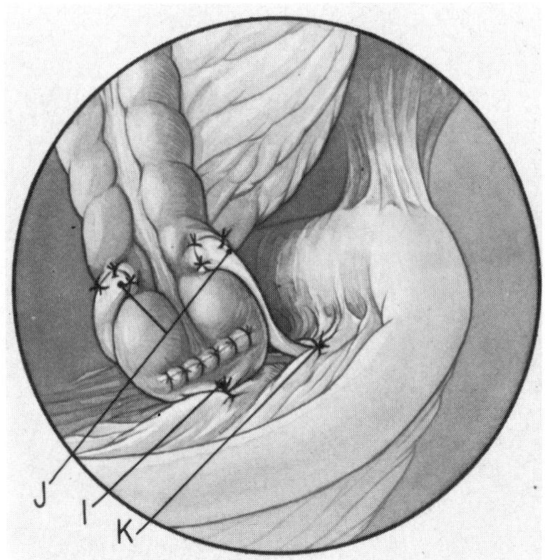

Figure 11–10. Technique of transverse colon conduit. *I,* Fixation of segment; *J.,* direct end-to-side (refluxing) ureterocolic anastomosis; *K,* retroperitonealization of anastomoses. Antireflux anastomoses are an alternative when using normal or minimally dilated ureters. (From Schmidt, J.D., et al.: Transverse colon conduit: a preferred method of urinary diversion for radiation-treated pelvic malignancies. J. Urol. *113*:308–313, 1975. Copyright © The Williams & Wilkins Co., Baltimore. Reproduced by permission.)

In our early experience we made no attempt to perform an antireflux anastomosis, because the transverse colon segment functions as a conduit and not as a reservoir. There may be an increased risk of ureteral obstruction if an antireflux ureterocolic anastomosis is performed in the standard technique as for ureterosigmoidostomy. In the last several years, however, we have successfully performed antirefluxing ureterocolic anastomoses (according to the modified Leadbetter technique) when dealing with normal or minimally dilated ureters. We continue to perform end-to-side (refluxing) anastomoses when the ureters are dilated to a diameter of 1 cm. or more. The use of ureteral stents continues to be individualized, based on factors such as renal function and degree of ureteral dilation.

The stomal end of the transverse colon segment is then brought out a full-thickness abdominal wall defect in either the right or left upper quadrant (Fig. 11–11). As for the

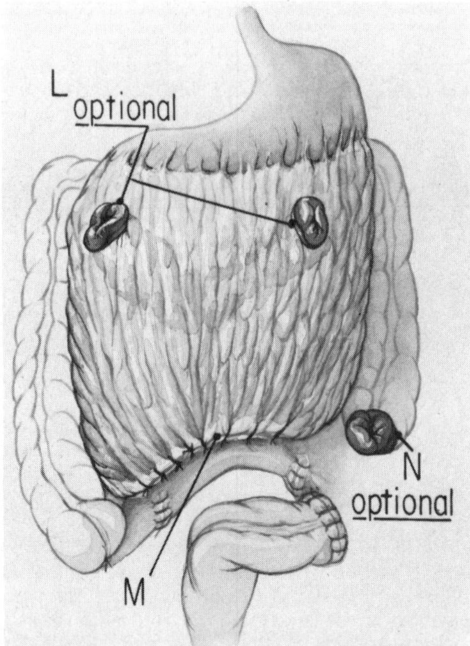

Figure 11–11. Technique of transverse colon conduit. *L,* Stomal position in either right or left upper quadrant. *N,* Optional sigmoid colostomy for total exenteration. *M,* Omental covering of viscera. (From Schmidt, J.D., et al.: Transverse colon conduit: a preferred method of urinary diversion for radiation-treated pelvic malignancies. J. Urol. *113*:308–313, 1975. Copyright © The Williams & Wilkins Co., Baltimore, Reproduced by permission.)

standard ileal conduit, the site of the stoma should be selected prior to surgery for optimal use of an external appliance. Formation of the stoma is similar to that of the ileal conduit in that the peritoneum and anterior fascia can be sutured to each other and then sutured to the seromuscular layer of the conduit. If desired, the peritoneum and anterior fascia can be sutured separately to the seromuscular layers. Either a "flush" or "rosebud" type of skin anastomosis is made with absorbable suture material.

If at all possible, a rosebud, protruding type stoma should be constructed. A fine chromic or polyglycolic acid suture is passed between the everted mucosa of the bowel segment and the adjacent subcuticular tissue. Interrupted suturing using this technique prevents unsightly skin scarring, reduces peristomal inflammation, and results in a stoma more easily cared for by both patient and nursing staff.

Examples of urographic studies in patients with diversions by the transverse colon conduit are shown in Figures 11–12 through 11–18.

Descending or Sigmoid Colonic Conduit. Either the descending or sigmoid portion of the left colon is available for use as a conduit for urine to the skin. In patients irradiated for genital cancers, the sigmoid and possibly a portion of the descending colon may have received high doses of radiation. The chance of postoperative complications when such a segment of bowel is chosen for a conduit is high (Figure 11–2).

If sufficient length of the descending colon above the field of irradiation can be obtained for a conduit, this can eliminate the colonic anastomosis. In this situation the terminal colostomy will be that portion of the colon just proximal to the proximal end of the colon selected for the conduit. Since the colon distal to the conduit segment is resected as part of a total exenteration, no bowel anastomosis is required.

The technique of ureterocolic anastomosis is essentially the same, except that the right ureter may have to be mobilized further in order to reach the colon. If at all possible, the colonic conduit length should be sufficient to minimize the amount of ureteral dissection. It is better in principle to bring the bowel to the ureters than the ureters to the bowel. Again, sites for the stoma should be made prior to surgery. We find that patients requiring both a colostomy and a urinary conduit do better with two appliances and belts at a different level than with two stomas at the same level, with overlapping of appliances and belts.

For the woman who requires only an anterior exenteration with a sigmoid colon conduit, reconstruction of the large bowel should be by two-layer closure. A sigmoid colon conduit stoma is pictured in Figure 11–19.

Intestinal Tract in Continuity (Intact Bowel)

Ureterosigmoidostomy

The main advantages of supravesical diversion via ureterosigmoidostomy are the use of the terminal colon as a reservoir

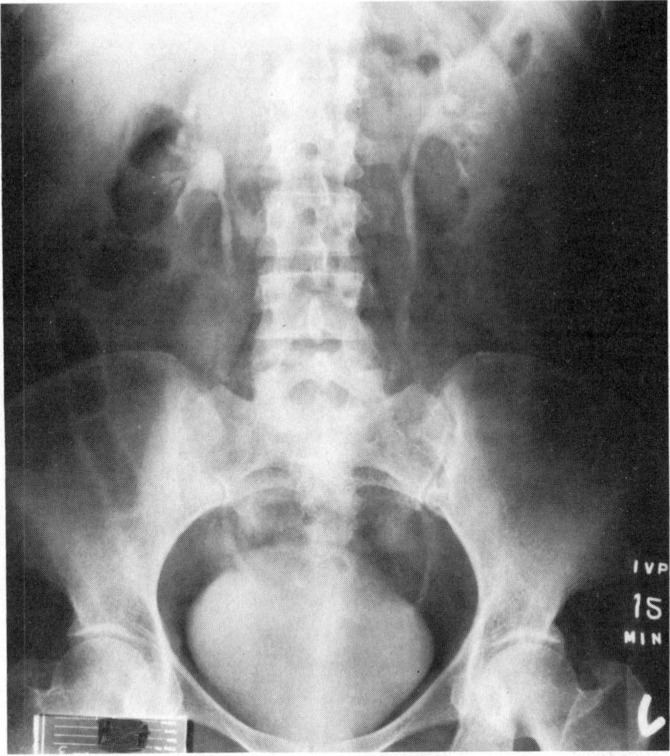

Figure 11–12. Normal upper urinary tracts on preoperative intravenous pyelogram of a 44-year-old patient with cervical cancer. (From Schmidt, J. D., et al.: Transverse colon conduit: a preferred method of urinary diversion for radiation-treated pelvic malignancies. J. Urol. *113*:308–313, 1975. Copyright © The Williams & Wilkins Co., Baltimore. Reproduced by permission.)

rather than as a conduit, the absence of a stoma and appliance, and the lack of a bowel anastomosis.

Contraindications. It must be emphasized that such a urinary diversion should *not* be performed in two specific situations:

(1) in the presence of pelvic irradiation, and

(2) with dilated, obstructed ureters.

In the first situation the consequences of poor healing with resultant urinary extravasation, fistula, abscess and renal impairment are a real danger and threat to the patient. In the second situation, the existing renal impairment is magnified by urine absorption across the rectosigmoid mucosa, causing a metabolic hyperchloremic acidosis, leading to progressive renal insufficiency, renal calculi, and pyelonephritis.

Preoperative Considerations. Thus, in the patient who will be treated with an anterior pelvic exenteration and has no history of radiotherapy, fairly normal ureters, and a normal rectosigmoid and anal sphincter, the ureterosigmoidostomy is an alternative form of diversion. A preliminary barium enema should be performed along with a proctoscopy, in a search for specific intestinal pathology that would make the procedure unwise. Also, the functional integrity of the anal sphincter should be carefully elucidated. The patient may have no trouble holding solid fecal material, but may have considerable difficulty holding a water or saline enema and thus be incontinent of urine per rectum after a technically successful operation.

As in the performance of a conduit operation using the large bowel, the patient should be prepared with mechanical cleansing and preoperative oral nonabsorbable antibiotics.

Surgical Technique. After the anterior exenteration has been performed, the mobilized proximal ureters are anastomosed end-to-side, in an antirefluxing manner, along the colonic taenia by one of several techniques. Often these anastomoses are stented, with the ureteral catheters passed through a large-caliber rectal tube. This tube drains the rectosigmoid and exits per rectum, carrying the ureteral catheters to drainage bags. Such ureteral stents are usually left in place 7 to 10 days.

If a patient later has trouble with a ure-

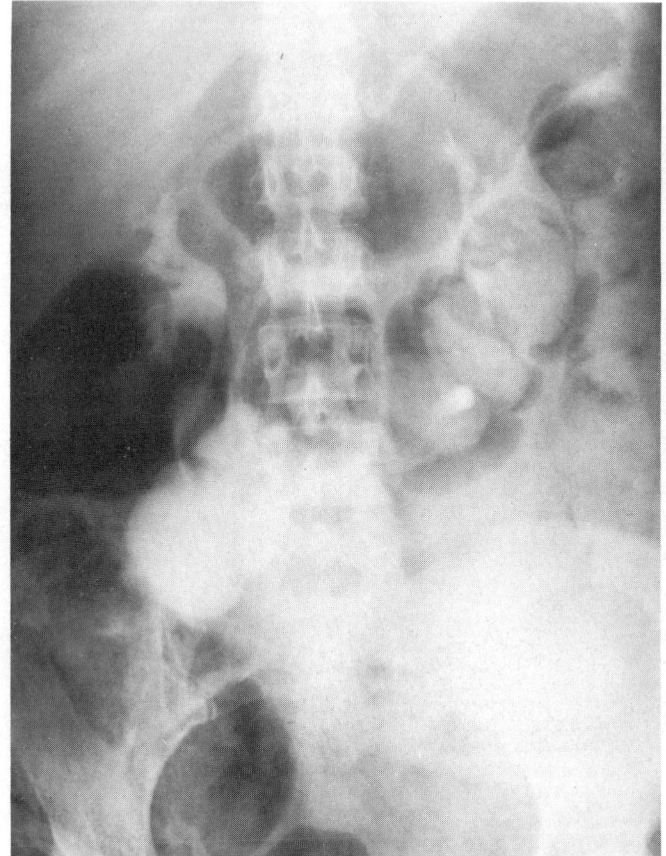

Figure 11–13. Normal upper urinary tracts on intravenous pyelogram two weeks following creation of transverse colon conduit and total exenteration. (From Schmidt, J.D., et al.: Transverse colon conduit; a preferred method of urinary diversion for radiation-treated pelvic malignancies. J. Urol. *113*:308–313, 1975. Copyright © The Williams & Wilkins Co., Baltimore. Reproduced by permission.)

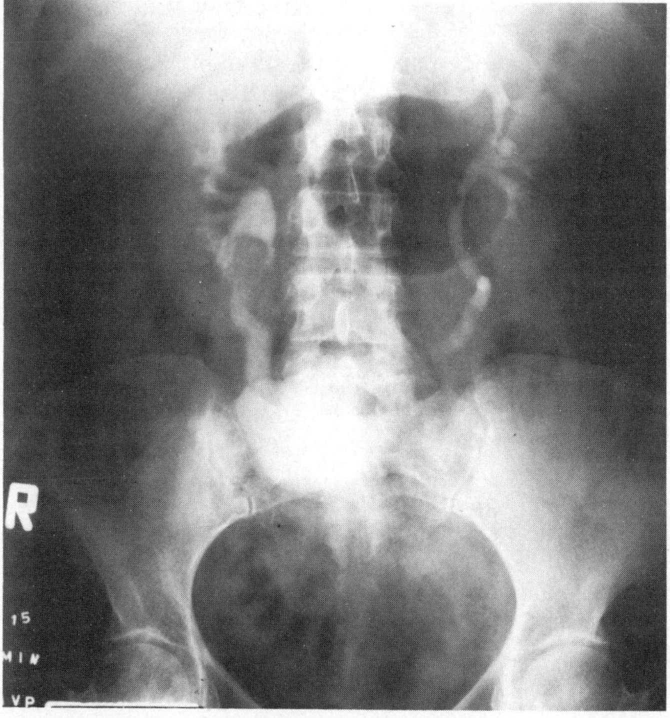

Figure 11–14. Same patient as in Figures 11–12 and 11–13. Normal upper urinary tracts on intravenous pyelogram two years after diversion by transverse colon conduit. (From Schmidt, J.D., et al.: Transverse colon conduit: a preferred method of urinary diversion for radiation-treated pelvic malignancies. J. Urol. *113*:308–313, 1975. Copyright © The Williams & Wilkins Co., Baltimore. Reproduced by permission.)

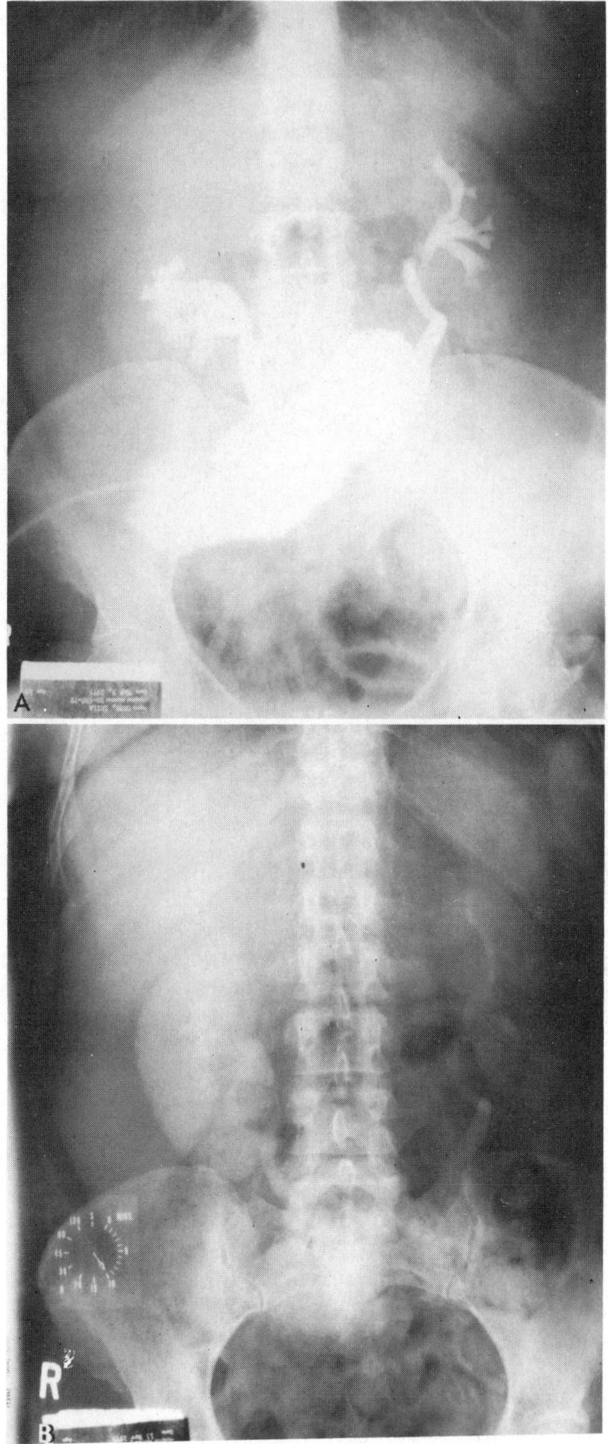

Figure 11–15. Same patient as in Figures 11–12 and 11–14. Conduitogram *(A)* and IVP *(B)* five years after diversion by transverse colon conduit and total exenteration. Upper urinary tracts remain normal in spite of reflux.

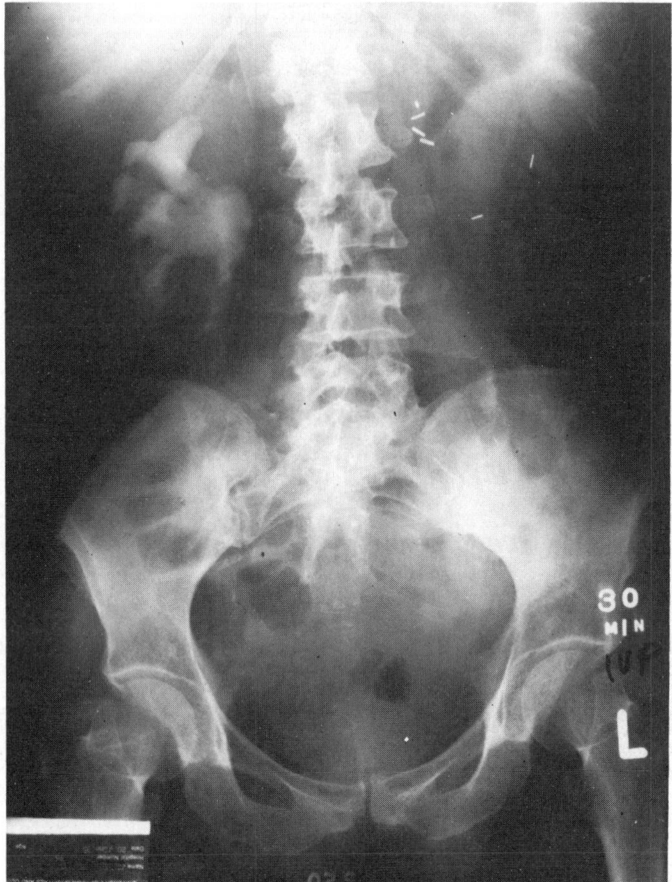

Figure 11–16. Excretory urogram three months following pyelo-transverse colic anastomosis and left nephrectomy in a 54-year-old woman with cervical cancer and vesicovaginal fistula following radiotherapy. Right hydronephrosis markedly improved compared to prediversion study. (From Schmidt, J.D., et al.: Transverse colon conduit for supravesicular urinary tract diversion. Urology *3*: 542–546, 1976. Reproduced by permission.)

terosigmoidostomy, because of rectal incontinence or progressive ureteral obstruction and infection, the diversion can be converted into an ileal or colonic conduit.

Variations. A variation of the ureterosigmoidostomy adds transection of the colon well above the level of the anastomoses and the making of an end colostomy of the proximal colon (rectal pouch). Thus, the patient wears an appliance for a colostomy, whereas urine enters the rectosigmoid as a reservoir emptied at will. An advantage of this variation is that with the diversion of the fecal stream away from the ureterosigmoidostomy reservoir, the chances of ascending infection and progressive renal deterioration are diminished.

If, in the performance of a ureterosigmoidostomy, it is seen that the right ureter is not of sufficient length to be mobilized safely to make an anastomosis to the colon, the technique of transureteroureterostomy may be applied. For this procedure, the right ureter is dissected proximally so that a sufficient length is available to pass retroperitoneally for direct end-to-side anastomosis to the left ureter well above the left ureterocolic anastomosis. This transureteroureterostomy may be difficult to stent. A watertight anastomosis should be performed with good extraperitoneal drainage (see Chapter 9).

Wet Colostomy. The main advantage of a wet colostomy is that the patient needs only a single appliance over a single stoma, the bowel, which acts as a cloaca. The procedure is technically simpler than the creation of a separate colonic conduit segment, since no bowel anastomosis is required. After total pelvic exenteration has been performed, the proximal mobilized ureters are sutured end-to-side to the segment of colon proximal to the end colostomy. Stenting for a period of 7 to 10 days is optional. The degree of urine absorption with resultant metabolic acidosis depends

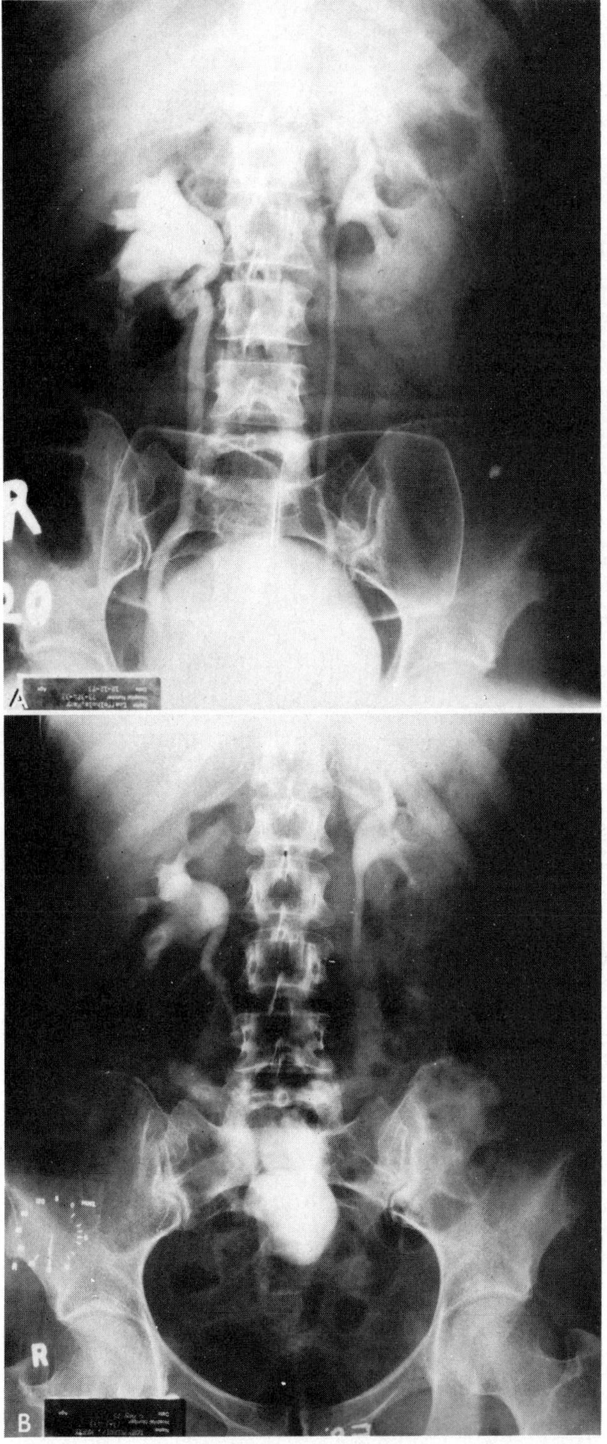

Figure 11–17. *A,* Preoperative intravenous pyelogram. Right hydroureteronephrosis in 40-year-old woman with cervical cancer and treated with irradiation. *B,* Normal upper tracts 18 months after transverse colon conduit diversion. (From Schmidt, J.D., et al.: Transverse colon conduit for supravesical urinary tract diversion. Urology *3*:542–546, 1976. Reproduced by permission.)

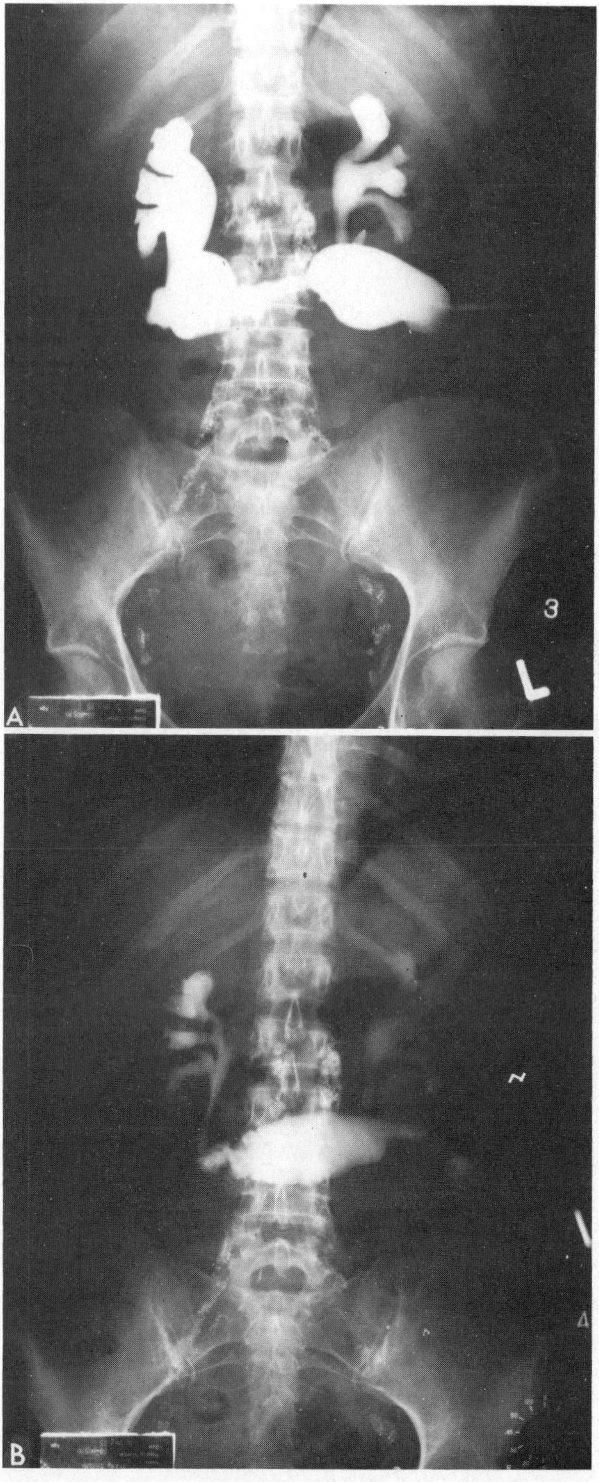

Figure 11–18. Conduitograms one year following transverse colon conduit diversion for radiation injury related to pelvic malignancy treatment in a 42-year-old woman. *A*, Overdistention produces "hydronephrosis" bilaterally. *B*, Drainage film demonstrates no obstruction. Intravenous pyelogram was normal. (From Schmidt, J.D., et al.: Transverse colon conduit for supravesical urinary tract diversion. Urology *3*:542–546, 1976. Reproduced by permission.)

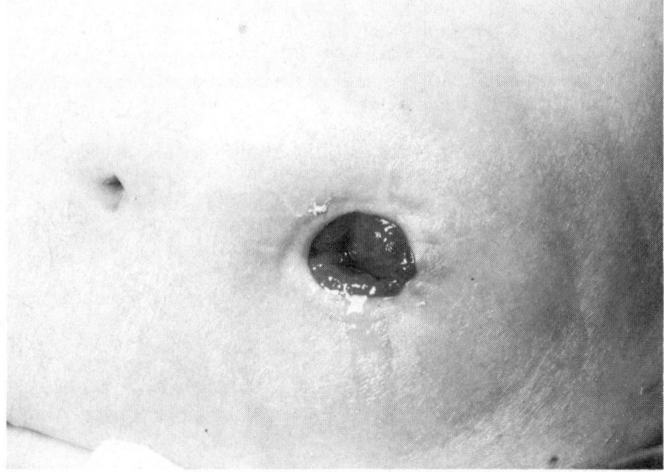

Figure 11–19. Mature stoma of sigmoid colon conduit in left lower quadrant. A few bits of adhesive remain near mucocutaneous junction.

on any existing renal disease as well as the amount of surface area available for such absorption.

Many patients have had a psychologic problem adjusting to a stoma that continually drains urine as well as intermittently draining fecal material. As might be expected, flushing enemas of a wet colostomy are hazardous, promoting ascending infection into the ureters and kidneys.

SUMMARY

For the patient with pelvic malignancy and prior irradiation therapy scheduled for exenteration, the transverse colon conduit is the method of choice for urinary diversion. In fact this method has wide application as a method of supravesical urinary diversion. Yet a knowledge of the various forms of and indications for urinary diversion will be of immeasurable help to the physician responsible for such patients. As Brunschwig (1970) said: "After doing some 800 bilateral ureteral diversions for various stages and forms of advanced pelvic cancer, I have come to the conclusion that there is no *one* method. The surgeon attacking those (problems) must be prepared to utilize any one of several methods, and we have used all of them."

REFERENCES

Altwein, J. E., and Hohenfellner, R.: Use of the colon as a conduit for urinary diversion. Surg. Gynec. Obstet. *140*:33, 1975.

Bricker, E. M.: Bladder substitution after pelvic evisceration. Surg. Clin. North Am. *30*:1511, 1950.

Brunschwig, A.: Some reflections on pelvic exenteration after twenty years' experience. *In* Sturgis, S. H., and Taymore, M. L. (eds.): Progress in Gynecology, Vol. V. New York, Grune and Stratton, 1970.

Brunschwig, A., and Daniel, W.: Pelvic exenteration operations: with summary of sixty-six cases surviving more than five years. Ann. Surg. *151*:571, 1960.

Douglas, R. G., and Sweeney, W.: Exenteration operations in treatment of advanced pelvic cancer. Am. J. Obstet. Gynecol. *73*:1109, 1957.

Dreschner, E. E., Goldstein, M. J., Melamed, M. R., et al.: A histological and kinetic study of an ileal conduit. Gastroenterology *64*:920, 1973.

Ellis, L. R., Udall, D. A., and Hodges, C. V.: Further clinical experience with intestinal segments for urinary diversion. J. Urol. *105*:354, 1971.

Ferris, D. O., and Odel, H. M.: Electrolyte pattern of the blood after bilateral ureterosigmoidostomy. J.A.M.A. *142*:634, 1950.

Goldstein, M. J., Melamed, M. R., Grabstald, H., et al.: Progressive villous atrophy of the ileum used as a urinary conduit. Gastroenterology *52*:859, 1967.

Harbach, L. B., Hall, R. L., Cockett, A. T. K., et al.: Ileal loop cutaneous urinary diversion: critical review. J. Urol. *105*:511, 1971.

Irvine, W. T., Yule, J. H. B., Arnott, D. G., et al.: Reduction in colonic mucosal absorption with reference to the chemical imbalance of ureterocolostomy. Proc. R. Soc. Med. *53*:1021, 1960.

Jensen, P. A., and Symmonds, R. E.: The rectosigmoid urinary reservoir with anterior pelvic exenterations: An evaluation. Obstet. Gynecol. *26*:786, 1965.

Kaplan, A. L., Hulme, G. W., Laskowski, T., et al.: The sigmoid conduit as a means of urinary diversion. South. Med. J., *60*:688, 1967.

Leadbetter, W. F., *In* Meigs, J. V., and Sturgis, S. H. (eds.): Progress in Gynecology, Vol. III. New York, Grune and Stratton, 1975, p. 713.

McConnell, J. B., and Stewart, W. K.: The long-term management and social consequences of ureterosigmoid anastomoses. Br. J. Urol. *47*:607, 1975.

Morales, P., and Golimbu, M.: Colonic urinary diversion: 10 years of experience. J. Urol. *113*:302, 1975.

Morales, P. A., and Whitehead, E. D.: High jejunal conduit for supravesical urinary diversion: report of 25 cases. Urology *1*:426, 1973.

Morley, G. W., Lindenauer, S. M., and Cerny, J. C.: Pelvic exenterative surgery in recurrent pelvic carcinoma. Am. J. Obstet. Gynecol. *109*:1175, 1971.

Nelson, J. H., Jr.: Atlas of Radical Pelvic Surgery. New York, Appleton-Century-Crofts, 1969, p. 181.

Nelson, J. H., Jr.: Personal communication, 1975.

Parsons, L., and Taylor, M.: Longevity following pelvic exenteration for cervical carcinoma. Am. J. Obstet. Gynecol. *70*:774, 1955.

Paull, D. P., and Hodges, C. V.: The rectosigmoid colon as a bladder substitute. J. Urol. *740*:360, 1955.

Ptacek, J. J.: Bowel damage after radiation therapy of carcinoma of the cervix. J. Iowa Med. Soc. *64*:510, 1975.

Rutledge, F. N., and Burns, B. C., Jr.: Pelvic exenteration. Am. J. Obstet. Gynecol, *91*:692, 1965.

Schmidt, J. D., Buchsbaum, H. J., and Jacobo, E. C.: Transverse colon conduit for supravesical urinary tract diversion. Urology *8*:542, 1976.

Schmidt, J. D., Flocks, R. H., and Arduino, L.: Transureteroureterostomy in the management of distal ureteral disease. J. Urol. *108*:240, 1972.

Schmidt, J. D., Hawtrey, C. E., and Buchsbaum, H. J.: Transverse colon conduit: a preferred method of urinary diversion for radiation-treated pelvic malignancies. J. Urol. *113*:308, 1975.

Schmidt, J. D., Hawtrey, C. E., Flocks, R. H., and Culp, D. A.: Complications, results and problems of ileal conduit diversions. J. Urol. *109*:210, 1973.

Schmitz, R. L., Schmitz, H. E., Smith, C. J., et al.: Details of pelvic exenteration evolved during an experience with 75 cases. Am. J. Obstet. Gynecol. *80*:43, 1960.

Smith, D. H., and Hinman, F., Jr.: The rectal bladder (colostomy with ureterosigmoidostomy): Experimental and clinical aspects. J. Urol. *74*:354, 1955.

Scott, W. W.: Methods of urinary diversion in radical pelvic surgery. Clin. Obstet. Gynecol. *8*:726, 1965.

Swan, R. W., and Rutledge, F. N.: Urinary conduit in pelvic cancer patients. A report of 16 years experience. Am. J. Obstet. Gynecol. *119*:6, 1974.

Symmonds, R. E., and Gibbs, C. P.: Urinary diversion by way of sigmoid conduit. Surg. Gynecol. Obstet. *131*:687, 1970.

Symmonds, R. E., and Jones, I. V.: Sigmoid conduit urinary diversion after exenteration. *In* Taymor, M. L., and Green, T. H., Jr. (eds.): Progress in Gynecology, Vol. VI. New York, Grune and Stratton, 1975, p. 729.

Symmonds, R. E., Pratt, J. H., and Welch, J. S.: Exenterative operations: experience with 118 patients. Am. J. Obstet. Gynecol. *101*:66, 1968.

Wrigley, J. V., Prem, K. A., and Fraley, E. E.: Pelvic exenteration: complications of urinary diversion. J. Urol. *116*:428, 1976.

12

POSTOPERATIVE BLADDER DRAINAGE

PAUL C. PETERS, M.D.

Postoperative urinary bladder drainage is indicated to prevent overdistention and subsequent infection. Muscular injury from overdistention in a patient obtunded by anesthesia, analgesics, or soporifics may greatly prolong the period required to regain normal bladder function and increase the likelihood of cystitis and pyelonephritis (Mehrotra, 1953; Lapides et al., 1968; Lapides et al., 1972). As stated by Campbell (1961), "Retention, rather than catheterization, is the thing to be feared." This is especially true if there is present superimposed partial denervation of the urinary bladder from a pelvic surgical procedure, such as radical hysterectomy by the abdominal (Wertheim) or vaginal (Shauta) route (vanNagell et al., 1972). Three degrees of injury to the pelvic plexus with resulting varying degrees of atony and lack of contractility of the urinary bladder have been characterized by Hohenfellner and associates (1980). The most severe degree of injury requires months for return of bladder function. Permanent residual atony and hypotonicity secondary to denervation are rarely associated with radical hysterectomy (Seski and Diokno, 1977).

SUPRAPUBIC TECHNIQUES

Bladder drainage can be carried out by the suprapubic route (Bonanno et al., 1970) (Figure 12–1*A*,*B*) or the transurethral route (Robertson, 1973). The author prefers suprapubic drainage with a soft No. 20 French Malecot catheter introduced into the bladder through an 8 or 9 mm. suprapubic incision made over a perforated male No. 20 French urethral sound (Shute and MacKinnon, 1970). The catheter is tied to a size 0 silk suture passed through the perforation in the male sound. The perforation is located about 5 mm. from the tip of the sound. The Malecot catheter is tied to the sound and pulled to the urethral meatus as the sound is withdrawn. There the suture may be visualized and cut, allowing the catheter to retract into the urinary bladder (Figure 12–2). The catheter is secured to the abdominal wall by means of a size 0 nonabsorbable suture and connected to sterile closed gravity drainage. A Foley catheter may be used instead of a Malecot or Pezzar type catheter, but because of the occasional discomfort and spasm associated with the balloon catheter (Foley, 1937), the author suggests the use of the Malecot catheter. We agree with Hodgkinson and Hodari (1966) that the cystotomy should be done at the start of the operative procedure.

Formerly, the author used a Lowsley curved prostatic retractor and cut down upon it suprapubically, forced the instrument through the cystotomy, opened its jaws, and then tightened them to grasp the catheter to be introduced, pulled the catheter into the bladder, disengaged it from the Lowsley retractor, closed the jaws of the Lowsley retractor, and withdrew it as one

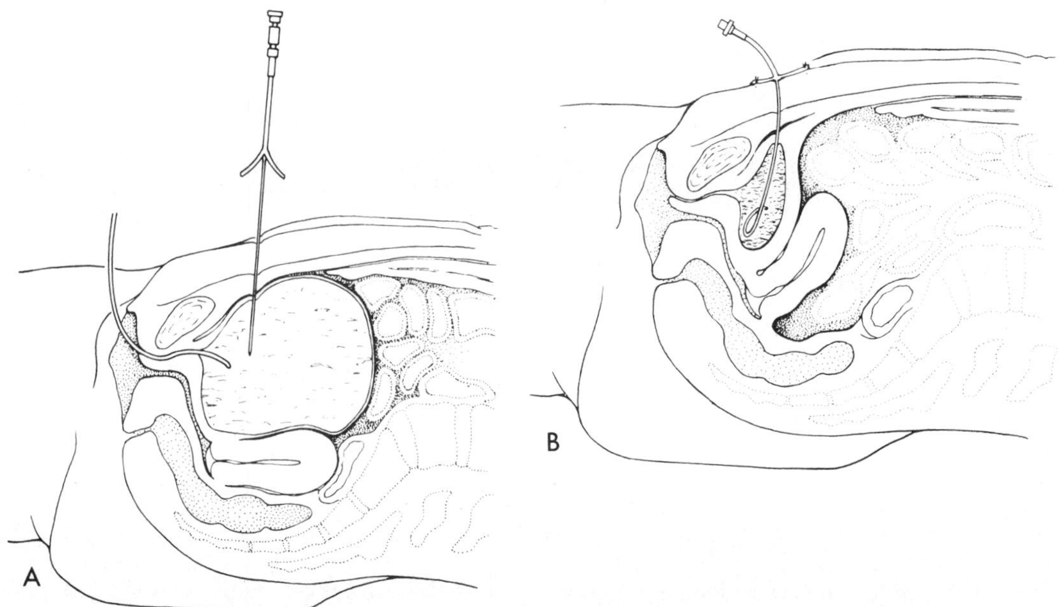

Figure 12–1. *A,* The No. 14 gauge Bonanno catheter, held straight within the lumen of a No. 18 gauge needle, is inserted into the distended bladder, with the patient in the supine position. *B,* Following removal of the intraluminal needle, the distal segment of the Bonanno catheter resumes its memory curve. Skin fixation is accomplished by taping or suturing the bifurcation sleeve to the skin. (Reproduced with permission from Bonanno, P. J., Landers, D. E., and Rock, D. E.: Bladder drainage with the suprapubic bladder needle. Obstet. Gynecol. *35*:807, 1970.)

would a urethral sound. For the past 10 years, the method originally suggested by Shute and MacKinnon (1970) using the perforated male urethral sound already described, has been preferred.

By a variety of transurethral techniques (Robertson, 1973), a No. 18 to 22 French catheter can be introduced through an 8 or 9 mm. incision, which usually closes functionally within 2 hours after the catheter has been removed even if it has been in place for weeks. Exceptions to this cause one to invoke the *"law of fistula,"* which states that "when the normal pathway is open, a fistula will close unless it is tuberculosis, completely epithelialized, contains a foreign body, or is the site of another infectious granuloma or a carcinoma." Persistent drainage means that either the normal pathway is not open or that one of the five previously described complications exists, and further inspection of the cystotomy site is warranted.

In the author's experience in 27 years of urologic surgery, the most common cause for a failure of a suprapubic sinus to close has been a previously unappreciated functional disturbance at the vesical neck or a urethral stricture. I have seen three cases of self-inflicted trauma to the sinus tract in mentally deranged patients resulting in a persistent vesicocutaneous fistula.

Infrequently, the transurethral route cannot be used, and one of the acceptable trocar methods is substituted to achieve suprapubic drainage (Hodgkinson and Hodari, 1966; Ingram, 1975). To minimize the risk of infection, the patient should connect the catheter to closed drainage using a leg bag when awake and a dependent bedside reservoir when asleep. It is unwise for the patient to sleep with the catheter connected only to a small leg bag, as back pressure on the upper tracts and reflux of possibly contaminated urine may occur if the bag becomes distended.

Even less frequently, a formal cystostomy is necessary in an individual who has had previous lower abdominal midline procedures. In such patients, loops of small bowel are adherent in the area of the symphysis pubis. A patient with a tiny, contracted, scarred bladder that cannot be distended to carry the peritoneal reflection to

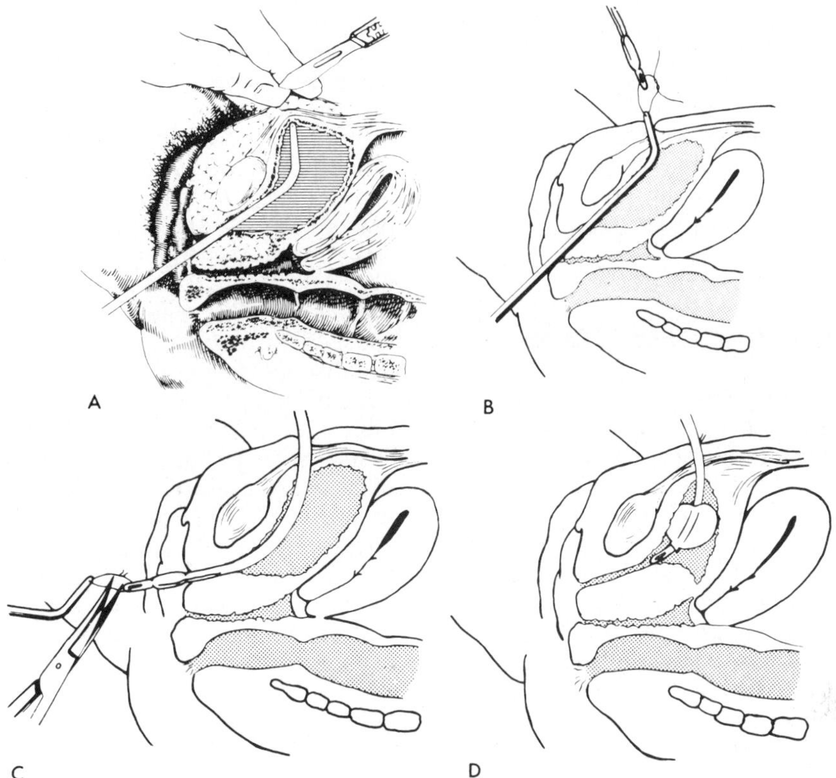

Figure 12–2. Suprapubic cystostomy by transurethral male sound. *A,* A scalpel is used to cut down on the easily palpable sound tip. *B,* The Foley catheter is tied through a 5 mm. hole in the sound. *C,* The catheter is drawn out of the urethra and the suture is cut. *D,* The catheter is then pulled into the bladder and the balloon is inflated. (Reproduced with permission from Wilson, E. A., Sprague, A. D., and vanNagell, J. R., Jr. Suprapubic cystostomy in gynecologic surgery: a comparison of two methods. Am. J. Obstet. Gynecol. *115*:991, 1973.)

the level of the symphysis will need an open exposure for formal cystostomy.

When one needs to perform a formal cystostomy, the abdominal incision should be made large enough to permit inspection of the surface of the urinary bladder (Figure 12–3). Usually an 8 to 10 cm. skin incision is adequate (either transverse or vertical). Avoid incising the periosteum of the pubis to minimize the risk of osteitis pubis. The rectus abdominis muscles are separated in the midline, and the extraperitoneal space is opened. The urinary bladder is usually identified by the large veins traversing its surface. Identification may be facilitated by distending the bladder with fluid introduced transurethrally or by passing a No. 20 French male urethral sound per urethra to palpate the tip of the sound within the bladder.

The author prefers to open the bladder by puncturing it with a tonsil hemostat, next spreading the tips of the clamp to enlarge the cystotomy opening to allow insertion of the index finger for exploration of the urinary bladder. One must be careful to identify the bladder and to ascertain that there are no loops of bowel adherent anteriorly before making the puncture wound. Bleeding from the urinary bladder will be much less if it is not cut with a knife but is opened with a puncture wound and enlarged by spreading the bladder muscles apart with the index fingers. A suitable suprapubic tube is inserted, usually a No. 20 French Malecot catheter, and a purse-string suture of 3-0 or 4-0 chromic gut is placed in the bladder musculature, but not through the mucosa, and tied to the catheter to secure it in place. Rarely, when the 3-0 chromic gut purse-string suture has not dissolved, the suprapubic tube can be removed by cutting the suture with a knife blade introduced alongside the suprapubic tube.

If possible, the suprapubic tube is brought through a separate stab wound in the bladder, and the original cystotomy is closed in three layers with 4-0 chromic gut to the mucosa, 3-0 chromic gut to the muscle layer, and 3-0 chromic gut to the adventitial layer.

TRANSURETHRAL TECHNIQUES

In considering the use of a transurethral Silastic retention catheter versus a suprapubic Malecot or a trocar catheter for postoperative bladder drainage, individual case judgment is applied. The author recommends a transurethral Silastic retention catheter of No. 18 to 20 French diameter when catheter drainage of less than 5 days is anticipated and little urethral repair work is to be done, i.e., simple hysterectomy or excision of a small urethral diverticulum. For prolonged catheter drainage, as is needed in patients with pelvic injuries following auto/pedestrian accidents, bladder or urethral ruptures, radical pelvic surgery, or pelvic exenteration, suprapubic drainage is preferred. The suprapubic tube should be placed high in the dome of the bladder, away from the trigone, and brought out obliquely through the abdominal wall (Figure 12–3). This minimizes the morbidity caused by a suprapubic tube, which is usually much more comfortable for the patient than an indwelling urethral catheter.

As there are no neurogenic vesical or obstructive urethral complications in over 95 per cent of gynecologic surgical procedures performed, many gynecologists prefer to use the Cystocath (Dow Corning). This kit allows one to use the suprapubic trocar method of insertion of a No. 12 French catheter of Silastic material, which

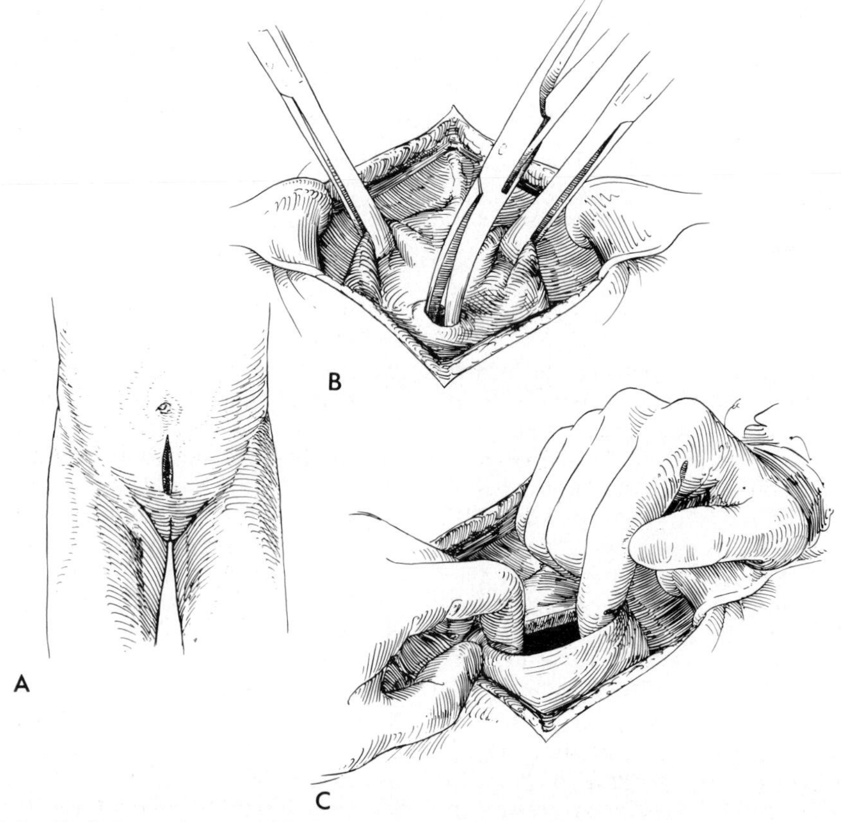

Figure 12–3. Technique of suprapubic cystotomy. *A,* A lower midline incision is made and the bladder is exposed. *B,* Between two Allis forceps a tonsil forceps is inserted quickly through the bladder wall. Failure to insert with quick sustained motion results in dissection of bladder mucosa from muscle and complicates bladder entry. *C,* Opposing index fingers open bladder bluntly, thereby minimizing bleeding.
Illustration continued on opposite page

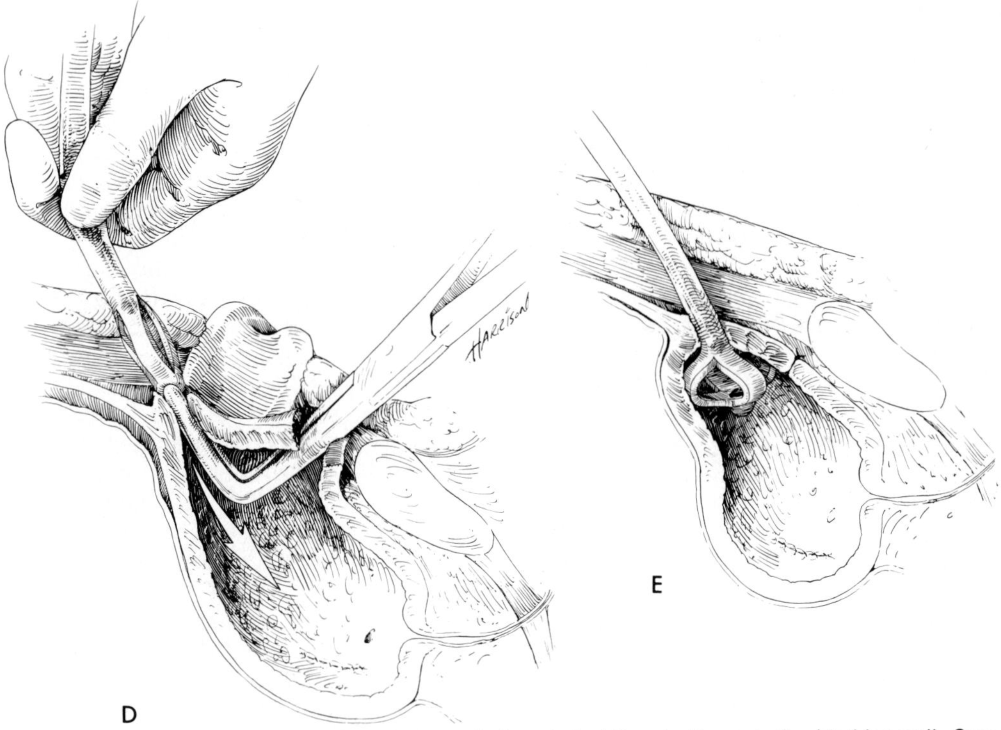

Figure 12-3 *Continued. D,* A Malecot catheter is inserted obliquely through the bladder wall. Care is taken to dissect the peritoneum free of the bladder dome to avoid bowel injury. *E,* A cystostomy tube is placed in oblique tunnel to decrease chance of fistula formation. (Reproduced with permission from Bright, T. C., III, and Peters, P. C.: Injuries to the bladder and urethra. *In* Harrison, J. H., Gittes, R. F., Perlmutter, A. D., Stamey, T. A., and Walsh, P. C. [eds.]: Campbell's Urology. 4th Ed. Volume 1. Philadelphia, W. B. Saunders Company, 1978, p. 911.)

is well tolerated by the patient for the 10 to 12 days of catheter drainage that are required. It may be used for longer periods of time if required. Short-term morbidity from a suprapubic tube is usually that of bladder spasms, particularly if there is troublesome bleeding for some reason following the cystotomy. The patient who complains of frequent bladder spasms must be suspected of having infection or a mucus plug or clot plugging the catheter. A properly draining suprapubic tube seldom causes bladder spasms. Occasionally, if the tube encroaches on the trigone or is pushed into the vesical neck by bladder contractions, the patient will develop a sense of urgency of micturition complicated by the bladder contractions. On occasion in patients with bladder infection, severe bladder spasms are seen, with forceful expulsion of the urine through the urethral meatus around an obstructing catheter.

CATHETER CARE

Eighty per cent of all gynecologic surgery requires catheter drainage of 5 days or less (vanNagell et al., 1972; Ingram, 1975; Peters and Thornton, 1980); urethral catheter drainage usually suffices. More than 98 per cent of female patients requiring postoperative bladder drainage have an adequate urethra for transurethral techniques of suprapubic catheter insertion (Peters and Thornton, 1980).

The suprapubic tube is comfortable for the patient, seldom becomes occluded, and can be left for weeks at a time without need for change. Need for change can be anticipated if one rubs the opposing walls of the catheter between the thumb and index finger and notes a gritty sensation, indicating that calcific deposition has begun. The author prefers to perform catheter change as infrequently as possible, emphasizing careful patient attention to personal hygiene and closed catheter drainage. The author has recorded an incidence of fever (0.5 to 4.0 per cent), diaphoresis, bacilluria, and sometimes positive blood culture following a catheter change, varying with the experience of the attendant performing the catheter change. Calcification can be minimized by assuring an adequate volume of acid urine.

Tidal drainage procedures and other methods of closed continuous irrigation have little place in the routine postoperative care of patients with drainage of clear urine from a urinary bladder. Renacidin (10 per cent) may be used as an irritant to dissolve calcifications in patients who do not have vesicoureteral reflux (Mulvaney and Henning, 1962), but it is seldom necessary in the short-term catheter drainage problems that are seen in the postoperative gynecologic patients.

Antibiotics should not be given to patients in the hope of preventing infection, as they will simply select out a more resistant organism and the patients soon are faced with undesirable side effects of the medication necessary to eliminate a more resistant organism (Kass, 1957; Kass and Schneiderman, 1957). Kass and Schneiderman (1957) demonstrated bacilluria in 96 per cent of patients tested after 4 days of urethral catheter drainage. Ingram (1975) reported a 21 per cent incidence of positive cultures and clinical cystitis in patients with suprapubic tubes as compared with 53 per cent in those patients with urethral catheters.

Most patients with bacilluria show no mucosal lesions. In our institution, of 100 patients with indwelling catheters who came to autopsy, only 30 per cent showed a demonstrable mucosal lesion due to bacterial injury, e.g., ecchymosis or change in the bladder epithelium. Lapides and associates (1968, 1972) have shown that the danger of bacilluria is greatest when overdistention of the bladder occurs. Bladder wall ischemia ensues, followed by mucosal invasion of microorganisms (Mehrotra, 1953; Lapides et al., 1968). Schoenberg and associates (1963) showed that no infection results when organisms are simply introduced into the bladder in the absence of previous mucosal injury. Cox and Hinman (1961) demonstrated that a normal urinary bladder completely eliminated potential pathogens within 48 hours, whereas a plastic bladder designed to empty completely (thereby eliminating residual urine, one of the major factors in persistent infection) allowed bacterial growth but not in a logarithmic phase. Patients with bladder dysfunction and persistent residual urine (e.g., paraplegics), who were inoculated with *Serratia marcescens*, had difficulty in clearing the organisms. Paraplegics were compared with normal medical students, who cleared the bladder of organisms within 48 hours. The study suggested that complete emptying per se is important, as the plastic bladder did have reduced (nonlogarithmic) bacterial growth, but that additional defense mechanisms other than complete emptying must be present if the urine is to be rendered sterile.

I feel that it is axiomatic to avoid giving broad-spectrum antibiotics to patients with a foreign body in the urinary tract, e.g., a suprapubic catheter. The principle should be to rid the urinary tract of the foreign body and then to attempt to sterilize the urine. Aside from the rare problem of latex allergy, simple irritation from an indwelling urethral catheter results in plugging of periurethral ducts with exudate. This irritation is less with a Silastic catheter. Bacteria migrate up the catheter, creating a suitable environment for infection to occur.

Long-term suprapubic drainage does have one major disadvantage, that of gradual reduction of bladder capacity, causing contracture of the urinary bladder, distortion of the ureteral orifices, vesicoureteral reflux, and subsequent pyelonephritis. Trabeculation and mucosal hypertrophy are part of this gradually developing picture.

Most patients requiring gynecologic surgery have no neurologic bladder instability (Peters and Thornton, 1980). An exception might be the diabetic patient coming to routine vaginal hysterectomy. Of 294 women subjected to vaginal hysterectomy and anterior and posterior repair by Peters and Thornton (1980), only two were found to have an unstable bladder by careful urodynamic studies, and these were so mild as to have escaped detection in the preoperative workup.

MANAGEMENT OF THE PATIENT WITH SUPRAPUBIC CATHETER

An important consideration in the management of the patient with an indwelling suprapubic catheter is the connection of the catheter in a sterile closed method to a large reservoir kept in the dependent position. A leg bag, such as a patient uses when awake and ambulatory, is a poor substitute for a large-reservoir, dependent bedside collection bag. High pressures may develop in a small-capacity bag if the patient falls asleep and the small leg bag becomes distended with urine. Overdistention of the leg bag may result in direct transmission of pressure to the bladder. This enhances the chances of overdistention of the bladder with mucosal ischemia and the chance of vesicoureteral reflux. These conditions provide a fertile ground for bacterial invasion.

Patients should be encouraged to connect an indwelling catheter in a sterile closed manner to a dependent bedside reservoir when they are going to sleep. The leg bag should be used only for short periods, usually less than 3 hours without emptying, and only when the patient is awake.

A Silastic suprapubic catheter is easily inserted and does not contribute to the development of a well-defined tract from the bladder to the abdominal wall. The low tissue reactivity and proliferative changes induced by the Silastic catheter are responsible for this. This is not a problem in patients requiring catheter drainage for 14 days or less. Latex allergy is encountered and can be effectively treated by removing the offending catheter and replacing it with a Silastic one. The latex catheter or other suprapubic catheters should be fixed at the skin level with a size 0 nonabsorbable suture. There is little skin reactivity to such a suture; it may remain in place for several weeks, which will suffice for more than 98 per cent of the gynecologic patients requiring suprapubic drainage. The Silastic catheter, despite the low reactivity, is nonetheless a foreign body in the urinary tract and calcific deposits do develop in its lumen, although this is less likely with Silastic catheters than with the indwelling latex catheters. When calcification does occur, management usually includes catheter change as noted previously, as well as maintenance of a large volume of urine.

The suprapubic tube may be clamped at any time to give the patient a trial of voiding. Ability of the bladder to contract can be predicted by bedside cystometry. The bladder is filled slowly through the suprapubic tube via an Asepto syringe. Contractions raising the fluid level in the syringe are noted. Residual urine can be easily checked after the patient voids with the tube clamped. The catheter can be removed when the residual urine volume is less than 100 ml and when capacity is greater than 300 ml. More than 95 per cent of patients will have zero residual volume.

Polypharmacy is of little help in the management of voiding problems after the catheter has been removed. Though the Urecholine test (Chapter 3) may give an indication of denervation by showing an exaggerated contractile response of the bladder to the pharmacologic agent (denervation hypersensitivity), drugs are of little help in getting the postoperative bladder to empty. Of all agents available for treatment of postoperative hypotonicity of the bladder, the combination of bethanechol (Urecholine), 25 mg every 6 hours, and phenoxybenzamine (Dibenzylene), 10 mg every 8 hours, has been found in the author's experience to be most beneficial. Results are dependent primarily upon the passage of time and nerve regeneration in the female patient recovering from partial denervation as a result of extensive pelvic surgery.

SUMMARY

If the need for more than 5 days of bladder drainage is anticipated, a suprapubic catheter is preferred to a urethral catheter. Prophylactic antibiotics have no place in the routine management of a patient with a suprapubic catheter. Their use simply results in selection of a more resistant organism. The proper time to give antibiotics to sterilize the urine is after the foreign body is removed. Closed drainage systems should always be used; aseptic techniques should be followed when catheter connections are changed. The neurologically unstable bladder is a rare finding in the preoperative gynecologic patient and in nearly all cases should be detected in the preoperative workup.

REFERENCES

Bonanno, P. J., Landers, D. E., and Rock, D. E.: Bladder drainage with the suprapubic bladder needle. Obstet. Gynecol. *35*:807, 1970.

Campbell, M. F.: Urologic complications of anorectal and colon surgery. Am. J. Proctol. *12*:51, 1961.

Cox, C. E., and Hinman, F., Jr.: Experiments with induced bacteriuria, vesical emptying and bacterial growth on the mechanism of bladder defense to infection. J. Urol. *86*:739, 1961.

Foley, F. E. B.: A self-retaining bag catheter. J. Urol. *38*:140, 1937.

Hodgkinson, C. P., and Hodari, A. A.: Trocar suprapubic cystostomy for postoperative bladder drainage. Am. J. Obstet. Gynecol. *96*:773, 1966.

Hohenfellner, R.: Personal communication, 1980.

Ingram, J. M.: Further experience with suprapubic drainage by trocar catheter. Am. J. Obstet. Gynecol. *121*:885, 1975.

Kass, E. H.: Bacteriuria and the diagnosis of infections of the urinary tract. Arch. Intern. Med. *100*:709, 1957.

Kass, E. H., and Schneiderman, L. J.: Entry of bacteria into the urinary tracts of patients with inlying catheters. N. Engl. J. Med. *256*:556, 1957.

Lapides, J., Costello, R. I., Jr., Zierdt, D. K., and Stone, T. E.: Primary cause and treatment of recurrent urinary infection in women: preliminary report. J. Urol. *100*:552, 1968.

Lapides, J., Diokno, A. C., Silber, S. J., and Lowe, B. S.: Clean, intermittent self-catheterization in the treatment of urinary tract disease. J. Urol. *107*:458, 1972.

Mehrotra, R. M. L.: An experimental study of the vesical circulation during distention and in cystitis. J. Pathol. Bacteriol. *66*:79, 1953.

Mulvaney, W. P., and Henning, D. C.: Solvent treatment of urinary calculi: refinements in technique. J. Urol. *88*:145, 1962.

Peters, W. A., III, and Thornton, W. N., Jr.: Selection of the primary operative procedure for stress urinary incontinence. Am. J. Obstet. Gynecol. *137*:923, 1980.

Robertson, J. R.: Suprapubic cystostomy with endoscopy. Obstet. Gynecol. *41*:624, 1973.

Schoenberg, H. W., Beisswanger, P., Howard, W. J., Walter, C. F., and Murphy, J. J.: Effect of lower urinary tract infection upon ureteral function. Surg. Forum *14*:483, 1963.

Seski, J. C., and Diokno, A. C.: Bladder dysfunction after radical abdominal hysterectomy. Am. J. Obstet. Gynecol. *128*:643, 1977.

Shute, W. B., and MacKinnon, K. J.: Postoperative restoration of micturition with suprapubic catheterization. Am. J. Obstet. Gynecol. *106*:943, 1970.

vanNagell, J. R., Jr., Penny, R. M., Jr., and Roddick, J. W., Jr.: Suprapubic bladder drainage following radical hysterectomy. Am. J. Obstet. Gynecol. *113*:849, 1972.

SECTION

3

URINARY INCONTINENCE AND FISTULA

13

URINARY STRESS INCONTINENCE: PATHOPHYSIOLOGY, DIAGNOSIS, AND CLASSIFICATION

T. H. GREEN, JR., M.D.

Until little more than a decade or two ago, the diagnosis of urinary stress incontinence in the female was, for the most part, made casually, primarily on the basis of the history given by the patient. The anatomic abnormality underlying the symptom was not precisely understood. Nor was it appreciated then that there might be individual variations in the underlying abnormal urethrovesical anatomic configuration, and that these variations could have an important bearing on the choice of surgical procedure most likely to completely and permanently correct the stress incontinence. In the ensuing years there have been important and fundamental additions to our understanding of the etiologic mechanisms involved in this common and troublesome disorder. Accurate diagnosis and effective management of stress incontinence depend on a correct understanding of the characteristic anatomic defect that produces it.

PATHOPHYSIOLOGIC FACTORS

It is generally agreed that the basic problem is one of inadequate support to the bladder base, vesical neck, and proximal urethra, with a resulting specific and rather characteristic distortion of the urethrovesical anatomy. In recent years, additional attention has been focused on certain other features of the anatomy and physiology of the continence mechanism in an attempt to explain stress incontinence. The following consideration of each of these several interpretations of the basic underlying abnormality should be helpful in clarifying our current understanding of the pathophysiology of stress incontinence.

Urethrovesical Pressure Relationships

Using direct urethrocystometry, a technique permitting simultaneous recording of the pressure within the bladder and urethra, the variations in these pressure relationships in patients with stress incontinence have been compared with normal, continent controls (Hodgkinson and Cobert, 1960; Enhorning, 1961; Beck and Maughan, 1964; and Toews, 1967). In all continent patients with normal urethrovesical anatomy, the pressure at some point in the urethra, invariably in the proximal half, always equals or exceeds that in the bladder. Furthermore, in these patients, sudden increases in intra-abdominal pressure resulting from cough or similar stresses are transmitted equally to the bladder and the proximal two thirds of the urethra, maintaining an intraurethral pressure equal to or greater than the intravesical pressure. On the other hand, in patients with stress incontinence, the intrinsic intraurethral pressure at rest tends to be lower (although still greater than resting intravesical pressure); coughing reverses the usual pressure differential between the urethra and the bladder, with vesical pressure equaling or exceeding urethral pressure.

Actually, the main conclusion of all these data seems obvious and hardly necessary to prove: If a patient has stress incontinence, it follows that during the interval in which the stress is applied the intravesical pressure has risen above the intraurethral pressure, elementary physics and pure logic rendering measurement unnecessary to prove this point. However, urethrovesical pressure studies have served to emphasize one important aspect of the present concept of the pathogenesis of stress incontinence. It is apparent that the normally supported proximal two thirds of the urethra is basically an intra-abdominal structure. Hence a sudden elevation of intra-abdominal pressure produces the same transmitted rise in pressure in the inner two thirds of the urethra as it does in the bladder. This concept clearly relates the disparity in intraurethral pressure in patients with stress incontinence to the fact that the poorly supported proximal urethra has been displaced and now lies outside the intra-abdominal field of force.

Urethral Length

A few years ago the possible significance of urethral length to the continence mechanism was again investigated. Lapides and co-workers (1960) even suggested the possibility that abnormal shortening of the urethra might be an important factor in the development of stress incontinence. They obtained their measurements of urethral length before and after operations for stress incontinence by using a calibrated inlying urethral catheter, exerting downward traction until it was believed that a meaningful measurement of urethral length was indicated by the reading noted on the distal end of the catheter. The accuracy possible with this method seems open to question, since the poorly supported urethra is prone to telescope within itself and undergo apparent shortening when placed under artificial tension-traction of this sort.

TABLE 13–1. CHANGES IN URETHRAL LENGTH AFTER SURGERY FOR STRESS INCONTINENCE (MEASUREMENTS ON PREOPERATIVE AND POSTOPERATIVE URETHROCYSTOGRAMS)

	336 Cured Patients	18 Failures
No change	166	7
Increase (cm.)		
0.1–0.5	88	6
0.5–1.0	71	4
1.0–2.0	11	1

On the other hand, with the beadchain technique of urethrocystography in which the urethral meatus is marked with a silver Duraclip, not only does telescoping never occur, but it is a simple matter to obtain extremely precise, undistorted measurements of urethral length both preoperatively and postoperatively. We have now accumulated such measurements in over 300 patients undergoing surgery for stress incontinence. As shown in Table 13–1, no change whatsoever occurs in urethral length in the majority of patients in whom operative repair has been successful in relieving stress incontinence. Hodgkinson and co-workers (1963) in a study of 105 patients, and Low (1964), in an analysis of 138 patients, made entirely similar observations and reached the same conclusion — that urethral length has no bearing on the problem of true, anatomic stress incontinence.

Urethrovesical Anatomic Relationships

The Posterior Urethrovesical Angle

Jeffcoate and Roberts (1952) were among the first to call attention to the importance of the anatomic configuration of the urethrovesical junction and proximal urethra to the continence mechanism. On the basis of their extensive studies using urethrocystography in large numbers of both continent women and patients with stress incontinence, they concluded that the presence of a normal posterior urethrovesical (PUV) angle was essential to the continence mechanism, and that in patients with stress incontinence it was characteristically absent. Hodgkinson (1953), employing the metallic beadchain technique of urethrocystography in similar studies on continent and incontinent women, reached essentially the same conclusions. It should be pointed out that the location of the bladder neck and urethra with respect to the public symphysis is not of direct importance, since many patients with marked bladder descent but a normal PUV angle are perfectly continent. In others with severe stress incontinence, the bladder and urethra remain normally positioned with respect to the symphysis, but the PUV angle is obliterated.

It is thus not the spatial location of the vesical neck and proximal urethra but the urethrovesical anatomic configuration as specifically manifested by the PUV angle that is involved in the continence mechanism. Urethrocystograms in normal, continent women reveal a flat bladder base and a sharply defined PUV angle (90 to 100 degrees). At least one third of the bladder base takes part in the formation of this angle (see Fig. 13–1). Even on cough the angle is maintained, and there is no funneling or posterior descent of the bladder neck.

Patients with stress incontinence, on the other hand, invariably exhibit complete or nearly complete loss of the PUV angle with resulting funneling and posterior descent of the vesical neck to the most dependent portion of the bladder.

Many studies (e.g., Barnett, 1969, 1970; Crist et al., 1969; Dutton, 1960; Low, 1964; and others) have verified this relationship

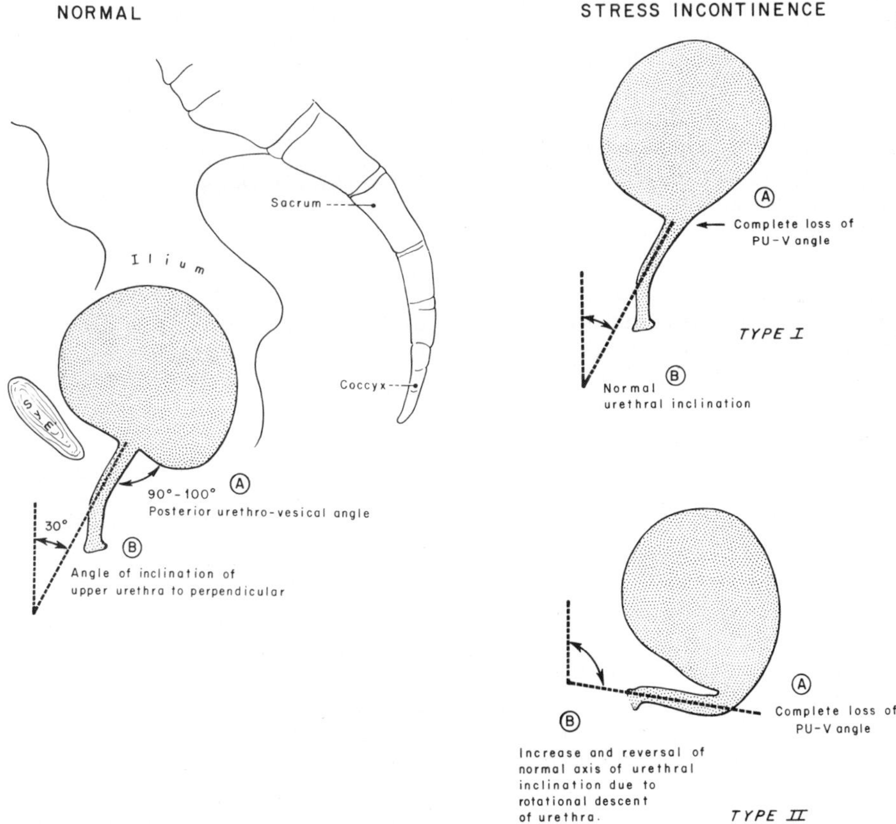

Figure 13–1. Anatomic configuration of the bladder in normal continent women and in women with stress incontinence. Drawn from urethrocystograms. (From Green, T. H., Jr.: Gynecology — Essentials of Clinical Practice. 2nd Ed. Boston, Little, Brown and Co., 1971. Chap. 18.)

between absence of the PUV angle and the occurrence of stress incontinence. Other evidence, direct and indirect, supporting the validity of this association, can be outlined as follows:

1. As a normal part of the voiding mechanism, momentary loss of the PUV angle produces conditions favorable to urine flow, even before the detrusor contraction begins to increase intravesical pressure. Obliteration of the PUV angle, with descent and funneling of the bladder neck immediately prior to detrusor contraction and actual micturition, is observed in normal continent women studied fluoroscopically (Muellner and Fleischner, 1949). Thus, the patient suffering from stress incontinence and exhibiting the characteristic loss of the PUV angle is, anatomically speaking, constantly in the preliminary phase of the voiding act; a sudden increase in intravesical pressure occasioned by cough or similar stress inevitably produces the same result that detrusor contraction achieves during normal micturition.

2. The vesical neck elevation test of Marchetti (1949), widely and successfully used as an aid in the diagnosis and management of stress incontinence, is based on the fact that the physician can temporarily prevent stress incontinence by manually restoring and maintaining the normal PUV angle and urethral axis during a pelvic examination.

3. In the operative procedures for stress incontinence that have been devised over the years, particularly those which have most consistently yielded successful results, it is apparent that the restoration of a PUV angle is the one important feature common to all. The original "Kelly vesical neck plication stitch" did it, although not nearly so effectively or permanently as do the procedures performed today (Barnett, 1969); a properly performed anterior colporrhaphy has this same effect (Chapter 15). The Marshall-Marchetti urethrovesical suspension (Chapter 16) and the fascial sling procedure (Chapter 19) do it best of all, reliably creating an adequate PUV angle as well as restoring a normal urethral axis.

4. Perhaps the most telling evidence is to be found in the many reported studies involving comparative preoperative and postoperative urethrocystograms in patients undergoing operations to correct stress incontinence (Bailey, 1954, 1956, 1963; Harer and Gunther, 1965; Hodgkinson, 1953; Schonberg et al., 1963; and many others). These studies clearly demonstrated that cure of the stress incontinence was always accompanied by restoration of a normal PUV angle and a normal urethral axis. Failures or recurrences were just as invariably associated with failure to create or maintain an adequate PUV angle and a normal urethral axis, as again revealed by the postoperative urethrocystograms.

5. Iatrogenic stress incontinence occasionally follows vaginal hysterectomy or anterior colporrhaphy, alone or in combination, resulting in numerous unplanned clinical experiments. In these instances, preoperative and postoperative urethrocystograms have clearly shown that a previously adequate PUV angle in a perfectly continent patient had been completely effaced as a result of the vaginal surgery, leading to the immediate development of stress incontinence postoperatively (see Figure 13–2).

The Urethral Axis

Although loss of the PUV angle is the most characteristic anatomic abnormality in patients with stress incontinence, urethrocystography often discloses a second important feature — distortion of the urethral axis, or angle of inclination between the proximal urethra and the bladder base.

The probable significance of the normal urethral axis in maintaining continence was first brought to light by the classic studies of Bailey (1954, 1956, 1963) in Manchester, England, whose continuing observations employing preoperative and postoperative urethrocystograms were made and reported during the decade 1954 to 1964. When Bailey's data, together with our own similar observations (Green, 1962) in a series of 90 patients, were analyzed carefully, it seemed apparent that, in addition to the characteristic loss of the PUV angle, there was one other variable feature of basic importance: the urethral axis, or angle of

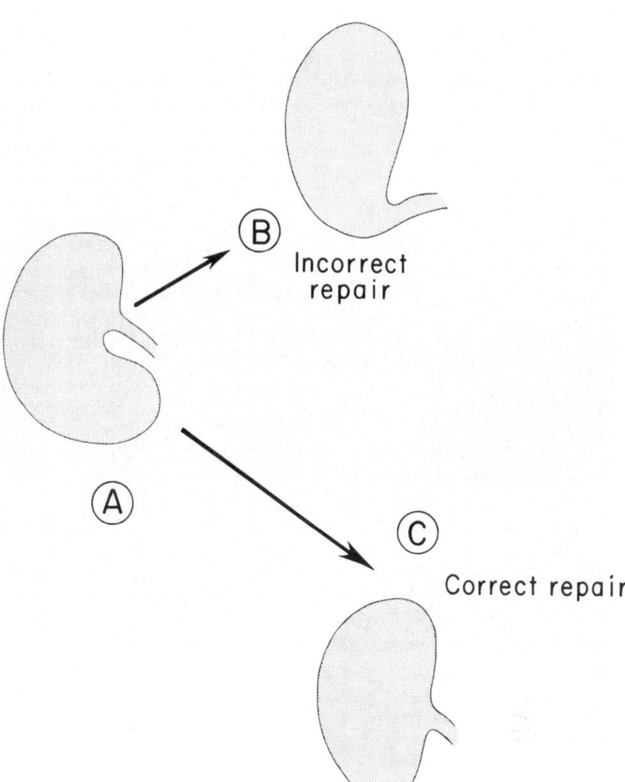

Figure 13–2. Probable mechanisms involved in the iatrogenic production of stress incontinence following improperly executed anterior colporrhaphy for cystocele. Drawn from urethrocystograms.

A, Anatomy of typical cystocele prior to anterior colporrhaphy.

B, Incorrect repair. Overzealous advancement of the bladder base combined with failure to repair the supporting structures beneath the vesical neck and the proximal urethra has produced the anatomic basis for the development of stress incontinence.

C, Correct repair. Proper correction of the cystocele and careful restoration of the posterior urethrovesical angle recreate normal urethrovesical support and also preserve the continence mechanism.

(From Green, T. H., Jr.: Development of a plan for the diagnosis and treatment of urinary stress incontinence. Am. J. Obstet. Gynecol. *83*:632, 1962.)

inclination of the proximal two thirds of the urethra.

Classification of Patients with Stress Incontinence

On the basis of these studies, it therefore seemed possible to define two basic types of anatomy in patients with stress incontinence (see Figure 13–1):

Type I. Complete or nearly complete loss of the PUV angle, but with the angle of inclination to the vertical of the urethral axis either normal (range, 10 to 30 degrees), or at least less than 45 degrees, as shown on the urethrocystogram in the lateral standing-straining view.

Type II. Loss of the PUV angle and, in addition, a definitely abnormal angle of inclination to the vertical of the urethral axis, the latter being greater than 45 degrees and often even completely reversed (greater than 90 degrees). Patients with this downward and backward rotational descent of the urethral axis invariably experience the most severe degree of stress incontinence; they are the most difficult to treat effectively and in the past have had the highest rate of failure after various operative procedures. Undoubtedly Type II stress incontinence represents the result of a more profound weakening of the supports of the proximal urethra and bladder neck.

DIFFERENTIATION FROM CYSTOCELE. A point worthy of emphasis is the importance of distinguishing the Type II stress incontinence anatomic configuration, with its characteristic downward and backward rotational descent of the urethra and bladder neck, from a cystocele. As clearly shown in Figure 13–3, the urethrovesical anatomy in a patient with a typical cystocele in no way resembles that of a patient with stress incontinence. In view of the persistence of a satisfactory PUV angle and a relatively normal urethral axis, it is not at all surprising that patients with cystoceles do not develop stress incontinence (see Figure 13–6). Thus, in spite of the superficial similarity in appearance of cystocele and Type II stress incontinence when pelvic examination is done with the patient in

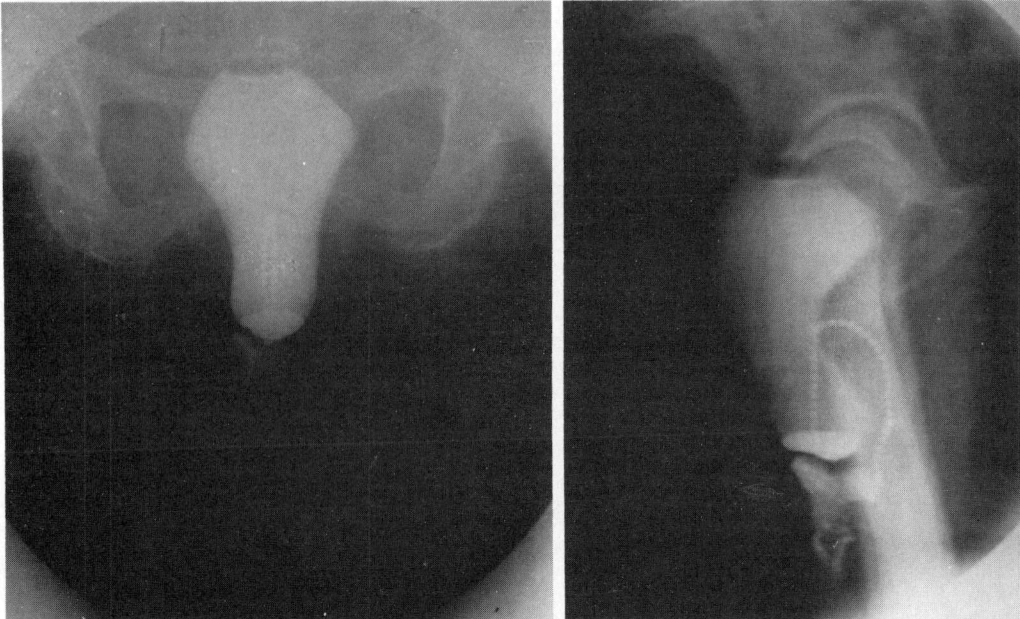

Figure 13–3. Urethrocystograms of a 57-year-old para III with a large cystocele and mild frequency, urgency, and nocturia but with no stress incontinence. Note that in spite of marked prolapse of the bladder base, the posterior urethrovesical angle is maintained and a relatively satisfactory urethral axis is preserved. (From Green, T. H., Jr.: Am. J. Obstet. Gynecol. *83*:632, 1962.)

lithotomy position, the two entities are different both anatomically and symptomatically, and the fundamental anatomy of each is well documented on urethrocystography (see Figures 13–1 and 13–4).

Physiologic Effects of Anatomic Abnormalities

The loss of the posterior urethrovesical angle and the downward and backward rotation of the urethral axis that so universally accompany stress incontinence can be interpreted as simply a reflection of poor urethral support. However, absence of the PUV angle seems important of and by itself. As Hodgkinson (1953) and Jeffcoate and Roberts (1952) first pointed out, loss of the anatomic configuration of the PUV angle results in displacement of the vesical neck to the most dependent portion of the bladder, thus positioning the internal urinary meatus at the point of maximum hydrostatic pressure. As illustrated in Figure 13–5, this anatomic funneling effect of the loss of the PUV angle renders impossible the equal transmission of sudden elevations of intra-abdominal pressure to the lumen of the proximal urethra via its walls and their supports. As a result, intravesical pressure in the region of the vesical neck rises more than intraurethral pressure just beyond it, and stress incontinence is the result.

In addition, as discussed above, patients with large cystoceles never suffer from stress incontinence, even though the vesical neck and proximal urethra have descended markedly and may even lie outside the introitus. Urethrocystograms in such patients demonstrate a normal posterior urethrovesical angle. As shown in Figure 13–6, this prevents intravesical pressure from exceeding intraurethral pressure during cough or similar stresses, despite the fact that the proximal urethra has completely lost its normal intra-abdominal location.

The tendency to rotational downward and backward descent of the urethral axis in many patients with stress incontinence likewise seems to be in itself important, above and beyond the fact that it is indicative of inadequate urethral support. Figure 13–7 illustrates diagrammatically the significance of this rotational descent in stress incontinence. The usual maximal transmission of stress-induced sudden elevations in

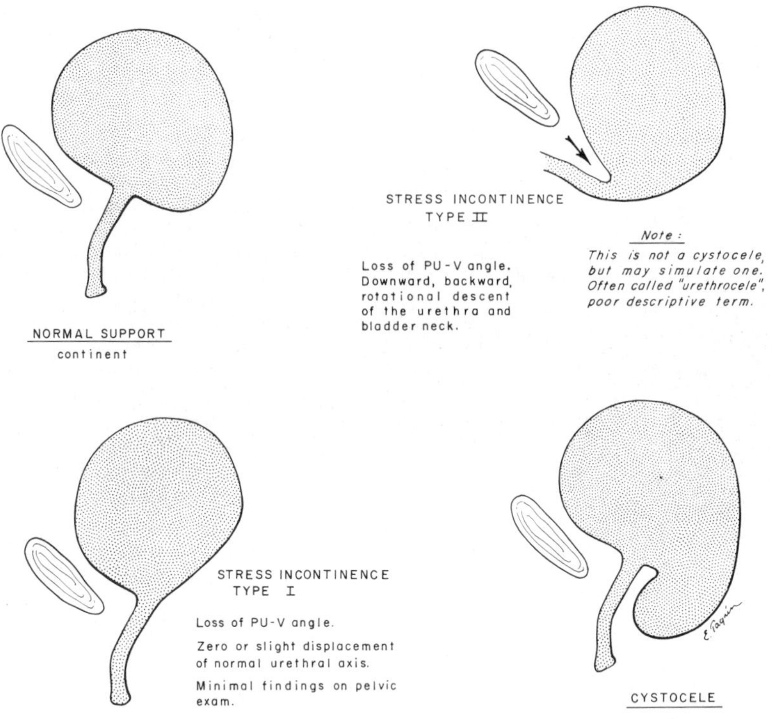

Figure 13–4. Anatomic configuration of the bladder in normal continent women and in women with stress incontinence and cystocele. Drawn from urethrocystograms. (From Green, T. H., Jr.: Gynecology — Essentials of Clinical Practice. 2nd Ed. Boston, Little, Brown and Co., 1971. Chap. 18.)

intra-abdominal pressure to the urethral wall and its surrounding soft tissue supports, which normally produces an increase in intraurethral pressure equal to the sudden rise in intravesical pressure, no longer occurs. This normal maximal pressure transmission depends on the urethra remaining in the fixed position. It is dissipat-

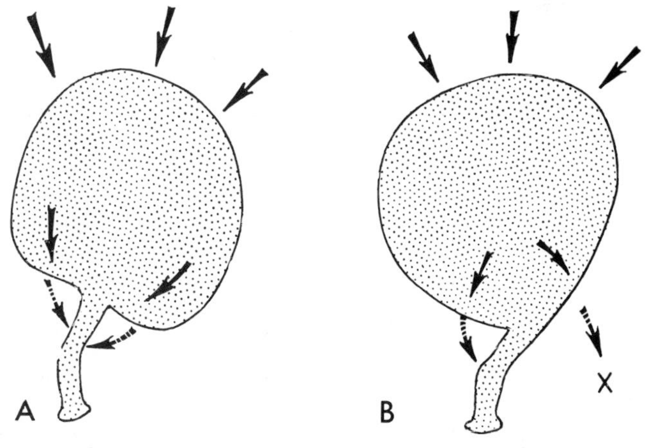

Figure 13–5. The importance of the posterior urethrovesical (PUV) angle to the continence mechanism.

A, Normal PUV angle permits maximal transmission (indicated by the dotted-line arrows), on all sides of the proximal urethra, of sudden increases in intra-abdominal pressure. Intraurethral pressure is maintained higher than the simultaneously elevated intravesical pressure, preventing loss of urine with sudden stress.

B, Loss of PUV angle results in displacement of the vesical neck to the most dependent portion of the bladder, the point of maximum hydrostatic pressure. The dotted-line arrow at X indicates the impossibility of effective transmission of pressure to the posterior aspect of the proximal urethra. Intravesical pressure in the region of the bladder neck thus rises considerably more than the intraurethral pressure, and stress incontinence occurs.

(From Green, T. H., Jr.: The problem of urinary incontinence in the female: An appraisal of its current status. Obstet. Gynecol. Surv. *23*:603, 1968. Copyright © The Williams & Wilkins Co., Baltimore.)

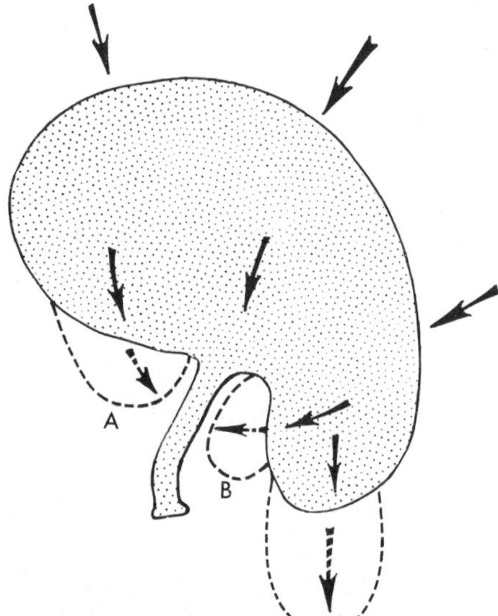

Figure 13–6. Mechanism of the preservation of continence with even a marked cystocele. The invariably normal posterior urethrovesical angle permits equal transmission of sudden increases in intra-abdominal pressure to the proximal urethra (indicated by the dashed-line arrows at *A* and *B*). In addition, the simultaneous increase in intravesical pressure may be rendered even less by the dissipating effect of the resultant further bulging-out of the cystocele (indicated by the arrow at *C*). (From Green, T. H., Jr.: Obstet. Gynecol. Surv. *23*:603, 1968. Copyright © The Williams & Wilkins Co., Baltimore.)

ed and greatly reduced by the effect of the rotational urethral descent that occurs in response to the sudden stress-induced increase in intra-abdominal pressure.

Thus, in patients with both abnormal urethral axis and absent PUV angle, there is an even greater disparity between the deficiently transmitted rise in intraurethral pressure and the much greater rise in intravesical pressure than there is in patients in whom loss of the PUV angle is not accompanied by any significant abnormality of the urethral axis.

Summary

The evidence is overwhelming that the specific urethrovesical relationships characterized by the posterior urethrovesical angle and the urethral axis are crucial to the etiology of stress incontinence. This concept is in no way incompatible with the observed alterations in urethrovesical pressure relationships. It is clear that the latter are in reality secondary to the more fundamental urethrovesical anatomic abnormalities.

An understanding of the various aspects of the pathologic anatomy has also proved valuable in the development of a more rational method of selecting the operative repair most likely to succeed for each individual patient.

DIFFERENTIAL DIAGNOSIS

Approximately one fourth of women with uncontrollable loss of urine do not have anatomic stress incontinence but instead have one of several other conditions that adversely affect the continence mechanism. Operations designed to correct stress incontinence never benefit and often aggravate these other disorders. Hence, a careful differential diagnosis of all the various abnormalities leading to urinary incontinence is extremely important before it is concluded that stress incontinence exists and that surgical correction is indicated.

The other causes of female urinary incontinence that must frequently be differentiated from true stress incontinence can be divided into the following five categories: (1) pure urgency incontinency, (2) bladder neuropathies, (3) urinary tract anomalies, (4) psychogenic incontinence, and (5) detrusor dyssynergia. The first three are usually fairly readily recognized during the course of a thorough diagnostic work-up, and psychogenic incontinence is extremely rare, so that these are only briefly noted. The fifth, detrusor dyssynergia, is not so

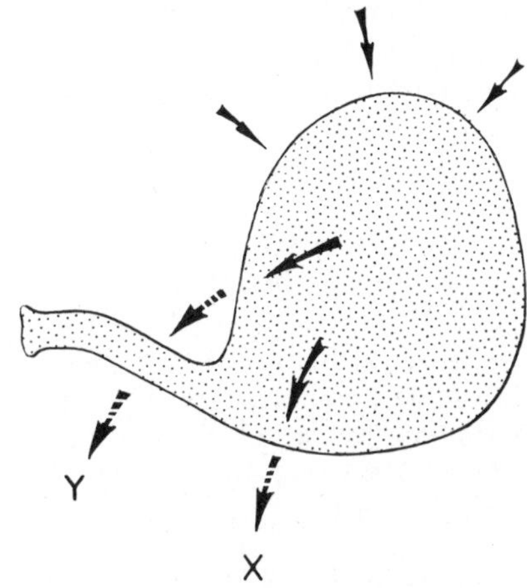

Figure 13–7. Mechanisms involved in Type II stress incontinence. Note characteristic loss of PUV angle (dashed-line arrow at X). Transmission of sudden increases in intra-abdominal pressure to the proximal urethra produces only a rotational descent of the urethra (dashed-line arrow at Y) rather than the maximum possible rise in intraurethral pressure, necessary to maintain continence. (From Green, T. H., Jr.: Obstet. Gynecol. Surv. *23*:603, 1968. Copyright © The Williams & Wilkins Co., Baltimore.)

straightforward or obvious in nature and often simulates stress incontinence closely enough to fool the unwary; hence, it is discussed in greater detail.

Pure Urgency Incontinence

Urgency incontinence may accompany urethritis, trigonitis, or cystitis, as well as other intrinsic lesions of the bladder and urethra. In the case of acute inflammations, the diagnosis is usually obvious, and the triad of urgency, frequency, and dysuria accompanying the episodes of urgency leakage renders confusion with stress incontinence highly unlikely. Similar symptoms are also often seen in association with acute vaginitis and in the early postoperative phase following certain pelvic operations.

In chronic inflammatory conditions of the urethra and trigone, pain is usually absent, and the history should be taken with care to elicit the important clue that frequency and a sudden urgency underlie the episodes of leakage, not a sudden stress such as coughing or laughing.

Finally, painless urgency of urination, with an urgency type of incontinence, may have a purely psychosomatic background in some women. As emphasized by Frewen (1972), such patients may experience intervals of this symptomatology during periods of psychosocial and environmental stress, with wide variations in the duration and severity of the symptoms. These intervals are usually of transient though recurring nature, and often respond promptly to bladder antispasmodics and sedatives, in contrast to the chronicity of the disorder of detrusor dyssynergia (discussed below).

Bladder Neuropathies

Bladder neuropathies may be due to fundamental neurologic disorders affecting either the central or the peripheral nervous system such as multiple sclerosis or diabetic neuritis, to name the two most frequently encountered. The resulting incontinence may be either of the overflow or of the urgency or uninhibited detrusor type (Chapter 23).

Congenital or Acquired Urinary Tract Anomalies

Ectopic ureter, urethral diverticulum, urethrovaginal or vesicovaginal fistula, and other anomalies produce abnormal leakage of urine. Occasionally the diagnosis is not as obvious as one would expect. Some urethral diverticula and some very tiny vesicovaginal fistulas (Chapter 21) may leak urine only with sudden stresses. Careful examination and a thorough diagnostic study program should readily establish the correct diagnosis.

One other anomaly that frequently mimics true anatomic stress incontinence is the so-called "short urethra-total incontinence" syndrome. Occurring as the result of congenital anomalies or acquired through obstetric or surgical trauma, a truly short urethra, less than 2.0 cm. in length, may be the cause of severe urinary incontinence. Such patients, although they may exhibit leakage of urine on stress as well, actually have total urinary incontinence and note almost continuous loss of urine, even at rest in the recumbent position. This is quite obviously a distinctly separate type of urinary incontinence, once quite different from that presented by the typical patient with true stress incontinence. Leadbetter (1964) has thoroughly discussed the problem of total urinary incontinence secondary to the short urethra and has devised a highly successful procedure for its surgical correction. Leadbetter's operation consists of reimplanting both ureters higher up on the bladder floor, thus making available four or five centimeters of bladder wall above the vesical neck, which is plicated to form a muscular tube, effectively restoring adequate length to the urethra.

Psychogenic Urinary Incontinence

This type of incontinence is extremely rare. The accidental loss of urine, emphasized by Hodgkinson (1970), is always produced by a voluntary effort, however unconscious of its voluntary nature the patient and her physician may be. This condition, which is probably similar to the disorder of enuresis of childhood, is usually of long duration and is basically a psychogenically induced abnormal habit pattern of voluntary bladder emptying at the wrong time and place, the initiation of which the patient is not conscious of. It is thus entirely different from the involuntary detrusor incontinence of the fifth and final category; however, psychogenic incontinence can also be recognized by the technique of direct electrourethrocystometry, provided that a rectal lead is incorporated into the system to permit documenting voluntary detrusor contraction effort.

Detrusor Dyssynergia

This is fundamentally a chronic, painless, urgency-frequency type of incontinence, sometimes with a "pseudo-stress" incontinence aspect. It is psychosomatic and functional in origin at least 50 to 80 per cent of the time. It results from involuntary detrusor activity and thus differs completely from the rare entity of psychogenic incontinence due to undisciplined voluntary detrusor action.

During the past decade, largely through the insights and careful studies of Hodgkinson and his colleagues (1960, 1963, 1969), and more recently by the investigations of the group at the Middlesex Hospital in London (Arnold et al., 1973; Bates et al., 1973), it has become apparent that detrusor dyssynergia is the second most common cause of urinary incontinence in the female. It results from sudden, uninhibited detrusor muscle activity, variously termed "detrusor irritability," "detrusor instability," or, perhaps more accurately, "detrusor dyssynergia." Prior to a general awareness of the existence of this syndrome, many of the patients who would now be assigned to this category were classified as having "urgency incontinence," since urgency and frequency are usually prominent symptoms of so-called detrusor incontinence. Moreover, the symptoms in some of these patients closely simulate true stress incontinence and often resulted in their erroneous inclusion in the group with anatomic stress incontinence. It is now obvious that even in the absence of any anatomic abnormalities of urethral and vesical neck support, the detrusor dyssynergia syndrome may have a symptomatic element of functional stress incontinence. For, as several authors have noted (Hodgkinson, 1970; Jeffcoate and Francis, 1966), stresses that suddenly increase intra-abdominal pressure may also precipitate uninhibited detrusor activity in these women, presumably by sudden stimulation of hyperirritable stretch receptors in the trigonal area with immediate activation of a hyperactive reflex arc controlling detrusor contraction. Thus, a sudden stress may set off uninhibited detrusor contractions and result in an actual voiding, rather than a leaking, type of incontinence. However, it should be carefully noted that detrusor incontinence occurs several seconds after the stress, not simultaneously, as is the case with true stress incontinence.

Approximately 10 per cent of all patients complaining of urinary incontinence suffer from pure detrusor dyssynergia, and roughly half of these women have this type of functional stress incontinence without abnormalities of anatomic support. On the other hand, true anatomic stress incontinence accounts for 75 to 80 per cent of female urinary incontinence. Thus, among all patients complaining of abnormal urinary leakage, 85 per cent have a history of stress incontinence; 90 to 95 per cent of this group have true, anatomic stress incontinence; and 5 to 10 per cent are suffering from detrusor dyssynergia. It is very important to distinguish this latter group, since operations designed to correct anatomic stress incontinence fail to alleviate and usually increase the severity of the symptoms in patients with detrusor dyssynergia.

Symptoms

A correct diagnosis of detrusor dyssynergia can often be established without complicated studies by the astute physician who takes the time to survey the patient's overall state and to elicit in detail the characteristics of the abnormal urinary leakage. The symptomatic hallmarks of detrusor dyssynergia are:

1. Urgency, frequency, and painless urgency incontinence are often prominent.
2. When a pseudo-stress type of incontinence is the more prominent component, there is a latent period of several seconds between the physical stress and the onset of leakage. The latter then occurs over a protracted interval of several seconds.
3. A large volume of urine is lost (actual uninhibited involuntary voiding is occurring).
4. Leakage may occur in any position, and often follows a change in position.
5. Running and walking may trigger detrusor incontinence; coughing, sneezing, and laughing are less likely to do so.
6. Symptoms tend to disappear at night.
7. A consistently observed difference between patients with detrusor dyssynergia and women with anatomic stress incontinence is that the former are unable to stop their stream during normal voiding whereas the latter invariably can.
8. Finally, an underlying generalized anxiety state is often discernible in patients with detrusor dyssynergia.

Confirmation of Diagnosis

Electronic Urethrocystometry. The above-listed clinical guides often make the elaborate and not yet widely accessible urethrovesical pressure measurements unnecessary to confirm the diagnosis of detrusor incontinence. If accessible, this diagnostic technique should certainly be used in doubtful cases, especially if it is suspected that the patient may be one of the relatively small group of women who have both anatomic stress incontinence and detrusor dyssynergia. Here, a hasty decision to operate should be avoided at all costs.

First introduced by Hodgkinson and Cobert (1960), direct electronic urethrocystometry involves continuous and simultaneous monitoring of urethral and vesical pressures as the bladder is allowed to fill naturally from a completely empty to as full a state as is tolerated by the patient. Even minor pressure variations in the bladder and urethra are readily detected, and with a rectal pressure lead incorporated into the system, the involuntary pressure changes seen in detrusor dyssynergia are readily distinguished from rises in pressure produced by voluntary actions that elevate overall intra-abdominal pressure.

Cystometrography. If direct electro-urethrocystometry is not readily available, simple water manometer cystometrograms remain a useful alternative. When done in the supine position, a routine cystometrogram study permits recognition of spontaneous, involuntary detrusor contractions as well as the abnormal detrusor activity typical of dyssynergia, triggered by coughing, heel jouncing, or suprapubic tapping, as the bladder is allowed to fill.

Precautions in Management

Above all, it is most important to remember that attempts at surgical repair in these patients are decidedly ill-advised and invariably make them worse. In those few patients who may have both detrusor dyssynergia and some degree of anatomic stress incontinence, if the former predominates, it is wiser to withhold surgery. Obviously, it is particularly important to be on the lookout for an underlying, previously unrecognized detrusor dyssynergia in any patient who has failed to be relieved of presumed anatomic stress incontinence by one or more prior operative procedures. As documented by Bates and his associates (1973), a high percentage of such so-called failures will be found on urethrocystometric study to have detrusor dyssynergia rather than stress incontinence. Needless to say, a proper preoperative differential diagnosis avoids unnecessary surgery.

Differential Diagnostic Studies

It is thus apparent that in the management of patients who seem to be suffering from stress incontinence, the first step is to obtain definite, objective proof of the presence of true, anatomic stress incontinence and to exclude the possibility that some other disorder causing abnormal urinary leakage is merely simulating it. In addition to a careful history and detailed physical examination, other studies helpful in revealing incontinence due to intrinsic pathology of the urinary tract or neurologic disturbances affecting bladder function include urinalysis and culture, intravenous pyelography, cystoscopy and urethroscopy, cystometrograms, and measurement of postvoiding residuals. Invariably all of these studies are normal in the patient with true, anatomic stress incontinence.

If detrusor dyssynergia is suspected, it may be possible to establish this diagnosis on the basis of the typical symptom complex alone, especially if there is no clinical or x-ray evidence of the abnormal anatomy of stress incontinence. However, in doubtful cases, and in reevaluating patients in whom previous surgery for alleged stress incontinence has failed to relieve the incontinence, electronic direct urethrocystometric studies may be very important and helpful in definitely determining whether or not abnormal, involuntary detrusor contractions are occurring.

Vesical Neck Elevation Test

The so-called vesical neck elevation test (see Figure 13–8) is also useful in tentatively establishing that an anatomic abnormality is responsible for the symptom of stress incontinence, and that it is potentially correctible by reparative surgery. Marchetti's extensive experience with this test, together with that of many other institutions including our own, indicates that, with occasional exceptions, it is highly reliable. Low (1964) found it to be universally confirmatory in his analysis of the clinical characteristics of 138 patients with stress incontinence.

Urethrocystography

The most decisive and helpful study of all continues to be metallic beadchain urethrocystography. The procedure is greatly facilitated by the preparation of sterile kits, each containing the necessary items (Figure 13–9). The technique is as follows:

1. The patient voids and any residual urine is removed by catheter and the amount recorded. Where indicated a specimen is submitted for culture.
2. Exactly 150 ml. of 12 per cent sodium iodide solution warmed to body temperature is instilled slowly into the bladder, followed by 15 ml. of warm Lipiodol solution, the latter settling to the bottom of the bladder and providing optimum visualization of the vesical neck area.
3. Almost the entire length of the metallic beaded chain is then inserted into the bladder, employing a longitudinally bisected urethral catheter. A short strip of umbilical tape fastened to the protruding end of the chain prevents its inadvertent loss within the bladder.
4. After disengaging the chain, the bisected urethral catheter is removed.
5. Standard x-ray exposures are then made in the anteroposterior and lateral views, first with the patient standing relaxed, then during maximum straining while performing the Valsalva maneuver. The lateral, standing-straining view is by far the most significant one, revealing as it does the principal urethrovesical relationships.

Urethrocystograms provide the only truly objective means of accurately visualizing and classifying the abnormal anatomy associated with stress incontinence, and

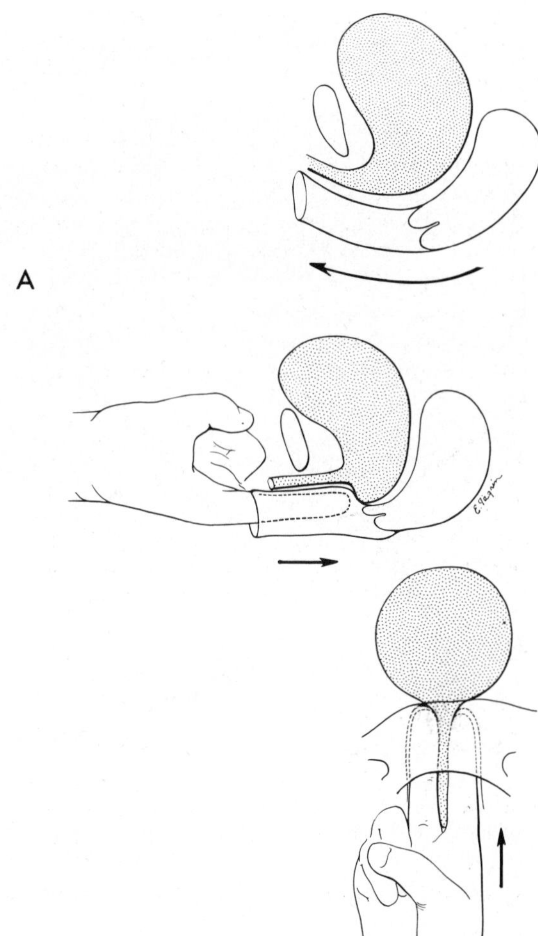

Figure 13-8. Vesical neck elevation test (Bonney-Kead-Marchetti).

A, Patient in lithotomy position, straining with full bladder, demonstrates incontinence as bladder neck descends.

B, Elevation and support of bladder neck by fingers of examiner prevents descent, and incontinence does not occur.

(From Green, T. H., Jr.: Gynecology—Essentials of Clinical Practice. 2nd Ed. Boston, Little, Brown and Co., 1971. Chap. 18.)

their use has led to a better understanding of these anatomic disturbances and how they may best be corrected. A uniform technique in all aspects of these radiologic studies markedly enhances their value. Accurate comparisons in pre- and postoperative films in each patient are thus possible and are of great help in determining the reasons for success or failure in the individual case. Furthermore, valid correlations of the radiologic changes in large numbers of patients treated by the various surgical procedures are also feasible, if all are studied by a consistent technique.

Radiologic study of urethrovesical relationships confirms the presence and precisely demonstrates the extent of the anatomic defect responsible for the symptoms in patients with true stress incontinence. In addition, a normal urethrocystogram positively identifies patients with abnormal urinary leakage of some other cause.

ANATOMIC CLASSIFICATION AND SELECTION OF OPERATIVE PROCEDURE

As already described in the section on pathophysiology, the use of urethrocystograms to accurately study the precise urethrovesical anatomic abnormalities encountered in women with true stress incontinence permits classification of these patients into two basic types of abnormal anatomy, based on the urethral axis factor (Type I and Type II). This classification has proved to be of great importance in the selection of the proper operative repair for the individual patient.

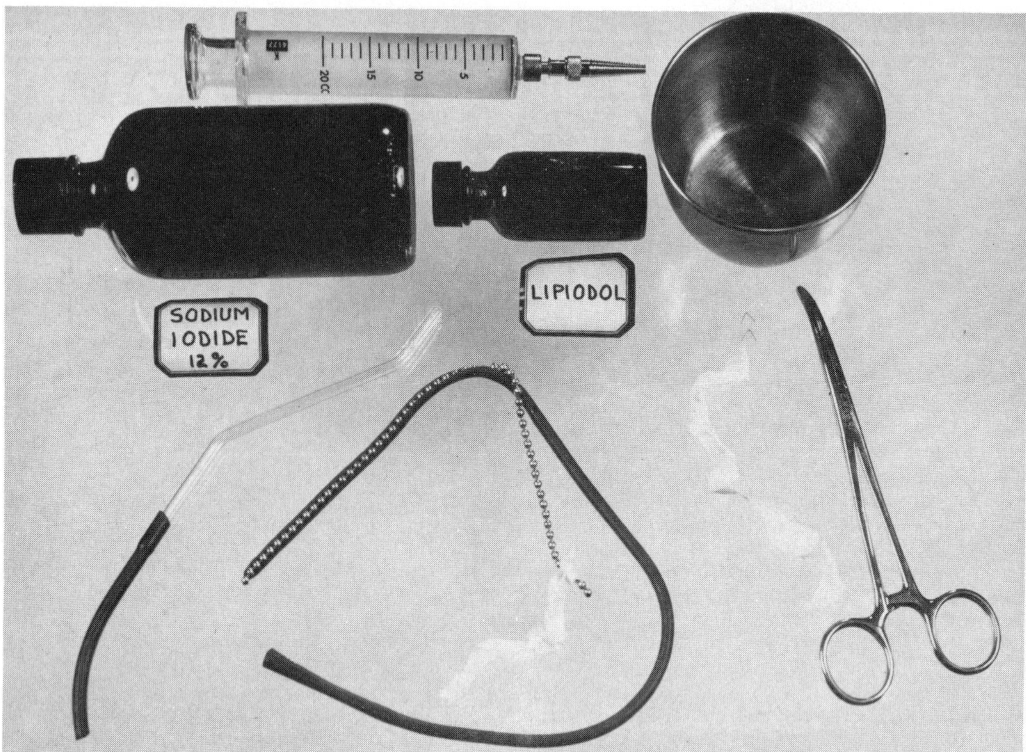

Figure 13–9. Items included in sterile Cystogram Kits prepared for use in the technique of urethrocystography described in text. (From Green, T. H., Jr.: Urinary stress incontinence. *In* Davis' Gynecology & Obstetrics, Vol. II. New York, Harper & Row, Chap. 56.)

Bailey had found by 1956 that vaginal repair alone, although yielding highly satisfactory results in the Type I patient, produced cure of stress incontinence in no more than half of the Type II patients. However, the introduction and subsequent use of his "modified colporrhaphy" (a retropubic suspension combined with the standard vaginal repair) in the management of patients with Type II stress incontinence had resulted in a 90 per cent 5 to 10 year cure rate in these cases by the time of his 1963 report. Clinical experience at our institution has been entirely in accord with Bailey's observations.

In an early report (Green, 1962), retrospective analysis of our material 5 years previously had revealed that a careful vaginal operation had successfully relieved the stress incontinence in 90 per cent of the Type I patients but had failed to correct effectively or permanently the abnormal anatomy or relieve the symptoms of incontinence in over 50 per cent of the Type II patients. However, use of the Marshall-Marchetti suprapubic urethrovesical suspension in the management of 28 women with Type II stress incontinence resulted in a 93 per cent 5 year cure rate. The significance of the abnormal urethral axis has subsequently been confirmed in a number of other reports (Barnett, 1969, 1970; Crist et al., 1969; Pereyra and Lebherz, 1967; and others).

Basic Surgical Approaches

This preliminary clinical experience suggested using the anatomic classification as a basis for selecting the appropriate operative procedure. A variety of operations to correct stress incontinence have been devised over the years. However, nearly all can be categorized as one of the following:

(1) A vaginal approach — an attempt to reconstruct normal urethrovesical anatomy

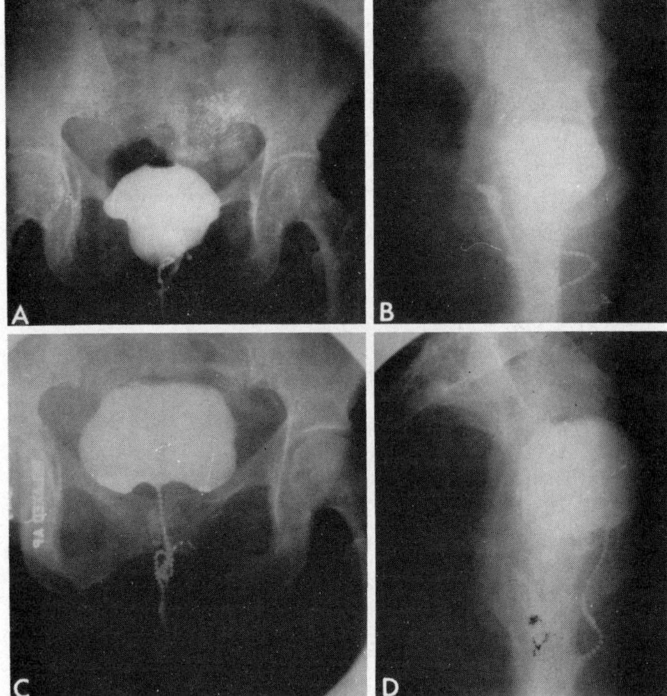

Figure 13–11. Urethrocystograms of a 47-year-old para IV with Type II stress incontinence of three years' duration, with associated uterine prolapse, successfully treated by vaginal hysterectomy and repair combined with suprapubic urethrovesical suspension. She has been completely relieved of stress incontinence during an 18-year follow-up period.

A and *B*, Preoperative anteroposterior and lateral straining views, showing a typical Type II configuration.

C and *D*, Postoperative anteroposterior and lateral straining views. Note that the PUV angle and urethral axis are effectively restored to normal, actually exhibiting the "overcorrected" pattern characteristic of the anatomy following a Marshall-Marchetti repair.

(From Green, T. H., Jr.: Am. J. Obstet. Gynecol. *83*:632, 1962.)

high rate of success can be obtained in the Type II patients by the addition of a supplementary suprapubic urethrovesical suspension to the overall surgical procedure. Among 110 patients undergoing corrective surgery during the period of 1953–1957, the overall cure rate was only 80 per cent, but with adoption of this plan of management in

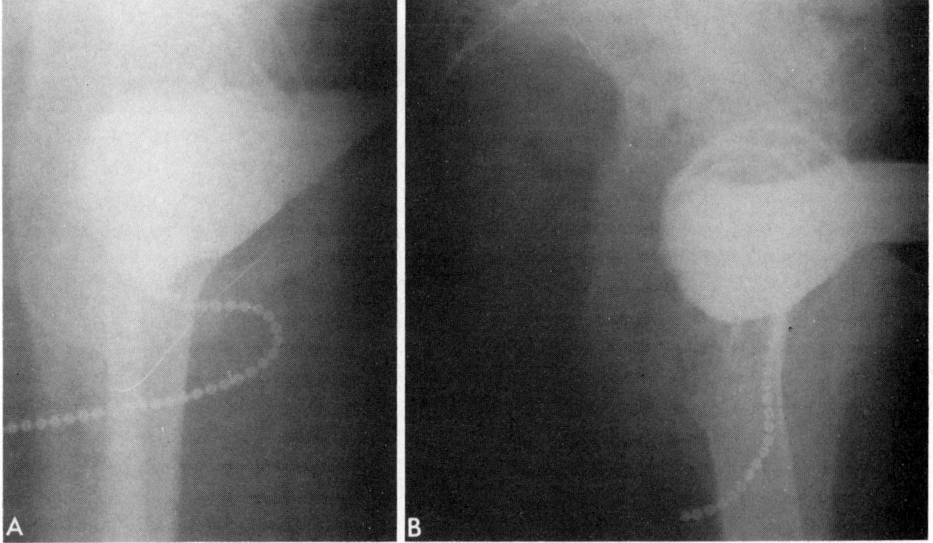

Figure 13–12. Urethrocystograms in Type II stress incontinence. *A*, Preoperative film; *B*, postoperative film following the Marshall-Marchetti suprapubic urethrovesical suspension operation. Note restoration of normal posterior urethrovesical angle and the normal urethral axis of inclination postoperatively, with relief of stress incontinence. (From Green, T. H., Jr.: Gynecology — Essentials of Clinical Practice. 2nd Ed. Boston, Little, Brown and Co., 1971. Chap. 18.)

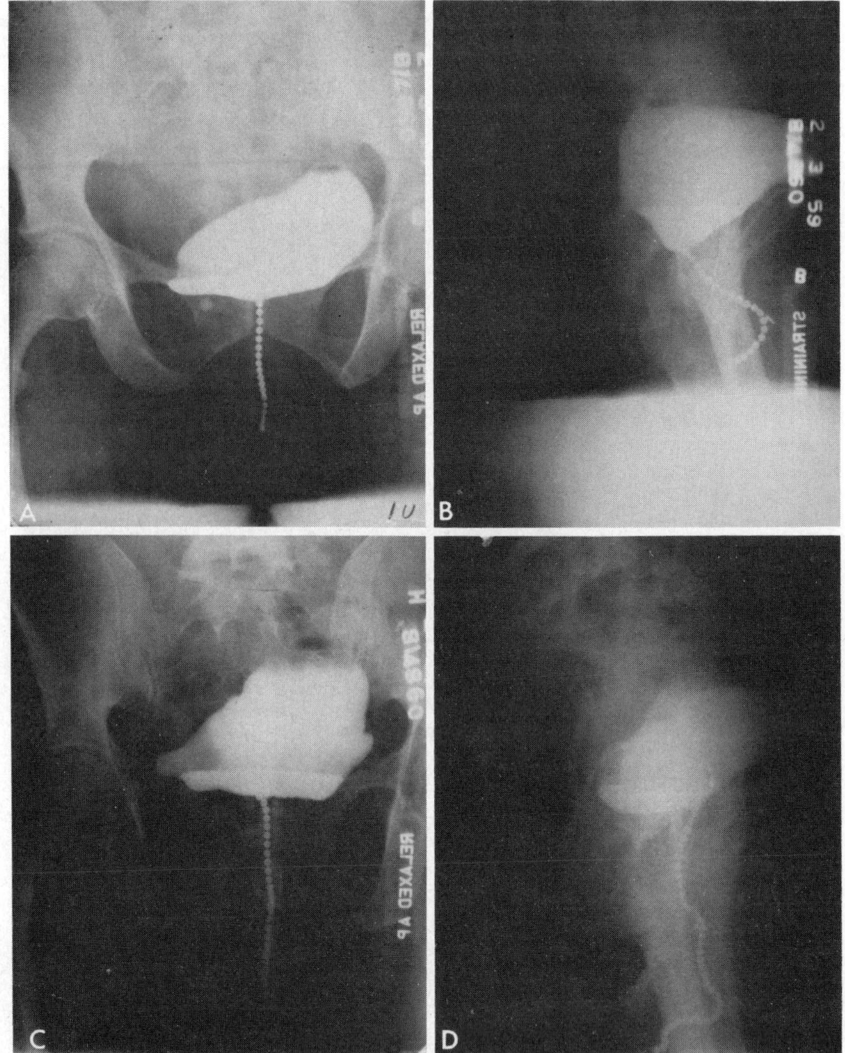

Figure 13–13. Moderate Type II stress incontinence: Treatment by Marshall-Marchetti procedure with abdominal hysterectomy, in a 40-year-old para II with a fibroid uterus and stress incontinence of five years' duration.

A and *B,* Preoperative urethrocystograms revealing a Type II configuration with complete loss of the PUV angle and rotational descent of the urethra, producing an angle of inclination of 60 degrees. Total abdominal hysterectomy combined with a suprapubic urethrovesical suspension was performed.

C and *D,* Postoperative urethrocystograms showing satisfactory repair: Note the typical "overcorrection" of both PUV angle and urethral axis rotation characteristic of the Marshall-Marchetti operation, with no significant increase in urethral length. The patient has remained free of stress incontinence during a 16-year-follow-up period.

(From Green, T. H., Jr.: Am. J. Obstet. Gynecol. *83*:632, 1962.)

1957, the permanent cure rate in subsequent years has risen to 96 per cent.

As reported 15 years ago (Green, 1968) and again more recently (Green, 1975), we continue to employ this program of management based on the anatomic classification at our institution, and analysis of the end-results achieved by this approach offers further convincing evidence for its success. As shown in Table 13–2, 341 patients were treated during the period 1957–1970 and have now been followed for a minimum of 5 years. In addition to the routine preoperative metallic beadchain urethrocystogram, all patients had one or more postoperative urethrocystograms.

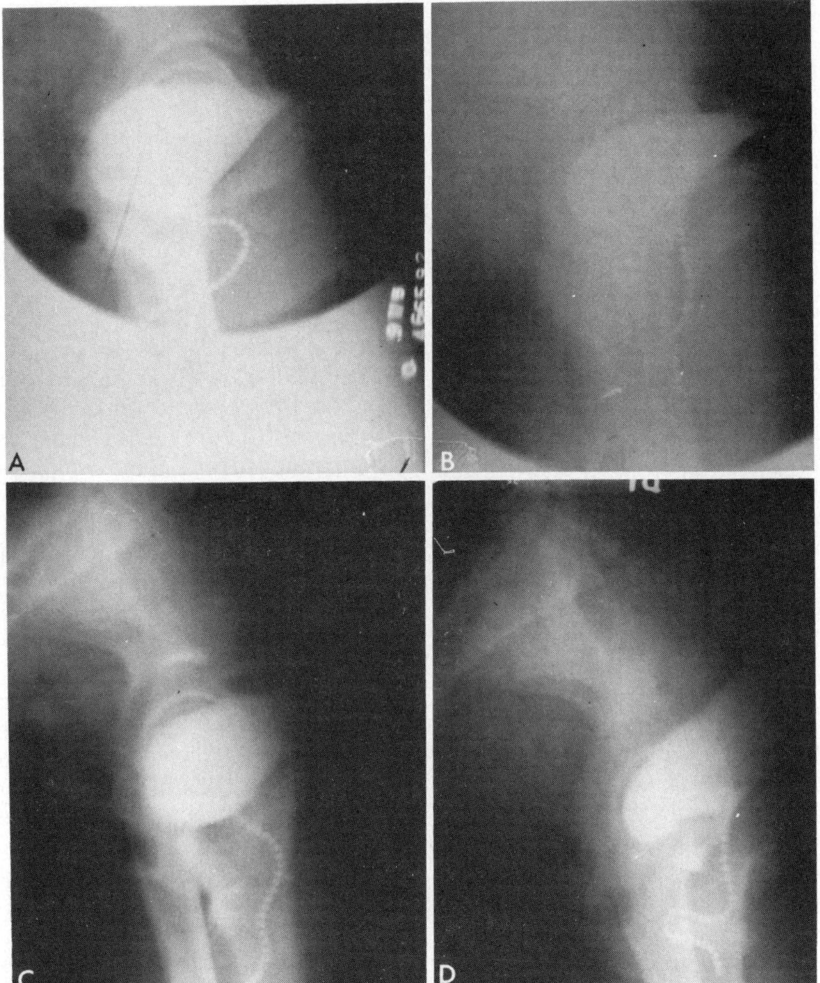

Figure 13–14. Urethrocystograms showing Type II stress incontinence: Recurrence after initial Marshall-Marchetti procedure, with eventual cure by fascial sling operation, in a 46-year-old obese para VI with a history of abdominal hysterectomy nine years previously and increasing stress incontinence of several years' duration.

A, Typical Type II findings.

B, Apparently satisfactory correction achieved by the initial suprapubic urethrovesical suspension.

C, Symptoms suggestive of recurrent stress incontinence appeared eight months later and became worse during the next six months. Note progressively increasing rotational descent of the urethra and widening of the PUV angle.

D, Final postoperative urethrocystogram. A combined abdominovaginal rectus fascial sling operation was done nearly 1½ years after initial Marshall-Marchetti procedure. There was immediate relief of stress incontinence, and the patient has remained free from symptoms during the 13 subsequent years of follow-up observation.

(From Green, T. H., Jr.: Am. J. Obstet. Gynecol. *83*:632, 1962.)

Without exception, x-ray studies demonstrated the typical abnormal urethrovesical anatomy preoperatively, and of equal significance, patients cured of stress incontinence presented and continued to retain normal-appearing urethrocystograms postoperatively. On the other hand, operative failures were accompanied by reappearance of the characteristic abnormal urethrovesical anatomy on the postoperative films. Type I anatomy was present in 77 patients (22 per cent of the total series), and a primary cure rate of 95 per cent was obtained in this group. Two additional pa-

TABLE 13–2. RESULTS OF STRESS INCONTINENCE TREATMENT PROGRAM MASSACHUSETTS GENERAL HOSPITAL, 1957–1970

Anatomic Type	Number of Patients	Primary Cure	Secondary Cure	Final Cure Rate	Persistent Failure Rate
I	77 (22%)	73 (95%)	2	75 (97%)	2 (3%)
II	264 (78%)	240 (91%)	15	255 (96%)	9 (4%)
Totals	341	313 (92%)	17	330 (97%)	11 (3%)

(Duration of Follow-up: 5–18 Years)

tients were cured by a second operation, yielding a final cure rate of 97 per cent over the 5 to 18 year follow-up period. The Type II abnormal anatomic configuration was present in 264 patients (78 per cent of the total series), and a 91 per cent primary cure rate was achieved by the initial operation. An additional 15 patients in this group were relieved of stress incontinence by a second operation, yielding a final cure rate of 96 per cent over the 5- to 18-year interval of postoperative observation. The final cure rate for the entire group of patients followed 5 to 18 years postoperatively was thus 96 per cent.

As indicated in Table 13–3, the vast majority (68 of 77) of the patients with Type I anatomy underwent primary vaginal procedures, with a cure rate of 96 per cent for the vaginal approach. There was also one failure in the group of nine undergoing a Marshall-Marchetti procedure; this represents an obvious technical failure, since this patient was completely cured by a repeat Marshall-Marchetti operation.

TABLE 13–3. RESULTS OF OPERATION FOR TYPE I STRESS INCONTINENCE IN 77 PATIENTS

Primary Cure	
Vaginal repair, with or without hysterectomy	65
Abd. hyst. and MM	7
MM alone	1
	73 (95%)
Primary Failure	
Vaginal repair	3
Abd. hyst. and MM	1
	4 (5%)
Cured by Second Operation	
MM (failed vaginal repair)	1
Repeat MM (failed abd. hyst. and MM)	1
	2
Persistent Failure	
MM (failed vaginal repair)	1
No further surgery	1
	2

Abd. hyst. = abdominal hysterectomy
MM = Marshall-Marchetti procedure

Table 13–4 presents the results of the various procedures employed in patients with Type II anatomy. It is of considerable interest from the standpoint of one technical point (should hysterectomy usually accompany a Marshall-Marchetti operation?), and also emphasizes again the relative inability of the standard vaginal approach alone to correct stress incontinence of the Type II anatomic variety. In the group of 149 patients undergoing the Marshall-Marchetti procedure with concomitant abdominal hysterectomy, 144 were cured (97 per cent). Thirty-seven of 41 patients who had undergone prior hysterectomy for other causes and who were then treated by us for stress incontinence by the Marshall-Marchetti operation were cured (90 per cent). On the other hand, in 40 patients in this series, the uterus was left in place at the time the Marshal-Marchetti operation was done, and the cure rate was only 82 per cent. (One of the failures is illustrated in Figure 13–15). This experience strongly suggests, and in fact has led us to adopt, a policy of concomitant hysterectomy whenever a Marshall-Marchetti operation is performed for Type II stress incontinence. An exception is made when there is a good reason to avoid removal of the uterus — e.g., in occasional younger patients in whom preservation of child-bearing function is desired, or in occasional elderly patients for whom the addition of hysterec-

TABLE 13–4. RESULTS OF OPERATION FOR TYPE II STRESS INCONTINENCE IN 264 PATIENTS

Cured		Failed	
MM + hyst.	144	MM + hyst.	5
MM alone	33	MM alone	7
MM (previous hyst.)	37	MM (previous hyst.)	4
Vag. hyst. + rep.	3	Vag. hyst. + rep.	3
Vag. hyst. + MM	9	Vag. rep. alone	2
Fascial sling operation	14	Fascial sling operation	3
	240 (91%)		24 (9%)

MM = Marshall-Marchetti procedure
Vag. hyst. = vaginal hysterectomy
Hyst. = abdominal hysterectomy
Vag. rep. = vaginal repair

tomy might unnecessarily increase the operative risk or morbidity.

That concomitant hysterectomy need not be mandatory is obvious from the reasonably satisfactory cure rate of 82 per cent observed in this series when the Marshall-Marchetti procedure alone was done. In addition, Marchetti and co-workers (1957) reported that after this operation, a number of young women later conceived and underwent vaginal delivery without subsequent recurrence of their stress incontinence. Nevertheless, it seems apparent that if conditions are favorable and there is no valid reason to preserve the uterus, concomitant hysterectomy increases the permanent, long-term cure rate of the Marshall-Marchetti suprapubic urethrovesical suspension.

That the standard vaginal approach is relatively ineffective in correcting Type II stress incontinence is also emphasized in Table 13–4. A small number of patients were selected for vaginal procedures because they were relatively poor candidates for abdominal surgery, despite the knowledge that their urethrovesical anatomic abnormality was of the Type II configuration.

TABLE 13–5. RESULTS OF SECONDARY OPERATION FOR TYPE II STRESS INCONTINENCE IN 24 PATIENTS (9%)

Primary Procedure		Secondary Procedure		Cured	Failed
MM with abd. hyst.	(5)	Fascial sling	(4)	3	1
		No further surgery	(1)	0	1
MM alone	(7)	Vag. hyst. + fascial sling	(4)	4	0
		Vag. rep. + fascial sling	(1)	0	1
		No further surgery	(2)	0	2
MM (previous abd. hyst.)	(4)	Fascial sling	(3)	3	0
		No further surgery	(1)	0	1
Vag. hyst. with rep.	(3)	Fascial sling	(1)	1	0
		MM	(2)	2	0
Vag. rep. alone	(2)	MM + abd. hyst.	(2)	2	0
Fascial sling	(3)	MM + vag. rep.	(1)	0	1
		Vag. rep. + MM + vaginal sling	(1)	0	1
		No further surgery	(1)	0	1
TOTALS	(24)			15	9

MM = Marshall-Marchetti procedure
Vag. hyst. = vaginal hysterectomy
Abd. hyst. = abdominal hysterectomy
Vag. rep. = vaginal repair

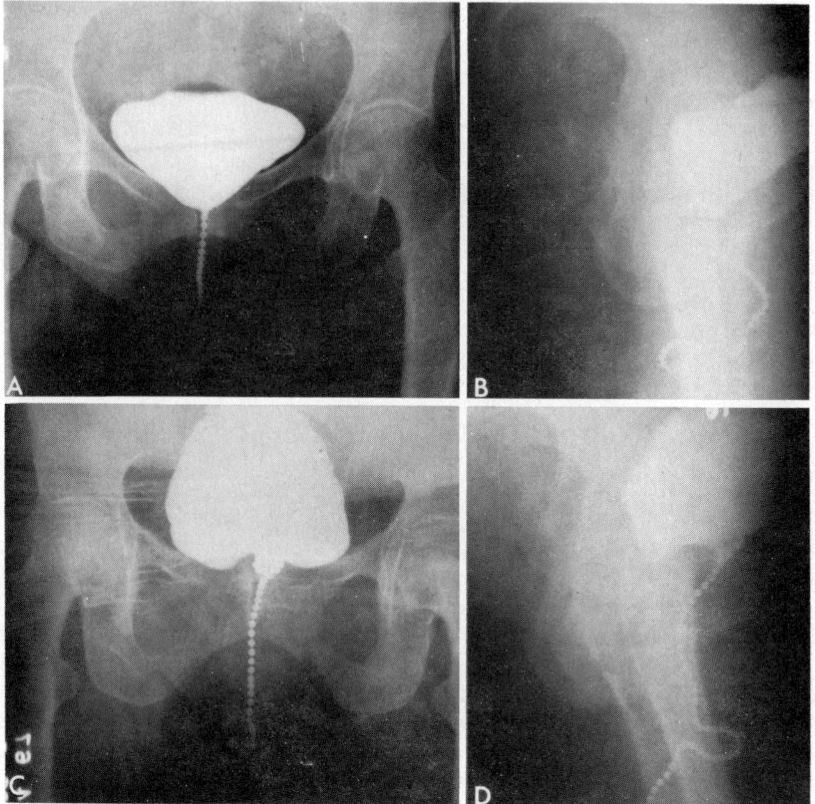

Figure 13–15. Urethrocystograms demonstrating failure of the Marshall-Marchetti operation alone to relieve stress incontinence when a relatively poorly supported uterus is allowed to remain.

A and *B*, Upper anteroposterior and lateral views, showing the anatomic situation six months following the initial Marshall-Marchetti procedure. The patient continued to suffer severe stress incontinence.

C and *D*, Lower anteroposterior and lateral views, demonstrating the restoration of a normal urethrovesical anatomic configuration achieved by the second operation, a combined vaginal hysterectomy and rectus fascial sling procedure. The patient has been completely cured of stress incontinence. (From Green, T. H., Jr.: The problem of urinary stress incontinence in the female: an appraisal of its current status. Obstet. Gynecol. Surv. *23*:603, 1968. Copyright © The Williams & Wilkins Co., Baltimore.)

Six underwent vaginal hysterectomy with anterior and posterior colporrhaphies, and, predictably, only three were cured. The 50 per cent cure rate was identical to that noted by Bailey (1954, 1956) and also reported in our own previous series (Green, 1962). Two patients underwent anterior and posterior colporrhaphies alone, leaving the uterus in place, and neither was relieved of her stress incontinence. It is of further interest to note in Table 13–5 that all five of these initial failures were later cured by a properly selected second operation — by a Marshall-Marchetti in two and by a fascial sling in the third of the three failures following vaginal hysterectomy and repairs; and by hysterectomy plus a Marshall-Marchetti in the two failures following vaginal repairs alone. An example of failure to cure Type II incontinence by a vaginal approach and subsequent successful correction by a Marshall-Marchetti procedure is shown in Figures 13–16 and 13–17. In contrast, and also listed in Table 13–4, nine patients with uterine prolapse accompanying their Type II stress incontinence underwent vaginal hysterectomy with concomitant Marshall-Marchetti urethrovesical suspension as their primary operation, and all nine were completely cured of their stress incontinence.

As noted in Tables 13–4 and 13–5, the fascial sling operation was used 30 times in this series of 341 patients. It was employed as the primary operation for Type II anatomy in 17 patients who were obese and asthmatic, with 14 cures (82 per cent), and on 13 occasions as the second operation

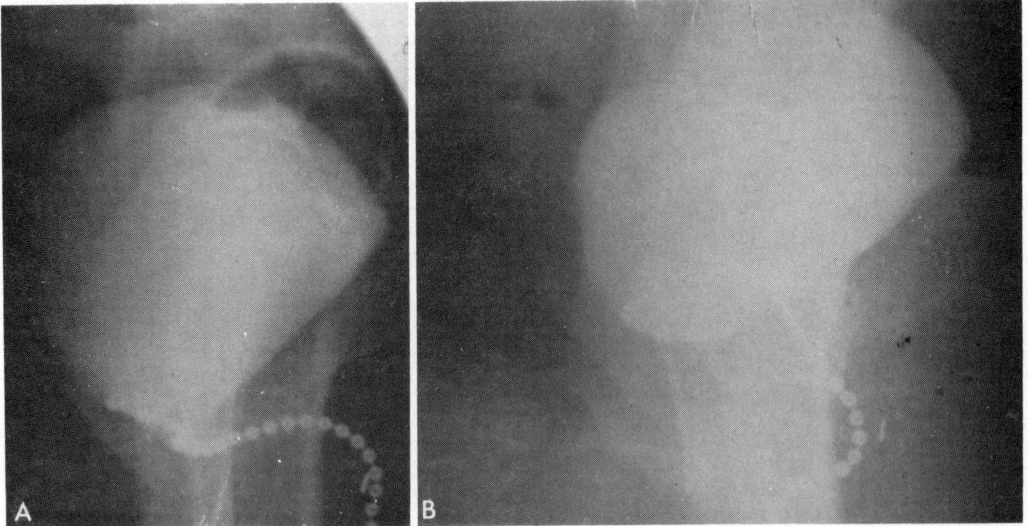

Figure 13–16. Type II stress incontinence and inadequate surgical correction. The significance of the rotational descent of the urethral axis in this patient was not appreciated prior to the initial operation.

A, Urethroystogram before vaginal hysterectomy and anterior colporrhaphy.

B, Urethrocystogram made 10 days after vaginal operation, which shows apparently satisfactory restoration of a normal posterior urethrovesical angle. On closer inspection, however, the PUV angle is rather "short," and the urethral axis remains partially rotated. As would now be predicted, incontinence recurred within six months.

(From Green, T. H., Jr.: Development of a plan for the diagnosis and treatment of urinary stress incontinence. Am. J. Obstet. Gynecol. *83*:632, 1962.)

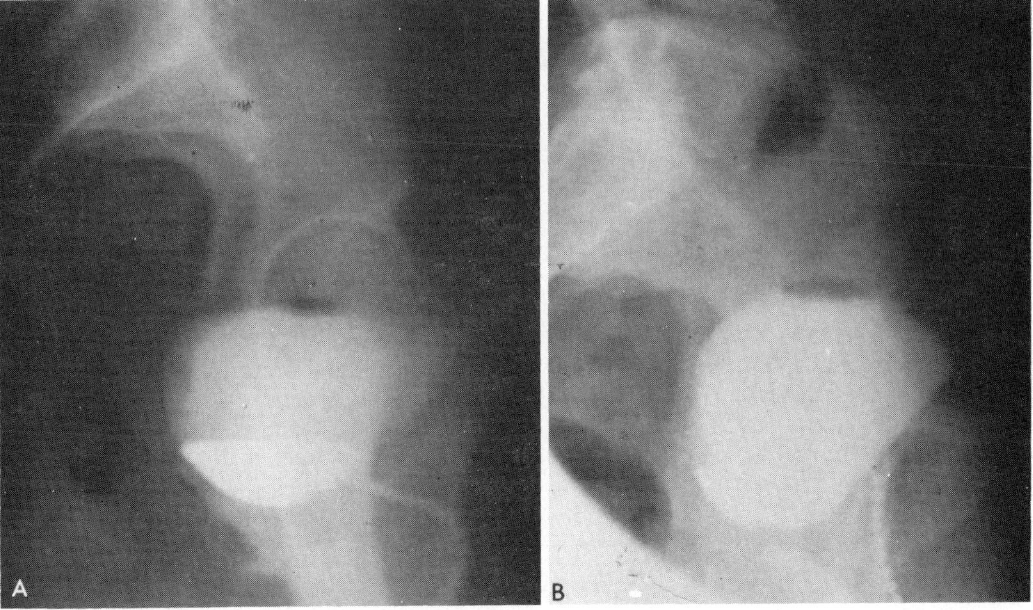

Figure 13–17. Recurrence of Type II stress incontinence six months after vaginal repair, with ultimate correction by Marshall-Marchetti procedure.

A, Urethrocystogram made following failure of vaginal repair; return of stress incontinence shows increasing loss of PUV angle and abnormal rotation of urethral axis.

B, Urethrocystogram made after successful suprapubic urethrovesical suspension; a complete cure of stress incontinence.

(From Green, T. H., Jr.: Development of a plan for the diagnosis and treatment of urinary stress incontinence. Am. J. Obstet. Gynecol. *83*:632, 1962.)

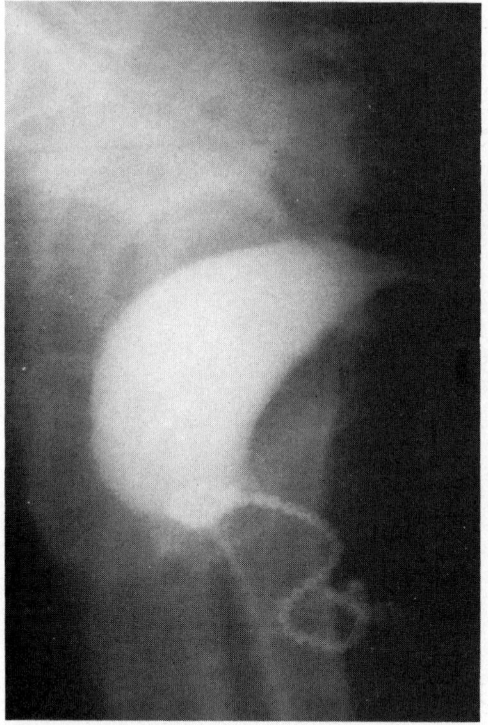

Figure 13–18. An example of persistent failure to relieve stress incontinence in a 50-year-old, obese diabetic who had undergone subtotal hysterectomy eight years previously, and who was first seen in 1962 with Type II stress incontinence. Vaginal cervicectomy, anterior and posterior colporrhaphies with repair of enterocele, and a concomitant Mersilene urethral sling operation were done in May 1962, with initial relief of stress incontinence for two years and then partial return of the symptom. Because of sinus formation and chronic suppuration around the Mersilene sling, it was removed in November 1965, with resulting increased severity of stress incontinence.

A Marshall-Marchetti procedure was done in May 1966, with only transient improvement; a suburethral myoplasty and vaginal obliteration in September 1966 also failed to relieve the incontinence. As clearly demonstrated in the lateral urethrocystogram obtained following her last operation and shown here, the reason for the persistent stress incontinence lies in the failure of her multiple surgical procedures to permanently restore normal urethrovesical anatomy, not in some obscure, hypothetical, as yet undiscovered cause for this type of abnormal leakage of urine.

(From Green, T. H., Jr.: The problem of urinary stress incontinence in the female: an appraisal of its current status. Obstet. Gynecol. Surv. *23*:603, 1968. Copyright © The Williams & Wilkins Co., Baltimore.)

following an initial failure, with cure resulting in 11 (85 per cent). A number of these patients experienced prolonged voiding difficulties, a few requiring catheter drainage for 3 to 6 months. Thus, the fascial sling procedure, though a somewhat more complicated and extensive procedure than the Marshall-Marchetti operation, has yielded very satisfactory results when used selectively in situations where the latter either has already failed or seems less likely to be effective.

Finally, Table 13–5 also reveals that there were a few persistent failures, some of them undergoing multiple unsuccessful operative procedures, often initially with apparent relief of their stress incontinence, only to have recurrence develop a few months later. (Such a case is illustrated in Figure 13–18.) Perhaps there will always be a small percentage of intractable cases in any sizable series, possibly primarily due to the poor quality of the tissues with which to work in some patients. The significant feature of the failures in this series is the fact that the repeated urethrocystograms following each unsuccessful operation clearly demonstrated that the characteristic abnormal urethrovesical anatomy of stress incontinence had recurred each time, despite our determined efforts to correct it surgically. Unsatisfactory clinical results, in patients who have been carefully studied and shown to have true, anatomic stress incontinence, are invariably due to technical failure of the operation rather than to treatment based on erroneous concepts of the cause of stress incontinence.

REFERENCES

Arnold, E P., Webster, J. R., Loose, H., et al.: Urodynamics of female incontinence: factors influencing the results of surgery. Am. J. Obstet. Gynecol., *117*:805, 1973.

Bailey, K. V.: A clinical investigation into uterine prolapse with stress incontinence. Treatment by modified Manchester colporrhaphy. J. Obstet. Gynaecol. Brit. Emp., Part I, *61*:291, 1954; Part II, *63*:663, 1956; Part III, *79*:947, 1963.

Barnett, R. M.: The modern Kelly plication. Obstet. Gynecol. *34*:667, 1969.

Barnett, R. M.: Ball combined cystopexy. Obstet. Gynecol. *36*:547, 1970.

Bates, C. P., Loose, H., and Stanton, S. L. R.: The objective study of incontinence after repair operations. Surg. Gynecol. Obstet. *136*:17, 1973.

Beck, R. P., and Maughan, G. B.: Simultaneous intraurethral and intravesical pressure studies in normal women and those with stress incontinence. Am. J. Obstet. Gynecol. *89*:746, 1964.

Burch, J. C.: Cooper's ligament urethrovesical suspension for stress incontinence. Am. J. Obstet. Gynecol. *100*:764, 1968.

Crist, T., Shingleton, H. M., and Roberson, W. E.: Urethrovesical needle suspension: postoperative loss of vesical neck support demonstrated by chain cystography. Obstet. Gynecol. *34*:489,.1969.

Dutton, W. A.: The urethrovesical angle and stress incontinence. Canad. M. Assoc. J. *83*:1242, 1960.

Enhorning, G.: Simultaneous recording of intravesical and intraurethral pressure: a study on urethral closure in normal and stress incontinent women. Acta Chir. Scand., Suppl. *276*:1, 1961.

Frewen, W. K.: Urgency incontinence. J. Obstet. Gynaecol. Br. Commonw. *79*:77, 1972.

Green, T. H., Jr.: Development of a plan for the diagnosis and treatment of urinary stress incontinence. Am. J. Obstet. Gynecol. *83*:632, 1962.

Green, T. H., Jr.: Urinary stress incontinence. *In* Meigs, J. V., and Sturgis, S. H. (eds.): Progress in Gynecology, Vol. IV. New York, Grune and Stratton, Inc., 1963, pp. 531–556.

Green, T. H., Jr.: The problem of urinary stress incontinence in the female: an appraisal of its current status. Obstet. Gynecol. Surv. *23*:603, 1968.

Green, T. H., Jr.: Operative management of urinary stress incontinence. *In* Cooper, P. (ed.): The Craft of Surgery. Boston, Little Brown and Co., 1971, Chap. 118.

Green, T. H., Jr.: Gynecology — Essentials of Clinical Practice. 2nd Ed. Boston, Little, Brown and Co., 1971.

Green, T. H., Jr.: Urinary stress incontinence: Differential diagnosis, pathophysiology, and management. Am. J. Obstet. Gynecol., *122*:368, 1975.

Harer, W. B., Jr., and Gunther, R. E: Simplified urethrovesical suspension and urethroplasty. Am. J. Obstet. Gynecol. *91*:1017, 1965.

Hodgkinson, C. P.: Relationships of the female urethra and bladder in urinary stress incontinence. Am. J. Obstet. Gynecol. *65*:560, 1953.

Hodgkinson, C. P.: Stress urinary incontinence — 1970. Am. J. Obstet. Gynecol. *108*:1141, 1970.

Hodgkinson, C. P., and Cobert, N.: Direct urethrocystometry. Am. J. Obstet. Gynecol. *79*:648, 1960.

Hodgkinson, C. P., and Morgan, J. E.: Basic pressures of voiding in the adult female. J. Obstet. Gynecol. *103*:755, 1969.

Hodgkinson, C. P., Ayers, M. A., and Drukker, B. H.: Dyssynergic detrusor dysfunction in the apparently normal female. Am. J. Obstet. Gynecol. *87*:717, 1963.

Hodgkinson, C. P., Drukker, B. H., and Hershey, G. J. G.: Stress urinary incontinence in the female—VIII, etiology, significance of the short urethra. Am. J. Obstet. Gynecol. *86*:16, 1963.

Ingelman-Sundberg, A.: Plastic repair of the pelvic floor with a report of 31 cases of stress incontinence. Acta Obstet. Gynecol. Scand. *30*:318, 1950.

Jeffcoate, T. N. A., and Francis, W. A. A.: Urinary incontinence in the female. Am. J. Obstet. Gynecol. *94*:604, 1966.

Jeffcoate, T. N. A., and Roberts, H.: Observations on stress incontinence of urine. Am. J. Obstet. Gynecol. *64*:721, 1952.

Jeffcoate, T. N. A. and Roberts, H.: Stress incontinence of urine. J. Obstet. Gynaecol. Br. Emp. *59*:685, 1952.

Jeffcoate, T. N. A., and Roberts, H.: Effects of urethrocystopexy for stress incontinence. Surg. Gynecol. Obstet. *98*:743, 1954.

Lapides, J., Ajemian, E. P., Stewart, B. H., et al.: Physiopathology of stress incontinence. Surg. Gynecol. Obstet. *111*:224, 1960.

Leadbetter, G. W., Jr.: Surgical correction of total urinary incontinence. J. Urol. *91*:261, 1964.

Low, J. A.: Clinical characteristics of patients with demonstrable urinary incontinence. Am. J. Obstet. Gynecol. *88*:322, 1964.

Marchetti, A. A.: The female bladder and urethra before and after correction for stress incontinence. Am. J. Obstet. Gynecol. *58*:1145, 1949.

Marchetti, A. A.: Urinary incontinence. J.A.M.A. *162*:1366, 1956.

Marchetti, A. A., Marshall, V. F., and Shultis, L. D.: Simple vesicourethral suspension for stress incontinence of urine. Am. J. Obstet. Gynecol. *74*:57, 1957.

Muellner, S. R., and Fleischner, F. G.: Normal and abnormal micturition; study of bladder behavior by means of the fluoroscope. J. Urol. *61*:233, 1949.

Nichols, D. H.: The Mersilene mesh gauze-hammock for severe urinary stress incontinence. Obstet. Gynecol. *41*:88, 1973.

Pereyra, A. J.: A simplified surgical procedure for the correction of stress incontinence in women. West. J. Surg. *67*:223, 1959.

Pereyra, A. J., and Lebherz,.T. B.: Combined urethrovesical suspension and vaginourethroplasty for correction of stress incontinence. Obstet. Gynecol. *30*:537, 1967.

Schonberg, L. A., Wentzel, G. M., and Higgins, L. W.: Urethrocystography, a practical office procedure in the evaluation and treatment of stress incontinence. Am. J. Obstet. Gynecol. *86*:995, 1963.

Shingleton, H. M., Barkley, K. L., and Talbert, L. M.: Management of stress urinary incontinence in the female. Use of the chain cystogram. South. Med. J. *59*:547, 1966.

Steinhausen, T. B., Kariher, D. H., Sherwood, C. E., et al.: Chain urethrocystography before and after urethrovesical suspension for stress incontinence. Obstet. Gynecol. *35*:405, 1970.

Te Linde, R. W.: The urethral sling operation. Clin. Obstet. Gynecol. *6*:206, 1963.

Toews, H. A.: Intraurethral and intravesical pressures in normal and stress-incontinent women. Obstet. Gynecol. *29*:613, 1967.

14

EVALUATION OF URINARY INCONTINENCE

SHLOMO RAZ, M.D.

INTRODUCTION

Continence in the female results from a complex interaction of several factors. The factors that combine to result in a perfectly competent mechanism may be categorized into four main groups: (1) functional length of the urethra; (2) closing pressure of the urethra; (3) anatomic position of the bladder neck and urethra; and (4) transmission of intra-abdominal pressures to the urethra. Each of these factors will be discussed separately. A full discussion of urodynamics is included in Chapter 4.

Functional Length of the Urethra

The female urethra measures approximately 4 cm. in length. Functional length is defined as the area of the urethra that exerts pressure above intravesical pressure, or the section that maintains the continence mechanism. In the past, length was believed to be one of the most crucial factors affecting continence. Now, with more modern urodynamic studies available, we have learned that this is not the case (Figure 14–1). More than 50 per cent of patients who are judged to be cured with a procedure for urinary stress incontinence maintain the same functional urethral length. Also, it is well known that patients who have undergone excision of the distal half of the urethra because of tumor or diverticulum can remain continent with a urethra of 1 cm. or less. In the normal female, the average functional urethra is 28 mm. long (Figure 14–2). In patients with urinary stress incontinence due to sphincter incom-

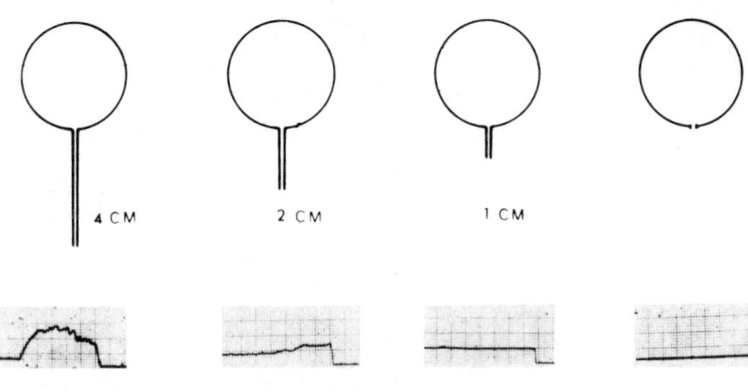

Figure 14–1. Experimental model using the female dog showing (top) diagrams of the urethra with incisions at differing lengths and distances from the bladder neck. On the far right, incision of the bladder neck itself is shown. The graphs (bottom) show the gradient pressures from urethra to the bladder. When the urethra is incised 4 cm. from the bladder neck, the bladder is competent, maintaining the capacity to hold urine. Similarly, when the urethra is incised at 1 cm. and 2 cm. for the neck, the remaining short segment of the urethra is capable of maintaining continence; but when the bladder neck itself is incised, incontinence occurs, and the ability to maintain the pressure gradient is lost. This experiment demonstrates that anatomically shortened urethral segments are capable of maintaining continence regardless of length.

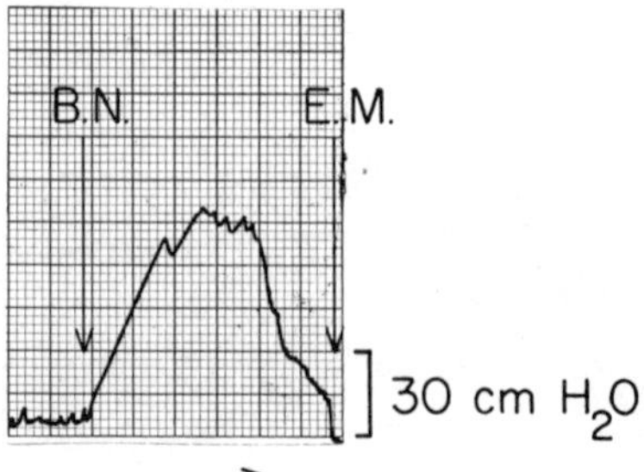

Figure 14–2. Normal urethral pressure profile in a woman, showing functional length of 28 mm. and anatomic length of 30 mm. When urinary stress incontinence due to sphincteric incompetence occurs, functional length decreases but anatomic length may remain unchanged. B.N., Bladder neck; E.M., external meatus.

petence, the functional length decreases to an average of 20 to 22 mm. But other patients can maintain continence with short functional urethras. It would, therefore, appear that functional length alone is not the factor that determines continence.

Closing Pressure of the Urethra

Factors involved in maintaining urethral pressures in the female are complex and, despite extensive investigation, not completely understood. The components of urethral pressures may be divided into factors that include the contribution of the smooth muscle, vascular (Beck and Maughan, 1964), and submucosal tissue, and those affecting extraurethral pressure, including skeletal muscle (Rudd et al., 1980) and the transmission of intra-abdominal pressure to the urethral lumen (Constantinou and Govan, 1980).

Flexibility, or compliance, of the urethra is important in determining the contribution of each of these various components. The urethra is composed of three sphincteric layers, the first being the mucosal-submucosal layer. In the well-vascularized premenopausal urethra, the mucosal layer functions as a seal, because it contains the features of infolding and cross-apposition (Figure 14–3) (Zinner et al., 1980). This arrangement results in a tight closure of the urethral lumen when voiding is not actually occurring. Thus, this layer functions much in the manner of a washer on a faucet, i.e., as a seal. The maintenance of normal urethral mucosal and submucosal layers is hormonally dependent (Raz and Caine, 1973; Van Geelen, 1980). Estrogen is responsible for maintaining a rich submucosal cavernosum similar to the corpora cavernosa in the male. Loss of estrogen with menopause or following bilateral oophorectomy may result in a decrease in thickness of this spongy tissue layer. Using sensitive urethral pressure profilometers, urethral pulsations can be recorded in premenopausal women (Figure 14–4) (Bruskewitz and Raz, 1979). In women with postmenopausal urethral mucosal and submucosal atrophy, it is occasionally possible to see a return of urethral pulsation following estrogen or progesterone administration.

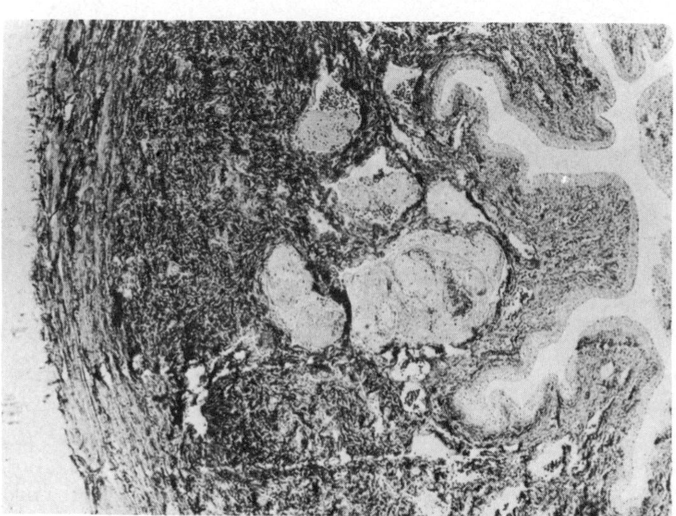

Figure 14–3. Transverse section of female urethra demonstrates infolded mucosa with rich submucosal vascular supply and a small ring of smooth muscle externally. The inner layer acts as a seal; continence is maintained with a minimal amount of external pressure. The mucosa and submucosa are estrogen-dependent.

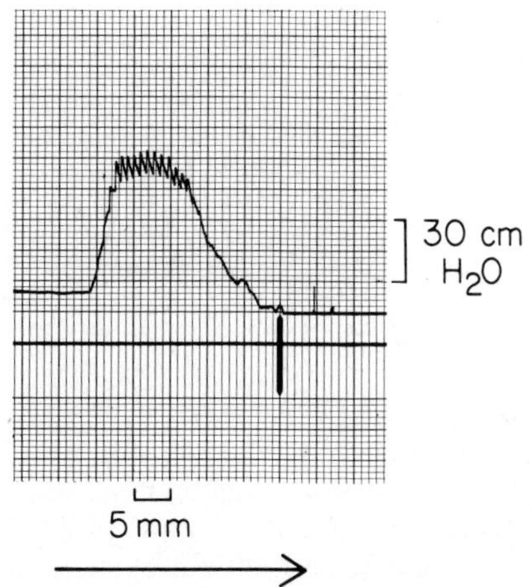

Figure 14–4. Urethral pressure profile in young woman (performed with microtip transducer) demonstrates vascular pulsations parallel to electrocardiographic changes. Postmenopausal patients do not demonstrate these pulsations.

It should be emphasized that the mucosal-sphincteric mechanism does not exert "true" pressure on the urethra, but exists primarily as a seal when the urethra is collapsed. The submucosa, however, may exert pressure.

A second component of urethral pressure is contributed by the smooth muscle layer. The smooth muscle is arranged within the urethral wall in two layers: the internal longitudinal layer, a continuation of the layers of bladder detrusor and trigone; and an external circular layer, which is in part a continuation of external detrusor fibers. Longitudinal layers predominate in an 8:1 ratio over circular fibers, signifying the regular occurrence of a small amount of circular smooth muscle fibers capable of exerting a true sphincteric action on the urethra (Figure 14–5).

It is believed that for a female to achieve continence, the true muscle fibers must be oriented properly and be of an appropriate length to assume a maximum length-tension relationship similar to that achieved by cardiac fibers with regard to Starling's law of the heart.

An important factor in maintaining intraurethral pressures is a layer of skeletal muscle situated adjacent to the female urethra. The heaviest concentration adja-

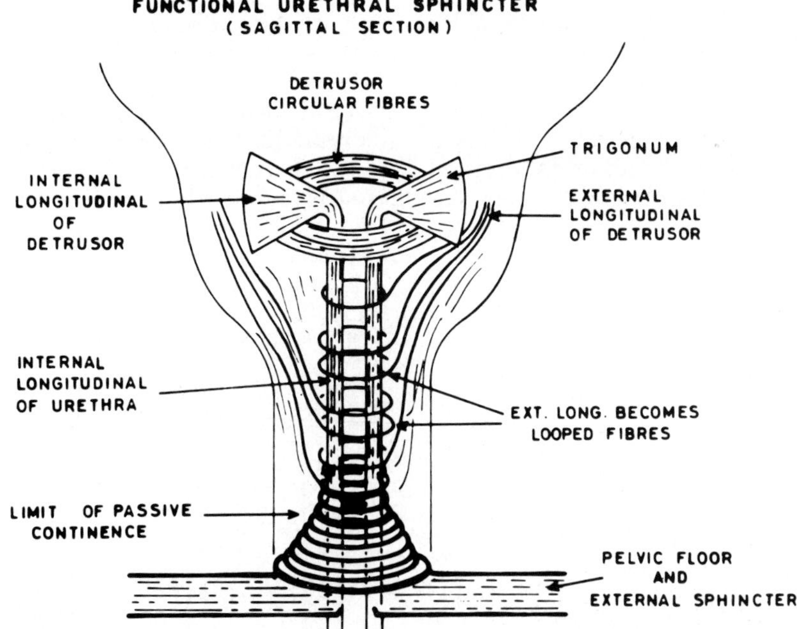

Figure 14–5. Diagram of smooth muscle and external sphincter muscles in a continent woman. Two layers of smooth muscle are present: an inner layer of longitudinal fibers, which is a continuation of the trigone and inner layers of the detrusor, and external looped fibers, which are a prolongation of external longitudinal fibers of the detrusor muscle. The external sphincter does not completely enclose the distal third of the urethra. (From Raz, S.: Pathophysiology of male incontinence. Urol. Clin. North Am. 5:295, 1978.)

EXTERNAL SPHINCTER/PELVIC FLOOR

1. Elasticity of skeletal muscle.

2. Basic tonus -- (Neurogenic integration: gamma loop).

3. Voluntary active contraction.

Figure 14–6. The female external sphincter has three functions: (1) the elasticity of the skeletal muscle, which encloses the smooth muscle and vascular tissue, improves continence; (2) the basic tonus is regulated neurogenically by the gamma loop (gamma and alpha fibers of the anterior neurons in the area of S2-S4); and (3) voluntary contractions.

cent to the urethra is at the level of the urogenital diaphragm, which has a slight proximal extension. It does not fully encircle the urethra, however, but inserts fibers posteriorly, between the urethra and vagina.

Pelvic floor muscles contribute, along with the urogenital diaphragm, to urethral closing pressure (Figures 14–6 to 14–8). This component may be demonstrated by measurement of urethral pressure before and after pudendal nerve block spinal anesthesia or by the administration of skeletal muscle blockers, such as curare or succinylcholine, with general anesthesia (Plante and Sussett, 1980).

Urethral pressure measurements done before and after the block show a drop in pressure of 30 to 50 per cent. In older patients with impairment of periurethral function (from childbirth, hysterectomy, and so forth), the external sphincter component is much less important; this is a factor in the clear decrease in urethral closing pressure, as is seen in older patients.

Anatomic Position

The bladder base and urethra are supported by structures similar to those supporting the cervix — the sacrouterine ligaments, the cardinal ligaments, and the pubocervical ligaments (Figure 14–9).

The largest group of patients suffering sphincteric insufficiency has anatomic abnormalities of the bladder base and urethra. Anatomic abnormalities are related primarily to multiple deliveries, hysterectomy, and diminished estrogenic influence on the urethra. Childbirth, especially when it has been traumatic and per vaginam, damages the pubocervical ligament and the support of the bladder base and urethra. This in turn contributes to a tendency to sphincteric insufficiency, because the urethra and the bladder base have prolapsed. Hysterectomy, especially vaginal hysterectomy, will also alter the support of the bladder base and urethra. The cardinal ligaments, the sacrouterine ligaments, and the pubocervical fascia maintain the uterus and bladder base in their anatomic positions. Surgical incision of this support during hysterectomy, particularly vaginal hysterectomy, contributes to a tendency toward posterior rotation of the bladder base, leading to the anatomic abnormality of urethral and blad-

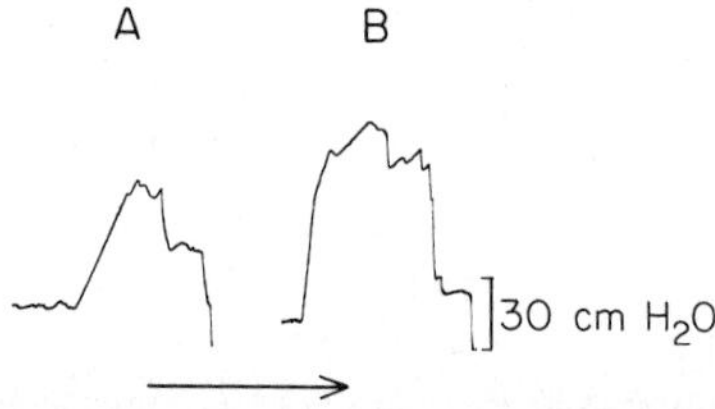

Figure 14–7. Urethral pressure profiles before (*A*) and during (*B*) active contraction of pelvic floor. During voluntary activity, urethral closing pressure increases by more than 30 cm. of water, and some lengthening occurs.

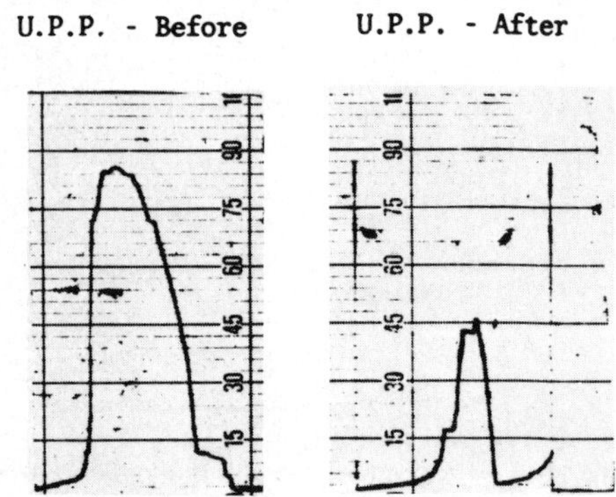

Figure 14–8. Urethral pressure profiles (UPP) before and after pudendal block in a young woman. Closing pressure decreases by 50 per cent following block.

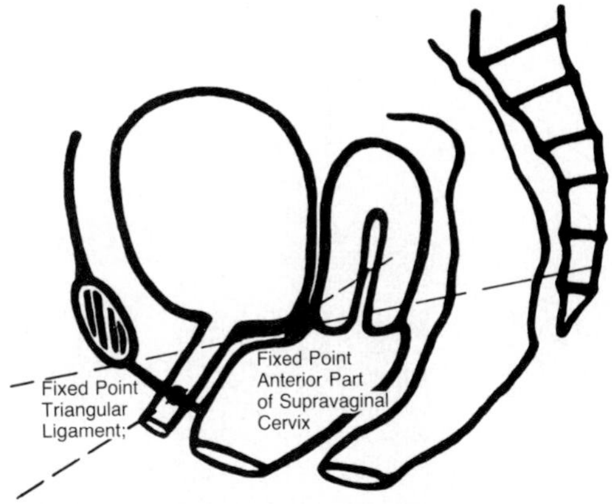

Figure 14–9. Urethra and bladder base are fixed at two points: (1) the triangular ligament of the urogenital diaphragm, and (2) the anterior point of the supravaginal cervix.

der base prolapse. This then contributes to a tendency toward urinary stress incontinence.

Anatomic defects of the bladder base and urethra are discussed in greater detail in the section on radiologic evaluation (Chapter 4).

Transmission of Intra-abdominal Pressures

The fourth factor that is important in maintaining continence in the female is the effect of sudden changes in intra-abdominal pressure on urethral pressure.

As mentioned earlier, the urethra is supported in a fashion similar to the cervix. Since the proximal two thirds of the urethra is an intra-abdominal structure, any acute change in intra-abdominal pressure during coughing or straining is transmitted equally to the proximal urethra and abdomen (Figure 14–10). Another phenomenon occurs during coughing or straining: during the sudden change in abdominal pressure, there is a cough reflex, a sudden contraction of the pelvic floor which stretches the urethra and increases closing pressures (Figure 14–11). This event is called a defense reflex or reflex contraction during cough. The significance of this cough reflex is that it defends the urethra and increases pressure to protect the patient from leakage. As mentioned, the occurrence of anatomic changes and the lack of support of the urethra and bladder neck produce a detrimental alteration in the position and support of the urethra. Hypermobility of the urethra will occur during coughing and straining, and a different transmission in urethral pressure will ensue.

The cough reflex is important in patients with sphincteric incontinence because damage to the external sphincter musculature in aging multiparous patients also damages the cough reflex. Patients then develop a loss of capability of the normal urethra to compensate for this sudden increase in intra-abdominal pressure and thus are unable to maintain continence.

Summary

Ideally, the four factors just described should balance each other. If one factor is deficient, the others should compensate. For example, a patient whose distal urethra has been excised due to carcinoma may be left with a urethra of only 1 cm. But if this urethra is in good anatomic position, and maintains good closing pressure, the patient should still be continent. On the other hand, if this patient has had damage to the intrinsic mechanism of the urethra or has

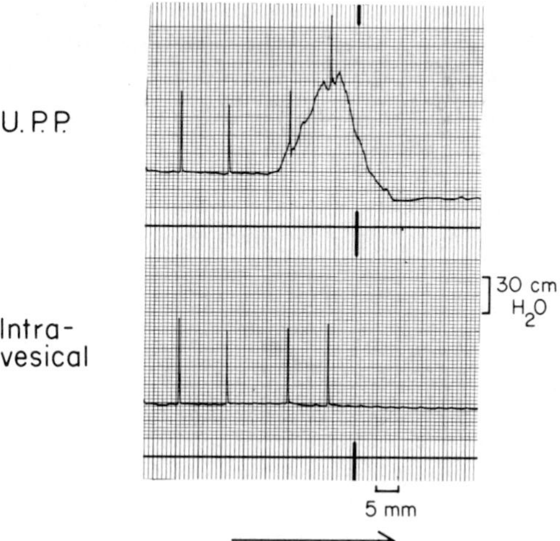

Figure 14–10. Simultaneous recordings of urethra (UPP) and intravesical pressures during coughing or straining. Stress produces a parallel increase of bladder and urethral pressure because the intraabdominal position of the bladder and proximal two thirds of the urethra are displayed.

poor anatomic support, incontinence occurs.

It is also true that many patients with anatomic abnormalities are perfectly continent. If the functional length is adequate, and the closing pressure of the remaining segment is intact, these factors will ensure continence. A patient with anatomic abnormality and poor compensation by the other factors (poor closing pressure or short functional urethra) will develop urinary incontinence.

Urinary incontinence, therefore, is the result of a balance among the four factors discussed previously. Urinary incontinence and an incompetent sphincter are the result of damage to one or more of these factors and the inability of the other mechanisms to compensate.

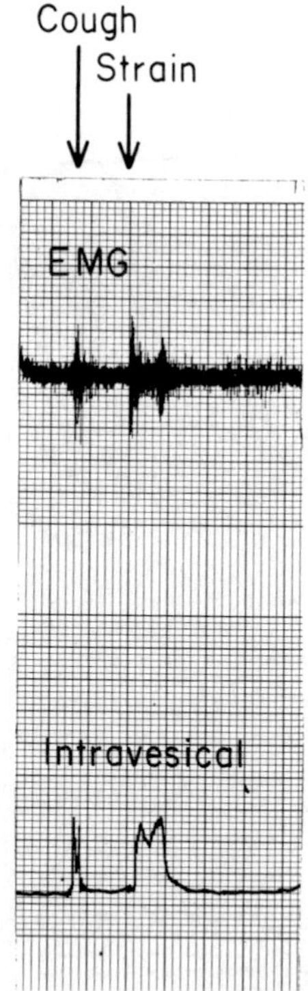

Figure 14–11. Simultaneous recordings of electromyographic (EMG) activity of pelvic floor and intravesical pressure during coughing and straining. Pelvic floor electromyographic activity increases, as does the urethral closing pressure (cough reflex).

CHARACTERISTICS OF FEMALE URINARY INCONTINENCE

Urinary incontinence is defined as the involuntary loss of urine through the urethra (Bruskewitz, in press). This must be distinguished from urinary leakage, which is primarily related to extraurethral reasons for losing urine e.g., fistula, congenital abnormality, and ectopy.

The several types of urinary incontinence are defined symptomatically, beginning with a categorical division between bladder incontinence and urethral incontinence.

Bladder incontinence includes all the aspects of urgency incontinence, hyperreflexia, and bladder instability. Bladder incontinence also may occur when patients retain large residuals of urine. Aspects of bladder incontinence will be discussed at length in the section on cystometric evaluation of the urinary tract.

There are two basic types of *urethral incontinence:* urethral insufficiency and urethral instability. The former occurs in typical cases of stress incontinence, that is, when the mechanism of continence is partially competent and can maintain continence in the resting situation (when the patient is supine). But sudden increases in abdominal pressure brought on by coughing and straining produce loss of urine because the mechanism is unable to compensate for such sudden increases. Incontinence of nonresistance occurs when the loss of urine is constant and there is no significant residual urine.

Urethral instability is a newly defined entity. When bladder filling produces sudden relaxation of the pelvic floor, without any change in detrusor pressure, there is loss of urine. This is accompanied by an inability to contract the pelvic floor at the time urine is lost and is an extremely rare condition.

Incontinence arising from sphincteric insufficiency is the most prevalent situation facing the practitioner. The largest group of females with problems in this category is the group with concomitant anatomic abnormalities of the bladder base and urethra relating primarily to multiple deliveries, hysterectomy, and diminished estrogenic influence on the urethra.

HISTORY AND PHYSICAL EXAMINATION

Despite increasing reliance on laboratory examination, a careful history of symptoms and a thorough physical examination are fundamental to the evaluation of female urinary incontinence (Bruskewitz and Raz, 1979). A meticulous workup can not only aid in diagnosing the problem, but it also allows the physician to select appropriately from the ever-increasing number of diagnostic studies. Whereas a history and physical examination are not in themselves infallible, they do lend direction and order to the complete evaluation of female incontinence.

In addition to determining that the loss of urine is through the urethra (see earlier), it is important to establish the degree of urine loss in making a diagnosis of incontinence. A large percentage of nulliparous young adult women admits to having a very mild and occasional degree of stress incontinence (Nemir and Middleton, 1954). Incontinence that occurs regularly and progresses to a degree that causes personal discomfort or embarrassment is worthy of investigation.

Urinary incontinence in the young girl, in addition to being a problem in its own right, may have a bearing on incontinence in the adult woman as well. It is estimated that about 75 per cent of primary enuresis persisting into late childhood or young adulthood will develop into bladder hyperreflexia (Whiteside and Arnold, 1975).

Green (1968) has estimated that 95 per cent of premenopausal women complaining of stress-type urinary incontinence have had pregnancies that progressed into the final stages of labor. Green also notes that, contrary to widespread opinion, vaginal delivery is not a necessary precursor to this type of incontinence. Radiographic studies performed during labor show pelvic stretching and the development of relaxation, despite the fact that cesarean section ultimately took place (Malpas et al., 1949).

Previous surgical procedures in the pelvis or involving the bladder, urethra, or vagina should be noted (Bruskewitz, in press). Although prolonged labor with difficult delivery represents the most common cause of vesicovaginal fistula for women in underdeveloped countries, iatrogenic vesicovaginal fistula heads the list in developed countries (Turner-Warwick, 1979). Ureterovaginal fistula, while less common, is often associated with a history of previous pelvic surgery and a stormy postoperative course characterized by flank pain, fever, or pyelonephritis believed to be secondary to ureteral ligation, with subsequent leakage of urine per vaginam (Leary et al., 1976). In addition to pelvic surgical procedures that can cause direct damage to the bladder, urethra, or vagina, injury of the pelvic nerves may result in bladder denervation, with subsequent overflow incontinence manifested by elevated postvoid residual urine or full-blown urinary retention (Bruskewitz, in press). Previous neurologic surgery or injury involving spine or brain should be carefully noted. Postlaminectomy adhesive arachnoiditis, in addition to causing persistent, often severe low back and extremity pain, may lead to dysfunction of the spinal cord or cauda equina. Injury incurred below vertebral body L1 (cauda equina injury) may result in an atonic bladder. Higher cord injuries damage the pyramidal and reticulospinal tracts.

Significant cord injury results in bladder hyperreflexia with or without concomitant sphincter dyssynergia (Bruskewitz, in press). Injury to the brain may cause bladder hyperreflexia or the inability to initiate micturition. In a different fashion, prolonged use of vaginal pessary for prolapse may lead to pudendal nerve injury and in that way compromise pelvic floor function, or it may lead to associated paravaginal anesthesia, decreased anal sphincter tone, worsening of prolapse, and incontinence.

Abdominal or perineal surgery may lead to pelvic or pudendal nerve injury, with resulting voiding dysfunction. Occult development of benign or malignant tumors within the distal spinal canal involving the nerve roots (cauda equina) (Figure 14–12) may result in marked pelvic floor relaxation, urinary retention, and associated overflow or stress-type urinary incontinence. Metastatic extradural lesions above L1 in the area of the cord can lead to hyperreflexia. Bowel dysfunction, particularly dysfunction of the rectum and defecation difficulty, parallels urinary tract

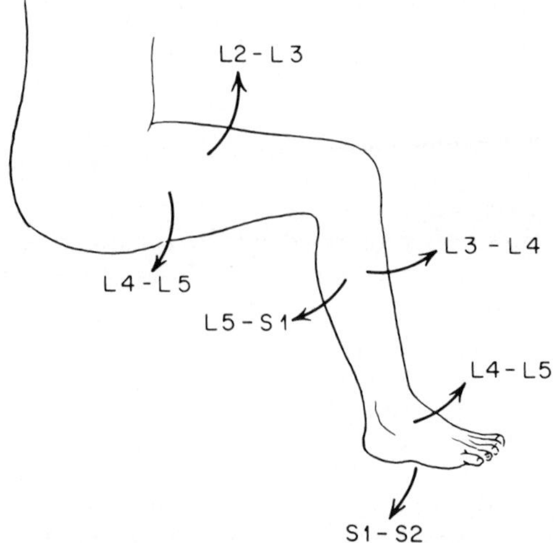

Figure 14–12. Diagram of root distribution of sacral and lumbar output. (From Raz, S., and Bradley, W. E.: Neuromuscular dysfunction of the lower urinary tract. *In* Harrison, J. H., et al.: Campbell's Urology. 4th Ed. Philadelphia, W. B. Saunders Co., 1979).

dysfunction (Godec and Cass, 1980). Constipation may be found with pelvic nerve or spinal cord injury, whereas rectal urge and fecal incontinence are associated with neurogenic hyperreflexic bladders.

A careful neurologic history should be taken, including notation of focal anesthesia, gait disturbance, lower extremity spasticity, visual or speech disturbance, nystagmus, or loss of hand or lower extremity coordination, to name several (Bruskewitz, in press). Congenital neurologic and acquired neurologic diseases must be considered. Tethered spinal cord or spinal cord canal stenosis may rarely lead to the development of voiding dysfunction at adolescence, but it should be considered if incontinence develops at the onset of menses. In females, occult multiple sclerosis leading to subsequent full-blown neurologic dysfunction is a leading cause of neurogenic bladder.

Long-term indwelling catheters may result in extreme urethral and bladder neck dilatation, with incontinence around the catheter.

In broad terms, drugs which as their primary mode of action affect the sympathetic or parasympathetic nervous system or function as striated muscle relaxants are capable of altering bladder and urethral function. Many drugs that affect the autonomic nervous system secondarily must be considered for their effect on the lower urinary tract.

Related psychogenic problems, mental retardation, and the development of urinary incontinence as an attention-getting device are additional causes of incontinence.

An adequate physical examination should also accompany an investigation of the symptom triad of urgency, frequency, and nocturia to rule out causes other than urge incontinence and bladder hyperreflexia. Possible bases for this symptom triad would include increased sensory activity arising from inflammation of the bladder secondary to irritation. When increased postvoid residual is present, urinalysis, urine culture, and objective measurement of the residual also become mandatory. If the triad of symptoms described here occurs in the face of large voiding volumes, polyuria must be suspected, as well as psychogenic water intake, renal failure, diabetes mellitus, diabetes insipidus, or the increased intake of fluids for any reason. The various edematous states, including those resulting from congestive heart failure, primary aldosteronism, or chronic renal failure, must be ruled out. When nocturia occurs without accompanying daytime frequency, a reversal in the normal diurnal pattern of fluid excretion must be suspected.

A full pelvic examination, including examination with the speculum and rectovaginal examination, should be done on the female with urinary incontinence (Bruskewitz, in press). Initial observation should be made of pubic hair distribution; paucity of hair may reflect previous irradiation of the pelvic area. A well-estrogenized introitus appears moist, pink, and well-vascularized. Lack of estrogen production through ovarian involution, as a result of aging or previous bilateral oophorectomy, may be associated with decreasing urethral compliance, and the onset or exacerbation of stress-type urinary incontinence. Examination of the perineal body behind the posterior vaginal wall and the rectum and the rectovaginal septum should be conducted simultaneously by palpating the septum through the rectum and vagina. Rectocele may be associated with splinting — the pa-

TABLE 14–1. QUESTIONNAIRE—SUBJECTIVE DATA REGARDING UROLOGIC HISTORY

	Yes	No
Incontinence		
1. Do you lose urine during the day?	____	____
2. Do you accidentally leak urine? If yes, answer the following questions.	____	____
3. Do you awaken as you are losing urine at night?	____	____
4. How many years have you had leakage of urine? State number.	____	____
5. Do you ever lose urine at night while sleeping?	____	____
6. Do you ever lose urine when lying down and awake?	____	____
7. Do you wear pads to absorb lost urine? (Number of pads ____)	____	____
8. Do you lose urine with (check appropriate answers)		
running?	____	____
walking?	____	____
laughing?	____	____
lifting?	____	____
straining?	____	____
coughing?	____	____
sudden movement?	____	____
quick change in position?	____	____
9. Do you usually have a sense of urgency prior to loss of urine?	____	____
10. Do you realize that urine is being lost at the time it runs out?	____	____
11. Do you lose urine from the vagina?	____	____
12. Did leakage begin immediately after the birth of a child?	____	____
13. Did you wet the bed as a child? (Until what age? ____)	____	____
14. After you lose urine, is there urine left in your bladder?	____	____
15. Can you pass urine with a good stream?	____	____
16. How much urine can you pass at one time? State number of ounces. ____		
17. Do you have to strain to void?	____	____
18. Do you feel you empty your bladder completely?	____	____
19. Do you have a warning that you are going to lose your urine?	____	____
20. Do you continue to dribble at the end of urinating?	____	____
21. Are you able to stop the flow of urine at will?	____	____
22. Are you able to detect when your bladder is full?	____	____
23. Do you lose urine in small amounts or large amounts (emptying your bladder)? Small ____ Large ____		
24. Do you lose urine in spurts just at the time of coughing or straining, or do you continue to lose urine well beyond the time of coughing, etc.? ____		
25. Was your incontinence a direct result of previous surgery?	____	____
26. Do you lose urine with coughing or straining while lying down?	____	____
27. When you turn on a faucet, do you have an urge to void or leak urine?	____	____
28. When you drink fluid do you have an urge to void or leak urine?	____	____
29. How many times in 24 hours do you lose urine quickly? (Number ____)		
30. Was your incontinence treated previously?	____	____
Name of medicine ____		
31. Have you had surgery to correct the leakage of urine?	____	____
32. Through the vagina?	____	____
33. Through the abdomen?	____	____
Date of operation	____	

TABLE 14–1. QUESTIONNAIRE—SUBJECTIVE DATA REGARDING UROLOGIC HISTORY *(Continued)*

	Yes	No
34. Result of surgery:		
Partial improvement	_____	_____
Helped only for awhile (Number of months _____)	_____	_____
Did not make any difference	_____	_____
After surgery you were worse	_____	_____
Frequency and Urgency		
35. How often do you need to empty your bladder?		
Every 6–8 hours	_____	_____
Every 4–6 hours	_____	_____
Every 2–4 hours	_____	_____
Every hour	_____	_____
Every 30 minutes or less	_____	_____
36. Do you often get up at night to void?		
Every hour or less (average)	_____	_____
Once a night	_____	_____
Two or three times	_____	_____
Four to six times	_____	_____
Never	_____	_____
37. Every time you void urine, the amount is:		
Large	_____	_____
Small	_____	_____
Variable	_____	_____
38. Do you have more frequency when you		
Stand?	_____	_____
Sit?	_____	_____
Lie down?	_____	_____
Walk?	_____	_____
39. Is urination painful?	_____	_____
If yes, answer the following:		
Pain every time you void	_____	_____
Pain only occasionally during voiding	_____	_____
Pain only when you have a urinary infection?	_____	_____
40. Do you have frequency only when you have pain?	_____	_____
41. When you feel the need to void:		
Can you hold urine for a long time?	_____	_____
Can you hold only for a few minutes?	_____	_____
Can you hold for a few seconds, and if there is no available bathroom do you leak urine?	_____	_____
Are you unable to hold back at all? (Urine comes immediately.)	_____	_____
42. Have you ever had an infection of the urinary tract?	_____	_____
If yes, answer the following:		
43. Have you ever had a kidney infection?	_____	_____
Right?	_____	_____
Left?	_____	_____
Both?	_____	_____
44. How many times?	______________	
45. Have you suffered kidney damage?	_____	_____
46. Have you had infections in childhood?	_____	_____
47. As an adult?	_____	_____

TABLE 14–1. QUESTIONNAIRE—SUBJECTIVE DATA REGARDING UROLOGIC HISTORY *(Continued)*

	Yes	No
48. How many infections?	______	
49. Have the infections been diagnosed by urine culture?	___	___
50. Do they occur one or two days after intercourse?	___	___
51. Are they associated with burning, frequency, or bleeding?	___	___
52. Do the infections respond quickly to antibiotics?	___	___
Stones		
53. Have you ever had kidney stones?	___	___
54. Have you had operation(s) for removal of stones?	___	___
55. How many stones?	______	
56. Has the cause of your stone problem been fully diagnosed?	___	___
57. Are you presently on medication or diet to prevent stones?	___	___
Hematuria		
58. Have you recently had blood in your urine? If yes, answer the following:	___	___
59. Does bleeding occur frequently (daily) or occasionally?	______	
60. Is bleeding painful?	___	___
61. Do you have pain in your side? Right ___ Left ___	___	___
Tumor		
62. Have you ever had a tumor in your bladder?	___	___
63. Have you ever had a tumor in your kidney?	___	___
64. Elsewhere?	___	___
65. Have tumors been removed from your bladder?	___	___
Gynecology		
66. Are you pregnant?	___	___
67. Have you ever had a venereal infection?	___	___
68. Are you presently on birth control?	___	___
Pill?	___	___
Diaphragm?	___	___
IUD?	___	___
Foam?	___	___
69. How long has it been since your last Papanicolaou smear? Number of months ___	Years ___	
	Yes	No
70. Are you still having menstrual periods? If yes, answer the following:	___	___
71. Is the flow normal in amount?	___	___
Number of pads or tampons	______	
Number of days	______	
72. Is the flow normal in duration?	___	___
73. Is menstruation painful?	___	___
74. At what age did menstruation begin?	______	
75. If you are not having periods, answer the following:		
76. Are you past your menstruating years?	___	___
77. At what age did menstruation stop?	___	___
78. Did your menstruation never start?	___	___
79. Start and then stop?	___	___
80. How many times have you been pregnant?	______	

TABLE 14–1. QUESTIONNAIRE—SUBJECTIVE DATA REGARDING UROLOGIC HISTORY *(Continued)*

	Yes	No
81. How many deliveries through the vagina?	______	
82. How many cesarean sections?	______	
83. If you are in menopause, are you having symptoms (hot flashes, etc.)?	______	______
Irritative Symptoms		
84. Is it painful to urinate?	______	______
85. Is there pain in the lower abdomen even without urinating, and with the bladder empty?	______	______
86. Do you get up to urinate at night?	______	______
87. How often? Number of times ______		
88. Do you urinate more often than normal during the day?	______	______
89. How often? Number of times ______		
90. Is sexual intercourse painful?	______	______
Pain		
91. Have you ever had pain related to voiding urine? If yes, answer the following:	______	______
92. Do you have pain during voiding urine?	______	______
93. Before you even start to void?	______	______
94. Mainly after you finish?	______	______
95. Is the pain mainly between two voidings?	______	______
96. Does the pain increase when the bladder is filling and decrease after voiding?	______	______
97. Is there pain only when an infection is found?	______	______
98. Does pain disappear with infection?	______	______
99. Is pain unrelated to infection?	______	______
100. The pain is located in:		
The bladder area	______	______
Along the urethra	______	______
Goes to the back	______	______
Goes to the legs	______	______
101. Is the pain continuous?	______	______
Obstruction		
102. Do you have difficulty in passing urine? If yes, answer the following:	______	______
103. Does it take a long time to start urinating?	______	______
104. Do you need to push and strain to start?	______	______
105. Do you need to press on your lower abdomen with your hand to start?	______	______
106. When the stream starts, is it		
Strong and steady?	______	______
Poor?	______	______
Starting and stopping?	______	______
Thin?	______	______
Sprayed?	______	______
Flowing when you push and stopping when you stop pushing?	______	______
107. At the end of voiding, does urine continue to flow?	______	______
108. When you finish, do you feel that you are empty?	______	______
109. Do you know if you are totally emptying your bladder?	______	______

TABLE 14–1. QUESTIONNAIRE—SUBJECTIVE DATA REGARDING UROLOGIC HISTORY *(Continued)*

	Yes	No
Retention		
110. Have you ever been or are you now unable to void at all? If yes, answer the following:	_____	_____
111. Have you been unable to pass urine at all?	_____	_____
112. For how long?	__________	
113. Did you ever have a catheter in your bladder?	_____	_____
114. For how long?	__________	
115. Do you presently have a catheter in your bladder?	_____	_____
116. While using the catheter, have you had		
Bleeding?	_____	_____
Fever and chills?	_____	_____
Obstructed catheter?	_____	_____
Leakage of urine around the catheter?	_____	_____
Pain/bladder spasm?	_____	_____
117. Have you taken any of the following for urinary retention? Urecholine?	_____	_____
Duvoid?	_____	_____
Dibenzyline?	_____	_____
No medication?	_____	_____
118. Did surgery help your retention of urine?	_____	_____
119. Are you doing self-catheterization?	_____	_____
120. Is the self-catheterization tolerated well?	_____	_____
121. What catheter are you using?	__________	
Diagnostics		
Have you ever had		
122. Kidney x-ray?	_____	_____
123. Bladder x-ray?	_____	_____
124. Cystoscopy (an instrument looks inside the bladder)?	_____	_____
125. Urethral dilatation (stretching of the urinary channel)?	_____	_____
126. Bladder dilatation under anesthesia (stretching the bladder while you were asleep)?	_____	_____
Treatment		
127. List medications you presently take.	_____	_____
128. List previous surgeries, with dates.	_____	_____
129. List allergies.	_____	_____

tient's need to introduce a finger into the vagina to redirect a stool into the anal canal during defecation.

Complete neurologic examination is indicated when the female patient presents with suggestions of neurologic dysfunction (Raz and Bradley, 1979). Long-standing and pronounced hypertension, and its association with cerebrovascular accident, or a history of meningitis and encephalitis would deserve such an investigation (Bruskewitz, in press). Likewise, multiple sclerosis, parkinsonism, diabetes mellitus, spinal cord injury, or meningocele mandates such an examination. Basal ganglia dysfunction, as seen in Parkinson's disease, is associated with slow movement and resting tremors. Spinal cord injury above the level of L1, the level at which the spinal cord ends in adults, is associated with extreme spasticity and hyperreflexic tendon reflexes, progressing to clonus. Depending upon the level of injury, both upper and lower extremity paraplegic involvement may be noted. An associated sensory deficit generally is noted below the injury. Although the majority of spinal cord injuries are partial, during pelvic examination a sensory examination of the genitalia is in order. In the female, the genitalia are innervated entirely by the somatic pudendal nerve below the levels S2 to S4. Perineal sensation may be examined by light touch with a pin. Motor function and the integrity of the sacral arc are examined by using the clitoral (bulbocavernosus) reflex and by examining for intact anal tone. It is important to remember that approximately 10 per cent of normal adults do not have a bulbocavernosus reflex that can be elicited. A deep tendon reflex using the knee and ankle jerk and the Babinski test should be performed, particularly in patients with neurologic dysfunction. These are tests of corticospinal function and are useful in identifying both the presence and level of neurologic dysfunction. The back should be checked for extensive surgical scarring.

In our urodynamic unit, I have found it helpful to involve our female patients by having them provide detailed urologic histories. Before coming in for evaluation, each patient returns a questionnaire to our office (Table 14–1).

REFERENCES

Beck, R. P., and Maughan, G. B.: Simultaneous intraurethral and intravesical pressure studies in normal women and those with stress incontinence. Am. J. Obstet. Gynecol. *89*:746, 1964.

Bruskewitz, R.: Female incontinence: signs and symptoms. *In* Raz, S. (Ed.): Female Urology. Philadelphia, W. B. Saunders Co., in press.

Bruskewitz, R., and Raz, S.: Urethral pressure profile using microtip catheters in females. Urology *14*:303, 1979.

Constantinou, C. E., and Govan, D. E.: Contribution and timing of transmitted and generated pressure components in the female urethra. Presented at the Eighth International Continence Society Meeting, Los Angeles, 1980.

Godec, C. J., and Cass, A. S.: Comparison of pressure measurements in the lower urinary and lower fecal pathways. J. Urol. *123*:58, 1980.

Green, T. H.: The problem of urinary stress incontinence. Obstet. Gynecol. Surv., *23*:603, 1968.

Leary, F. J., Bass, R. B., and Symmonds, R. E.: Water vaginal discharge in a young woman. J. Urol. *122*:226, 1976.

Malpas, P., Jeffcoate, T. N. A., and Lister, V. M.: Displacement of bladder and urethra during labour. J. Obstet. Gynaecol. Br. Emp. *56*:949, 1949.

Nemir, A., and Middleton, R. P.: Stress incontinence in young nulliparous women: A statistical study. Am. J. Obstet. Gynecol. *68*:1166, 1954.

Plante, P., and Sussett, J.: Studies of female urethral pressure profile. Part I. The normal urethral pressure profile. J. Urol. *123*:64, 1980.

Raz, S., and Bradley, W. E.: Neuromuscular dysfunction of the lower urinary tract. *In* Harrison, J. H., Gittes, R. F., Perlmutter, A. D., et al. (Eds.): Campbell's Urology. 4th Ed. Vol. 2. Philadelphia, W. B. Saunders Co., 1979, pp. 1215–1270.

Raz, S., and Caine, M.: The role of female hormones in stress incontinence. Communication to 16th Congress of International Society of Urology, Amsterdam, 1973.

Rud, T., Andersson, K. E., Asmussen, M., et al.: Factors maintaining the intraurethral pressure in women. Invest. Urol. *17*:343, 1980.

Turner-Warwick, R.: Urinary fistulae in the female. *In* Harrison, J. H., Gittes, R. F., Perlmutter, A. D., et al. (Eds.): Campbell's Urology. 4th Ed. Vol. 3. Philadelphia, W. B. Saunders Co., 1979, pp. 2499–2517.

Van Geelen, J. M.: The influence of hormonal changes during the menstrual cycle on the urethral pressure profile in normal women. Presented at the Eighth International Continence Society Meeting, Los Angeles, 1980.

Whiteside, C. G., and Arnold, E. P.: Persistent primary enuresis: a urodynamic assessment. Br. Med. J. *1*:364, 1975.

Zinner, N. R., Sterling, A. M., and Ritter, R. C.: Role of inner urethral softness in urinary incontinence. Urology *16*:115, 1980.

15

ANTERIOR COLPORRHAPHY

BRUCE H. DRUKKER, M.D.

Anterior colporrhaphy, whether performed as a separate procedure or combined with other forms of gynecologic surgery, is a common gynecologic operation. For many years it was the definitive operation for correction of urinary stress incontinence (USI). During the past two decades, the place of anterior colporrhaphy in gynecologic surgery has been re-examined carefully, and it has become evident that there are rather specific indications for its use. Particular care in the selection of operative candidates is mandatory for optimal long-lasting results.

As discussed in Chapter 13, the gynecologic surgeon can no longer assume correctness of the old adage for treating USI: "First do a vaginal operation for stress incontinence; if there is anatomic failure or recurrence of symptoms, then do an operative procedure by the abdominal route, that is, a retropubic urethrovesical suspension operation." Proper evaluation of patients with stress incontinence will help in choosing the appropriate method of management, so that disappointing postoperative results can be avoided.

A major purpose of this chapter is to reacquaint the gynecologic surgeon with the criteria that make anterior colporrhaphy the procedure of choice for correction of stress incontinence associated with vaginal relaxation. Careful attention to the guidelines for selection, plus precision of operative technique, will ensure that anterior colporrhaphy remains a valuable reparative procedure.

Anterior colporrhaphy as it is known today has a venerable history. The principal operation dates back to 1870. The classic description was published by Kelly in 1913. This operative technique, which included plication sutures in the torn fascia of the urethra and bladder, was modified by Kennedy in 1937. Subsequently, numerous minor modifications have been reported. These have been correlated by Barnett (1969). Contemporary thinking has emphasized the increased importance of developing correct urethrovesical relationships in addition to adequate fascial plication (Chapter 13).

RELATED ANATOMY

The performance of anterior colporrhaphy requires a precise knowledge of the anatomic location and function of significant structures in the pelvic floor. The anatomic structures that must be identified include:

1. Vaginal mucosa
2. Vesicouterine peritoneum
3. Pubovesical-cervical fascia — a portion of the levator fascia
4. Bladder muscularis
5. Urethrovesical junction
6. Urethra
7. Veins of the uterovaginal plexus

Vaginal Mucosa

The vaginal mucosa must be carefully scrutinized for evidence of pathologic processes that would contraindicate performance of colporrhaphy. A Papanicolaou smear from the cervix or vagina must be taken and interpreted as normal. Vaginitis of any type should be treated if present. The correction of decreased estrogen effect noted in the vaginal mucosa is advantageous prior to surgical repair of vaginal relaxation. A firm, thickened, well-cornified mucosa is a salutary factor. Estrogen effect can be readily produced by the use of intravaginal estrogen creams on a daily basis for 2 to 3 weeks before the operation. Healthy vaginal mucosa decreases problems of tearing at the time of dissection and may reduce bacterial contamination.

Vesicouterine Peritoneum

The approximate location of the reflection of vesicouterine peritoneum along the lower segment of the uterus is of prime importance, particularly when anterior colporrhaphy accompanies vaginal hysterectomy. This anatomic point is well delineated and can be readily recognized as a small triangular portion of peritoneum. It can be easily identified when traction is placed on the cervix and the bladder base has been reflected off the most distal portion of the cervix. Identification of this small inverse white triangular point allows ready access to the peritoneal cavity (Figure 15–1). Opening the edge of the triangular reflection eliminates the possibility of inadvertent bladder entry.

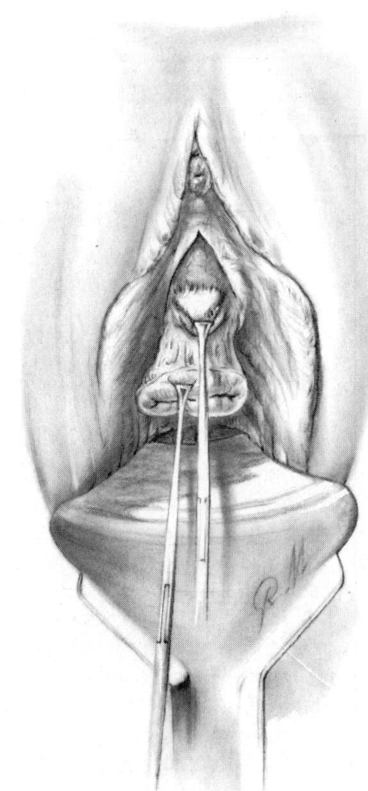

Figure 15–1. Triangular edge of peritoneum with Allis clamps, showing vesicouterine fold of peritoneum.

Pubovesical-Cervical Fascia

The interrelationship of the suspensory ligaments of the bladder as they relate to the cervix and the vesicouterine peritoneum is important. Delineation of the edge of the pubovesical-cervical fascia is necessary if accurate correction of the cystocele is to be achieved. The supporting structures of the pelvis are weakened during childbirth and with the aging process. The fascia may be separated or attenuated or lose inherent tone, but it is not absent. It can be located beneath the vaginal mucosa.

Bladder Muscularis

The interrelationships of the pubovesical-cervical fascia to the muscularis of the bladder, as well as to the vaginal mucosa, are important. Failure to identify this layer, with its sharp separation from the vaginal mucosa, will lead to deficiencies at the time of repair, resulting in failure 12 to 36 months following operation. The interdigitating smooth muscle fibers of the bladder with their prominent vascular supply are readily apparent to the discerning surgeon. Awareness of these muscular anatomic characteristics prevents inadvertent bladder penetration.

Urethrovesical Junction

The importance of locating the urethrovesical junction cannot be overemphasized. The key to good urinary control following colporrhaphy is, in large part, related to adequate elevation and correction of the urethrovesical angle (Chapter 13). If the urethrovesical junction is not identified, the placement of periurethral supporting sutures may be inaccurate and lead to potential failure.

Urethra

The urethra must also be identified. It is noted to be much more adherent to the vaginal mucosa than that portion of vaginal mucosa located directly over the bladder. Vaginal mucosa must be dissected laterally away from the urethra to gain access to the periurethral fascia. The presence of a urethral diverticulum should also be considered at this time.

Uterovaginal Venous Plexus

Some of the veins of the uterovaginal venous plexus are located beneath the vaginal mucosa lateral to the urethra, particularly distal to the urethrovesical junction. These veins are especially prominent adjacent to the muscles of the pelvic diaphragm next to the pubic rami. Knowledge of their presence, along with care during dissection, will decrease unnecessary and occasional heavy bleeding from these veins.

INDICATIONS

The indications for anterior colporrhaphy are generally considered in two main categories:

1. Evidence of anterior vaginal wall relaxation with minimal to marked cystocele formation.
2. Urinary stress incontinence associated with moderate cystocele.

Anterior vaginal wall relaxation is frequently associated with uterine prolapse. In this clinical situation, anterior colporrhaphy is considered necessary in addition to vaginal hysterectomy to return the anatomic relationships of the vagina and its supporting structures to a normal status. Cystocele per se is not universally associated with urinary stress incontinence. In fact, the patient with a large cystocele may have difficulty emptying the bladder and may not be able to void unless she manually places the prolapsed anterior vaginal wall back into the vaginal canal.

PREOPERATIVE EVALUATION

Symptomatology

Patients with anterior vaginal wall relaxation are subject to the stress of gravity. They present primarily with symptoms of pelvic pressure, particularly when standing for an extended period of time, or associated with physiologic movements producing increased intra-abdominal pressure, with concomitant pressure transmitted to the muscles and fasciae of the pelvic diaphragm.

Symptoms of urinary urgency and urinary stress incontinence occasionally may accompany moderate anterior vaginal wall relaxation with cystocele formation. Urinary stress incontinence does not accompany every cystocele. It is not uncommon for a patient with a marked cystocele to have excellent continence. In this situation surgical correction, if injudicious, with excessive elevation of the bladder base and creation of an obtuse posterior urethrovesical angle, will create incontinence. Adequate evaluation of the extent of relaxation is a crucial factor guiding the degree of operative correction.

Objective Findings

The patient presents with bulging vaginal mucosa at the introitus. Although this may not be marked initially, on Valsalva maneuver the anterior vaginal wall relaxation produces a prominent, ballooning effect at the introitus with occasional protrusion through the introitus. Urethrocele may also be present. If the patient has uterine prolapse, the cervix will appear at or through the introitus in conjunction with the anterior vaginal wall relaxation. Posterior vaginal wall relaxation frequently accompanies anterior wall changes, as does vault weakness if prior hysterectomy has been performed. These areas require careful evaluation to determine need for corrective surgery in conjunction with anterior colporraphy.

Radiologic Evaluation

In addition to a complete history and physical examination, it is particularly important to have documented radiographic evidence of the degree of anterior vaginal wall relaxation. This evaluation affords precise anatomic information relating to the degree of cystocele, as well as anterior vaginal wall descent. The relationships of the urethra to the bladder and the urethra and bladder to the symphysis pubis become apparent, and the urethrovesical angle is identified. This radiologic evidence is also of value in the selection of the appropriate operative procedure.

Other radiographic studies done routinely include intravenous pyelography, which is useful to exclude upper urinary tract disease, particularly hydroureter and hydronephrosis. These abnormalities are observed on occasion in patients with severe vaginal wall relaxation in which the anterior vaginal wall in actuality protrudes through the vagina in both the straining and nonstraining states. Detection of this degree of relaxation is particularly important since in these patients, alteration in the position of the ureters has been noted (Hodgkinson et al., 1964).

All patients should undergo preoperative beadchain radiographic evaluation of the bladder and urethra (discussed later). This well-established procedure provides documented evidence of the degree of vaginal wall relaxation, as well as demonstrating relationships between the urethra and bladder. Postoperative beadchain radiographs should also be completed. These provide the operator with documented information concerning the adequacy of the surgical procedure. Review of postoperative films showing the characteristics of the urethrovesical angle and the degree of correction of anterior wall relaxation will permit prognostic estimation of long-term results and correlate with changes of symptoms.

Beadchain Urethrocystography

The general technique of beadchain urethrocystography is described in Chapter 13. Considerations especially pertinent to evaluation prior to anterior colporrhaphy are presented here.

After the dye and the beadchain have been inserted, an ample amount of radiopaque vaginal paste* is placed in the vagina to ensure a coating of the vaginal mucous membrane. The patient is then evaluated radiographically, in both the anteroposterior and the lateral projections. Films are taken with the patient standing and the feet approximately 16 inches apart. Initial projections are taken in the anteroposterior projection, first with the patient standing erect and not straining. Films are then repeated straining down. The patient is then placed in the lateral position with the feet 16 inches apart, and lateral radiographs are obtained in both the nonstraining and the straining situations.

An analysis of these radiographs is undertaken to evaluate the urethrovesicopubic relationships. If the inferior margin of the bladder on the straining anteroposterior radiograph is seen to lie 4 cm. below the inferior margin of the symphysis pubis, adequate correction utilizing the technique of anterior colporrhaphy can generally be accomplished. The aim of adequate anterior colporrhaphy includes not only adequate plication of the pubovesical-cervical fascia and urethra, but also and probably of more importance, appropriate elevation and correction of the urethrovesical angle to a degree compatible with continence. This critical point must be appreciated if the operation is to be successful.

Utilization of the straining anteroposterior radiographs is helpful in determining the technical capability of elevating the urethrovesical angle. When the descent of the bladder base below the inferior margin of the symphysis on straining is less than 4 cm., it is often difficult to obtain adequate, long-lasting angle elevation by vaginal operation. In such a situation, a primary retropubic operation should be considered.

Figure 15–2 demonstrates anteroposterior beadchain cystourethrography in the preoperative evaluation. Note the marked descent of the inferior margin of the bladder below the inferior margin of the symphysis pubis. The beads of the chain can be seen coiled at the base of the bladder. The urethrovesical junction is located at the midpoint between the bladder base and upper margin of the bladder noted on the radiograph.

Figure 15–3 shows preoperative and postoperative radiographs for the same patient. Note the elevation and correctness of the urethrovesical angle in the postopera-

*Esophotrast. Barnes-Hinds Diagnostics, Canovanas, Puerto Rico.

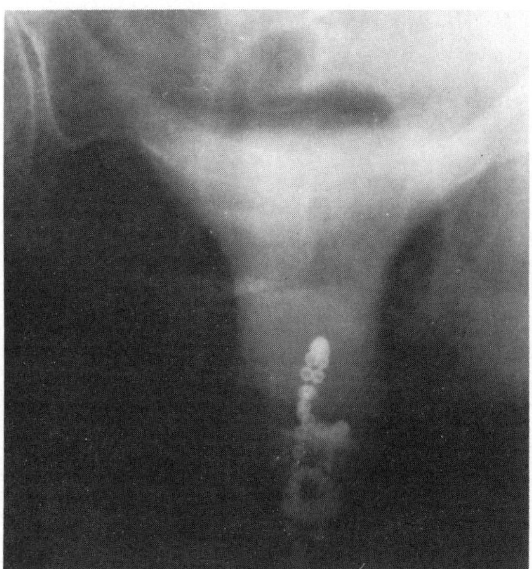

Figure 15–2. Preoperative cystourethrograms showing base of bladder more than 4 cm. below inferior margin of symphysis pubis. See text.

tive film. A "mini-cystocele" is retained to allow some posterior rotation of the bladder, which is salutary to good angle elevation. A flat bladder base can occur as a result of overzealous cystocele correction. This will significantly reduce the success of operative correction and contribute to recurring or possibly new symptoms of stress incontinence.

Figure 15–4 demonstrates lateral and anteroposterior beadchain radiographs taken before operative correction of total uterovaginal prolapse. This patient had complete bladder eversion, was totally continent and could not void unless she manually compressed the anterior vaginal wall into the vaginal canal. Note the urethra exiting from the upper surface of the bladder (arrow). Careful vaginal hysterectomy with anterior and posterior colporrhaphy corrected this problem, and the patient remained continent postoperatively.

PROCEDURE

Anterior colporrhaphy can be carried out as a separate operation, in conjunction with vaginal hysterectomy and posterior colporrhaphy, or in association with enterocele repair and posterior colporrhaphy. Additionally, in unusual circumstances, a

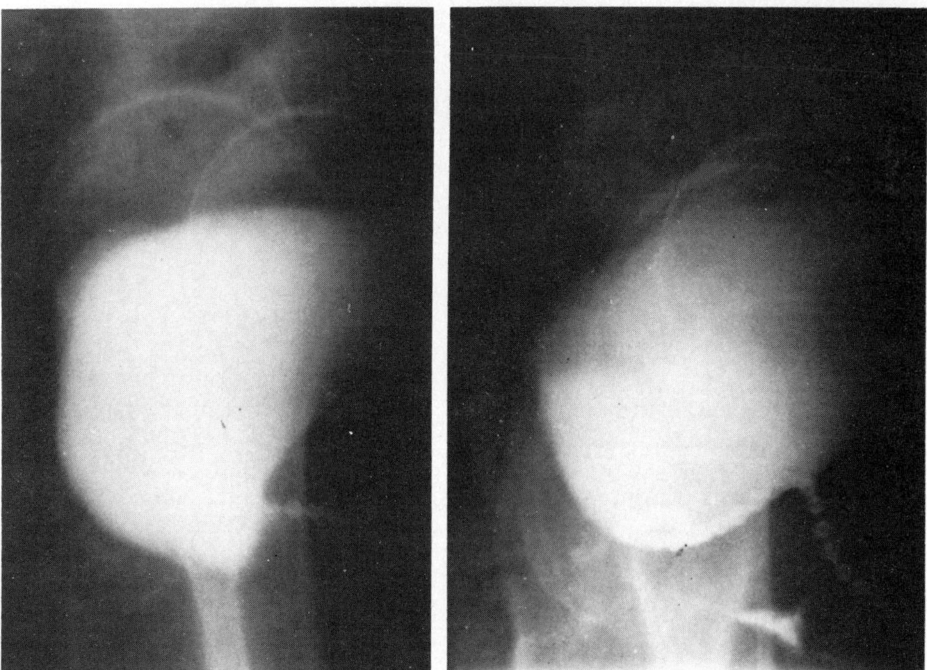

Figure 15–3. Pre- and postcolporrhaphy lateral radiographs. The urethrovesical angle is securely elevated. See text.

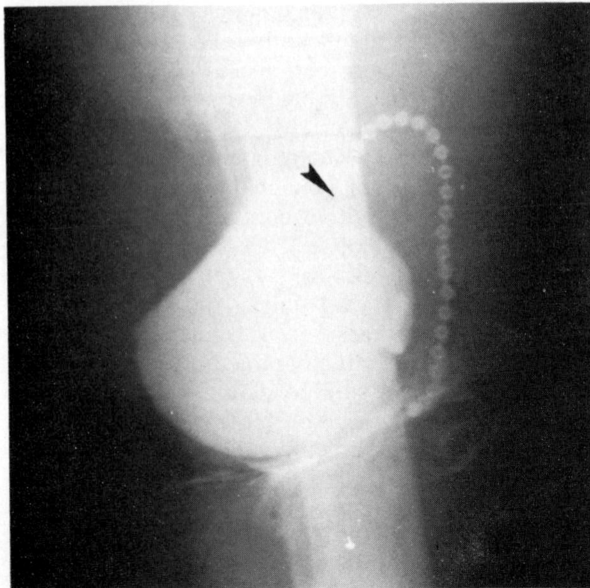

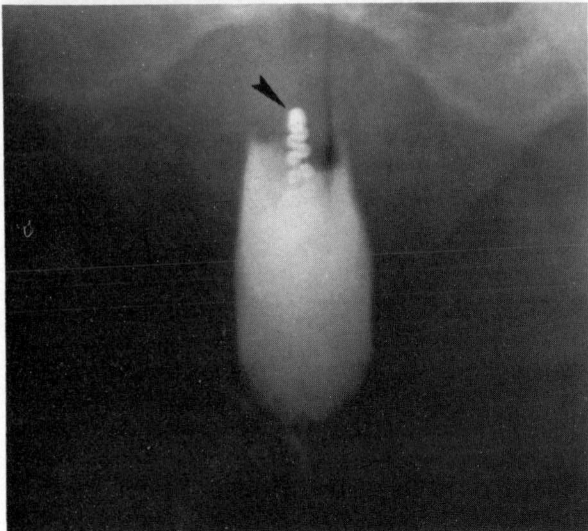

Figure 15–4. Complete bladder prolapse. Urethra exits from superior surface of bladder (arrows). See text.

minimal anterior colporrhaphy can be accomplished following retropubic urethral suspension.

The patient is placed in the dorsolithotomy position, and the vagina and perineum are cleansed with a povidone-iodine solution. All dissection is sharp, utilizing a Beaver scalpel* and blade. An injection solution containing saline (100 ml.) and epinephrine (0.5 ml. of 1:1000) is utilized to improve hemostasis and to delineate tissue planes. If vaginal hysterectomy has been accomplished prior to anterior colporrhaphy, the incision is begun at the upper portion of the vaginal hysterectomy incision (Figure 15–5). If anterior colporrhaphy is done alone or is accompanying enterocele repair, the incision is made as high in the apex of the vagina as possible, with the apex being drawn to the introitus, using Allis clamps placed lateral to the site of incision.

After the point for initial incision has been identified, the vaginal mucosa is infiltrated with the saline-epinephrine solution.

*Available through Rudolph-Beaver, Incorporated, Belmont, Massachusetts.

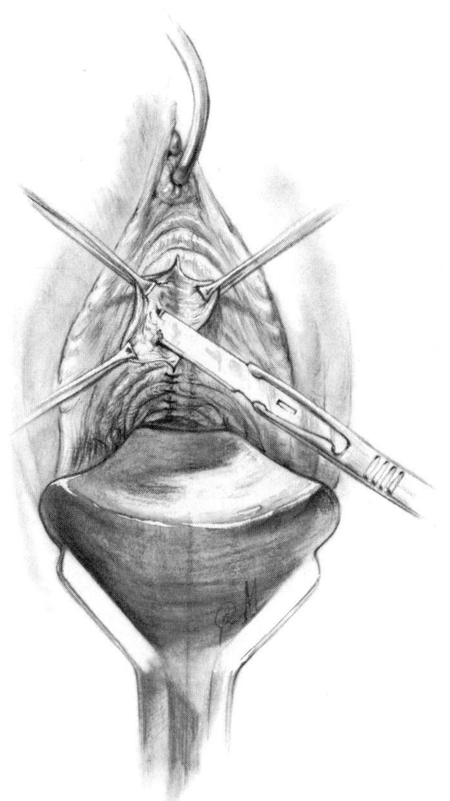

Figure 15–5. Start of anterior colporrhaphy following vaginal hysterectomy. Anterior vaginal mucosa has been incised.

A vertical incision is made through the mucosa extending in a stepwise fashion from the apex of the vagina to the urethral meatus. The incision is not completed in its entirety at the onset, but rather is extended 5 to 6 cm. at a time, with the edges of the vaginal mucosa being elevated with Allis clamps and the fascial layer sharply dissected from the inner surface of the vaginal mucosa (Figure 15–6). Particular care must be taken to carefully remove the fascia from the inner surface of the vaginal mucosa and to demarcate the appropriate plane. Dissection in this plane will be relatively avascular and affords healthy fascia for closure and correction of the cystocele.

The dissection is continued until the entire vaginal wall has been separated from the fascia. Particular care must be taken in the area of the urethrovesical junction and in the periurethral area. Here the vaginal mucosa is more adherent than it is over the bladder. The periurethral area laterally contains large venous plexuses that must be carefully separated from the mucosa of the vagina to avoid lacerating the veins.

Following dissection of the fascia, the No. 14 French Foley 5 cc. bulb catheter that has been previously placed in the bladder is drained. The urethrovesical junction is supported using 0 chromic catgut sutures placed parallel to the urethra. These are placed through the fascia beginning initially at the urethrovesical junction. The sutures, so-called "twin stitches," are tied in the midline utilizing one arm from each side, with the remaining arm being tied after the sutures are snugged together, and the urethrovesical angle is elevated by approximation of the fascia in the midline (Figure 15–7). Two or three subsequent twin stitches are placed more distally beneath the urethra, imbricating the fascia and minimally constricting the urethra. The catheter should be snug in the urethra at the conclusion of the imbrication process.

The remaining portion of the cystocele is then corrected, beginning at the urethrovesical junction and utilizing 2–0 interrupted chromic sutures. The fascia is closed in the midline from the urethrovesical junction to the apex of the incision. Following approximation of the fascia, the suture line of the corrected cystocele is carefully oversewn, using continuous 2-0 chromic catgut for additional support. The use of polyglycolic sutures is perfectly acceptable for this type of repair. The vaginal mucosa is then appropriately trimmed, removing redundant and excess mucosa, and closed using a continuous 2-0 chromic catgut suture. Care should be taken to obliterate the dead space between the fascia and vaginal mucosa. Drainage of the area is not routinely necessary.

Following completion of anterior colporrhaphy, if the operation is to be terminated, an intravenous tubing attached to a 500 ml. bottle of normal saline is attached to the Foley catheter, and the bladder is filled with 500 ml. of saline. Suprapubic catheterization is then carried out to establish urinary drainage. The Foley catheter is removed at the termination of the operative procedure. Vaginal packing is not routinely necessary. If, however, a minimal amount of venous ooze occurs, a 2-inch rolled moistened gauze packing impregnat-

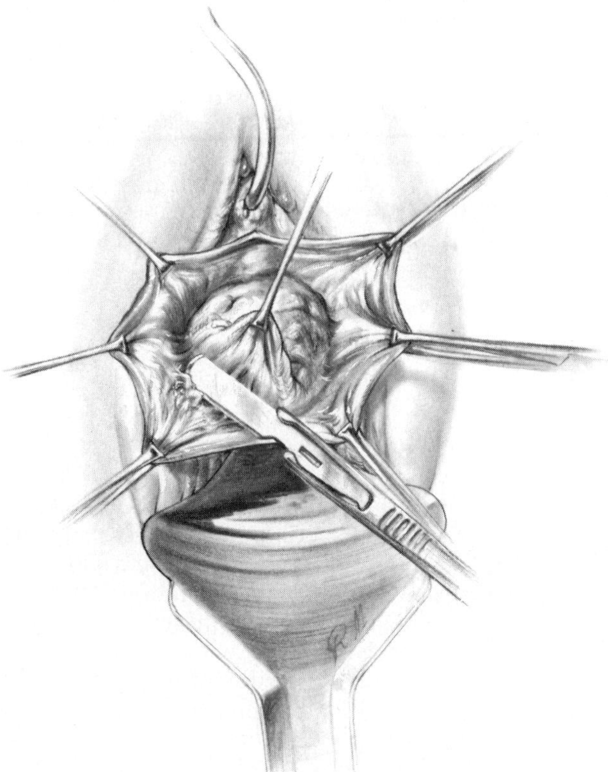

Figure 15–6. Separation of fascia from vaginal mucosa, with bladder apparent.

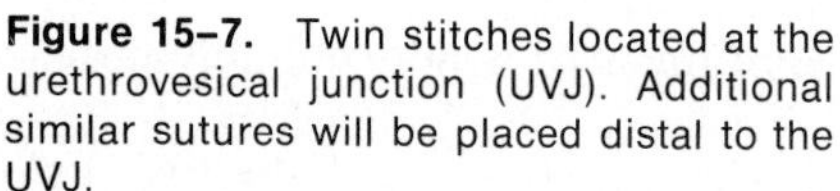

Figure 15–7. Twin stitches located at the urethrovesical junction (UVJ). Additional similar sutures will be placed distal to the UVJ.

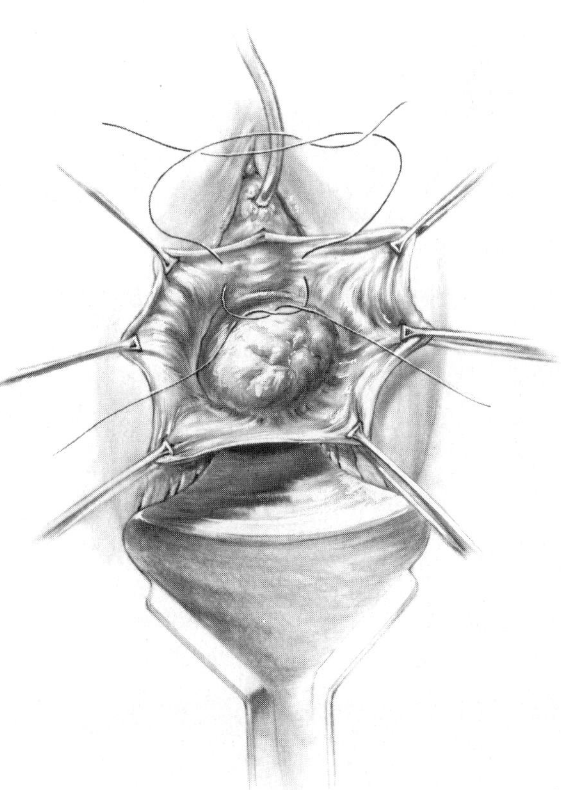

ed in a mild povidone-iodine/saline solution can be used for the first 18 to 24 postoperative hours. This will afford sufficient pressure to terminate minimal venous oozing. As a rule of thumb, if a vaginal pack is inserted and the patient bleeds sufficiently to completely soil the packing within 1 to 2 hours following its insertion, one can assume that bleeding is excessive, and that the site of bleeding must be determined and hemostasis achieved.

Intraoperative Complications

The major problems that can occur during the procedure of anterior colporrhaphy are vesical laceration and hemorrhage.

Vesical Laceration

Vesical laceration, although infrequent, is more prone to occur in patients who have had previous vaginal operative procedures producing scarring of the anterior vaginal wall. This problem can be avoided by a meticulous sharp dissection of the fascia from the inner surface margin of the vaginal mucosa. Should vesical laceration occur, the site of the aperture into the bladder usually is easily identified. The defect can be closed with two or three layers of interrupted 3-0 chromic catgut, or interrupted sutures followed by a continuous layer of 3-0 chromic catgut sutures. Hemostasis must be adequate and there must be no tension on the suture line. Following repair of the bladder, the efficacy of the repair can be determined by utilizing dilute sterile infant formula injected gently into the Foley catheter. If no milk is visible at the site of laceration repair, the integrity of the repair is obvious.

Hemorrhage

Hemorrhage is not a great problem if meticulous attention has been paid to sharp dissection of the fascia from the vaginal mucosa. The periurethral venous plexus is the major concern. Excessive bleeding from the venous plexus is often difficult to control with routine clamping procedures. Rather than clamping, bleeding can be controlled utilizing a continuous 2-0 chromic catgut suture on a through-and-through basis. If this fails, one can attempt to place interrupted figure-eight 2-0 chromic sutures through the vaginal mucosa external to the venous plexus, approximating the vaginal mucosa to the venous plexus and fascia. The dead space between the vaginal mucosa and fascia is thus obliterated. This compresses the venous plexus and results in hemostasis.

Postoperative Care

The immediate care of the patient following colporrhaphy includes adequate monitoring of vital signs and urinary output. Urinary output should be monitored carefully, with production of 700 to 1000 ml. of clear urine in the first 24 hours considered satisfactory. If the suprapubic catheter does not appear to be functioning correctly, it should be irrigated with normal saline to eliminate the possibility of blood clots or the problem of a misplaced catheter. Patients are encouraged to ambulate on the night of surgery and frequently thereafter.

Following operation the bladder is drained by suprapubic catheter gravity drainage for 5 days. On the fifth postoperative day the catheter is clamped and the patient is allowed to begin voiding spontaneously, with residual urine monitored every 4 hours. A "gynecologic cath routine" is followed. If residual urine is greater than 150 ml., the residual is checked in 4 hours; if 100 to 150 ml., residual is checked in 6 hours; if 75 to 100 ml., residual is checked in 12 hours; if less than 50 ml., residual is checked in 24 hours. If the patient is comfortable and the residual 24 hours later is again 50 ml. or less, a normal voiding pattern has been re-established. In most patients this end point occurs by the seventh or eighth postoperative day. Prolongation of return to normal voiding is provoked by excessive urethral catheterization or by the development of urinary tract infection, particularly cystitis, trigonitis, or urethritis. The use of postoperative medications with anticholinergic actions such as imipramine-HCl or diazepam, as well as postoperative tissue edema, will delay normal voiding.

When normal voiding patterns have been

established, postoperative beadchain radiographs are obtained and the suprapubic catheter is removed. Postoperative films unequivocally demonstrate the degree of operative success. If the urethrovesical angle is not acute and not elevated above the bladder base, delayed recurrence is probable. The judgment of success should not be made immediately, for only the gravitational stress of normal life will test the durability of correction obtained by anterior colporrhaphy. Estimation of success should be delayed until at least 18 months after surgical repair. Postoperative attenuation of pelvic fascia is gradual, and recurrent relaxation and recurrent urinary stress incontinence occur gradually. The traditional concept of an 85 per cent success rate of vaginal repairs has been eroded and not substantiated by recent evaluations (Chapter 13). Low (1967) found the failure rate of vaginal plastic operations to be as disturbingly high as 50 per cent.

POSTOPERATIVE PROBLEMS

Infection within tissue planes dissected during anterior colporrhaphy has not been carefully evaluated. General opinion would, however, indicate that this is not a significant problem when colporrhaphy alone is the operative procedure. When anterior colporrhaphy is associated with vaginal hysterectomy, an increase in postoperative morbidity in certain special risk groups has been identified. The use of prophylactic antibiotics in these patients has been shown to decrease postoperative morbidity significantly (Ledger et al., 1975*a*). A report by Ledger and coworkers (1975*b*) has called attention to the rather high occurrence, 60.8 per cent, of both aerobic and anaerobic organisms in the vagina prior to vaginal operations. Anaerobic organisms and aerobic organisms occurred either alone or in combination in 95 of 97 patients undergoing preoperative vaginal culture. If the patient is in a category associated with a significant risk, prophylactic antibiotics should be considered as a preoperative, intraoperative, and short-term postoperative adjunctive therapy. Sufficient antibiotics should be given to permit adequate tissue concentrations at the time of operation. Cephaloridine has been effective for this purpose.

Hodgkinson and Hodari (1966) reemphasized the techniques of suprapubic cystostomy as a means of postoperative bladder drainage for all types of operative procedures related to urinary stress incontinence. Many investigators have subsequently confirmed the benefits of this method, i.e., reduced frequency of urinary tract infection, increased patient comfort and a reduction in nursing care. Transurethral catheterization, whether continuous or intermittent, with its attendant high occurrence of urinary tract infection, can be completely abolished when using a suprapubic urinary drainage apparatus. Three major commercial suprapubic catheterization kits are available. Each is convenient, easy to use and efficacious. Occasional utilization problems include minimal skin irritation at the site of skin fixation and, infrequently, lumen obstruction by small blood clots if hematuria is present owing to the operative procedure or suprapubic catheter installation. Occasional calcareous encrustations will occur in any suprapubic catheter that must be left indwelling for an extended period of time.

Postoperative tissue swelling delaying voiding is a very infrequent occurrence. Should this be an apparent problem, systemic corticosteroids for a short period, 7 to 10 days, with a tapering dosage regimen will often correct the problem.

SUMMARY

Anterior colporrhaphy is a significant operative procedure. However, it must be chosen with great care and related specifically to the symptomatology of stress incontinence and prolapse. Anatomic guidelines for selecting the procedure should be utilized. The use of pre- and postoperative beadchain radiographs provides this invaluable information. With adherence to these principles, and the use of meticulous technique including sharp tissue plane dissection and attention to precise hemostasis, anterior colporrhaphy will continue to be a durable operative procedure, efficacious for a specific group of women requiring corrective surgery for urinary stress incontinence or vaginal relaxation.

REFERENCES

Barnett, R. M.: The modern Kelly plication. Obstet. Gynecol. *34*:667, 1969.

Hodgkinson, C. P., Eyler, W. R., and Ayers, M. A.: Dynamic topography of the lower ureter in vaginal hysterectomy. Am. J. Obstet. Gynecol. *89*:111, 1964.

Hodgkinson, C. P., and Hodari, A. A.: Trocar suprapubic cystostomy for postoperative bladder drainage in the female. Am. J. Obstet. Gynecol. *96*:773, 1966.

Kelly, H. A.: Incontinence of urine in women. Urol. Cutan. Rev. *17*:291, 1913.

Kennedy, W. T.: Incontinence of urine in the female. Am. J. Obstet. Gynecol. *33*:19, 1937.

Ledger, W. J., Carol, G., and Lewis, W. P.: Guidelines for antibiotic prophylaxis in gynecology. Am. J. Obstet. Gynecol. *121*:1038, 1975*a*.

Ledger, W. J., Norman, M., Lee, C., et al.: Bacteremia on an obstetric and gynecologic service. Am. J. Obstet. Gynecol. *121*:205, 1975*b*.

Low, J. A.: Management of anatomic urinary incontinence by vaginal repair. Am. J. Obstet. Gynecol. *97*:308, 1967.

16

THE MODIFIED MARSHALL-MARCHETTI-KRANTZ OPERATION AS A PRIMARY PROCEDURE IN URINARY STRESS INCONTINENCE

R. A. LEE, M.D.

In an attempt to reduce the frequency of recurrent stress incontinence, various surgical approaches have undergone critical evaluation. In past years urinary incontinence was treated with a vaginal operation, which, if it failed (as it did in 20 to 40 per cent of the patients followed for 5 and 10 years), a retropubic operation was undertaken. While we still favor the vaginal approach in patients with mild stress incontinence and associated pelvic relaxation, it is now apparent that certain groups of patients may be better managed with a primary retropubic operation. It appears that the more substantial tissue used in this approach provides more satisfactory and permanent control in patients with severe, complex, and recurrent stress incontinence.

SELECTION OF PATIENTS

Selection of the appropriate operation for a patient with stress incontinence is based on the history, physical examination, and findings on urologic investigation.

History

Most surgeons dealing with urinary stress incontinence agree that a careful history is of critical importance in the differential diagnosis and treatment. The history should relate time of onset, severity, type of incontinence, and associated symptoms of urgency, frequency, and nocturia. One should be alert to associated medical conditions that adversely affect the incontinent patient, such as chronic lung disease, gross obesity, and diabetes mellitus. Specific occupations requiring heavy lifting or straining or unusual athletic interests that may stress an operative repair should influence the surgeon in choosing a surgical procedure. The time of onset of incontinence or an adverse effect after a previous surgical procedure may point to the underlying cause and suggest a surgical approach.

Physical Examination

Important factors in the physical examination include: (1) the degree of musculofascial weakness as demonstrated by rotational descent of the bladder neck and urethra; (2) the presence of scarring or distortion of the vagina secondary to laceration or previous surgical procedure; (3) the presence of cystocele or rectocele; (4) the degree of uterine descensus; and (5) the quality of the pubococcygeus and perineal muscles.

General Urologic Investigation

Cystourethroscopic studies permit evaluation of bladder sensation, the degree of relaxation of the vesical neck, and the tone and length of the urethra. In addition, the volume of fluid required to produce the initial urge to void, bladder capacity, presence of residual urine, bladder-wall trabeculation, and expulsive force can be studied. The presence of inflammatory incontinence and fistulas can be eliminated.

SPECIAL DIAGNOSTIC CONSIDERATIONS

The neck of the urinary bladder is thought to be the most important structure in maintaining urinary continence. Various anatomic abnormalities, such as alterations in urethral length, urethrovesical angular relationships, and intraurethral pressure, have been implicated as the cause of incontinence.

Urethral Length

Lapides and co-workers (1960) declared that the cause of stress incontinence was an actual or functional shortening of the urethra to a length of less than 30 mm. Their concept was based on the principle that the resistance of the urethra varies directly with the inherent tension of the wall of the urethra and the length of the urethra, and inversely with the radius of the urethral lumen. Although postoperative measurements suggest a trend toward lengthening the urethra by both retropubic and vaginal procedures, a successful outcome does not appear to depend solely on this factor. The longer urethra with its greater resistance may compensate for a slightly atonic and patulous vesical neck. Conversely, 1 cm. of proximal urethra with excellent smooth muscle tone that maintains a lumen of zero will be more effective than a 5 cm. atonic funneled or scarred urethra. Unfortunately, this distinction cannot be made simply by measuring the length of the urethra. Most agree that successful operative procedures are associated with an increased functional length in the urethra, whereas the anatomic length usually is not significantly changed.

Urethrovesical Angle

Jeffcoate and Roberts (1952) emphasized the importance of the urethrovesical angle as an underlying factor in stress incontinence. With cystourethrography, it is possible to demonstrate urethrovesical relationships, dependency of vesical junction, and positional changes with stress. Lateral x-ray views taken with a catheter or beadchain in the urethra frequently confirm the loss of urethrovesical angles in patients with stress incontinence. Based on exhaustive studies, Green (1968) and Hodgkinson (1970) have concluded that a beadchain cystography is essential in diagnosing stress incontinence and in the choice of an operative procedure. On this basis, Green (1968) established rather strict criteria suggesting a specific operative approach.

Unfortunately, correlation between the quantitative determinations of the degree of relaxation and the presence or severity of stress incontinence appears to be inconsistent. In fact, if improperly interpreted, these rather static anatomic findings may result in inaccurate diagnosis, inappropriate operation, and persistent or recurrent stress incontinence. Yet, a high retropubic position of the vesical neck is usually accomplished in successful operations, regardless of the specific technique employed.

Urodynamic Investigation

Enhörning (1961) showed conclusively that urine would not be lost from the bladder because of stress so long as the pressure in the urethra equaled or exceeded that in the bladder. Patients with pure stress incontinence have consistently lower intraurethral pressure than those with normal continence. Hodgkinson (1970) suggested that poor pelvic supports result in a low resting intraurethral pressure and permit the urethra to assume a position in direct line with the intra-abdominal thrust, resulting in loss of urine.

Urodynamic investigations are assuming a more important role in the ongoing search to better understand urinary control and the causes of urinary incontinence. Technical advances have improved the accuracy and reproducibility of various urodynamic modalities. Yet, in some instances of normal voiding or attempts to control leakage, this rather sophisticated equipment may record data that are poorly understood or incorrectly interpreted. Further, there exists the temptation to perform a urodynamic investigation and the shun the time-consuming and sometimes frustrating clinical evaluation of the patient. We believe it is clearly impractical and unnecessary to have all patients with disorders of micturition undergo sophisticated urodynamic studies. For instance, the typical patient with a combined syndrome of symptomatic uterovaginal prolapse with loss of urine only with activities of stress should not be required to undergo urodynamic investigation. Naturally, if the patient has associated nocturia, symptoms of urgency, or urge incontinence, some suspicion of an unstable bladder must be considered and investigation carried out.

McGuire and co-workers (1976, 1980), while emphasizing that the low urethral pressure profile and a short effective urethral length were significant criteria in the assessment of anatomic stress incontinence, were quick to emphasize that there are frequent exceptions. They also demonstrated that involuntary destrusor contractions in patients with stress incontinence may complicate but do not contraindicate the surgical management. Beck (1976) and Parker and associates (1979) both reported that in approximately 60 per cent of patients with mixed stress incontinence and unstable bladder symptoms the problems were corrected with a sling operation. We favor a nonoperative medical approach for patients whose symptoms are mainly that of an unstable bladder. However, extreme care must be taken in making this diagnosis, for it may result in denying operation for the patient who could obtain complete urinary control.

Interpretation of urodynamic data has not reached the point where it can replace wide clinical experience and good surgical judgment. Until that time, we need to pursue conscientious clinical assessment of the individual patient and selectively incorporate urodynamic investigation.

INDICATIONS

Approximately one third of patients (192 of 600) undergoing Marshall-Marchetti-Krantz (MMK) procedures at the Mayo Clinic have the procedure as the primary operation for correcting stress incontinence. Whereas this retropubic procedure usually is reserved for patients with recurrent stress incontinence after a previous vaginal repair, careful analysis suggested that most failures with initial vaginal procedures occurred in the more severe or complex forms of stress incontinence. It was apparent that a primary retropubic operation should be considered for:

1. Patients with severe degrees of incontinence out of proportion to the degree of rotational descent of the urethra and vesical neck;
2. patients with complicating medical factors, such as chronic lung disease, asthma, gross obesity, and diabetes;
3. patients with iatrogenic incontinence after vesical neck resection, urethral fulguration, or operative procedures such as the Le Fort operation, partial or total vaginectomies, excisions of portions of the urethra, diverticular repair, and radical hysterectomy (resulting in partial denervation of the bladder);
4. patients with strenuous occupations or those participating in vigorous athletic exercises;
5. patients with associated pelvic pathologic findings requiring a lower midline incision; and
6. patients with poor pelvic tissues, such as those who are elderly or debilitated.

Although one is somewhat hesitant to advocate the more complex retropubic approach, in these selected patients a much more satisfactory long-term cure rate with elimination of many of the failures after primary vaginal repair can be anticipated. The tenuous tissues approximated with the vaginal repair should not and cannot be expected to give satisfactory long-term results in the obese hard-working farmer's wife with severe incontinence and chronic bronchitis.

SURGICAL TECHNIQUE

Through a lower abdominal midline incision, the bladder and urethra are displaced from the posterior surface of the rectus muscle and symphysis pubis. In the absence of previous retropubic operation, adhesions and scarring are not encountered, and this space is developed in a few moments. Periurethral tissue and perivesical fatty tissue are gently removed, and the central vein is clamped, cut, and tied. The dome of the bladder is opened longitudinally to permit direct visualization and palpation of the tone and quality of the bladder neck and proximal urethra and to facilitate accurate placement of the suspending sutures, as previously noted by Symmonds (1972). With experience, this becomes an accurate intraoperative method of assessing the tone, length, and quality of the incontinent and perhaps much operated-on urethra, and it allows one to visualize the alterations produced by the surgical procedure (Figure 16–1).

A second glove is then placed on the surgeon's hand, and the left index and middle fingers are inserted into the vagina to permit accurate placement of the periurethral permanent sutures. This maneuver is preferred over a sponge stick, a retractor, or an assistant's finger to elevate the vaginal wall and to identify the urethra. We use the index finger to identify the urethral catheter and the middle finger to push up the vaginal wall just lateral to the urethra (Figure 16–2). This not only aids in determining the thickness, quality, and mobility of the anterior vaginal wall and the most appropriate position for its suspension to the pubic symphysis but also permits accurate location of the urethra, which can then be avoided in the placement of the sutures.

After accurate identification of the periurethral region, one to three nonabsorbable sutures are inserted lateral to the urethra, and placed so that almost the entire thickness of the anterior vaginal wall is included with each suture (Figure 16–3). The number of sutures used is governed by the length of the available urethra (Figure 16–4). Sutures are placed securely and deeply in fibrocartilage of the symphysis,

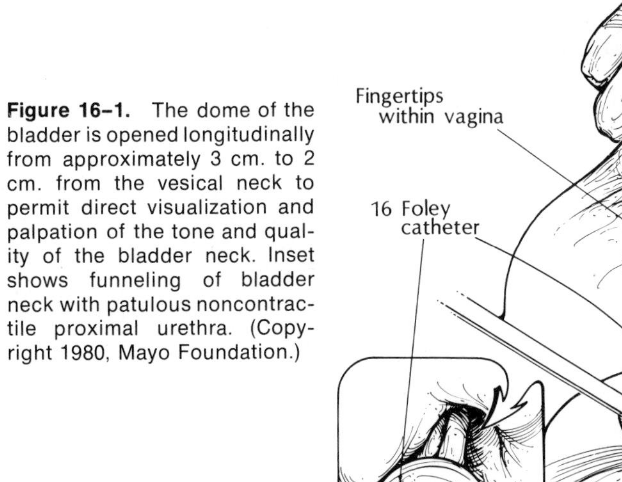

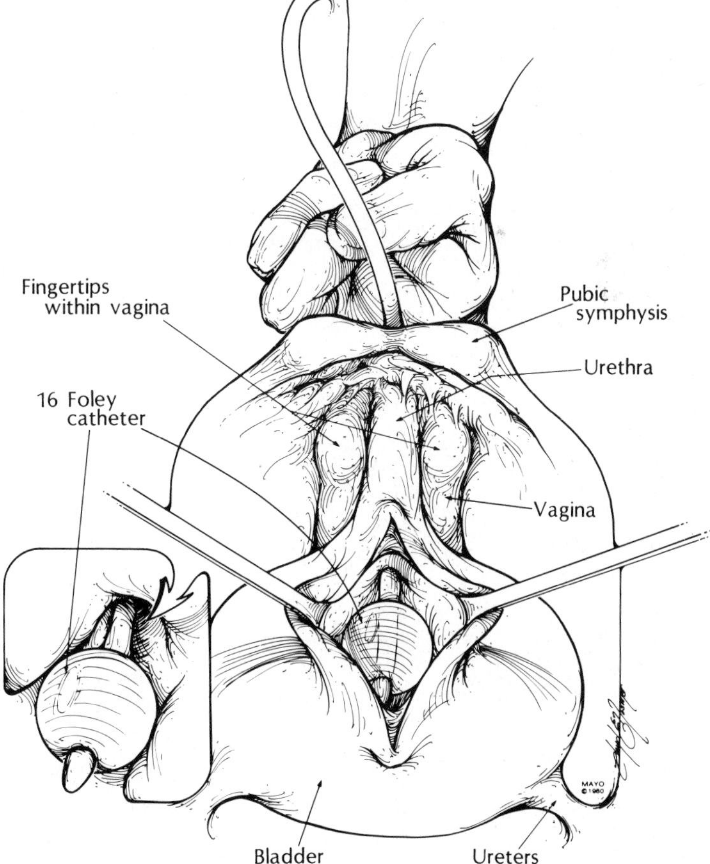

Figure 16–1. The dome of the bladder is opened longitudinally from approximately 3 cm. to 2 cm. from the vesical neck to permit direct visualization and palpation of the tone and quality of the bladder neck. Inset shows funneling of bladder neck with patulous noncontractile proximal urethra. (Copyright 1980, Mayo Foundation.)

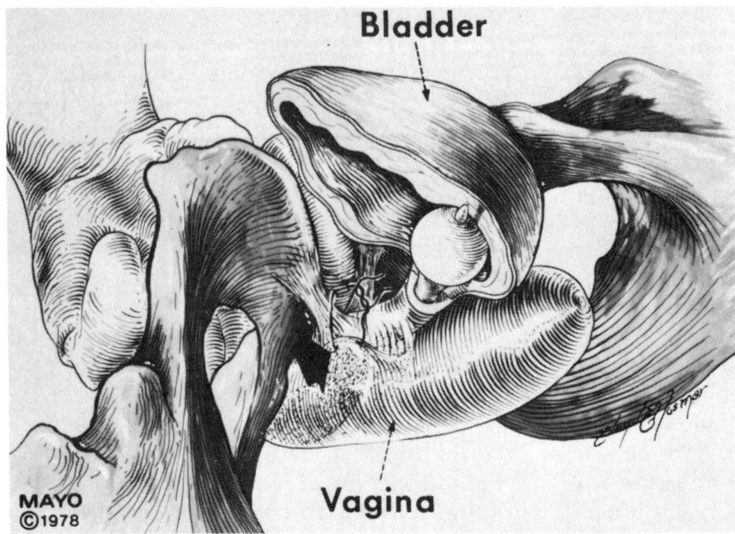

Figure 16–2. First suture on left side of urethra is placed. The midline finger of the surgeon's left hand is used to identify the urethra and to aid in determining the depth of penetration into the vaginal wall. (From Lee, R. A.: Correcting recurrent stress incontinence. Contemporary OB/GYN *12*:33, August, 1978.)

not the periosteum, with a sturdy No. 6 Mayo needle (Figure 16–5). A lighter needle will not permit deep penetration into the cartilage of the symphysis without risk of breakage. Periurethral sutures placed too far lateral to the urethra will not provide the desired support, and some degree of incontinence may persist. Conversely, if sutures are inserted too close to the urethra, mechanical urethral and bladder neck obstruction may occur, causing long-term urinary retention (Figure 16–3). The proper placement of the titration sutures (closest to bladder neck) is facilitated by their insertion under direct vision with the bladder open (Figure 16–4).

After all suspending sutures have been placed, they are tagged with an instrument and held laterally. Both gloves are changed at this time, and the bladder sutures are tied

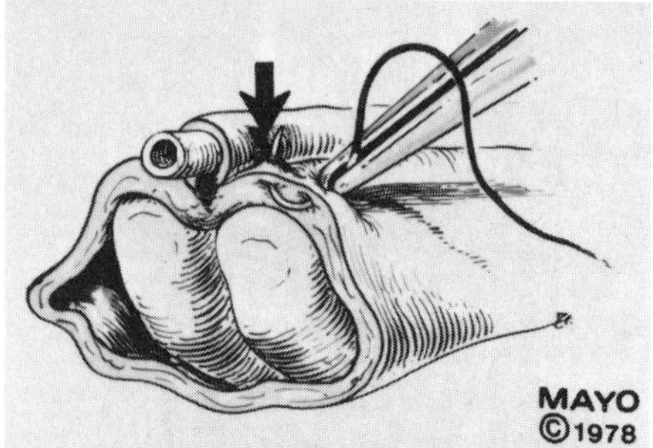

Figure 16–3. Almost the entire thickness of vaginal wall is included in the suturing, with the needle close to the urethra (3 to 5 mm.) (arrow). (From Lee, R. A.: Correcting recurrent stress incontinence. Contemporary OB/GYN *12*:33, August, 1978.)

(Figures 16–6 and 16–7). As previously reported (Lee, 1976), urethral plication and vesical neck support are emphasized in this approach, with no attempt to suture the bladder to the anterior abdominal wall.

In numerous observations of the normally continent bladder neck, invariably the proximal urethra has contracted tightly about a size 16 or 18 urethral catheter. Conversely, direct observation of the incontinent bladder neck almost always has revealed a significant and rather impressive degree of urethral atonicity. Often the urethra will permit insertion of an index finger alongside the catheter, and the finger can be inserted almost to the external meatus without encountering significant resistance.

After the suspending sutures have been tied and the urethral catheter has been removed, the vesicourethral junction should appear tight, with no discernible aperture or lumen. The neck of the urethra should provide considerable resistance to the insertion of the tip of the little finger. At this point, intraurethral pressures are obtained 1, 2, and 3 cm. from the vesical neck by means of a 3 ml. water-filled balloon attached to a mobile two-channel Sanborn recorder-electromanometer-transducer unit. This permits immediate revision or adjustment of the urethral or vesical neck supports in order to obtain optimal correction of urinary incontinence and yet eliminate overcorrection and postoperative urinary retention.

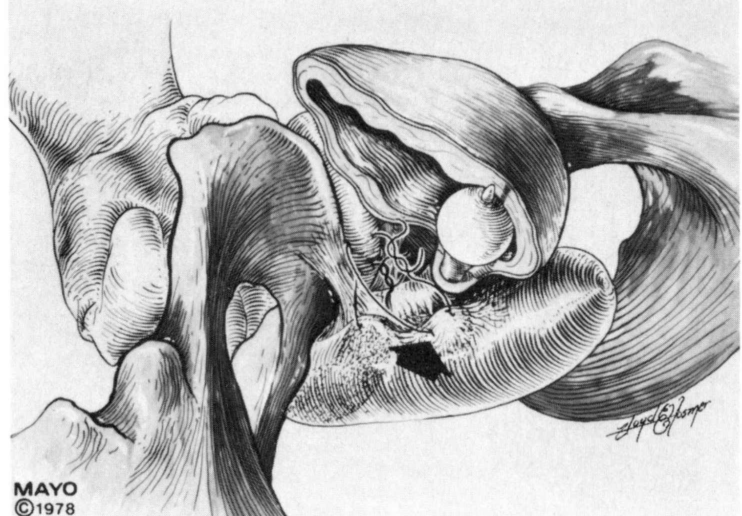

Figure 16–4. Relative position of second suture (in this case, the suture closest to vesicle neck), with its placement into the cartilage of the symphysis pubis. (From Lee, R. A.: Correcting recurrent stress incontinence. Contemporary OB/GYN *12*:33, August, 1978.)

A No. 16 French Silastic Foley suprapubic catheter is then brought out through a stab wound lateral to the midline incision, and the cystotomy is closed with two rows of continuous 2-0 chromic catgut. Loss of blood is minimal, and hemostasis is adequate once the suspending sutures are tied. In primary retropubic operations, a Hemovac drain is infrequently required but, in selected patients, it may be placed in the retropubic space and brought out through a stab wound lateral to the midline incision in order to avoid formation of a hematoma or infection.

POSTOPERATIVE MANAGEMENT

Patients usually receive antimicrobial therapy with sulfisoxazole (Gantrisin) after operation and for 1 week after removal of the suprapubic catheter. Urine cultures are obtained as indicated in the postoperative period and at the time the catheter is removed. Anticoagulant therapy with sodium warfarin (Coumadin), used regularly in the past, is no longer begun after an uncomplicated primary retropubic operation. Instead, early ambulation is relied on to avoid thrombophlebitis and pulmonary embolism, which has been reported as the cause of death associated with this procedure. The Hemovac suture catheter, when used, is removed after 48 hours, during which time 50 to 100 ml. of serosanguineous drainage is usually collected.

The suprapubic catheter is initially clamped on the seventh postoperative day. Once the patient is voiding, the volume of residual urine is determined by opening the suprapubic catheter. What constitutes satisfactory voiding and when to remove the

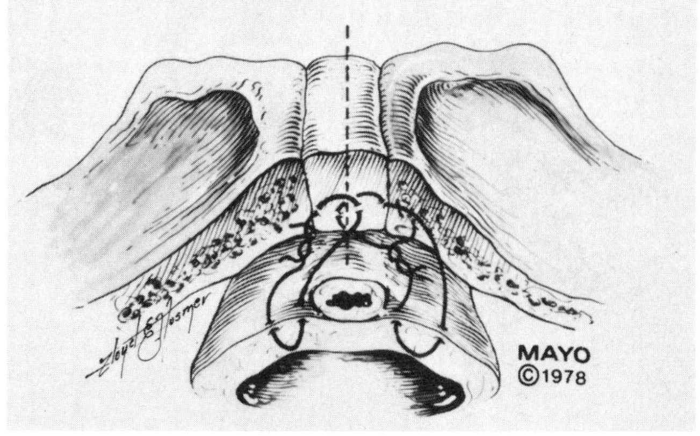

Figure 16–5. Demonstration of the relative position of a pair of sutures adjacent to the urethra securely placed into the cartilage of the symphysis pubis. (From Lee, R. A.: Correcting recurrent stress incontinence. Contemporary OB/GYN *12*: 33, August, 1978.)

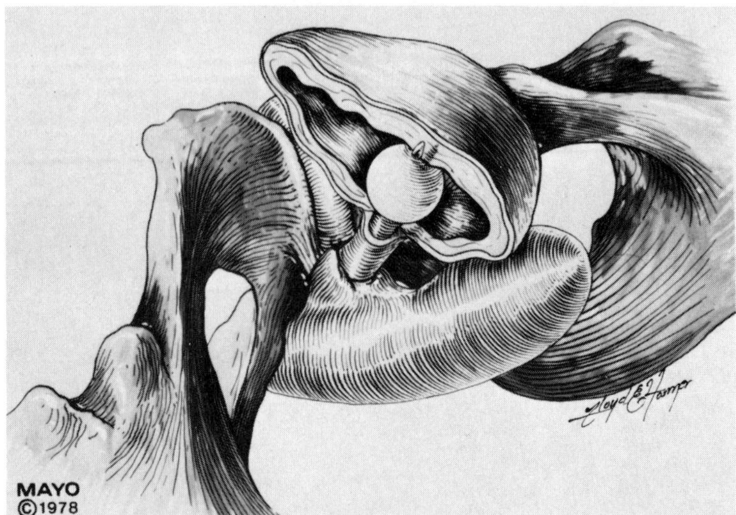

Figure 16–6. First set of sutures (immediately adjacent to posterior pubourethral ligament) have been tied. (Copyright 1978, Mayo Foundation.)

catheter depend on the volume of urine voided and the residual volume (usually less than 100 ml.). Urinary retention can follow any operation (thoracotomy, cholecystectomy, and so forth), but prolonged urinary retention (more than 2 weeks) is best managed by careful preoperative explanation and postoperative patience and reassurance. The patient and the relatives are comforted to know that it is only a matter of time before spontaneous voiding begins and the catheter will be removed. "Tincture of time" is far more valuable than bladder irritants or stimulants in an already irritable bladder. We would caution against urethral dilatation and would never suggest vesical neck resection "to loosen it up a little," lest urethral support be lost and total urinary incontinence result.

COMPLICATIONS AND RESULTS

The MMK operation, particularly the primary type, has been found to be a remarkably effective and safe operation, associated with minimal morbidity and no mortality. The complications noted by others such as osteitis pubis, prolonged

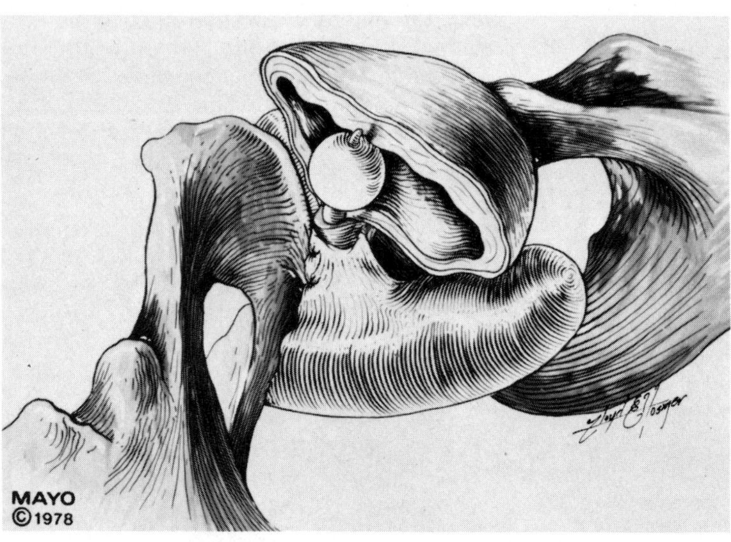

Figure 16–7. Placing of second set of sutures has resulted in a high retropubic position of the vesicle neck with a tight (hammock) effect on the entire urethra. (From Lee, R. A.: Correcting recurrent stress incontinence. Contemporary OB/GYN *12*:33, August, 1978.)

urinary retention, thrombophlebitis, and enterocele formation have been infrequent in Mayo Clinic experience. Osteitis pubis was found in 5, thrombophlebitis in 5, and enterocele in 6 of 231 patients. The suprapubic catheter is usually removed in 10 days (mean time, 10.2 days). Three patients had a degree of overcorrection requiring the standing position to accomplish successful voiding. One patient had a suture through the urethral catheter requiring reoperation for its removal. (This occurred before our present open bladder technique.) No fistulas or vesical stones have formed. The condition of all patients has been determined 2 years or more after the MMK operation, with a mean time of 7.8 years.

Proper evaluation of the present status of the incontinent patient necessitated a personal interview and examination whenever possible. When personal contact was not possible, questionnaires or telephone interview or both were used to differentiate stress from residual urgency or frequency incontinence. Stress incontinence was corrected in 215 of 231 patients (93 per cent); and of the 215 patients who are continent, 28 had concomitant plication of the proximal urethra and bladder neck.

Also of interest is the fact that in 14 patients the urethral length permitted only one pair of periurethral sutures to be placed at operation; however, 5 of our 15 failures occurred in this group. Three of these patients did undergo a later vaginal Kelly-Kennedy plication with successful correction. At least in this group of patients, a combined Ball suprapubic and vaginal approach may have been preferable at the original operation.

SUMMARY

Surgical correction of stress incontinence in the female remains a complex and distressing problem. After a complete evaluation of the patient (history, physical examination, and ancillary urologic evaluation), a primary retropubic operation for selected patients will produce improved long-term results and will eliminate many of the failures that follow the Kelly-Kennedy repair.

We continue to favor the less complex Kelly-Kennedy vaginal repair combined with vaginal hysterectomy for the usual patient with minimal to moderate stress incontinence and associated pelvic relaxation. However, deserving of special consideration are those patients whose severe incontinence (perhaps aggravated by a medical condition such as chronic lung disease or obesity); those with apparently good vesical support (e.g., a snug vagina with minimal anterior rotational descent of the bladder); and those with associated intra-abdominal disease that requires suprapubic incision. The added stress of these conditions, plus the wear and tear of time and menopausal attenuation of tissues, eventually results in loss of the support provided by vaginal repair and in recurrence of incontinence.

The primary retropubic urethral suspension, which relies on more substantial tissues, would appear to provide a more permanent urethral support and lasting control of symptoms in the patient with a complex and severe type of urinary stress incontinence. It is hoped that this will diminish the distressing incidence of "recurrent" stress incontinence.

REFERENCES

Beck, R. P.: Urinary stress incontinence. Ob./Gyn. Digest, pp. 19–37, November, 1976.

Enhörning, G.: Simultaneous recording of intravesical and intra-urethral pressure: a study on urethral closure in normal and stress incontinent women. Acta Chir. Scand. (Suppl.) *276*:1, 1961.

Green, T. H., Jr.: The problem of urinary stress incontinence in the female: an appraisal of its current status. Obstet. Gynecol. Surv. *23*:603, 1968.

Hodgkinson, C. P.: Stress urinary incontinence — 1970. Am. J. Obstet. Gynecol. *108*:1141, 1970.

Jeffcoate, T. N. A., and Roberts, H.: Observations on stress incontinence of urine. Am. J. Obstet. Gynecol. *64*:721, 1952.

Lapides, J., Ajemian, E. P., Stewart, B. H., et al.: Physiopathology of stress incontinence. Surg. Gynecol. Obstet. *111*:224, 1960.

Lee, R. A.: Recurrent stress incontinence of urine: preoperative assessment and surgical management. Clin. Obstet. Gynecol. *19*:661, 1976.

McGuire, E. A., Lytton, B., Pepe, V., and Kohorn, E. I.: Stress urinary incontinence. Obstet. Gynecol. *47*:255, 1976.

McGuire, E. A., Lytton, B., Kohorn, E. I., and Pepe, V.: The value of urodynamic testing in stress urinary incontinence. J. Urol. *124*:256, 1980.

Parker, R. T., Addison, W. A., and Wilson, C. J.: Fascia lata urethrovesical suspension for recurrent stress urinary incontinence. Am. J. Obstet. Gynecol. *135*:843, 1979.

Symmonds, R. E.: The suprapubic approach to anterior vaginal relaxation and urinary stress incontinence. Clin. Obstet. Gynecol. *15*:1107, 1972.

17

THE MODIFIED PEREYRA PROCEDURE

A. J. PEREYRA, M.D.
THOMAS B. LEBHERZ, M.D.

It is no longer customary today in the field of gynecologic urology to look upon anatomic stress urinary incontinence as the end result of pubourethral support failure. Equally uncommon is the idea of directing attention first to restoring the integrity of these supports in surgical treatment of this type of incontinence. Yet there is abundant and compelling evidence to show that elongation of these supports usually is the basic cause of such incontinence and that correction of this defect restores continence. The modified Pereyra procedure is the result of over 20 years of study to perfect an operation that can relieve women suffering from this incontinence and permit surgical correction of the associated vaginal defects that often accompany the condition without need for wide abdominal exposure or repositioning of the patient. A second objective has been to assure durability of the repair. Many methods of accomplishing this already exist, and some show early high success rates. With time, however, the percentage of failures progressively increases. It is our conviction that this is an inevitable result of dependence of these procedures on weakened supporting tissues. Accordingly, our efforts have been directed to strengthening and utilizing the natural supports provided rather than circumventing them.

CURRENT CONCEPTS

Anatomic stress urinary incontinence has been defined by Zacharin (1972) as "the sudden and involuntary loss of a small volume of urine consequent upon a sudden rise in intra-abdominal pressure. Immediately following the loss of control, control can be restored, preventing further loss." Prolapse of the urethrovesical (UV) junction outside the environment of intra-abdominal pressure commonly is associated with this incontinence (Green, 1978; Hodgkinson, 1953; Jeffcoate and Roberts, 1952). Elevation of the junction back to its orthotopic position usually restores continence (Marshall et al., 1949).

Loss in elevation often follows difficult vaginal childbirth that leaves the supporting structures stretched. These supports consist of the pubourethral ligaments that lie supraurethrally (Krantz, 1978; Zacharin, 1972; Langreder, 1956) and the endopelvic fascia in the vaginal canal wall (Kegell and Powell, 1950) lying lateral to the urethra. Many operative methods for correcting UV junction prolapse have been devised. Most of them depend on elevating this stretched fascia, which is located superficially in the anterior vaginal wall, protected only by a thin layer of epithelium. In consequence of this position, it is exposed to considerable stretching in childbirth. Often, it is left paper-thin.

Such attenuated fascia lacks the body and strength necessary to impede pull-out of the suspensory sutures attached to it. These sutures are subjected to considerable strain with increases in intra-abdominal pressure. It is not surprising, therefore, that some of the sutures affixed to the thin fascia pull out. As a result, in time, depending on the residual strength of the fascia, UV junction prolapse recurs and incontinence returns.

Notwithstanding this evident deficiency in the fascia, operations utilizing the periurethral tissues to elevate the UV junction continue to be used without any attempt to reinforce the attenuated fascia contained by them that is the main source of their strength. Meanwhile, the much stronger pubourethral ligaments have been little employed for this purpose. The relative difficulty of access to these ligaments has, no doubt, contributed to their neglect.

DEVELOPMENT OF MODIFIED PEREYRA PROCEDURE

In 1949, Marshall, Marchetti, and Krantz demonstrated relief of urinary incontinence by use of their procedure (Marshall-Marchetti-Krantz or MMK), which restores UV junction elevation with sutures inserted into the periurethral tissues and anchored to the posterior pubic periosteum. Unfortunately, in our hands, these sutures sometimes cut through the pubic periosteum or pulled out of the periurethral tissues. Occasionally a painful periostitis developed. To prevent suture pull-out from above, the senior author (Pereyra, 1959) substituted the rectus fascia for the often thin pubic periosteum to anchor the suspensory sutures. With this change, it became possible to secure these sutures to the fascia through a small suprapubic abdominal skin incision. Thus, UV junction elevation and the vaginoplasty often required in patients with anatomic incontinence could be accomplished without repositioning the patient.

A special ligature carrier instrument was developed to transfer the sutures retropubically. In 1959, a combination pointed cannula and stylet needle was introduced for this purpose. However, it was replaced by a single sliding needle in 1975 (Figure 17–1).*

This left unresolved the problem of preventing suture pull-out from the periurethral tissues below. Such suture pull-outs were found in failed MMK, Burch, and the original Pereyra procedures. Stalactite-shaped fibrous extensions from above were found joined to stalagmite-like fibrous cones formed below by stretched fibrous strands containing the detached sutures.

Many modifications in technique, including interpositioning of baffles between the sutures and endopelvic fascia in the periurethral tissues, were tried without success. A combination Kelly procedure (Kelly and Dumm, 1914), using the suprapubic suspensory sutures as already described, delayed but failed to prevent suture pull-out (Pereyra and Lebherz, 1967). Ultimately, reinforcement of the stretched endopelvic fascia or substitution of stronger urethral tissue supports, or both,

*Pereyra Ligature Carrier Instrument, '75. Manufactured and distributed by El Rey Industries, P. O. Box 791, Upland, CA 91786.

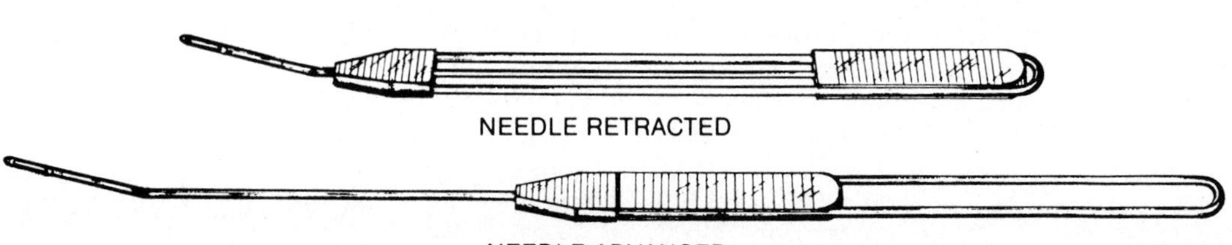

Figure 17–1. Pereyra Ligature Carrier, '75.

appeared to be the only possible enduring solution.

REINFORCEMENT OF THE ENDOPELVIC FASCIA

In 1974, an operation was carried out in which the endopelvic fascia, denuded of anterior vaginal wall epithelium, was freed from its anterolateral attachments to the inferior borders of the pubic rami. The freed ends were ruffled together with a helical suture to form a thickened mass better capable of resisting suspensory suture penetration. This was elevated retropubically using the new Pereyra Ligature Carrier '75 needle. The four suture ends were tied together over the suprapubic midabdominal fascia. Observations over a period of 3 years postoperatively showed a marked improvement in results, which were reported in the first edition of this book.

INCLUSION OF PUBOURETHRAL LIGAMENTS

More importantly, freeing the endopelvic fascia from the pubis exposed the retropubic spaces bilaterally. Now, the much tougher posterior pillars of the pubourethral ligaments came clearly into view and became readily accessible. For years, these ligaments have been esteemed to be the main supports for the urethra and the urethrovesical junction by Zacharin (1963, 1968), Krantz (1951), Nichols and Randall (1976), Milley and Nichols (1971) and others (Figure 17–2).

In 1974, the posterior pillars of the pubourethral ligaments were included in the suspensory sutures used to reinforce and elevate the endopelvic fascia. Both pubourethral supports are thickened, providing optimal resistance to suture pull-out, thus assuring enduring elevation of the UV junction.

In 1976, Pereyra reported his early results with this modification of the original procedure, which involves binding the posterior pillars of the pubourethral ligaments and the reinforced pelvic fascia before elevation. In 1978, he published his 3-year follow-up results using the modified procedure in 29 patients. In 1981, Pereyra and co-workers published the results of their operations with this modified procedure in 82 patients followed for 36 to 60 months. During this period, the technique described and illustrated in this chapter has been followed.

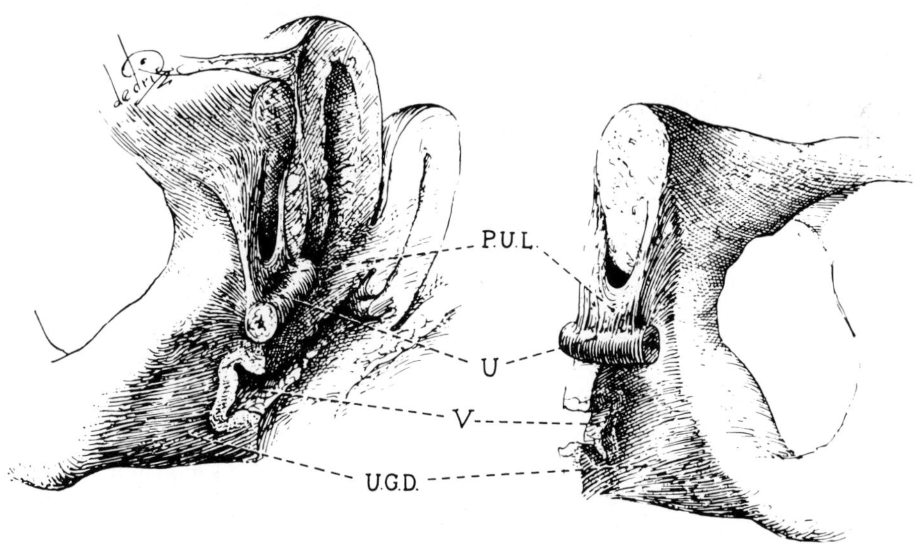

Figure 17–2. The pubourethral ligaments. Sagittal section showing pubourethral ligaments (P.U.L.), urethra (U), vagina (V), and urogenital diaphragm (U.G.D.). (From Milley, R. S., and Nichols, D. H.: The relationship between pubourethral ligaments and urogenital diaphragm in the human female. Anat. Rec. *170*:281, 1971. Reproduced with permission of the Wistar Press.)

TABLE 17–1. PREOPERATIVE EVALUATION OF PATIENTS

NAME:__________ AGE:______ PARA:______ DATE:______

Factors recommended for review in patients with anatomic stress urinary incontinence (ASUI) under consideration for this operation:

	METHODS USED	CONFIRMED YES : NO
1. *Symptomatic confirmation* of ASUI:	Hodgkinson's questionnaire	___ : ___
(In ASUI, patient can stop urine, etc.)		___ : ___
2. *Prolapsed urethrovesical (UV) junction*:	Chain urethrocystogram	___ : ___
(Junction descends 15 mm. + with strain):		___ : ___
(PUV angle > 110 degrees without cystocele):		___ : ___
3. *Urethral pressure* < than vesical pressure: (Mid-intraurethral pressure lower on straining)	Urethrocystometrogram	___ : ___
4. *Absence of anatomic urinary tract defects:*	IVP	___ : ___
5. Absence of intrinsic UV pathology (check if present): a. Urethrocystitis e. Polyp urethra/bladder b. Stricture urethra f. Fistula urethra or bladder c. Diverticula g. Limited bladder capacity d. Atrophic urethritis h. Other:______	Cystoscopy	___ : ___
6. Absence of unstable bladder: (Characterized by following, check if present) a. Low midurethral pressure b. Low bladder filling resistance c. Low bladder capacity (note amount) d. Detrusor dyssynergia e. Controlled with drugs—list drug used:______	Urethrocystometrogram	___ : ___
7. Absence of atonic or hypotonic bladder:	Urethrocystometrogram	___ : ___
8. Increased rotation urethral axis (degree of rotation__):		___ : ___
9. Adequate estrogen level:	Vaginal smear	___ : ___
10. Absence of cervical or endometrial carcinoma:	Papanicolaou smear	___ : ___
11. Absence of vaginal pathogens:	Vaginal smear	___ : ___
12. Absence of systemic diseases (list below if present): a. Neuropathic______ b. Metabolic______ c. Cardiopulmonary______	Clinical evaluation	___ : ___
13. Absence of pregnancy:	UCG test and pelvic examination	___ : ___
14. Other anatomic pelvic defects present and in need of surgical correction (list)______		
15. Prior pelvic surgery (list dates and names of operations):______		

PREOPERATIVE EVALUATION

Great care must be taken to exclude those patients who lose urine as a result of causes unrelated to anatomic stress urinary incontinence. These patients will not be benefited by the modified Pereyra procedure. To help exclude such patients with urinary incontinence, the following preoperative evaluation form is proposed for regular use in each woman with urinary incontinence who is under consideration for surgical correction of her problem by use of this procedure (Table 17–1).

INTERPRETATION OF RESULTS (PREOPERATIVE EVALUATION)

Item No. 1 relates to a complete *symptomatic evaluation* of the patient with regard to conditions under which involuntary loss

TABLE 17–2. URINARY INCONTINENCE RECORD

NAME ______________________ AGE ________ DATE ____________

SUMMARY OF HISTORY AND TREATMENT ______________________

CURRENT MEDICATIONS ______________________

UROLOGIC QUESTIONNAIRE*

Group 1

1.	Have you had treatment for urinary tract disease such as stones, kidney disease, infections, tumors, injuries?	YES	NO
2.	Have you had repeated bouts of pyelitis?	YES	NO
3.	Is your urine ever bloody?	YES	NO
4.	Is the volume of urine you usually pass large, average, small, very small? (Underline correct one)		
5.	When you lose urine accidentally, are you ever not aware that it is passing?	YES	NO
6.	Do you always have a severe sense of urgency before you lose your urine?	YES	NO
7.	Do you lose urine as a constant drip from the vagina?	YES	NO
8.	Did you have difficulty holding urine as a child?	YES	NO
9.	Is it usually painful or difficult to pass your urine?	YES	NO

Group 2

1.	As a child did you wet the bed?	YES	NO
2.	Do you wet the bed now?	YES	NO
3.	Have you ever had paralysis, polio, multiple sclerosis, a serious injury to your back, cyst or tumor on your spine? (If yes, check proper one)	YES	NO
4.	Does the sound, sight or feel of running water cause you to lose urine?	YES	NO
5.	Is your loss of urine a continual drip so that you are constantly wet?	YES	NO
6.	Are you ever not aware that you are losing, or are about to lose, control of your urine?	YES	NO
7.	Is your clothing slightly damp, wet, or soaking wet, or do you leave puddles on the floor? (If yes, check proper one)	YES	NO
8.	Have you had an operation on your spine, brain or bladder?	YES	NO
9.	Do you find it frequently necessary to have your urine removed by means of a catheter because you are unable to pass it?	YES	NO

Group 3

1.	Do you lose urine by spurts during coughing, sneezing, laughing, lifting? (Underline)	YES	NO
2.	Do you lose urine when you are lying down?	YES	NO
3.	Do you lose urine when you are sitting or standing erect?	YES	NO
4.	When you are urinating, can you usually stop the flow?	YES	NO
5.	Did your urine difficulty start after delivery of an infant?	YES	NO
6.	Did it follow an operation?	YES	NO
7.	Circle the type of operation: Hysterectomy, abdominal incision; hysterectomy, removed through the vagina; removal of a tumor, abdominal incision; vaginal repair operation; suspension of the uterus; cesarean section.		
8.	If your menstrual periods have stopped, did the menopause make your condition more severe?	YES	NO
9.	Is your control of urine good unless you cough, sneeze, laugh, lift, or strain?	YES	NO
10.	Do you have difficulty holding urine if you suddenly stand erect from a sitting or lying down position?	YES	NO
11.	Do you find it necessary to wear protection because you get wet?	YES	NO

*From Hodgkinson, C. P.: Stress urinary incontinence. Table I, Three-part questionnaire. Am. J. Obstet. Gynecol. *108*:1149, 1970. Reprinted with permission.

of urine occurs, which is prerequisite to performing related objective tests. We have found the Hodgkinson's three-part "Urologic Questionnaire" (Table 17–2) to be very helpful for this purpose. Affirmative answers to questions contained in the first section suggest the presence of intrinsic urinary tract disease. Affirmative answers to questions in the second section suggest malfunction of the neuromuscular system as it pertains to the urinary tract. Affirmative answers to the third group support the concept of physical defects as the cause of the stress urinary incontinence. "Yes" answers to this group of questions imply that the patient has symptomatic anatomic stress urinary incontinence.

Item No. 2 in the form calls for a check mark in the "Yes" column if the *chain urethrocystogram* performed as described by Steinhausen and co-workers (1970) shows UV junction descent of 15 mm. or more on straining by the patient and often an increase in posterior pubourethral angle of 110 degrees or more (in the absence of a cystocele).

Item No. 3 justifies a check mark in the "Yes" column if the urethrocystometrogram performed as described by Raz (1979) shows a mid-intraurethral pressure equal to or lower than that obtained intravesically on straining.

Item No. 4 is checked "Yes" if intravenous pyelography fails to detect any physical defects along the entire urinary tract that could affect successful outcome of the operation.

Item No. 5 is checked "Yes" if cystoscopy fails to reveal any intrinsic pathology that could affect successful results, complicate the operative procedure, or require prior or concurrent medical or surgical treatment of lower urinary tract defects.

Item No. 6 is checked "Yes" if a urethrocystometrogram performed as described by Raz (1979) shows absence of an *unstable bladder* if there are no check marks denoting presence of any of the items in subsections *a* to *e* in this part of the form.

Item No. 7 is checked "Yes" if the urethrocystometrogram shows normal intravesical pressure adequate to empty the bladder.

Item No. 8 is checked "Yes" if a cotton-tipped applicator or stick or swizzle stick inserted in the urethra rotates upward more than 30 degrees on straining.

Item No. 9 is checked "Yes" if a fresh recent vaginal smear reveals an adequate *estrogen index*. Absent or low estrogen levels will affect firm, lasting repair and usually require indefinite postoperative estrogen therapy.

Item No. 10 is checked "Yes" if a *Papanicolaou cervical smear* taken within a month of surgery is reported as Class 1, negative.

Item No. 11 is checked "Yes" if a fresh, *recent vaginal smear* shows absence of *Candida* or *Trichomonas vaginalis* infection. If venereal disease or the presence of chlamydia or other pathogens is suspected, culture and treatment should be accomplished before surgery.

Item No. 12 is checked "Yes" if the patient is free of *systemic diseases,* such as (1) multiple sclerosis or other neuropathology; (2) diabetes mellitus or other metabolic diseases; (3) bronchitis, emphysema, or other pulmonary or cardiac disease.

Item No. 13 is checked "Yes" if pelvic examination, urine chorionic gonadotropin (UCG) test, and menstrual history do not support a *diagnosis of pregnancy*.

On completion of this form to this point, all check marks should be in the "Yes" column, indicating that the patient is a suitable candidate for the modified Pereyra procedure, insofar as the factors covered are concerned. Absent, questionable, or "No" check marks should be reevaluated and reviewed with the patient before scheduling her for this procedure.

In Item No. 14, if there are other physical *pelvic defects* present, a recommendation for concurrent surgical correction should be discussed with the patient and an additional signed informed consent obtained for such surgery.

Item No. 15 is important. The surgeon should be well informed regarding prior pelvic surgery, which may lead to complications or require modification of the technique described and illustrated below.

TECHNIQUE OF THE MODIFIED PEREYRA PROCEDURE

1. Preparing the Patient for Operation

With the patient in the dorsal recumbent position (patient on back, with lower limbs slightly flexed and rotated outward) the head of the operating table is dropped 30 degrees.

A No. 18 Foley catheter is inserted through the urethra, the 5 ml. catheter bulb is inflated, and the bladder is drained dry.

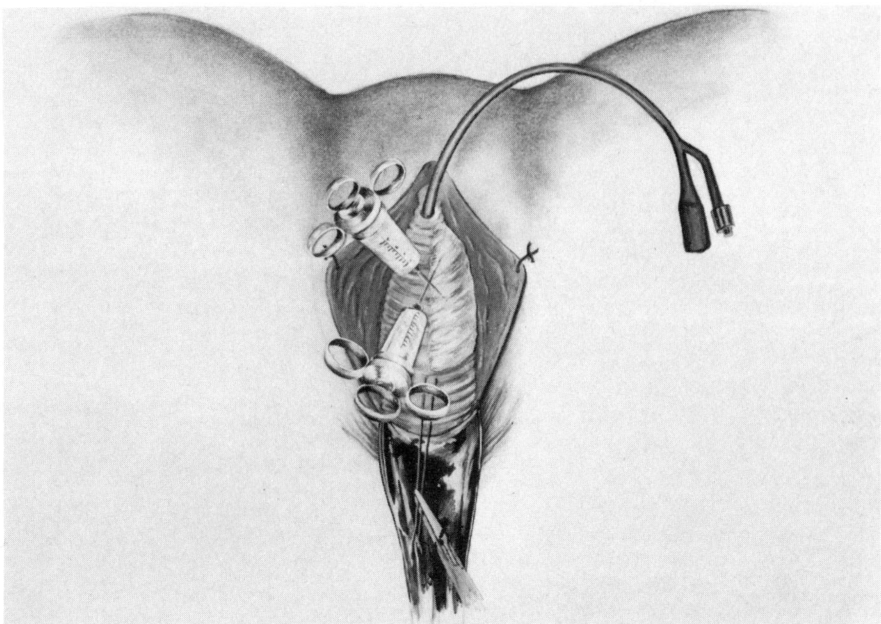

Figure 17–3. Injection of saline subepithelially to facilitate dissection.

The catheter end is elevated but not clamped, so that bladder filling and need for further drainage are noted by spill of urine or the appearance of hematuria will warn the surgeon of possible bladder, urethral, or ureteral injury.

2. Freeing Epithelium from Anterior Vaginal Wall

Traction is made on the Foley catheter, causing its balloon to impinge against the internal orifice of the urethra. This approximates the location of the UV junction. An ectal suture is transfixed to the underlying epithelium to mark this junction. Sterile normal saline solution is injected subepithelially from the level of the junction to 2 cm. behind the urinary meatus (Figure 17–3). The injection is continued laterally on each side of the urethra to the pubic rami. This detaches the epithelium from the underlying endopelvic fascia and its enclosed levator ani muscle complex.

3. Denuding Anterior Surfaces of the Endopelvic Fascia

A half-circle incision is made through the freed epithelium 2 cm. around the lower urethral meatus (Figure 17–4). A vertical incision is made through the freed epithelium over the urethra, beginning at the middle of the half-circle incision and extending down to the marker suture (Figure 17–5). Using Metzenbaum scissors, the epithelium is dissected free laterally on each side to the sites of insertion of the endopelvic fascia into the pubis.

4. Entering the Space of Retzius

A fingertip pointed against the inferior posterolateral pubic rami is inserted through the endopelvic fascia at its site of attachment to the rami 3 to 4 cm. lateral to the UV junction on each side (Figure 17–6).

Sometimes, owing to fibrous tissue formation (a residual from prior failed surgery) the points of a pair of Metzenbaum scissors may be required to penetrate the fascia. Under these circumstances, the possibility of the bladder being involved in such adhesions must be kept in mind and even greater care taken to keep the points bearing firmly against the inferior posterolateral pubic rami.

5. Exposing the Space of Retzius

Once a proper opening into the space of Retzius is made, the retropubic space is

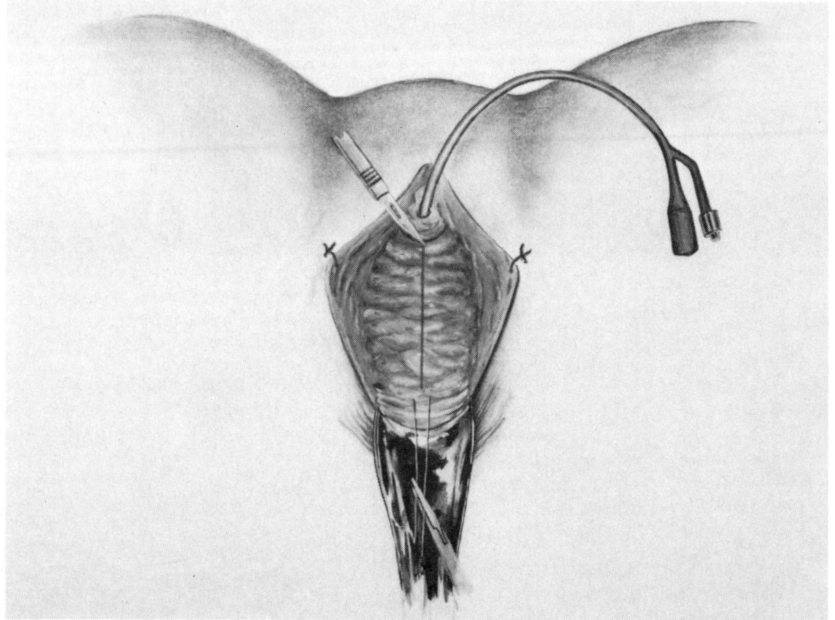

Figure 17–4. Incising the freed anterior vaginal epithelium.

explored with an index finger, which is extended upward so that the tip is palpable through the skin suprapubically (Figure 17–7). The finger is rotated medially as far as the urethra and laterally down to the level of the UV junction (arrow). Any adhesions bound to the bladder, the urethra, or posterior pubis are noted.

The same procedure is carried out on the opposite side. The operator's right index

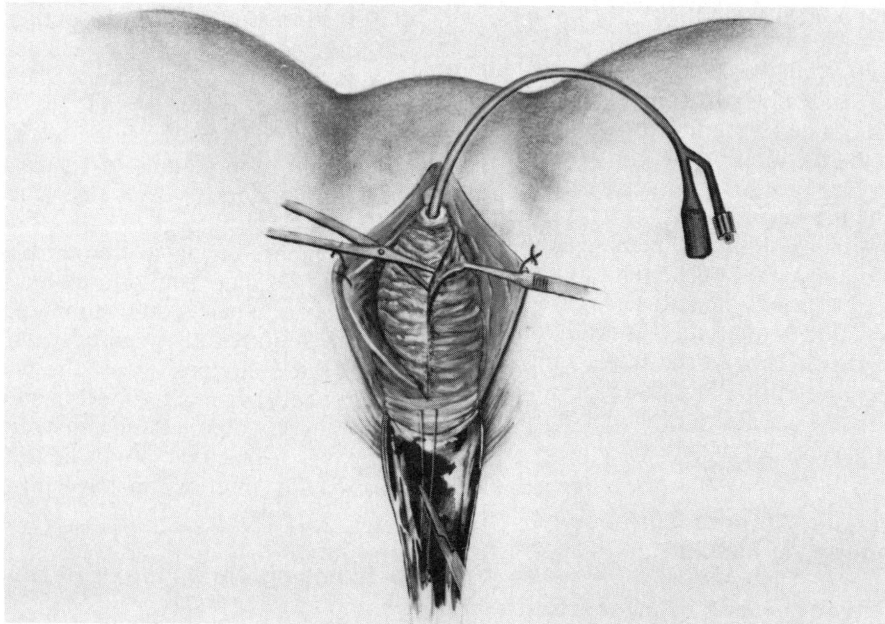

Figure 17–5. Dissecting the epithelium from the endopelvic fascia.

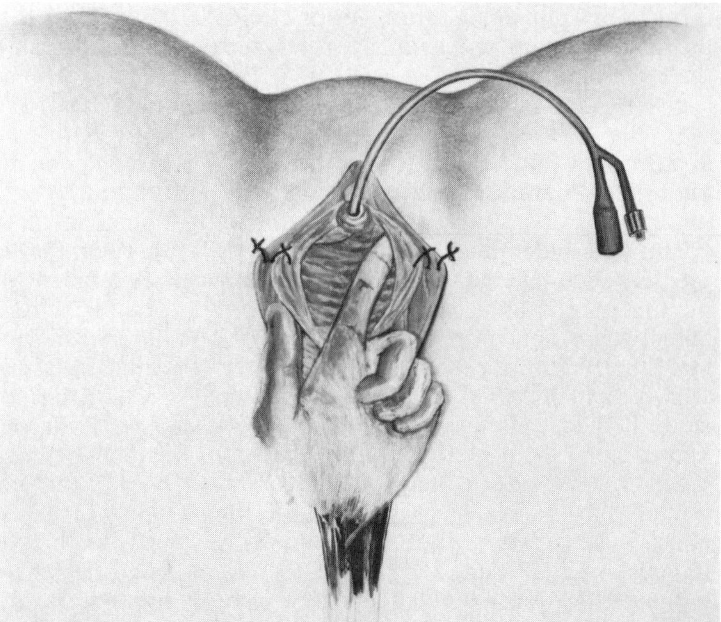

Figure 17–6. Perforating the endopelvic fascia at the attachment to the pubis.

finger is used to expose the patient's right space of Retzius and the left finger to expose the patient's left space of Retzius. With the retropubic spaces thus widely exposed on each side, the operator frees any adhesions found, whether or not these are tense. (Lax fibrous bands when left in have been found to tighten on filling of the bladder, causing traction on the UV junction and interference with proper functioning of the closing mechanism in the vesical neck.) Rarely, as in the case of firm supraurethral adhesions, suprapubic entry must be made to free such scar tissue

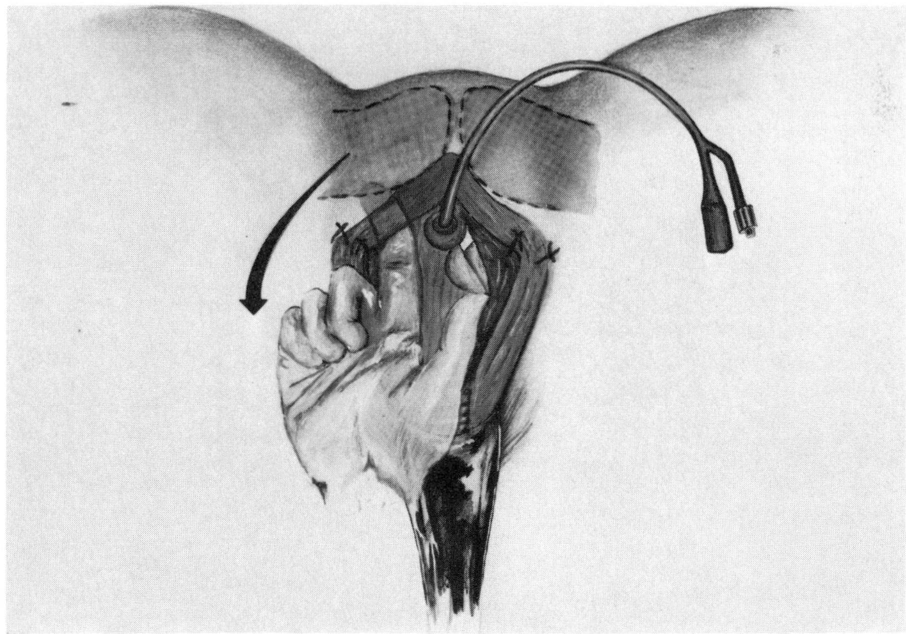

Figure 17–7. Rotating the penetrating finger to widen the opening.

formations remaining from prior failed operations before proceeding further with the procedure.

6. Locating Pubourethral Ligament Posterior Pillars

The right index finger is extended along the left side of the exposed retropubic urethra until it abuts against the catheter bulb, which has been drawn toward the inner urethral orifice by traction on the catheter and deflected to the patient's right side. The fingertip is flexed medially to hook around the posterior pillar of the ligament on that side (a narrow Deaver retractor aids in exposing the edge of the pillar). The pillars are grasped with Allis forceps and held aside (Figure 17–9). The left index finger is extended along the right side of the retropubic urethra in a similar manner to locate and grasp the right posterior pillar (Figure 17–8). Both posterior pillars lie immediately in front of the catheter bulb in the bladder. In patients with true anatomic incontinence, the fingertip, when flexed, enters the triangular space, separating both posterior pillars supraurethrally.

7. Uniting the Pillars to the Endopelvic Fascia

A size 0 Prolene suture,* 30 inches (76 cm.) long, is introduced once or twice through one pillar near its attachment to the urethra. The suture then is inserted three or four times in a helical fashion transversely through the endopelvic fascia, each bite being taken further laterally (Figure 17–9). The two suture ends when drawn taut bundle the whole into a thick mass, leaving the denuded fascia and ligament pillar wrapped around the posterior pubic periosteum. A *sharp* pull on the two suture ends will establish whether the bound tissues will hold. If the suture cuts through, the suspension will fail. This usually indicates that the pubourethral ligament's posterior pillar was not grasped or that it is weak and requires reinforcement. In this event, further wider turns of the Prolene suture around the posterior pillar and endopelvic fascia are needed. The same procedure then is carried out with the posterior pillar and endopelvic fascia on the opposite side, using a second size 0 Prolene suture.

*Prolene (Polypropylene), size 0 suture (Ethicon, Somerville, New Jersey, 08876).

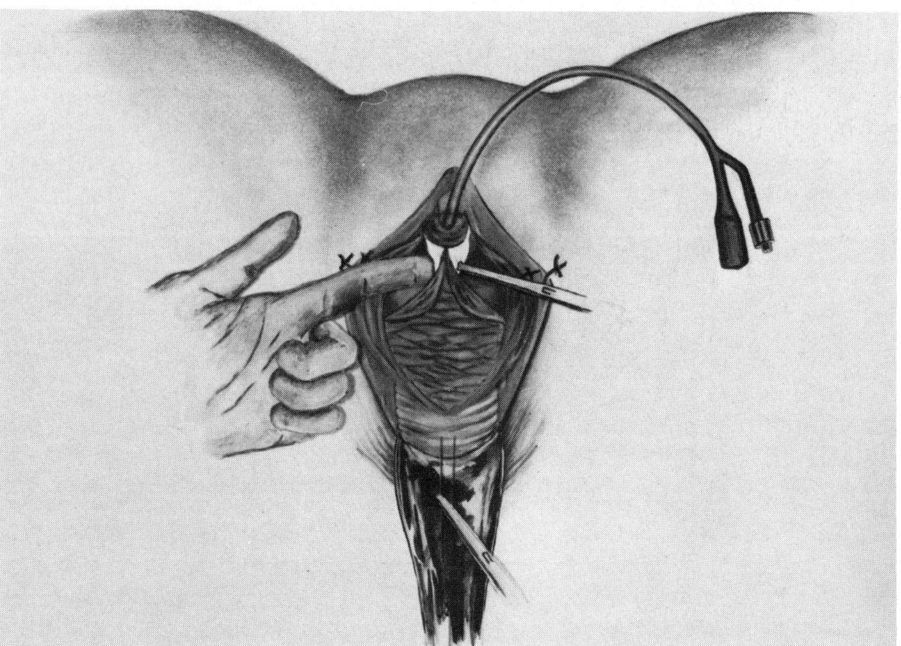

Figure 17–8. The finger identifies the posterior (white) pubourethral ligaments.

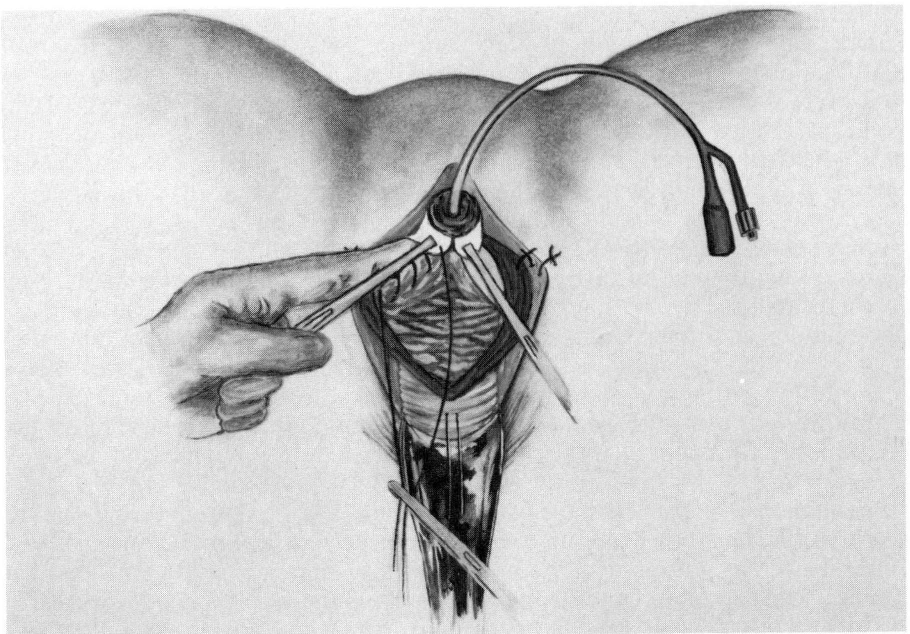

Figure 17–9. Allis forceps grasp the posterior pillars of the ligaments and helical sutures bind pillars and endopelvic fascia.

8. Passing Pereyra Ligature Carrier Needle Retropubically

A transverse suprapubic skin incision approximately 4 cm. wide is made 2 cm. above the symphysis pubis (Figure 17–10). With the needle in the instrument fully retracted within its brace and the triangular brace held with its serrated surface facing the posterior pubis, the needle point is

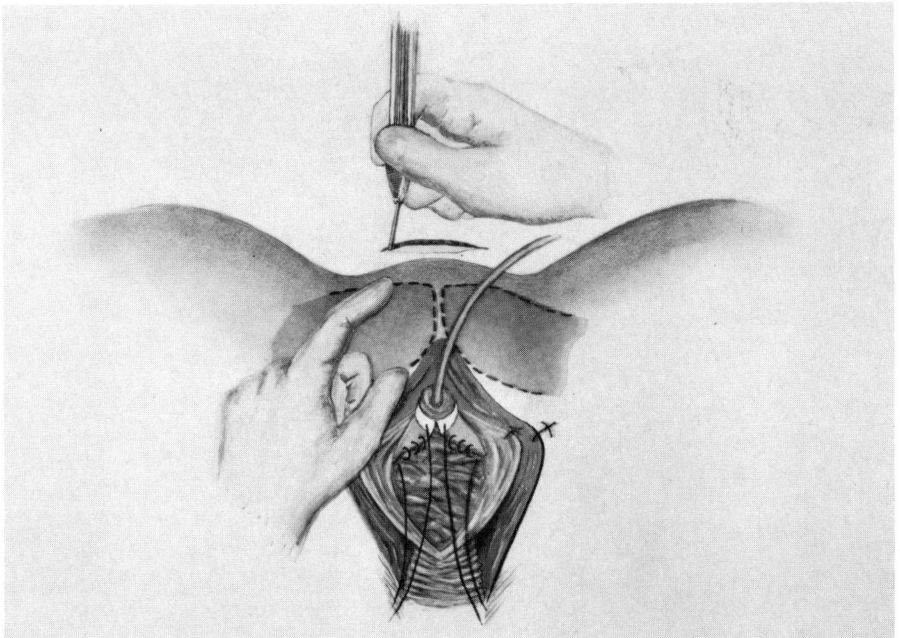

Figure 17–10. The needle is inserted behind the pubic crest.

introduced laterally through the right end of the incision. The angulated section of the needle protruding from the lower end of the brace must face toward the posterior pubis. The point at the end of this angulated section is advanced through the abdominal fascia where it attaches to the crest of the pubis, 3 cm. lateral to the symphysis pubis. A fingertip of the opposite hand placed on the skin overlying the site of fascial penetration assures that the needle stays behind the pubis and does not override its crest.

9. Retropubic Transfer of Needle and Suspensory Sutures

The operator inserts the left hand vaginally and extends the index finger up to the junction of the rectus muscle with the posterior pubis in the patient's right retropubic space. This finger serves as a guide to the site of penetration by the needle immediately back of the posterior pubis and helps hold the anterior upper edge of the bladder away from the needle. The fingertip caps the point of the needle as it is advanced by drawing down the elongated serrated handle attached to its upper end. This safeguards against penetration or trauma to bladder, urethra, or posterior pubic periosteum. The long needle shaft is advanced retropubically out through the vagina, where the elongated eye near the point is threaded with the two Prolene suture ends on the right (Figure 17–11). Enough slack should remain so that the sutures do not bind when pulled up. The ends of the sutures should extend at least 5 cm. (2 inches) beyond the eye of the needle so they do not slip out. The needle then is withdrawn suprapubically. The two suture ends are disengaged from the needle, clamped together with a curved Mayo forceps, and allowed to lie free on the abdomen.

Steps No. 8 and 9 are repeated on the patient's left side to bring the two left Prolene suture ends out through the left end of the suprapubic skin incision. These suture ends are clamped together with a straight Mayo forceps.

10. Elevating Pubourethral Supports

The pubourethral supports are elevated retropubically by pulling on both pairs of Prolene suture ends lying on the suprapubic

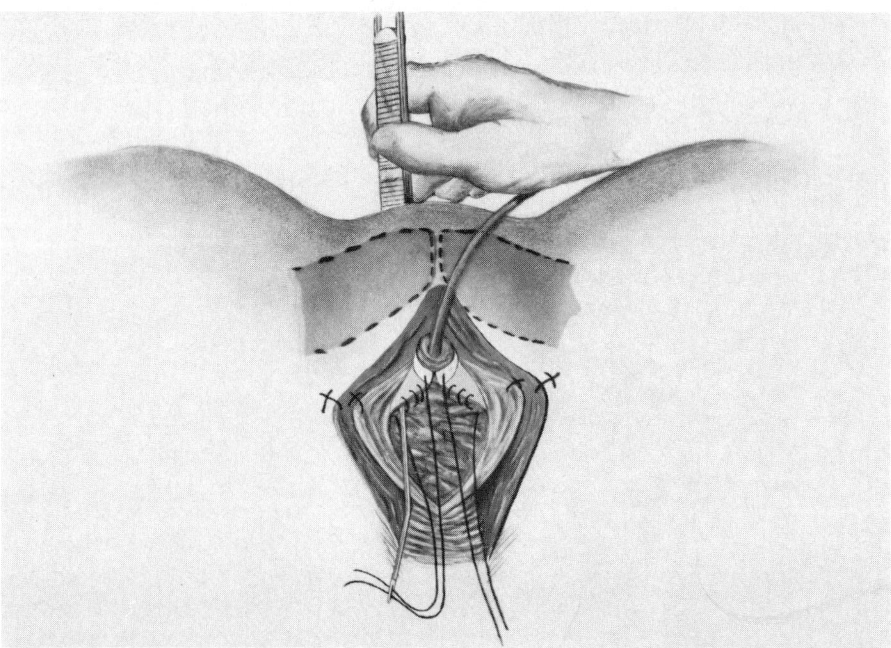

Figure 17–11. The needle is advanced out of the vagina and threaded with suture ends.

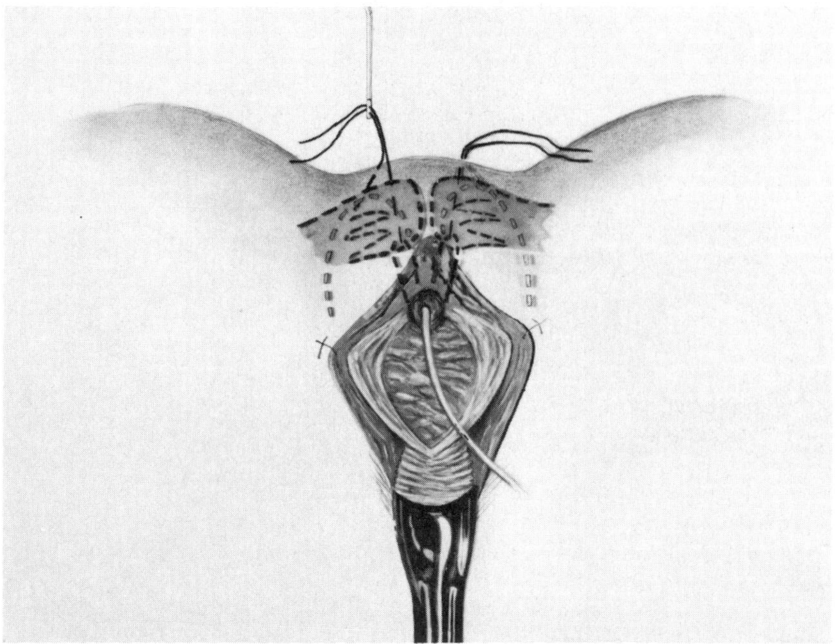

Figure 17–12. The suture ends are lifted out through the suprapubic skin incision.

abdominal skin (Figure 17–12). When a cystocele is present, this is repaired in the usual manner first, before the tissues are elevated. Following reduction in the cystocele, the opening in the anterior vaginal epithelium is closed.

11. Affixing Prolene Suture Ends to Abdominal Fascia

The Foley catheter is removed and a urethroscope is inserted by an assistant. The four suture ends are tied together over the suprapubic abdominal fascia when the lower edge of the urethral internal meatus begins to close, as observed by an assistant through the urethroscope (Figure 17–13).

The center of the abdominal fascia lying beneath the suprapubic skin incision is elevated with a Kocher forceps. Two of the tied Prolene suture ends are drawn transversely for 2.5 cm. beneath the midfascia with an aneurysm needle. The Kocher forceps then is removed. The two suture ends are disengaged from the needle and are tied a second time to the other pair of Prolene suture ends.

Before accomplishing this, the assistant makes a final check through the urethroscope to determine the correct level at which the transfixing of the abdominal fascia should be accomplished.

Testing the Closing Mechanism for Continence. The internal urethral orifice connected to an empty bladder presents a flattened inferior margin, as shown by Robertson (1978). Elevation and anchorage of the pubourethral supports to the suprapubic abdominal aponeurosis further appears to increase this flattening (Figure 17–13, left). Actually, what is happening is that the suspensory sutures are producing an upward rotation of the urethra. In consequence, as the inferior margin recedes back and up, the orifice presents a transverse sesamoid shape as viewed through the urethroscope. However, this only confirms that the forces of suture traction are being exerted on the UV junction.

It does not necessarily follow from this observation that the valvular mechanism is now functional and can close to effect continence. Such functional capacity can only be tested by filling the bladder and increasing intravesical pressure. This is done best by having the patient operated on under conduction anesthesia so that she can voluntarily produce an increase in intra-abdominal pressure when instructed to do

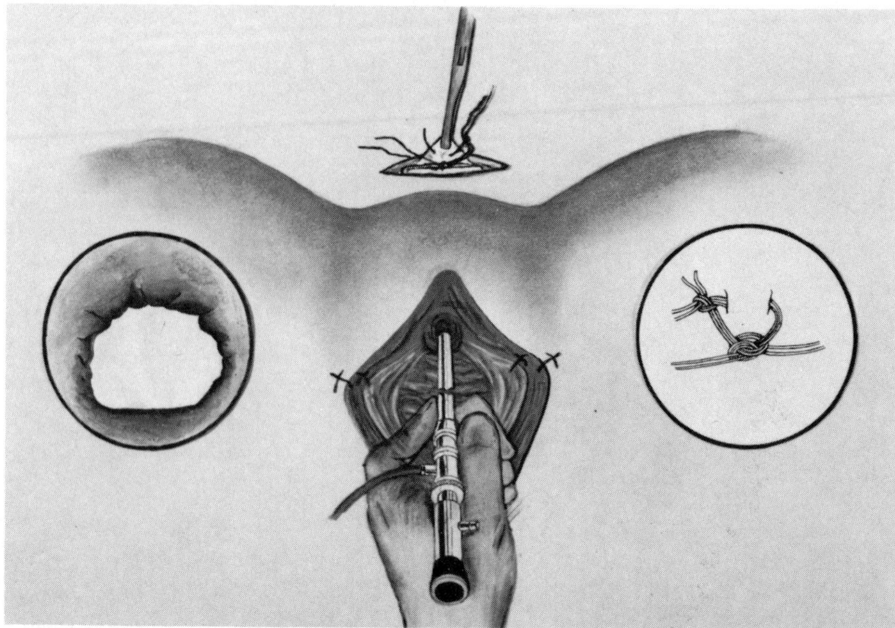

Figure 17–13. Four suture ends tied and transfixed to the abdominal fascia (detail at right). *Left,* Inferior margin of the internal meatus flattens slightly as viewed through urethroscope.

so by coughing. Prior to this, the bladder is filled with 350 ml. of sterile physiologic saline solution. With filling of the bladder, the curved folds of mucosa at the orifice respond by coming together. If the UV junction elevation is at the right height, the folds will evenly interdigitate to produce complete closure at the orifice. If the elevation is correct, the central point where the mucosal folds meet will move only slightly downward, if at all, with coughing by the patient. Should the patient undergo surgery under general anesthesia, the increase in intravesical pressure is effected by manual compression of the anterior abdominal wall. Such movement will not show separation of the folds, so the orifice remains closed. Following these adjustments, the excess suture ends are cut and the transverse suprapubic skin incision is closed

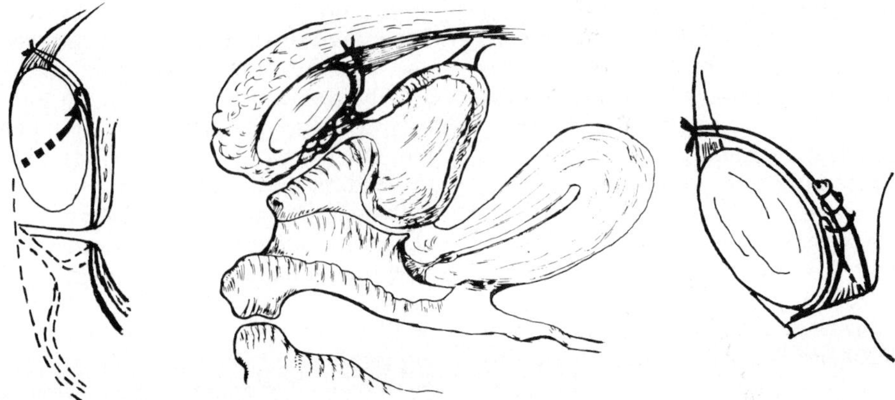

Figure 17–14. *Left,* The endopelvic fascia transposed to the upper posterior pubis. *Right,* The bound endopelvic fascia and pillars anchored to the abdominal fascia. *Center,* The completed modified Pereyra procedure.

(Figure 17–14). Thus, the success of the operation is established before the patient leaves the operating room.

12. Reaction of Pubourethral Supports to Increase in Intra-abdominal Pressure

Immediately following increase in intra-abdominal pressure, the Prolene sutures affixed to the abdominal fascia are tensed. This counteracts the tendency to downward displacement of the pubourethral supports by the force exerted against the urogenital diaphragm with increase in intra-abdominal pressure. As a result, the endopelvic fascia and posterior pubourethral ligament pillars are held in a relatively fixed position. The anchorage thus provided is wide, strong, and enduring.

MATERIAL AND METHODS

Previously published and tabulated results on 82 patients who underwent the modified Pereyra procedure and were followed 3 to 5 years (Table 17–3) revealed that the few failures observed occurred almost immediately after surgery (Pereyra et al., 1981). The same observation has been made with respect to other patients who underwent the modified Pereyra procedure, but these patients were not included in the 1981 report.

In view of these observations, we are including in our present results all patients operated on with the modified Pereyra procedure and observed for 1 year or longer postoperatively. With this limitation, a total of 162 women have undergone the modified procedure. All but one were parous women.

The average number of obstetric deliveries for this group was 3.1. Multiparity not uncommonly ranged from 10 to 20 vaginal deliveries in some of these patients.

Ages of the patients ranged from 26 to 95 years, with a median of 47.4 years. Most of the elderly women required regular external estrogen supplementation after the operation in order to maintain the turgor and tone of the urogenital tissues necessary to effect continence.

RESULTS

A total of 162 patients have been treated for anatomic stress urinary incontinence using the modified Pereyra procedure. One

TABLE 17–3. RESULTS IN PATIENTS WITH ANATOMIC STRESS URINARY INCONTINENCE OPERATED ON USING THE MODIFIED PEREYRA PROCEDURE

Duration of Postoperative Observation	No. of Patients	Markedly Improved*		Improved		Failed	
		Symp.	*Obj.*	*Symp.*	*Obj.*	*Symp.*	*Obj.*
36–47 months							
Primary operations	25	18	22	2	0	5	3
Secondary operations	8	7	8	1	0	0	0
Multiple operations	6	5	5	1	0	0	1
Total	39	30	35	4	0	5	4
48–59 months							
Primary operations	15	13	13	2	2	0	0
Secondary operations	6	4	5	1	0	1	1
Multiple operations	4	3	3	1	1	0	0
Total	25	20	21	4	3	1	1
60 months plus							
Primary operations	14	11	12	3	2	0	0
Secondary operations	4	3	3	1	1	0	0
Multiple operations	0	0	0	0	0	0	0
Total	18	14	15	4	3	0	0
TOTAL	82	64	71	12	6	6	5

*Symp., symptomatically; Obj., objectively.

hundred and eight were primary operations, 34 were done as a secondary procedure, and in 20 patients, two or more procedures for incontinence had been performed previously.

Table 17–4 depicts results in all patients treated with the modified Pereyra procedure and followed for 1 year or more. Of these patients, 143 were considered to have marked improvement objectively; that is, they had no evidence of stress incontinence in the supine or squatting position when straining and coughing. Eight patients were considered "improved;" that is to say, there was leakage of only a drop or two of urine, but the patients stated that this was no problem, and they were happy with the results. In 11 patients, the procedure was considered a failure.

One patient had sutures placed through the bladder. In this case, the operator, under training, performed a suprapubic cystotomy prior to passing the Pereyra needle. The bladder was tamponaded against the abdominal wall with the use of a Foley catheter and needle penetration was inevitable. These sutures were removed 10 days postoperatively and the patient went to another institution for a second procedure. Two patients were markedly improved for 2 months and 3 months, at which time stress incontinence returned. Both of these patients were in a group in which No. 2 Vicryl absorbable sutures were used to bind and elevate the pubourethral supports. In both patients a second Pereyra procedure was performed using size 0 Prolene suspensory sutures, and both patients now are asymptomatic. These cases are considered suture material failures.

Two patients in the Prolene suture group underwent corrective surgery initially, but 8 weeks and 10 weeks postoperatively the patients noted a return of incontinence. In one case, at reoperation, the suture was found to have pulled through the supporting fascia. It would appear that inadequate fascia had been grasped with a helical suture in the original operation. A repeat Pereyra procedure was successful in this patient. In the second case, at reoperation, it was noted that the knot had slipped, and the suture was found loose in the operative area. This latter case represents a problem with the Prolene material since it is a monofilament suture and will tend to slip. We recommend at least six throws in each Prolene tie when doing this procedure. This patient had a second Pereyra procedure and is presently continent.

Two patients early in the study developed outlet obstruction with residual urine and the sutures had to be removed. One patient had a second Pereyra procedure after removal of the first suture and is now considered markedly improved. The second patient had the suture removed at another institution and the outcome is not known.

One patient had three prior procedures for stress urinary incontinence as well as vesicourethral fistula when first seen for the problem. The fistula was repaired and a Pereyra procedure performed at the same time. She still has stress urinary incontinence and is being evaluated to decide what should be done.

Three patients state that they have not had improvement and refuse to return for further evaluation; no cause for failure can be stated in these cases.

It would appear that the modified Pereyra procedure is effective in 94 per cent of patients operated on for stress urinary incontinence. One third of these failures seem to be related to a suture problem. It is

TABLE 17–4. RESULTS IN PATIENTS WITH ANATOMIC STRESS URINARY INCONTINENCE OPERATED ON USING THE MODIFIED PEREYRA PROCEDURE, 1974–1979

Type of Procedure	Number of Patients	Markedly Improved	Improved	Failed
Primary	108	94	6	8
Secondary	34	32	1	1
Tertiary	20	17	1	2
TOTAL	162	143	8	11

hoped that the consistent use of size 0 Prolene at all times will favorably affect results.

Vicryl,* No. 2, 27 inches long, *absorbable* sutures were used to reinforce and elevate the urethral supports in most of the patients operated on in the West End San Bernardino County Hospitals, California. The patients operated on at UCLA Medical Center had size 0 Prolene *non-absorbable* sutures used for this purpose. A comparison of results shows that the corrective procedures performed using the nonabsorbable sutures had more dependable results. No foreign body reaction was noted requiring removal of these sutures. Accordingly, the use of absorbable sutures was discontinued.

Suprapubic cystotomy and bladder drainage through a No. 16 Foley catheter was performed routinely on patients operated on in the West End San Bernardino County Hospitals without complications other than subacute cystitis. Most of these patients were discharged with a catheter in place on the fifth to sixth postoperative day. The catheters usually were removed at the time of their first postoperative visit to the office, 1 to 2 weeks following discharge. The residual urine, checked immediately after voiding, was less than 30 ml.

At UCLA Medical Center, a No. 18 urethral Foley catheter with a 5 cc. balloon was introduced at surgery and was removed routinely by the third postoperative day. Following this, the patient was encouraged to void and was taught to use small, sterile disposable plastic catheters to drain the bladder afterward.† Using this technique, the patients usually began voiding sooner and the incidence of cystitis in these patients was lower. Barring concurrent surgery or disability, patients trained in self-catheterization were often discharged on the second, third, or fourth postoperative day.

One comment should be made concerning cystocele management at the time of the Pereyra procedure. If the patient has a cystocele with the prolapsed UV junction, this cystocele should be repaired at the same time. One must not be deluded by the apparent cystocele correction evident with elevation of the urogenital fascial dome. Two patients required a second procedure for correction of a cystocele because the operator believed a cystocele repair was not necessary at the time. In neither patient did stress incontinence persist, but both complained of a bulging discomfort due to the cystocele.

COMPLICATIONS

Prolonged catheter time was a problem early in the study and resulted from overcorrection. With the use of intraoperative urethroscopy and conduction anesthesia, average catheter time is now 3 days. Bladder perforation and outlet obstruction have already been discussed. A single urethral perforation occurred while preparing photographs for publication. The marked angulation present was not appreciated, and perforation resulted. This was repaired immediately and has produced no problems. One patient developed a suprafascial hematoma that was associated with some febrile morbidity, but this gradually resolved and the patient is well and continent at this time.

SUMMARY

Anatomic stress urinary incontinence results from prolapse of the UV junction. This occurs when the pubourethral ligaments and the endopelvic fascia in the periurethral tissues are weakened or lengthened. Both of these pubourethral supports are strengthened and shortened in a direct, highly effective manner by this procedure.

The modified Pereyra procedure is a suspensory-type operation. But, in contrast to other suspensory operations, this procedure accomplishes UV junction elevation without resorting to wide abdominal incision. Repositioning of the patient for abdominal entry after vaginoplasty is usually avoided. Nearly the entire surgical procedure is performed vaginally. In conse-

*Vicryl (Polyglactin 910), Ethicon, Somerville, New Jersey 08896.

†Mentor Self-Cath (Female Catheter 14 French, No. 240). Manufactured and distributed by Mentor Corporation, 1499 West River Road North, Minneapolis, Minnesota 55411.

quence, it is done in less time and with less trauma.

The posterior pillars of the pubourethral ligaments and the periurethral endopelvic fascia are exposed to view so that both can be clearly identified before being bound and elevated. There are no "blind" steps in this procedure, as occur in most suspensory-type operations, including the original Pereyra procedure of 1959 and the combined procedure described by Pereyra and Lebherz in 1967.

The retropubic space is exposed for exploration. It is most important that this be done, regardless of the procedure performed, in order to free adhesions remaining from prior surgery or inflammation. Neglect in freeing such adhesions formed near the UV junction may allow interference with closure of the valvular mechanism in the proximal urethra. This can result in failure to relieve the incontinence, no matter how perfectly the procedure is performed.

Opening of the anterior vaginal wall in this procedure permits retropubic transfer of the pubourethral supports and anchorage at a higher level on the pubis. A higher UV junction elevation thereby is possible, where necessary, than can be done with other vaginal procedures currently used to correct anatomic stress urinary incontinence. However, overcorrection must be guarded against.

Instead of depending on the small spotty fibrous tissue often formed about the sites of tissue penetration by sutures used to suspend the periurethral tissues in other operations, this procedure suspends the endopelvic fascia and the posterior pubourethral ligaments by broad anchorage to the suprapubic abdominal fascia.

Retropubic transfer of the suspensory sutures is readily accomplished by this procedure through a 2.5 cm. suprapubic abdominal skin incision by using the new Pereyra Ligature Carrier '75 instrument illustrated in Figure 17–1.

The single needle in this instrument provides the short, rigid, angulated, pointed tip needed to penetrate the tough abdominal fascia. A triangular handle set close to the needle end permits firm control of the point during its placement and penetration of the fascia.

The long, straight needle shaft held in a protective brace is attached to a sliding handle, which allows the needle to be advanced retropubically after the fascial barrier is penetrated. By capping the point with a fingertip immediately on its emergence below the rectus muscle, accidental penetration of the bladder or urethra is avoided. The eye at the point of the needle thus can be advanced safely so that it is well out of the vagina to facilitate threading with the suspensory suture ends.

The modified procedure is theoretically sound, technically precise, and readily performed under direct view throughout; in addition, its effectiveness is validated by over 300 patients followed independently for up to 5 years postoperatively by many surgeons both in the United States and in other countries. They have found it highly effective, durable, safe, reliable, and generally free from serious complications.

PRECAUTIONS

1. The needle point must always be capped with a fingertip during retropubic transfer to protect against bladder or urethral injury.
2. The serrated surfaces of the Pereyra Ligature Carrier '75 handles must always face the pubis during use of the instrument to assure that the angulated needle end is pointed anteriorly.
3. The bladder must be kept empty during the entire operation with an open *urethral* catheter in place.

CONTRAINDICATIONS TO PROCEDURE

A specific contraindication to this procedure is the presence of dense supraurethral or anterior bladder adhesions, usually residual from previous failed operations. Wide suprapubic abdominal exposure may be required in order to safely sever such adhesions by sharp dissection. Following freeing of the proximal urethra, the UV junction, and the anterior bladder wall, the abdominal fascial opening is closed with nonabsorbable sutures and the procedure is completed vaginally as outlined.

REFERENCES

Burch, J. C.: Cooper's ligament urethrovesical suspension for stress incontinence. Nine years' experience — results, complications, technique. Am. J. Obstet. Gynecol. *100*:764, 1968.

Green, T. H.: Development of a plan for the diagnosis and treatment of urinary stress incontinence. Am. J. Obstet. Gynecol. *83*:632, 1962.

Green, T. H., Jr.: Urinary stress incontinence. Pathophysiology, diagnosis, and classification. *In* Buchsbaum, H. J., and Schmidt, J. D.: Gynecologic and Obstetric Urology. Philadelphia, W. B. Saunders Co., 1978.

Hodgkinson, C. P.: Stress urinary incontinence. Table I. Three-part questionnaire. Am. J. Obstet. Gynecol. *108*:1149, 1970.

Hodgkinson, C. P.: Relationships of the female urethra and bladder in urinary stress incontinence. Am. J. Obstet. Gynecol. *65*:560, 1953.

Jeffcoate, T. N. A., and Roberts, H.: Stress incontinence of urine. J. Obstet. Gynecol. Br. Emp. *59*:685, 1952.

Kegel, A. H., and Powell, T. H.: The physiologic treatment of stress incontinence. J. Urol. *63*:808, 1950.

Kelly, H., and Dumm, W. M.: Urinary incontinence in women without manifest injury to the bladder: a report of cases. Surg. Gynecol. Obstet. *18*:444, 1914.

Krantz, K. E.: Anatomy, physiology, and embryological development of the urethrovesical junction in disorders of the female urethra and urinary incontinence. *In* Slate, W. G. (Ed.): Disorders of the Female Urethra and Urinary Incontinence. Baltimore, Williams & Wilkins, 1978, pp. 1–20.

Krantz, K. E.: The anatomy of the urethra and anterior vaginal wall. Am. J. Obstet. Gynecol. *62*:374, 1951.

Langreder, W.: Die weibliche Urethra, funktionelle Anatomie. Pathologie und Therapie des verschluss Mechanismus. Zbl. Gynaekol. *15*:561, 1956.

Marshall, V. F., Marchetti, A. A., and Krantz, K. E.: The correction of stress incontinence by simple vesicourethral suspension. Surg. Gynecol. Obstet. *88*:509, 1949.

Milley, P. S., and Nichols, D. H.: The relationship between the pubourethral ligaments and the urogenital diaphragm in the human female. Anat. Rec. *170*:281, 1971.

Nichols, D. H., and Randall, C. L.: Vaginal Surgery, the Urogenital Diaphragm, and the Pubourethral Ligaments. Baltimore, Williams & Wilkins, 1976, p. 15.

Pereyra, A. J.: The Pereyra Procedure Modified. Symposium on "Treatment of Disorders of the Urethrovesical Junction." Wilmington Medical Center, Wilmington, Delaware, November 10 and 11, 1976.

Pereyra, A. J.: The revised Pereyra procedure using colligated pubourethral supports. *In* Slate, W.: Disorders of the Female Urethra and Urinary Incontinence. Baltimore, Williams & Wilkins, Maryland, 1978.

Pereyra, A. J.: A simplified procedure for the correction of stress incontinence in women. Surg. Gynecol. Obstet. *67*:233, 1959.

Pereyra, A. J., and Lebherz, T. B.: Combined urethrovesical suspension and vaginourethroplasty for correction of urinary stress incontinence. Obstet. Gynecol. *30*:537, 1967.

Pereyra, A. J., Lebherz, T. B., Growdon, W. A., and Powers, J. A.: The pubourethral supports in perspective: A modified Pereyra procedure for stress urinary incontinence. Obstet. Gynecol. 1981 (in press).

Raz, S.: CO_2-urethral pressure profile in female incontinence. *In* Cantor, E. B. (Ed.): Female Urinary Incontinence. Springfield, Illinois, Charles C Thomas, 1979, pp. 128–140.

Robertson, J. R.: Genitourinary Problems in Women. Springfield, Illinois, Charles C Thomas, 1978, p. 84.

Steinhausen, T. B., Kariher, D. H., Shirwood, C. F., et al.: Chain urethrocystography before and after urethrovesical suspension for stress incontinence. Obstet. Gynecol. *5*:35, 1970.

Zacharin, R. F.: Stress Incontinence of Urine. New York, Harper and Row, 1972, p. 7.

Zacharin, R. F.: The anatomic supports of the female urethra. Obstet. Gynecol. *32*:754, 1968.

Zacharin, R. F.: The suspensory mechanism of the female urethra. J. Anat. Lond. *97*:423, 1963.

18

ENDOSCOPICALLY CONTROLLED URETHROPEXY

DANIEL A. NACHTSHEIM, M.D.

Renewed interest in the transvaginal approach to urethrovesical suspension of the bladder neck for urinary stress incontinence occurred when Stamey (1973) refined the original Pereyra (1959) operation (see Chapter 17) and added endoscopic control to the procedure. The proved success of transvaginal bladder neck suspension has spawned a variety of modifications of the Pereyra operation, which can effectively treat urinary stress incontinence.

PATIENT SELECTION

Endoscopic urethrovesical suspension is suitable for almost all patients with demonstrated urinary stress incontinence regardless of previous pelvic surgery or hysterectomy (see Chapter 20). Care must be taken to rule out a neurogenic cause for the incontinence, although patients with a mild degree of urgency incontinence associated with stress urinary loss are acceptable candidates.

Ideally, patients who have had prior suprapubic or abdominal operations or failure of the Marshall-Marchetti-Krantz operation are best suited for endoscopic suspension, since that approach obviates the need for dissection through the scarred area. Even patients who have had pelvic irradiation or pelvic fracture may be successfully treated by the endoscopic suspension.

In our experience, patients who have had previous vaginal surgery with extensive scarring and fibrosis limiting mobility of the bladder neck and urethra are best treated by a more extensive supravesical approach.

OPERATIVE PROCEDURE (AFTER STAMEY [1980, 1981])

Special Needles

Long needles with an eyelet specifically designed for endoscopic suspension are available* with 0, 15 and 30 degree angled tips (Figure 18–1). If these are not available, an orthopedic K wire with an eyelet drilled in the tip may also suffice. For large or obese patients the standard Stamey needle may be too short. Jacobo (1981) has

*Pilling Company, Delaware Drive, Fort Washington, Pennsylvania 19034.

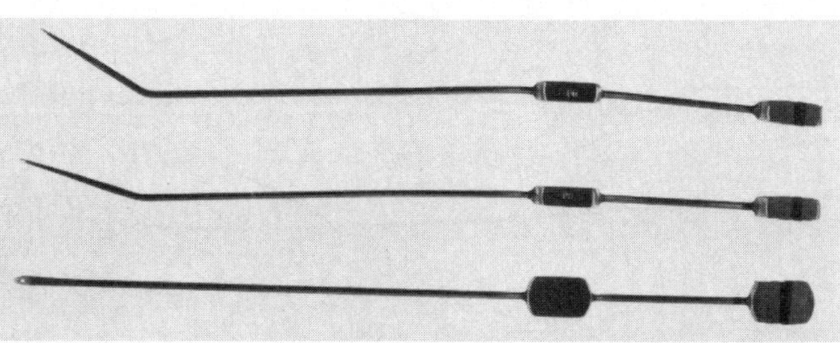

Figure 18–1. Stamey needles: 30 degree, 15 degree, and 0 degree angle tips with eyelet.

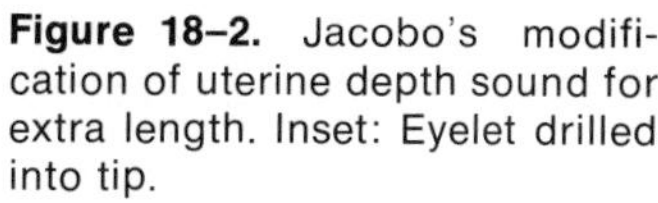

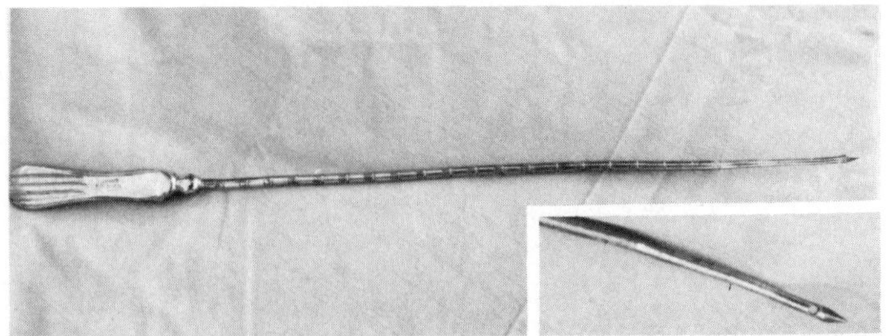

Figure 18–2. Jacobo's modification of uterine depth sound for extra length. Inset: Eyelet drilled into tip.

modified a uterine depth measuring sound by flattening the tip and making an eyelet (Figure 18–2), which may be useful when there is a thick abdominal wall.

Operative Procedure

Gentamycin (1 mg./kg.) or a cephalosporin is given the evening before the operation and again immediately preoperatively.

After the induction of anesthesia, either regional spinal or general, the patient is placed in the lithotomy position with the legs somewhat lowered. This flattens the suprapubic area and facilitates the incisions in this area. The abdomen is prepared from the umbilicus to the perineum, and a thorough vaginal preparation is accomplished with povidone-iodine. The rectum is draped from the field. A towel is draped across the suprapubic area midway between the umbilicus and pubis, and the vulva and the remaining suprapubic area are draped for cystoscopy. A drainage bucket is placed below the vagina for run-off cystoscopy fluid. The drape on the suprapubic area should be stable so that a suction apparatus and electrocautery probe can be positioned and room can be made to place the cystoscope on the lower abdomen during the operation.

A sterile side table is set for routine cystoscopy with panendoscope and foreoblique and right-angle lens.

Cystoscopy is done initially to evaluate bladder landmarks with the patient in this position. The bladder neck and ureteral orifices are noted, and the urethral length is measured with the cystoscope for future reference. The urethral length can also be measured with a No. 16 to 18 French Foley catheter by inflating the balloon in the bladder, gently pulling it down to the bladder neck, and clamping the side wall of the catheter (away from the balloon sidearm) at the meatus with a hemostat. The balloon is deflated and the distance from the clamp to the balloon edge is taken as the initial urethral length. This information is useful for estimating the length of the vaginal incision.

The labia majora are sutured in the midportion to the skin of the inner thigh with 2-0 silk for retraction, and a weighted posterior vaginal retractor is placed in the vagina. The Foley catheter is inserted into the bladder and inflated. It is clamped and the end is placed in the suprapubic area. A transverse incision is made in the anterior vaginal wall, approximately 1 cm. from the urethral meatus, and a plane is developed between the vaginal mucosa and the urethra (Figure 18–3). It is difficult to establish a plane under the mucosa immediately surrounding the meatus. Therefore, the incision is started somewhat proximally and the plane is developed with a Metzenbaum scissors and finger dissection back to the bladder neck and trigone, with palpation of the catheter along the way. The incision may be extended in a T fashion toward the vaginal apex at this point and the space around the urethrovesical angle widened slightly laterally. The endopelvic fascia around the urethra remains intact. Active bleeding may be encountered in this area and is controlled with electrocautery.

Extreme care should be taken in dissecting off the vaginal mucosa, if previous surgery has scarred the area, to avoid entering the bladder or urethra. If a small rent is made, it can be closed with fine interrupted sutures of chromic gut or polyglycolic acid and the operation continued.

Once the vaginal plane is established, a moist gauze sponge is inserted into the

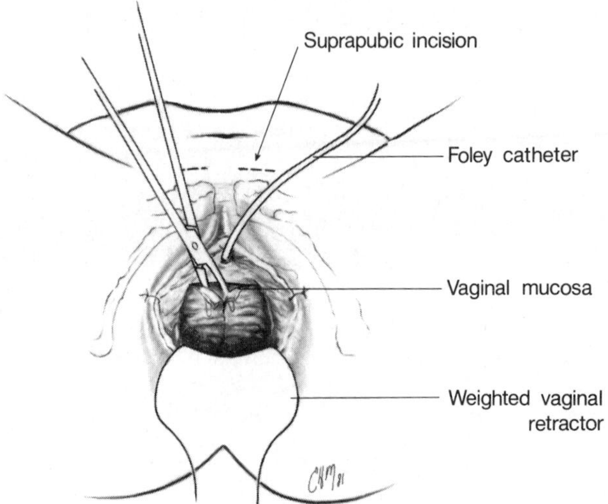

Figure 18–3. A horizontal incision is made 1 cm. from the urethral meatus and a plane is developed under the vaginal mucosa with scissors. The incision is bisected to expose the urethrovesical junction.

vaginal incision and suprapubic incisions are made. These are transverse incisions approximately 3 cm. in length made 2 to 4 cm. from the midline and 1 to 2 fingerbreadths above the superior pubic symphysis (Figure 18–3). A hemostat clears the fat down to the anterior rectus fascia. It is through these incisions that sutures will be looped down to the paraurethral fascia and back and then tied over the rectus fascia. The weighted vaginal speculum is removed and the bladder emptied.

Suture placement is accomplished by passage of an unthreaded special needle (Figure 18–1). The needle is passed perpendicularly from the medial aspect of the incision down through the rectus fascia and into the retropubic space. The base of the needle is tilted toward the patient's head, so that the tip identifies the pubic bone. The base of the needle is then elevated so that the needle tip travels down behind and parallel to the pubic bone (Stamey, 1981). While the needle is advanced, the free hand palms the urethral catheter. The index finger elevates the urethrovesical junction to meet the tip of the needle and guide it into the vagina just distal to the Foley balloon (Figure 18–4). The catheter is then removed and the cystoscope, with 30 and 90 degree lenses, is inserted into the urethra to ascertain that the needle has not perforated the bladder and is not lying just submucosally. If the needle is improperly positioned, it is withdrawn, the bladder is emptied, and the needle is passed again. The straight needle is usually the initial choice, but 15 or 30 degree needles should be tried if repeated perforations into the bladder occur. Once the needle is successfully passed, a to-and-fro motion of the needle with the urethra under cystoscopic vision will ascertain its correct position at the urethrovesical junction (Figure 18–5).

The suture material (No. 2 nylon or 0 polypropylene) is then passed through the eye of the needle projecting into the vagina. The needle is pulled up. One end of the suture is allowed to remain in the vagina and the other exits the suprapubic incision. A hemostat may be placed at each end; the Foley catheter is reinserted and the bare

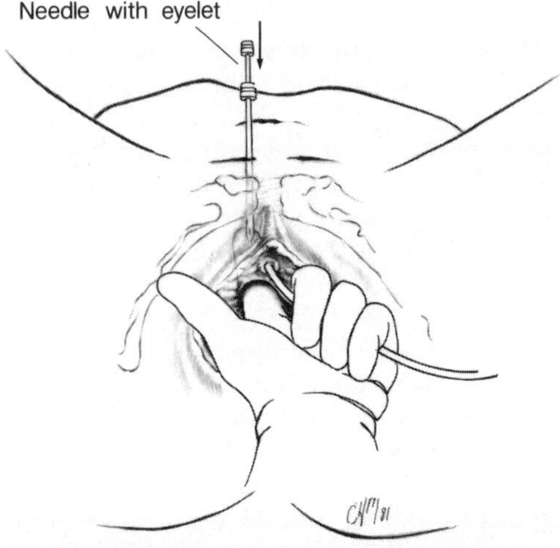

Figure 18–4. The hand palms the catheter and the index finger pushes up at the urethrovesical junction to meet the needle tip behind the pubis and guide the needle into the vaginal incision.

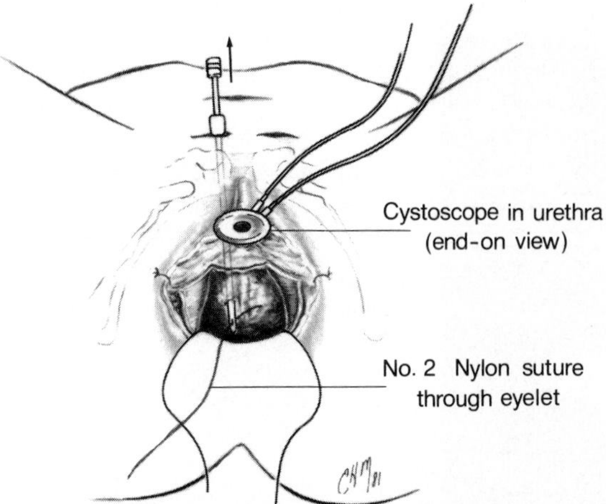

Figure 18–5. The cystoscope verifies the correct position of the needle. One end of the suture is passed into the eyelet and the needle is pulled up, bringing the suture into the suprapubic area.

needle is again placed through the same suprapubic incision on its lateral aspect. The point of the needle on this passage should start 1 to 2 cm. from the first needle entry suprapubically and enter the vagina about 1 cm. distal to the first needle tract and slightly lateral to the urethra (Figure 18–6). The position is again checked cystoscopically. If there is suspicion that the needle has pierced the detrusor muscle on any passage and lies submucosally, the suture material can be pulled through and the area viewed again. If the dark-colored suture material is visible submucosally, it should be pulled out and the needle repositioned.

When the needle is in position near the distal urethra, a 1 to 2 cm. segment of knitted Dacron 5 mm. vascular graft is threaded over the suture before it is put into the eye of the needle. This will act as a bolster to prevent the suture from cutting into the paraurethral tissue and will fix it in position. The needle is pulled up suprapubically, and care is taken not to twist the vascular graft bolster (Figure 18–6). An Allis clamp may be used to guide the bolster into correct position while the suture is being pulled up. A single loop is thus formed so that upward traction on the two free ends elevates the bladder neck and urethra.

The same procedure is performed on the opposite side of the urethra through the other suprapubic incision (Figure 18–7). It is not uncommon to pass the needle several times on either side during the procedure to accomplish perfect positioning and to avoid the bladder, particularly if there has been previous vaginal or suprapubic surgery.

When the two suture loops are in position, the vaginal mucosa is closed with 2-0 or 3-0 chromic gut. If the vagina is not

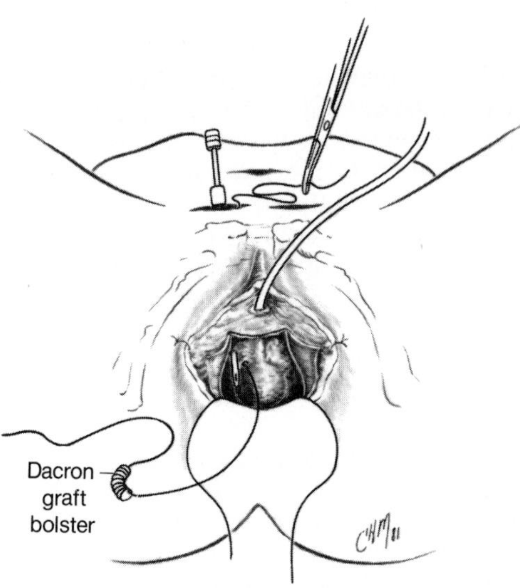

Figure 18–6. The needle has been passed again, entering the vaginal area 1 cm. distal and slightly lateral to the first entry. Dacron graft bolster is placed over the suture before inserting the suture material into eyelet.

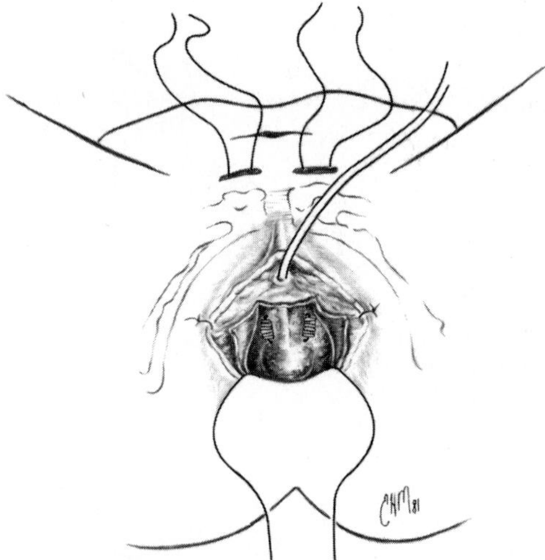

Figure 18–7. Bolsters are in position on each side of the urethrovesical junction. A loop has been formed on either side of the urethra, with a bolster over each of the sutures to prevent the sutures from cutting into the tissue. The free ends are seen in the suprapubic area.

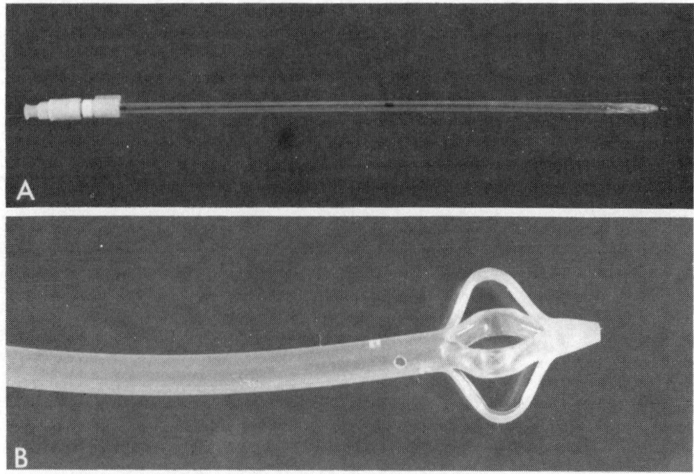

Figure 18–8. A 14 French silastic Malecot-type suprapubic tube (Vance Products). *A*, Obturator in place. There is Luer-Lok drainage at the end of the tube. *B*, Malecot tip with the obturator removed.

closed at this point it may be very difficult to close once the bladder neck and anterior vaginal wall have been pulled up.

A suprapubic "punch-type" catheter is placed in the bladder just before the vesical neck is elevated. We prefer to use the Stamey-type small Malecot plastic suprapubic tube with sharp-tipped obturator* (Figure 18–8). The bladder is filled and the suprapubic tube location checked endoscopically. With the suprapubic tube in place and the suspending sutures in proper position, the bladder neck is ready for elevation. The surgeon may view the vesical neck with the cystoscope in place and apply upward tension on one or both suspending sutures to ascertain the amount of tension needed on the suture that will allow the vesical neck to elevate and close (Figure 18–9). Once there is a feel for this, the sutures are individually tied with very light tension. In the past there has been a tendency to apply too much upward tension on these sutures, constricting the bladder neck. If the abdominal fascia is of poor quality, a small segment of the Dacron graft may be used under the suprapubic knot. The suprapubic incisions are closed with interrupted 3-0 chromic gut subcutaneous sutures and 4-0 Nylon skin sutures. Cotton vaginal packing saturated with triple sulfa cream is placed in the vagina and removed in 24 hours.

*Vance Products, Inc., 165 S. Main St., Spencer, Indiana 47460.

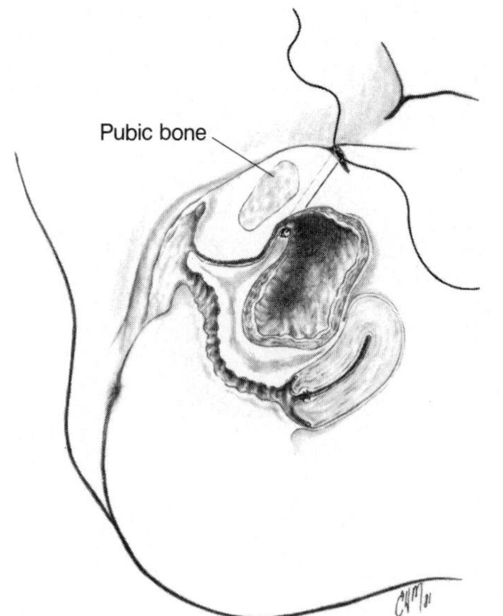

Figure 18–9. Lateral view of the pelvis. The vaginal mucosa has been closed. Ends of the sutures in the suprapubic area are lightly pulled up and tied over abdominal fascia, elevating the bladder neck.

POSTOPERATIVE CARE

The antibiotic that was started preoperatively is stopped after 48 hours and the patient is given no further antibiotics while the suprapubic tube is still in place.

The vaginal pack is removed on the first postoperative day. The suprapubic tube is clamped on the third or fourth postoperative day and the patient is encouraged to void. The volume of residual urine is checked by unclamping the suprapubic tube after voiding. When voiding is satisfactory and the residual urine is less than 20 per cent of the voided volume, the suprapubic tube can be removed. This usually is accomplished between the fifth and seventh postoperative days. Occasionally patients will be unable to void for a prolonged time postoperatively; in these cases they may be sent home with the suprapubic catheter. A urine culture should be obtained through the suprapubic tube just before it is removed. If there is significant bacterial growth, the patient should be placed on antibiotic therapy.

Stamey (1979) recommends the removal of only one of the suprapubic sutures (under a local anesthetic) after 6 weeks if it is suspected that the bladder neck has been pulled up too securely or that the detrusor muscle is too weak to accomplish voiding. Do not remove both sutures, for in this procedure the postoperative scarring around the bladder neck alone is insufficient to maintain continence.

MODIFICATIONS OF THE ENDOSCOPIC URETHROPEXY

The Mason and Sodenstrom Approach

Mason and Sodenstrom (1975) modified the endoscopic suspension procedure by placing an 8-inch No. 20 French Foley catheter suprapubically with the aid of a Lowsley retractor. A 2.7 mm. 0-degree Storz infant cystoscope lens is passed into a catheter whose tip has been cut off, allowing constant visualization of the bladder neck as the needles are being passed. The procedure is done in similar fashion to the Stamey technique, except that the needles are passed from the vaginal incision up into the suprapubic incisions, while an assistant continuously views the bladder neck area for correct positioning and avoidance of perforation (Figure 18–10).

The Double-Pronged Needle

Cobb and Ragde (1978) have designed a double-pronged needle with a 40 degree angle for use in the endoscopic suspension operation (Figure 18–11). The double-pronged needle is passed from the suprapubic incision and perforates the vaginal mucosa at the urethrovesical angle on one side of the urethra, and another paired needle is passed on the opposite side. The vaginal wall is not dissected. An incision is made over the tips of the prongs and the ends of the nylon suture are placed in the needle holes after a barrel knot is tied in the midportion of the suture. A small segment of Silastic catheter is placed over the knot. The suture is pulled up to the suprapubic area and tied. Endoscopic surveillance is also employed. Disadvantages of this approach to endoscopic suspension are that

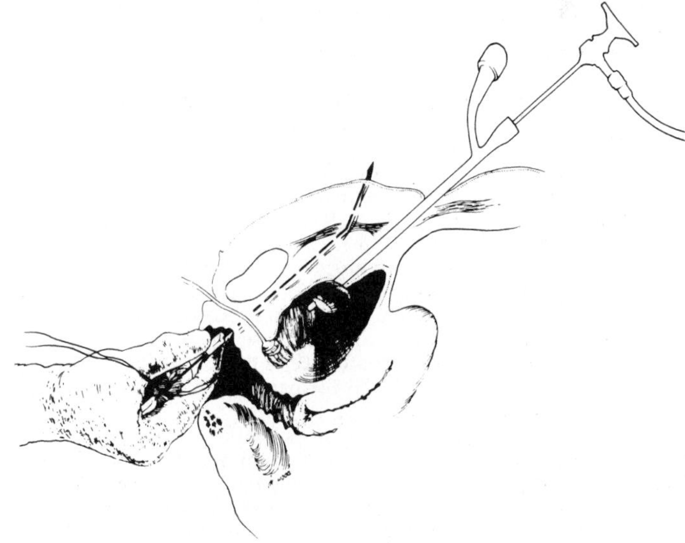

Figure 18–10. Mason procedure. An infant cystoscope in a short suprapubic catheter monitors the bladder neck while needles are passed from the vaginal incision to the suprapubic area. (From Mason, J. T., and Sodenstrom, R. M.: Suprapubic endoscopic evaluation of vesical neck suspension procedure. Urology *6*:233, 1975.)

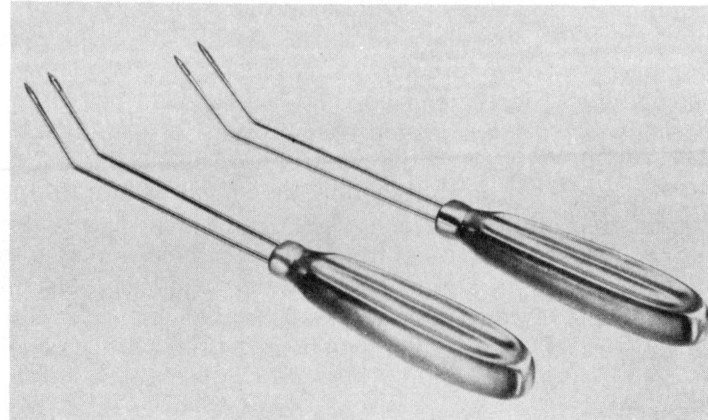

Figure 18–11. Cobb-Ragde needles. Overall length is 10 inches. The angle of the needle prongs is 40 degrees. (V. Mueller Co.)

the fixed position of the needles and their 40 degree angle limit mobility of the instrument and can compromise placement of the sutures.

RESULTS

Our results in over 40 patients are in agreement with those reported from Stanford (Stamey, 1980, 1981). Over 90 per cent of patients are rendered continent following endoscopically controlled urethropexy. One half of our patients were referred for surgery after previous failed vaginal or retropubic operative procedures. While endoscopic suspension is an excellent approach in these patients, we have used it as the primary operation for most, regardless of previous hysterectomy or other surgery.

We have not routinely measured pre- and postoperative urethral length but note Stamey's data (1981) indicating an increase in urethral length from 2.6 cm. preoperatively to 4.0 cm. postoperatively. This lengthening is apparently achieved by placing the bladder neck and urethra into a more cephalad position, allowing transmission of intra-abdominal pressure to the urethra and facilitating continence (Faysal et al., 1981). In addition, lengthening the urethra allows for maximal reflex contraction of its smooth muscle while under stress.

REFERENCES

Cobb, O. E., and Ragde, H.: Simplified correction of female stress incontinence. J. Urol. *120*:418, 1978.

Diagnosis and Treatment of Urinary Stress Incontinence. Urology Today, Third Program. Norwich, New York, Norwich-Eaton Pharmaceutical Company, 1981.

Faysal, M. H., Constantinou, C. E., Rother, L. F., et al.: The impact of bladder neck suspension on the resting and stress urethral pressure profile. J. Urol. *125*:55, 1981.

Jacobo, E. C.: Personal communication, 1981.

Mason, J. T., and Sodenstrom, R. M.: Suprapubic endoscopic evaluation of vesical neck suspension procedures. Urology *6*:233, 1975.

Pereyra, A. J.: A simplified procedure for the correction of stress incontinence in women. West. J. Surg. Obstet. Gynecol. *67*:223, 1959.

Stamey, T. A.: Endoscopic suspension of the vesical neck for urinary incontinence. Surg. Gynecol. Obstet. *136*:547, 1973.

Stamey, T. A.: Urinary incontinence in the female. *In* Harrison, J. H., Gittes, R. F., Perlmutter, A. D., et al. (Eds.): Campbell's Urology. 4th Ed. Volume 3. Philadelphia, W. B. Saunders Company, 1979, pp. 2272–2293.

Stamey, T. A.: Endoscopic suspension of the vesical neck for urinary incontinence in females: report on 203 consecutive patients. Ann. Surg. *192*:465, 1980.

Stamey, T. A.: Endoscopic suspension of the vesical neck for surgically curable urinary incontinence in the female. Monographs in Urology. Volume 2, Number 3. Research Triangle Park, North Carolina, Burroughs-Wellcome Company, 1981.

19

THE SLING OPERATION

R. P. BECK, M.D.

The sling operation is indicated for treating stress urinary incontinence when the support tissues in the bladder neck area are irreparably poor (a local tissue graft is necessary), or rarely when failure of the proper repair of reasonably normal support tissue is forecasted by potential extreme future stress (such as when the patient has severe uncontrollable coughing, as in chronic obstructive lung disease).

HISTORICAL BACKGROUND AND GENERAL CONSIDERATIONS

Selection of Sling Material

Muscle, fascia, and synthetic materials have been used as "straps" in the various sling operations described in the literature for treating urinary stress incontinence (Read, 1950; McLaren, 1957; Low, 1969; Morgan, 1970; and TeLinde, 1970). Muscular slings have fallen into disuse because of the difficulty in maintaining blood supply and mechanical problems of muscle bulk and length in accomplishing encirclement of the urethra. Mersilene strips and inert polypropylene (Marlex) mesh have been used, but because they are foreign bodies, the possibility of infection and excessive scar tissue reaction must be of prime concern to the surgeons who advocate their use (MacFarlane, 1970; Morgan, 1970; and Stallworthy, 1976).

Autogenous fascial strips probably stimulate less scar tissue reaction in most patients than does synthetic material currently available. If infection at the fascial sling site occurs, the surgeon is not faced with the specter of having to remove the sling, a disturbing consideration for those who use synthetic material. Fascia is pliable and is currently the easiest material to manipulate surgically. The Goebell-Frangenheim-Stoeckel procedure employed the use of a split vertical strip of rectus sheath with sutured plication of the ends under the urethra. The Aldridge modification of the former procedure utilized transverse strips of rectus sheath with the lateral ends being similarly plicated under the urethra (TeLinde, 1970). The Millin-Read procedure, utilizing a single strip of fascia, was designed to provide a similar fascial sling without entry into the vagina, thereby minimizing ascending infection from the potential field (Read, 1950). The latter procedure also obviated the mechanical disadvantages of suturing two ends of fascia strip at the critical point in the "hammock." Surgeons who advocate the use of fascia lata believe that such a fascial strip can be obtained quicker, with less incisional skin scar and with predictably better fascial tissue quality, than when anterior rectus sheath fascia is used.

The sling procedure used by Sir John Stallworthy, modified slightly and called by us the Oxford sling, utilizing fascia lata, involves a combined suprapubic and transvaginal approach (Zacharin, 1972; Stallworthy, 1976). Entry into the vaginal field introduces the possibility of infection, but this now theoretic problem is more than offset by avoiding injury to the urethra that could occur when urethral encirclement is attempted without entry into the vagina as with the Millin-Read procedure (Read, 1950). Without denigrating the importance of meticulous attention to proper surgical technique designed to minimize infection, modern antibiotics have rendered the need for a Millin-Read type of procedure obsolete when nonsynthetic sling material is used. Advocates of using synthetic material point to the fact that such a sling is not absorbed. A fascial sling may (or may not) be absorbed, and the long-term effectiveness of the procedure is maintained by a localized area of periurethral scar tissue, which closes the urethra (at the sling site) by a kinking effect at rest. This kinking effect is accentuated by an increased intra-abdominal pressure with stress. This scar tissue should not be extensive enough to interfere with the normal anatomic and physiologic changes that occur with micturition.

Anatomic and Physiologic Considerations

There are three requisites for urinary continence: (a) surface continuity of the urinary tract; (b) a proper pressure gradient between the urethra and bladder; and (c) a normal detrusor muscle. Urinary stress incontinence may be caused by an abnormality of either or both of the last two factors. Three types of urinary stress incontinence, equally common in our bladder physiology unit, can therefore be delineated by simultaneous intraurethral and intravesical pressure studies:

1. **A pressure equalization type,** in which the intravesical pressure becomes equal to the intraurethral pressure under the stress of increased intra-abdominal pressure from cough and similar forces (Beck and Maughan, 1964). This type is identical to anatomic or true stress incontinence, and its cause may be one or more of three anatomic changes: (a) poor periurethral support, (b) bladder neck descent, and (c) periurethral scar tissue formation.

2. **A detrusor overactivity type,** in which a sudden increase in intra-abdominal pressure triggers a hyperactive (irritable) detrusor muscle into contraction with subsequent urine loss (Beck et al., 1966).

3. **A combined type,** involving pressure equalization between the urethra and bladder, and involuntary detrusor contraction with the stress of increased intra-abdominal pressure.

Although these three types of stress incontinence are best identified by pressure studies, they can also be recognized by a proper history and careful observaton of the type of urine loss with stress (Chapter 13).

Pressure equalization (anatomic or true) stress incontinence is the type most amenable to surgical correction, whereas detrusor overactivity caused by infection or parasympathomimetic overactivity should be treated with appropriate medication. Funneling of the bladder neck in the resting state can render the detrusor muscle irritable, and surgical correction of such funneling is associated with an 80 per cent success rate in correcting detrusor overactivity in patients without infection and not showing a response to parasympatholytic drugs. Funneling of the bladder neck is a mandatory prerequisite to voiding in the dog and is one of four anatomic changes that occur immediately prior to voiding in the human female (Zacharin, 1972; Beck et al., 1976*a, b*). On the basis of the foregoing, one can appreciate the relationship between bladder neck funneling in the resting state and detrusor irritability.

In my opinion, surgical correction of stress incontinence should be considered only when pressure equalization (anatomic or true) stress incontinence exists. If detrusor overactivity coexists, this component of the patient's incontinence problem should be treated with appropriate medications. If infection does not exist and if the detrusor overactivity does not respond to parasympatholytic drugs, surgical correction of the anatomic (pressure equalization) component of the incontinence may be contemplated, with the realization that detrusor overactivity incontinence will persist in approximately 25 per cent of such cases following surgery (unpublished data, Bladder Physiology Unit, University of Alberta). If standard surgery for stress incontinence is done in the presence of detrusor overactivity without pressure equalization or an anatomic component to their incontinence, the results are dismal. Only 25 to 30 per cent of such patients show a satisfactory response (unpublished data, Bladder Physiology Unit, University of Alberta).

PATIENT ASSESSMENT

The routine assessment of any patient being investigated for urinary stress incontinence in our unit includes the following:

History

An incisive, directed history is one of the two most important aspects of patient assessment. The type of loss (drops, dribbles, spurts, gushes, or streams) should be ascertained (Chapter 13). Triggering factors for incontinence (such as coughing, laughing, sneezing, and jolting body movements) should be sought to determine that the urine loss is in fact due to stress. Inquiry in this area also helps to determine the degree of disability or inconvenience that the urine loss poses for the patient.

Whether or not the urine loss is subject to spontaneous exacerbations and remissions is an important question. A positive answer suggests detrusor overactivity stress incontinence. Accentuation of urine loss by such factors as the erect position, a full bladder, and neurogenic stimuli — such as the sound of running water and thermal stimulation (e.g., hot water or cold weather) also signifies detrusor overactivity. (Loss of urine in bed strongly suggests a fistula or neurogenic bladder.) Other symptoms frequently noted in stress incontinence also serve as clues to detrusor overactivity: bladder spasm, urgency incontinence, hesitancy, incomplete emptying urgency, and urinary frequency or dysuria. The severity of the incontinence, varying from occasional loss with hard coughing to continuous loss of urine requiring the constant use of sanitary napkins, must be determined. Continuous urine loss may be due to a fistula, to severe pressure equalization, or to combined pressure equalization and detrusor overactivity.

The history should endeavor to rule out a neurogenic bladder or psychotropic drugs (which pharmacologically produce a neurogenic bladder) as the cause of urine loss. If the patient has had previous surgery for stress incontinence, as much information as possible about the actual surgery performed and when incontinence occurred in relation to this surgery should be obtained. Precipitating factors, such as heavy lifting, violent coughing, or postoperative bleeding preceding recurrence of incontinence, suggest that poor local tissues may not be the reason for recurrence.

Physical Examination

A physical examination should be aimed at identifying significant chronic respiratory disease and any hint of neurologic disease. Normal anal sphincter tone is helpful reassurance that the patient does not have a neurogenic bladder.

Pelvic Examination

Careful pelvic examination, with the careful observation of the type of urine loss, constitutes the second of the two most important parts of the patient's assessment. The loss of a spurt of urine synchronous with and ending abruptly with stress is virtually diagnostic of pressure equalization or anatomic stress incontinence. Other types of loss suggest detrusor overactivity incontinence. Even when stress incontinence is demonstrated, the anterior vaginal wall should be inspected for the coexisting fistula. This latter examination is best done using Sims's specula with the patient in the Sims's left lateral position. The degree of cystocele or urethrocele and the amount of scar tissue along the anterior vaginal wall should be assessed. The existence of palpable defects in the pubocervical fascia rimmed with scar tissue should be sought. On palpation, these defects feel like the anterior fontanelles of a newborn's head. The degree of retrocession of the bladder neck and anterior vaginal wall from behind the symphysis pubis (Green type II stress incontinence) (Green, 1962) should be ascertained. The possibility of pelvic masses should be eliminated, since these may also cause stress incontinence.

Urethral Length and Residual Urine

The urethral length should be measured using a 5 cc. Foley catheter, and the amount of residual urine should be determined. Urethral shortening to less than 1 cm. total length is significant in planning surgery, but otherwise urethral length is of no clinical significance (Beck and Hsu, 1964). A residual volume of 30 ml. or more is almost always due to psychotropic drugs or a neurogenic bladder and rarely to cystocele formation, unless there is a marked kinking of the urethra by the cystocele. In nearly 4000 patients in our unit, a cystocele was found to be the cause of significant residual urine in only three cases (unpublished data, Bladder Physiology Unit, University of Alberta).

Urine Culture

A urine culture is an essential part of the investigation. Urinary stress incontinence may be the only symptom of urinary tract infection.

Bladder Capacity

The bladder capacity is measured at the point when the patient feels a distinct urge to void. The fluid (normal saline) should be warmed to body temperature and administered slowly (10 ml./minute) by urethral catheter to avoid premature detrusor reaction. A bladder capacity of less than 200 ml. is considered reduced; a capacity of 250 to 500 ml. is definitely normal. A reduced bladder capacity suggests the effect of a fistula, chronic interstitial cystitis, or severe stress incontinence. A reduced bladder capacity also provides a useful prognosis of when normal voiding will recur following surgery. A reduced bladder capacity or an atonic bladder (sensation of bladder fistulas felt beyond 500 ml.) indicates that delayed voiding and problems with residual urine can be anticipated following surgery and that substantial postoperative time will be required to rehabilitate the bladder.

Intraurethral and Intravesical Pressure Studies

Simultaneous intraurethral and intravesical pressure studies, in the standing and lithotomy positions, can determine the type of stress incontinence present, identifying pressure equalization or detrusor overactivity components (Beck and Maughan, 1964; Beck et al., 1966). Delineation of the type of pressure equalization stress incontinence can help the surgeon plan his surgical approach more effectively, with emphasis on one or all of the following procedures: tightening of the urethra, restoration of the bladder neck to proper position (1 cm. behind and 1 cm. above the inferior edge of the symphysis pubis), and correction of scar tissue effect (Beck et al., 1968, 1974).

Urethroscopic Examination

Urethroscopic examination (extended to cystoscopic examination when necessary) has become an integral part of our routine assessment since the introduction of the Robertson urethroscope.

Other Diagnostic Aids

Radiologic and dye studies and neurologic consultation are initiated when the preceding investigation fails to yield a definitive diagnosis.

INDICATIONS FOR SLING PROCEDURE

Indications for a fascia lata sling procedure include the following:

1. A major degree of pressure equalization or anatomic incontinence with or without detrusor overactivity.

2. Major interference with the patient's life style by the incontinence.

3. (a) The failure of two or more primary procedures to correct stress incontinence satisfactorily; *or*

(b) The failure of one previous operation to correct incontinence satisfactorily, with (i) postoperative breakdown of good urethral pressures created at surgery (diagnostic of irreparably poor local tissues) (Zacharin, 1972), (ii) extensive postoperative scar tissue along the anterior vaginal wall, or (iii) a postoperative palpable defect in the pubocervical fascia, as previously described; *or*

(c) Severe respiratory disease attended by recurrent violent bouts of coughing, or the existence of gross congenital support defects. These are the only two circumstances in which the author would consider using a sling as the primary procedure in treating stress incontinence. *A sling procedure cannot be justified as a primary operation in other circumstances because it is a far more extensive surgical exercise than anterior colporrhaphy or any of the ventral flexion procedures, and is attended by very significant postoperative complications and problems.* The author has never employed the sling operation as a primary procedure in treating urinary stress incontinence.

Contraindications

These specific conditions contraindicate a sling operation:

1. Detrusor overactivity stress incontinence without pressure equalization incontinence.
2. Coexistent bladder neck fistula.
3. Coexistent neurogenic bladder.

THE OBJECTIVE OF SURGICAL CORRECTION OF STRESS INCONTINENCE

In the author's opinion (Beck, 1980), the main mechanism for maintaining urinary continence with stress is via a urethral kinking effect, which occurs along the entire length of the urethra as the bladder base rocks downward and backward with increased intra-abdominal pressure and the urethra bends backward like a supple willow wand. The kinking effect in the urethra is the result of differentially better support to the urethra than to the base of the bladder by the pubocervical fascia. The kinking effect occurs in the urethra when the bladder base and, to a lesser extent, the urethra rotate downward and backward with stress. The objective of the sling procedure is not to occlude the urethral lumen at rest or with voiding, but rather to provide a segment of urethra with better support than that to the bladder base so that urethral kinking will effectively occur at the sling site with stress (see Figure 19–17).

OPERATIVE PROCEDURE

Preparation of Donor Site

The night before surgery, the thigh from which the fascial strip will be taken is washed with hexachlorophene lotion from the groin to midcalf. If large varicosities or

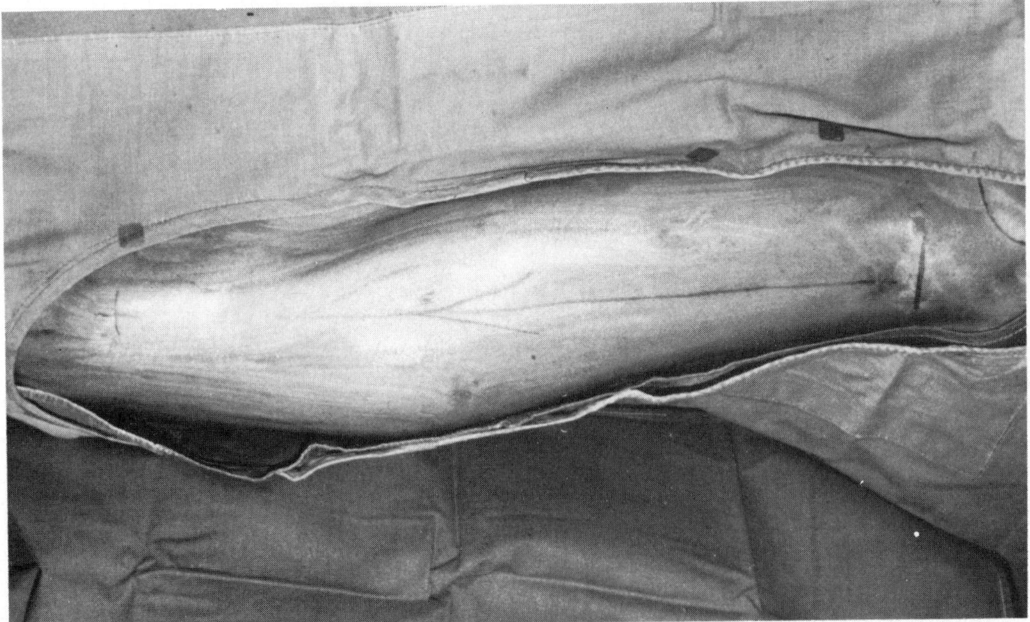

Figure 19–1. The thigh prepped and draped for the fascia lata stripping procedure. An incision 3 to 4 cm. in length should be made transversely over the iliotibial tract at a level just above the superior edge of the patella.

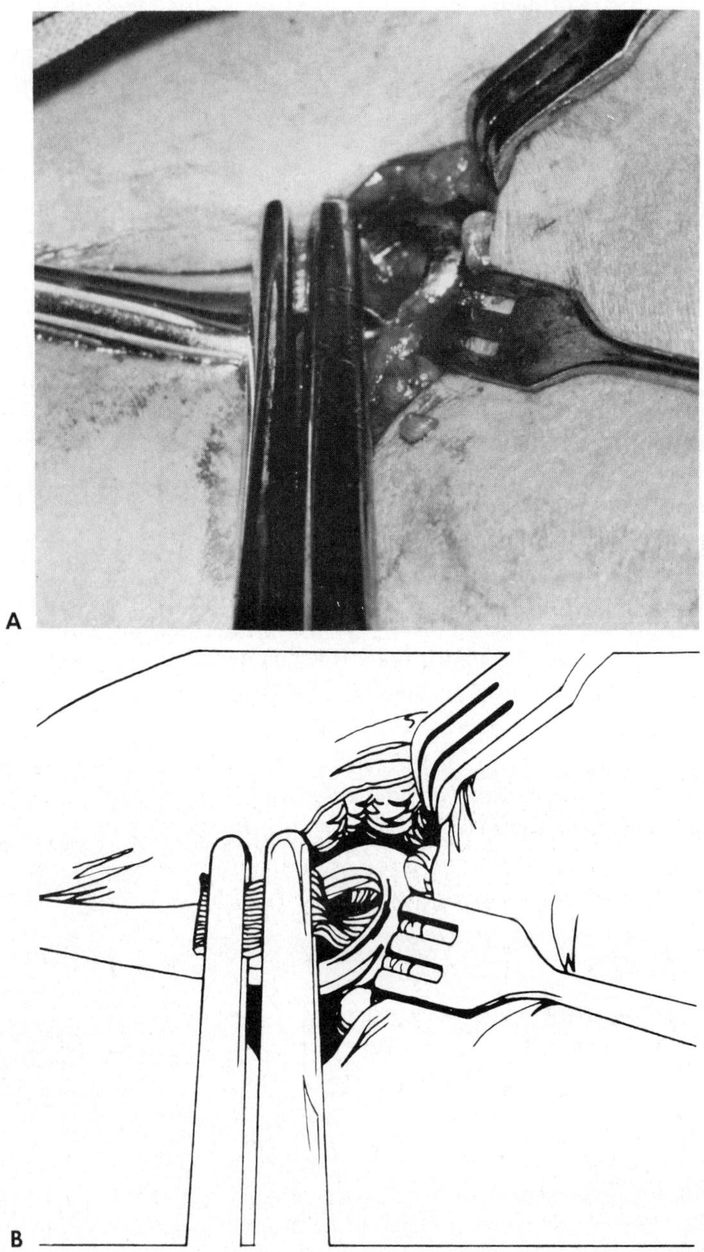

Figure 19–2. *A*, The fascial tab being pulled through the cutting aperture of a Wilson fascial stripper. *B*, Schematic representation.

external urethral meatus, extending on each side up to the bladder neck area, superficial to the pubocervical fascia.

Vaginal Skin Flap

A vaginal skin flap is established by peeling the vaginal mucosa off the underlying pubocervical fascia, up the vagina slightly beyond the bladder neck area (Figure 19–5). The vaginal skin flap can be cut transversely, leaving a triangular defect in the vaginal mucosa calculated to allow for easy closure without tension at the end of the procedure.

Dissection of Space of Retzius

If the patient has had a previous ventral suspension or sling operation, it is necessary to enter the space of Retzius and dissect the bladder from the posterior aspect of the symphysis pubis. If the patient has not had such previous surgery, this dissection is unnecessary. In these patients, the anterior rectus sheath is not opened, except for stab incisions designed to anchor each end of the fascial strip (discussed later). Figure 19–6 demonstrates a vertical incision through the anterior rectus sheath into the space of Retzius and the dissection of the bladder from the posterior aspect of the symphysis pubis in a patient who had had a previous ventral fixation procedure. This dissection is best performed with scissors and fingers, keeping the concave curvature of the scissor blades tightly applied to the posterior aspect of the pubic tubercle and symphysis pubis throughout the entire dissection. Whenever pressure is exerted during the finger dissection, it should be applied against the symphysis pubis rather than backwards towards the bladder. This procedure will minimize injury to the bladder.

Placement and Fixation of the Fascial Strip

Next a stab incision is made on each side of the urethra (using a urethral catheter as a guide) at the bladder neck junction through the pubocervical fascia (Figure 19–7). One end of the fascial strip is then pushed through one stab incision and the space of Retzius, using uterine packing forceps. These are kept closely applied to the posterior aspect of the symphysis to avoid injury to the bladder (Figure 19–8). The tip of the forceps is directed to a point 1 cm. superior to the symphysis pubis and 1 cm. lateral to the midline, and a vertical stab incision is

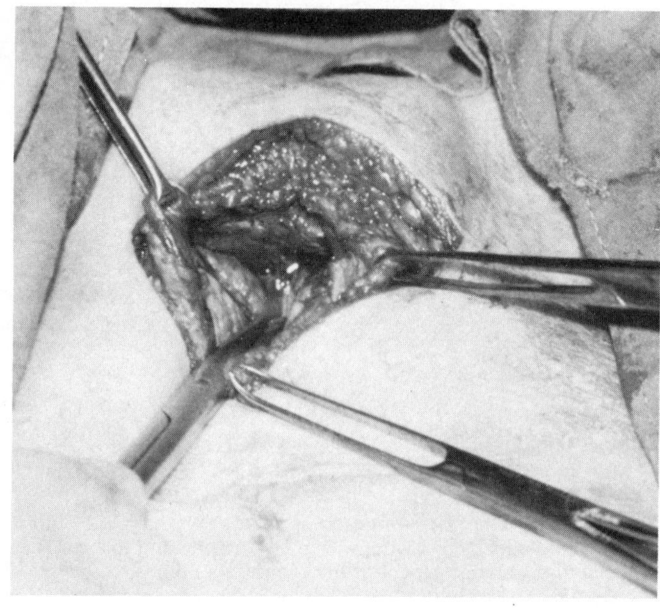

Figure 19–6. A vertical incision made through the anterior rectus sheath into the space of Retzius, and the dissection of the bladder from the posterior aspect of the symphysis pubis in a patient who had had a previous ventral fixation procedure.

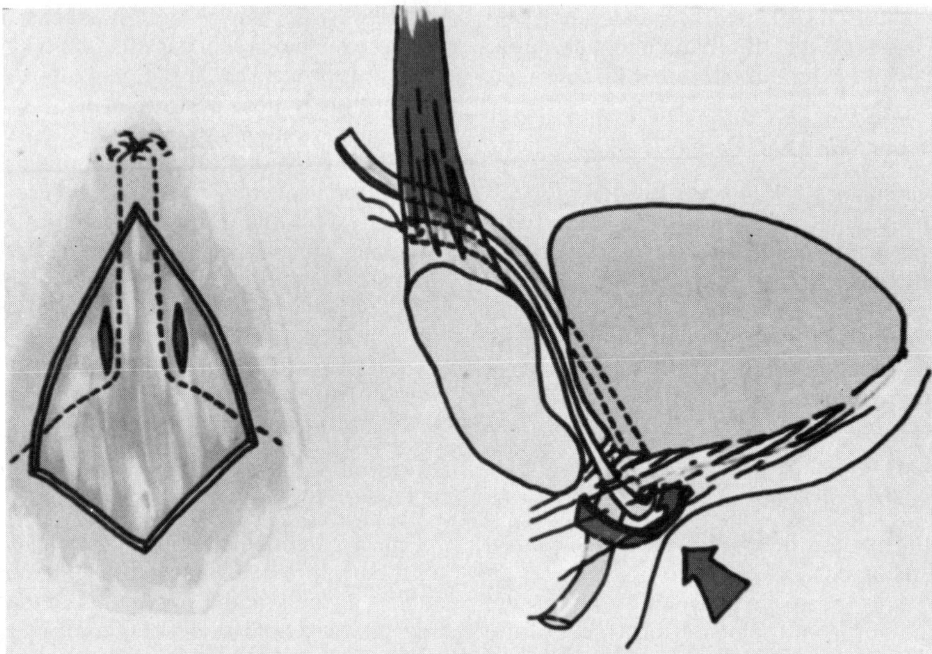

Figure 19–7. *Left,* The stab incision on each side of the urethra at the bladder neck junction. *Right,* Fixation of one end of the fascial strip to the anterior rectus sheath to the left of the midline. The other end of the fascial strip has been slung around the urethra, pushed through the space of Retzius and a stab incision in the anterior rectus sheath, and is ready for suturing, under proper tension, to the right of the midline.

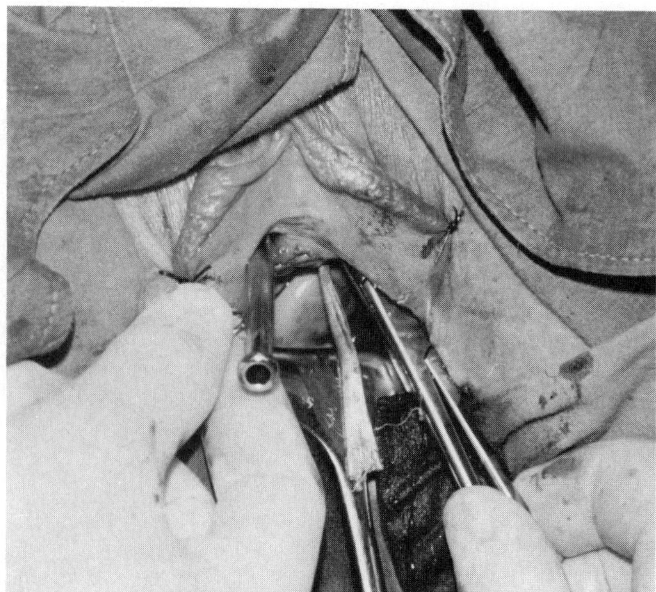

Figure 19–8. The fascial strip being pushed through the stab incision in the pubocervical fascia, to the left of the bladder neck area, with a uterine packing forcep. The end of the packing forcep is kept tightly against the posterior aspect of the symphysis pubis.

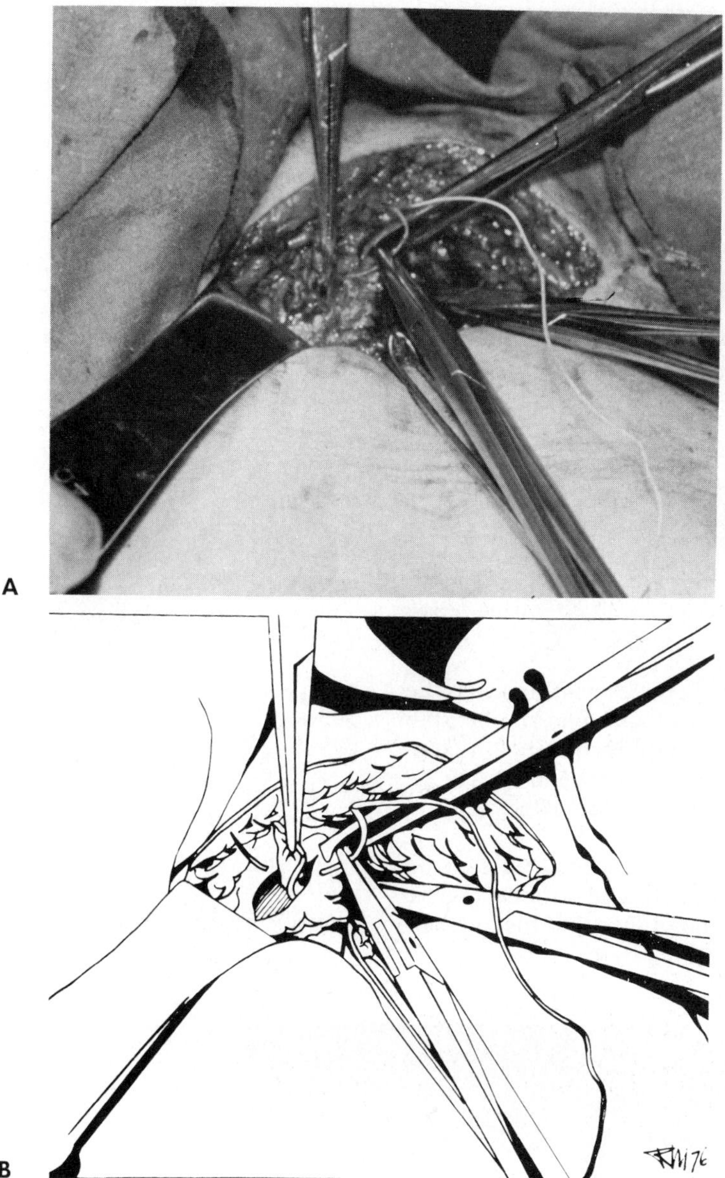

Figure 19–9. *A,* The first end of fascial strip being sutured to the anterior rectus sheath with chromic 1 catgut. The suture passes through rectus sheath, fascial strip, and rectus sheath in succession. *B,* Schematic representation.

then made down through the anterior rectus sheath, exposing the tip of the forceps and the end of the fascial strip.

The end of the fascial strip is then sutured to the anterior rectus sheath with chromic 1 catgut, with the suture passing through the rectus sheath, fascial strip, and rectus sheath in succession (Figure 19–9*A*). The suture is then tied on both sides of the fascial strip in order to avoid fraying of the vertical fibers of the fascial strip. Two similar additional sutures are used to firmly anchor the "first" end of fascial strip to the anterior rectus sheath.

The "second" end of fascial strip is then slung (see Figure 19–7) around the juncture of the urethra and bladder neck and is similarly pushed through the other stab

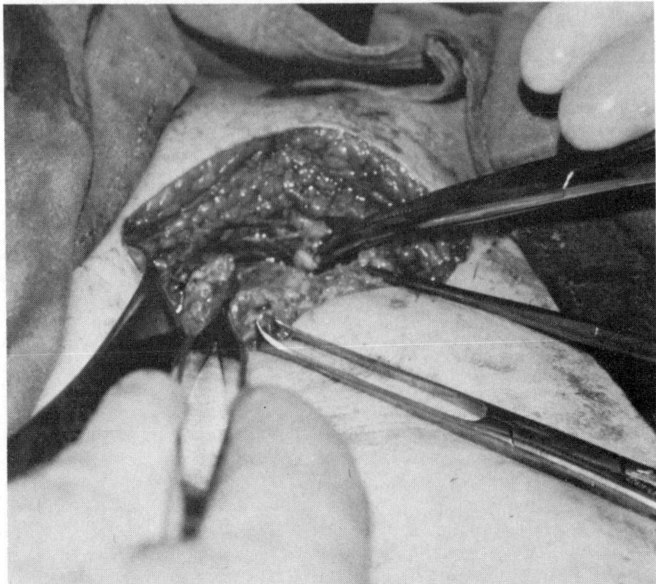

Figure 19–10. The second end of fascial strip being pushed up through the space of Retzius, ready for introduction into the stab incision in the anterior rectus sheath to the right of the midline.

incision in the pubocervical fascia, the space of Retzius, and a second similar stab incision in the anterior rectus sheath (Figure 19–10). The "second" end of fascial strip is then pulled up under proper tension to make the fascial "V" taut.

It is difficult to maintain proper tension on the second end of fascial strip during the suturing of this end of fascia to the anterior rectus sheath. Figure 19–11 shows the best method for maintaining steady traction on the sling during this procedure.

Confirming Proper Sling Tension

As shown in Figure 19–12, the second end of the fascial strip is sutured to the anterior rectus sheath to the right of the

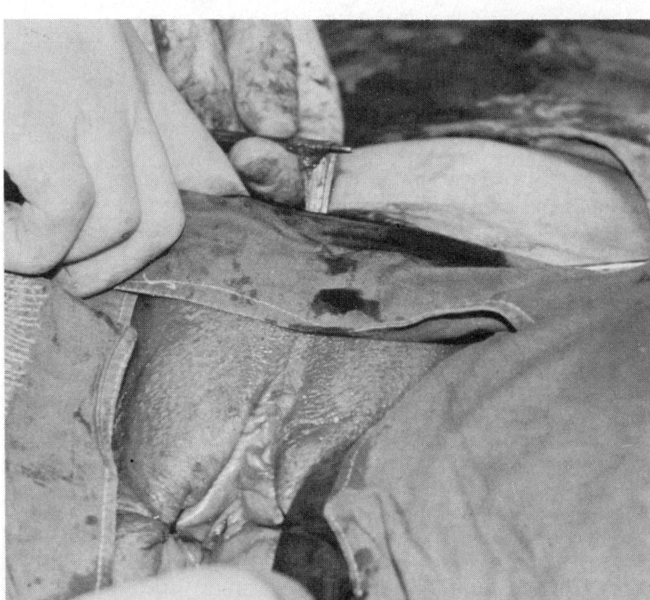

Figure 19–11. The best method for maintaining steady traction on the sling during the suturing of this end of fascia to the anterior rectus sheath.

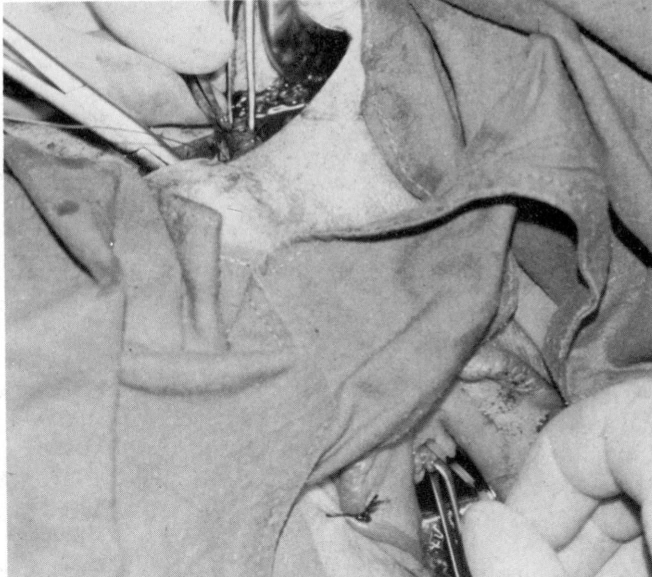

Figure 19–12. Suturing the second end of the fascial strip to the anterior rectus sheath to the right of the midline, with the pressure-recording catheter in place as a guide to obtaining proper tension on the sling in the upper 1 cm. of the urethra.

midline, with the pressure-recording catheter in place as a guide to obtaining proper tension on the sling in the upper portion of the urethra. If pressure-recording equipment is not available, the surgeon can use a No. 12 Foley catheter with 0.5 ml. water in the bag to test for the achievement of adequate intraurethral resistance at the sling site (Beck, 1980).

Figure 19–13 illustrates the measurement of intraurethral pressure in the upper urethra at the sling site during the process of suturing the second end of the fascial strip. The fascial strip is sutured so that a

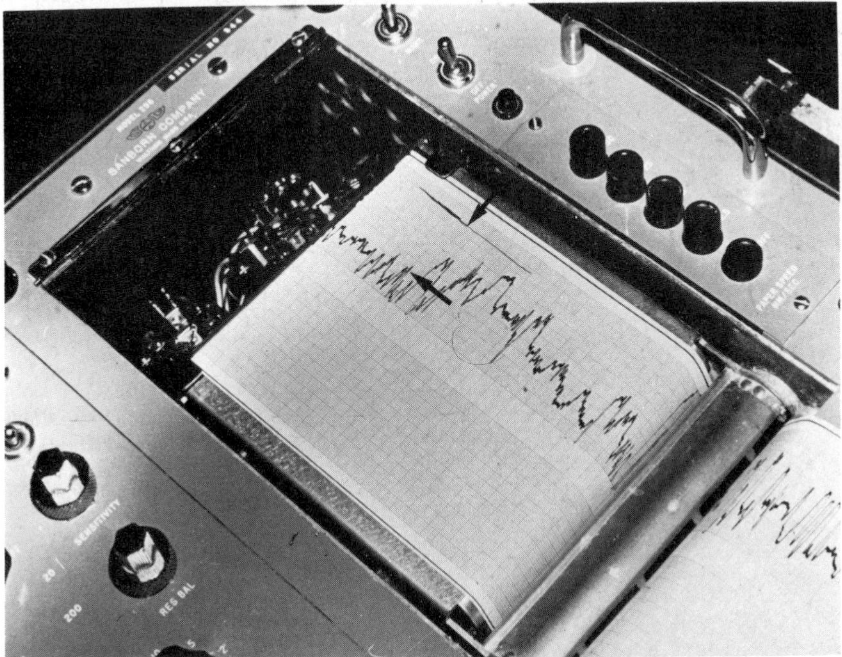

Figure 19–13. Cystometrograph showing the intraurethral pressure in the upper cm. of the urethra at the sling site during the process of suturing the second end of the fascial strip. See text.

pressure of 70 to 80 mm. of mercury is created, as indicated on the right side of the tracing. The baseline of the tracing is indicated by a horizontal pencil mark on the paper. The pressure swings on the left side of the tracing indicate the difficulty that can be experienced in obtaining the proper tension on the sling during the fixation of the second end of the fascial strip.

Drainage of Space of Retzius

As indicated in Figure 19–14, the author no longer drains the space of Retzius, suspecting the drain to be the cause of seroma formation. The vertical incision in the anterior rectus sheath is closed with interrupted chromic 1 catgut sutures. The fixed ends of the fascial strip can be seen on either side of the midline incision.

Suturing Fascial Strip to Pubocervical Fascia

The fascial strip should be sutured to the pubocervical fascia with 2–0 chromic catgut so that the sling is maintained in proper position at the upper 1 cm. of the urethra (Figure 19–15*A*). Placement of the suture is very awkward because of the extreme elevation of the bladder neck area that is accomplished with the sling procedure. In Figure 19–15*A*, the uterine sound points to the suture needle in the sling (glistening dot above suture) and pubocervical fascia, demonstrating the difficulty of access at this step in the procedure. The patient must be in extreme Trendelenburg position for correct placement of this important suture. The anterior vaginal wall is then closed with a continuous chromic 1 catgut suture. If the patient has a marked cystocele, it is important to correct it (but also to avoid overcorrection) in order to obviate an excessive kinking effect by the sling in the postoperative period, which might seriously interfere with voiding.

Figure 19–16 demonstrates the tremendous elevation of the bladder neck area that is accomplished with the sling procedure. With the patient in the lithotomy position, the anterior vaginal wall is not visible because of the bladder neck elevation.

POSTOPERATIVE CARE

Patients tolerate this extensive procedure very well and have minimal pain associated with the leg and suprapubic incisons. Any other pain in the surgical field suggests

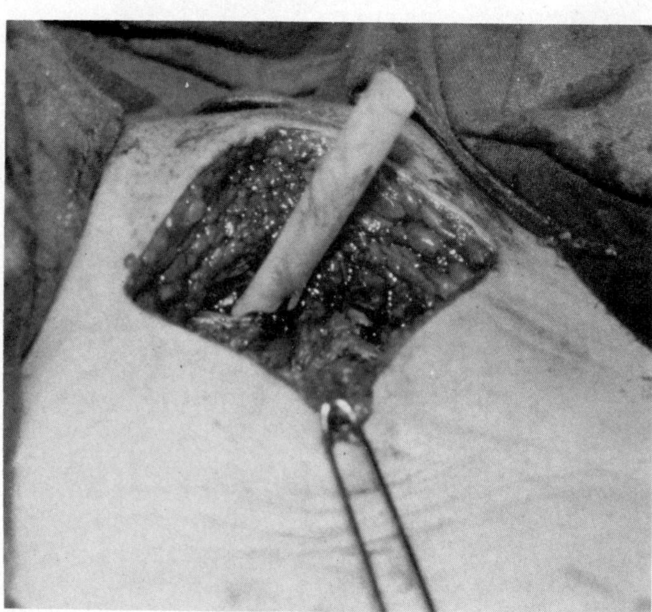

Figure 19–14. The Penrose drain in place, with the vertical incision in the anterior rectus sheath closed with interrupted chromic 1 catgut sutures. The fixed ends of the fascial strip can be seen on either side of the former midline incision. (The author has not used a drain in the last 36 cases, suspecting the drain as the cause of seroma formation.)

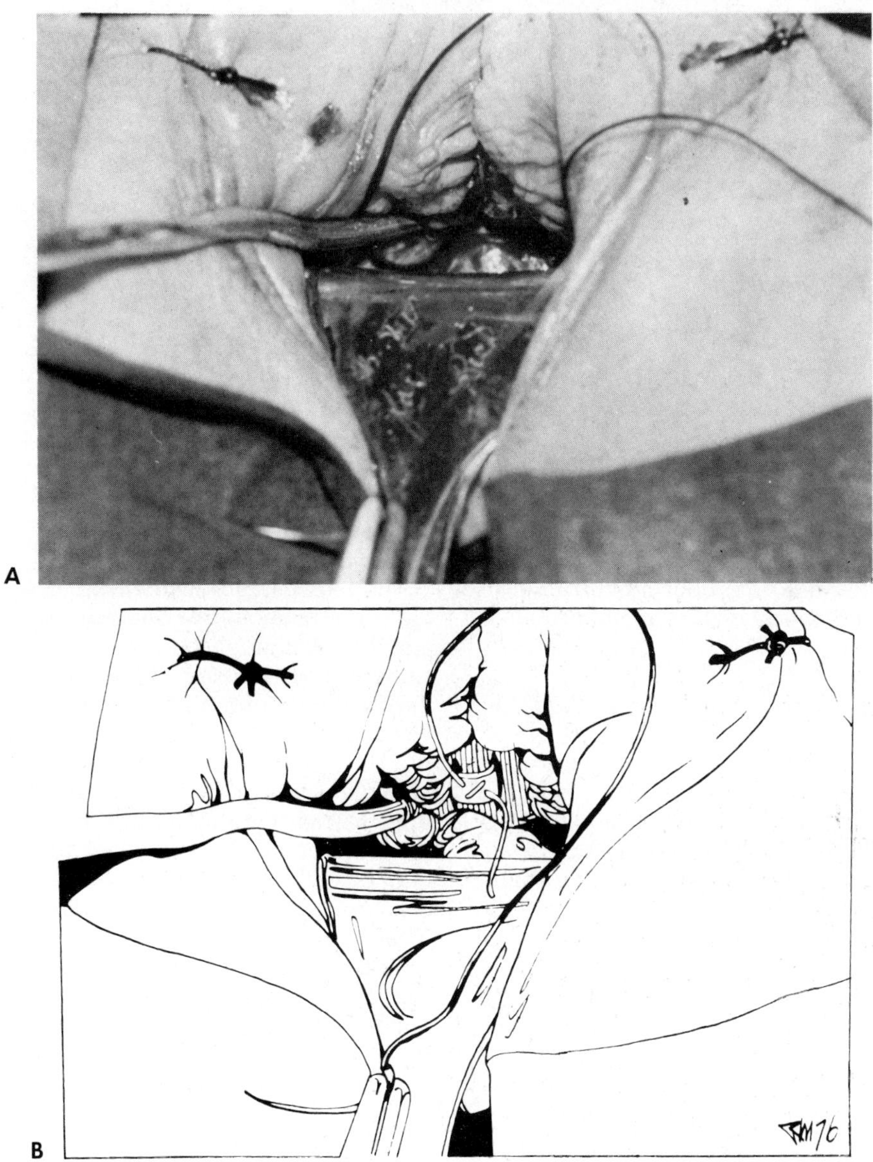

Figure 19–15. *A,* Suturing the fascial strip to the pubocervical fascia with 00 chromic catgut to maintain the sling in proper position at the upper 1 cm. of the urethra. The uterine sound points to the suture needle in the sling (glistening dot above suture) and pubocervical fascia. *B,* Schematic representation.

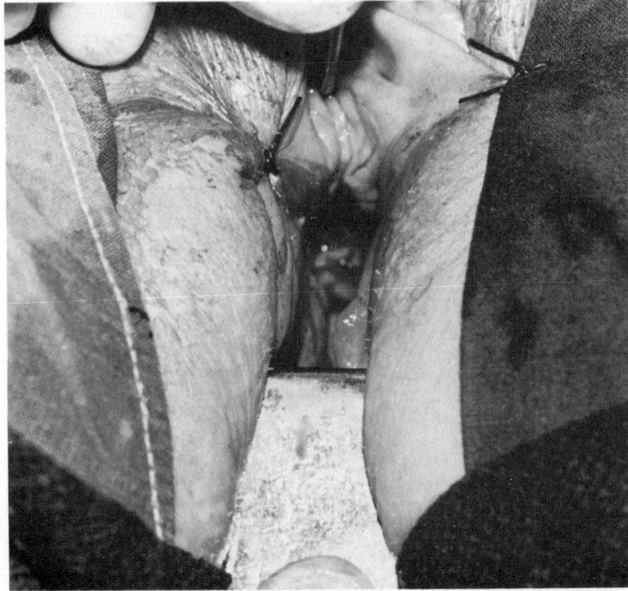

Figure 19–16. Note the tremendous elevation of the bladder neck area accomplished with the sling procedure.

bladder spasm, hematoma formation, or infection. Because the anesthesia is prolonged, attention to proper mobilization of the chest following surgery is important.

Leg Care

The temperature and color of the foot of the leg from which the graft was taken should be checked frequently for the first 24 hours following surgery to make certain that the tensor bandages are not too tight. These bandages should be kept snugly applied to the leg for one week, at which time they can be removed.

Mobilization of the limb should be encouraged as soon as the patient is conscious. The day after surgery, the patient should be out of bed and moving around the room for short periods, morning and afternoon. Mobilization is accelerated in an appropriate, graduated manner thereafter. The leg sutures should not be removed for 12 to 14 days, since the skin tension is great and the incisions will dehisce if nonabsorbable sutures are removed on the usual seventh postoperative day. Patients should have very little discomfort at the graft site and remarkably little tenderness along the donor tract.

Catheter Routine

The indwelling transurethral or suprapubic catheter should be allowed to drain, by gravity, continuously for 48 hours. The catheter is then clamped for 1 hour periods during the day for the next 48 hours, with continuous drainage at night. Subsequently, the catheter is clamped for 2 hour periods in a similar manner for another 48 hour period. On the seventh postoperative day, the catheter is attached to the stem end of a Y-shaped glass or plastic tidal drainage system. Approximately 1000 ml. of normal saline are administered every 24 hours in a drip through one upper arm of the Y. The other upper end of the Y is connected to a drainage tube that is pegged to a standard (similar to the high jump standard) at the patient's bedside, initially at the level of the bladder with the patient in the recumbent position.

The residual urine should be checked twice daily after a rush of urine into the urine receptacle. The patient should be instructed to empty her bladder immediately if she experiences any suprapubic discomfort. If the residual urine on each of the twice-daily estimations is less than 50 ml., the drainage arm of the catheter system should be elevated by 2.5 cm. If the residual urine is more than 100 ml., the level on the standard should be decreased by 2.5 cm. If the residual urine is 50 to 100 ml., the level of the drainage arm is left at the same height for the next 24 hours. When the patient is able to empty her bladder effectively against a 25 cm. gradient above the bladder level, the catheter can be removed, and the patient is nearly always able to void spontaneously.

Bethanechol chloride (Urecholine) can be used to enhance detrusor muscle power if progress in building up a gradient is slow. Doses of 12.5 mg., then 25 mg., then 50 mg., by mouth, four times daily, can be used as long as the patient does not develop side reactions to the drug. Overstimulation can produce incoordinated detrusor contractions, which should be suspected if bladder spasm or residual urine increase develops. It should be emphasized to nurses that if the bladder is allowed to become overdistended with urine volumes greater than 250 ml., progress in detrusor muscle rehabilitation can be retarded.

We recommend the use of prophylactic sulfonamide or urinary antiseptic administration while the catheter remains in the bladder. Bladder infection is inevitable if such therapy is not employed.

Delayed Voiding

Prior to surgery the patient should be told that the average interval from surgery to successful voiding is 3 to 4 weeks (mean of 40 days in our experience). The more severe the previous stress incontinence has been, the longer this interval will be. With severe stress incontinence, the bladder may become merely part of a conduit between the ureters and the external urethral meatus, so that it retains very little urine. As a consequence, the detrusor muscle undergoes disuse atrophy and the program of rehabilitation described earlier is required. During the postoperative period, the patient frquently becomes depressed and thinks she will never void again. Confident reassurance by nurses and doctors is required to buoy her spirits. Rehabilitation of the detrusor muscle, by the aforementioned catheter and tidal drainage routine, should be continued for 3 or 4 weeks following surgery.

If the patient is not voiding within 3 or 4 weeks of surgery, she goes home with instructions on the proper care of the suprapubic catheter, including the use of prophylactic sulfonamides or urinary antiseptic medication. When residual urine volumes are regularly 50 to 100 ml, the suprapubic catheter is removed. Failure to void in a completely satisfactory manner may be due to emotional disturbances, and the patient often responds well to a familiar home environment and release from hospital tensions.

The physiologic cause of delayed voiding is discussed in the following section.

Significant Residual Urine

Approximately one third of patients develop significant (greater than 30 ml.) residual urine one or more times during the first 2 years following surgery. Upon discharge from the hospital, the patient should be instructed to use postural changes (e.g., bending over or voiding in the reclining or standing positions) and suprapubic pressure to aid in bladder emptying. Some patients find hot baths to be of help. Alcoholic beverages or tranquilizers may interfere with voiding.

The cause of significant residual urine is basically the same as that of delayed voiding following surgery: ineffective detrusor contraction. The detrusor muscle may be acting in either a hypotonic or an incoordinate manner. Either of the latter dysfunctions may be caused by previous disuse atrophy of the detrusor muscle, excessive kinking of the bladder neck area by the sling, or interference with funneling of the bladder neck area by the sling. In our experience, bethanechol chloride (Urecholine) administration always corrects the problem when hypotonic detrusor activity is the cause, provided that there is proper bladder innervation. If the significant residual urine is due to hypertonic incoordinate detrusor contraction, the patient will complain of bladder spasm and will often indicate that the urine stream stops suddenly, which is followed by urgency. Such patients may respond to probantheline bromide (Pro-Banthine) or dicyclomine hydrochloride (Bentylol), or such medication may increase the hypertonicity of the detrusor muscle.

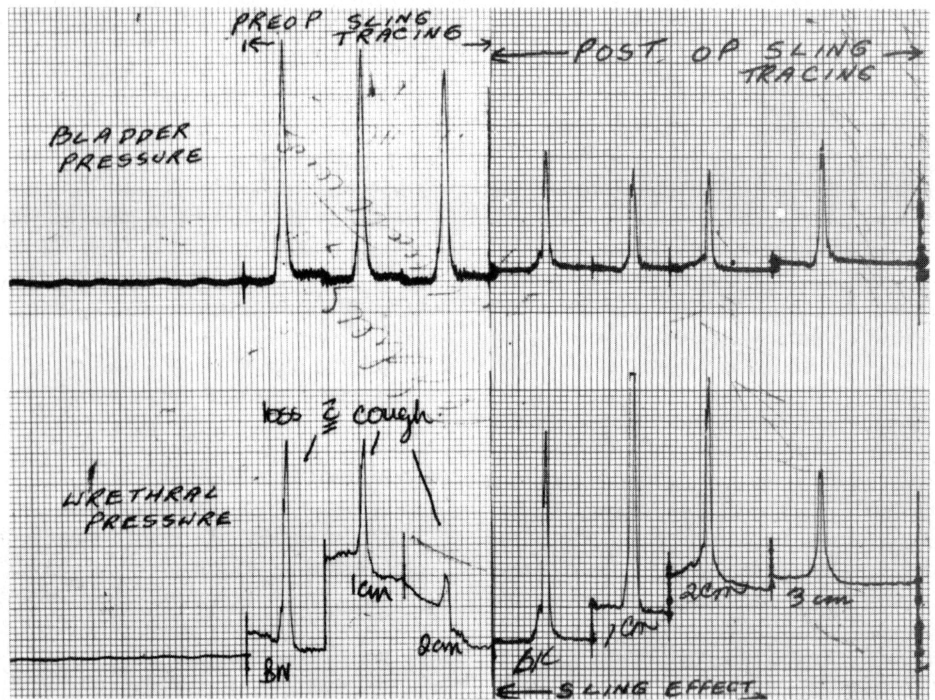

Figure 19–17. Effective postoperative urethral kinking at the sling site.
The preoperative urethrovesical gradient, showing pressure equalization with each cough pressure spike, is seen on the left. The postoperative gradient is seen on the right, demonstrating an excellent kinking effect in the urethra at the sling site with each cough, maintaining a higher overall pressure in the urethra than in the bladder—and resulting in continence of the patient. In the latter tracing note that there is reduced kinking effect in the urethra at 3 cm. from the bladder neck (B.N.) and distal to the sling effect.

TABLE 19–1. COMPLICATIONS OF SLING OPERATION: 83 CASES

	Cases
Delayed voiding of more than 7 days' duration	82 (mean, 39.9 days)
Residual urine >30 ml. (at 6 weeks up to 2 years)	21
Urinary tract infection	21
Pyrexia >100° F.	11
Hematuria	38*
Seroma	4
Entry into bladder at surgery	2†
Slough of sling	2
Fistula (with spontaneous closure)	1
Chest complications	4
Sling released 210 days postoperatively	1
Wound infection	3
Deep vein thrombosis	1
Peptic ulcer flareup	1
Gastric dilatation	1
Paralytic ileus	1
Change of suprapubic catheter	1

*Last 38 cases had a suprapubic catheter.
†Other than suprapubic catheter.

TABLE 19–2. DETRUSOR MUSCLE STATUS BEFORE AND AFTER SLING OPERATION: 83 CASES

Preoperative Status	Total Number of Patients	Postoperative Status *Normal*	*D.O.*	*D.I.*
Normal	50	46	3	1
D.O.*	20	15	2	3
D.I.†	13	1	9	3
	83			

*Detrusor overactivity, apparent only on tracing.
†Detrusor overactivity incontinence.

Long-term Follow-up

Approximately half of our "sling patients" have virtually no problems after leaving the hospital. Six weeks, 6 months, 1 year, and 2 years following surgery, they are checked in our unit for urine loss with a full bladder, urethrovesical pressure gradient, and residual urine. The remaining patients have trouble with residual urine and detrusor overactivity and must be seen when necessary, with careful attention to these problems. The problem of detrusor overactivity is discussed under Postoperative Complications.

POSTOPERATIVE COMPLICATIONS

Delayed voiding and *significant residual urine* are so common that they have been discussed under routine postoperative care.

Table 19–1 lists the complications encountered in 83 consecutive fascia lata sling procedures done in our unit. Five of these complications deserve special comment.

Entry into the Bladder at the Time of Surgery. Every effort should be made to avoid entry into the bladder and damage to the bladder wall at the time of surgery. Careful dissection of the bladder from the posterior aspect of the symphysis pubis is particularly important whenever a sling or retropubic fixation procedure has previously been employed. A laceration of the bladder can be easily repaired, but the surgeon must be concerned about subsequent breakdown of bladder and other damaged tissue at the site of surgical insult. The one **bladder fistula** (which closed spontaneously with continuous catheter drainage) and the two instances of **slough of the sling** into the bladder (with later passage per urethra) were recorded in patients in whom the bladder had been entered at surgery.

TABLE 19–3. PREVIOUS SURGERY FOR STRESS INCONTINENCE (MEAN OF TWO PROCEDURES) PERFORMED PRIOR TO SLING OPERATION: 83 CASES

Number of Previous Operations	Number of Patients	Procedure
1	2	M.M.*
	22	Ant. colp.† (+ radium one case)
2	18	M.M. + Ant. colp.
	20	Ant. colp × 2
	1	Ant. colp. + sling
3	8	M.M. + Ant. colp. × 2
	3	Ant. colp. × 3
	1	Ant. colp. × 2 + sling
	1	M.M. × 3
	1	Ant. colp. × 2 + fistula repair
4	2	M.M. + Ant. colp. × 3
	2	Ant. colp. × 4 (+ radium one case)
	1	Ant. colp. × 3 + 1 fistula repair
5	1	M.M. × 2 + Ant. colp. × 3

*M.M. = Marshall-Marchetti-Krantz procedure.
†Ant. colp. = Anterior colporrhaphy.

Seroma Formation. This problem can be avoided by not removing the drain too soon and by taking steps to ensure that the drain does not pull out prematurely. Unless the mass steadily increases in size, the temptation to incise and drain should be resisted in order to avoid infection. Local heat resolves the mass very effectively in 3 or 4 days. The author has now discontinued using the suprapubic drain and in the last 36 cases there have been no further cases of seroma formation.

Persistent Detrusor Overactivity. Table 19–2 shows the detrusor muscle status of our fifty patients before and after the sling procedure. These patients all had severe recurrent stress incontinence. (Table 19–3 indicates the previous surgical procedures in this group.) Only 50 of the 83 patients had normal detrusor muscle function prior to surgery. Six of the 33 patients who had mild detrusor overactivity or serious detrusor overactivity incontinence prior to surgery continued to have detrusor overactivity following surgery despite every effort to correct this problem by eliminating infection and using parasympatholytic drugs (probantheline bromide, 15 mg., or dicyclamine hydrochloride, 10 mg., four times daily for 3-week periods). In all six patients the sling had very effectively corrected the pressure equalization or anatomic component of stress incontinence. Every effort should be made to correct detrusor overactivity prior to surgery, and if it persists both the doctor and the patient should realize that it may continue even following surgery that cures the anatomic or pressure equalization component.

TABLE 19–4. RESULTS OF FACIA LATA SLING OPERATIONS IN 83 CASES (1968–1980)

	Number of Patients
Cure	73 (88%)
Improved	6 (7%)*
Failure	4 (5%)*

*In the first edition, reporting on 50 cases, there were 10 failures to cure. The 10 cases reported here are not all the same patients. Some patients in the first series have had improvement in their detrusor overactivity and one patient with pressure equalization incontinence has subsequently been cured as a result of spontaneously developed compensatory urethral kinking with progression of a cystocele.

TABLE 19–5. DURATION OF FOLLOW-UP IN 83 SLING CASES

	Number of Patients
6 Weeks	5
6 Months	9
1 Year	18
2 Years	51

RESULTS WITH THE FASCIA LATA SLING PROCEDURE

Tables 19–4 and 19–5 indicate the results and the length of follow-up in the 83 patients treated with a fascia lata sling procedure. Table 19–6 shows the time of recurrence and Table 19–7 explains the reason for recurrence. Three of the failures involved the sling itself. Two of these were due to an error in judgment regarding the technical approach, and occurred early in the series. The other sling failure was associated with a diminution of urethral resistance (pressure decrease) at the sling site, but this patient is happy with her result and does not require further surgery. The other seven failures to cure stress incontinence were due to persistent detrusor overactivity. Similar experience has been reported by McLaren (1957), who has stressed the problem of concurrent "urgency incontinence" persisting after "successful" surgery. Obviously some authors ignore the problem of detrusor overactivity or refuse

TABLE 19–6. TIME OF FIRST RECURRENCE OF INCONTINENCE IN 83 SLING CASES

	Type		Total Number
	*P.E.I.**	*D.I.*†	of Recurrences
6 Weeks	1	6	7
6 Months	1	0	1
1 Year	1	0	1
2 Years	0	1	1

*Pressure equalization incontinence.
†Detrusor overactivity incontinence.
(See also table 19–4.)

TABLE 19–7. REASON FOR RECURRENCE IN 83 SLING CASES

Patients	P.E.I.*	D.I.†
6 (improved)	1	5
4 (failures)	2	2

*Pressure equalization incontinence (sling failure).
†Detrusor overactivity incontinence.

to operate when pressure equalization or anatomic stress incontinence is complicated by detrusor overactivity.

SUMMARY

Every patient with urinary stress incontinence deserves a careful evaluation. The initial surgery to treat stress urinary incontinence should be performed with meticulous care by a competent surgeon who will continue the same care following surgery. Statistically the best chance of cure is with the first operation (Beck et al., 1968).

A patient with recurrent urinary stress incontinence requires even more careful evaluation and qualified care. The quality of the local support tissues should receive serious consideration. If the local tissues are weak, another primary procedure is doomed to failure. Too often the gynecologist mechanistically follows an anterior colporrhaphy with a ventral suspension or vice versa without asking, "Is this support tissue really reparable?" Lack of thought in this regard may be due to an egotistic belief that one can cure where others have failed, or to a slavish adherence to routine and ritual.

If careful consideration indicates that the local support tissues is irreparably poor, fascia lata can provide an ideal tissue graft. *Because of the extended operating time and the very significant postoperative problems, a sling operation should not be performed as a primary procedure unless it can be predicted that a well-done standard primary procedure will not withstand the stress of violent increase in intra-abdominal pressure, such as may occur with coughing in a patient with severe asthmatic bronchitis.* Surgeons who perform sling procedures must be prepared to "suffer" with their patients through the sometimes difficult postoperative period and to provide emotional support and prompt, intelligent, and sustained medical care.

REFERENCES

Beck, R. P.: Urinary stress incontinence. S. Afr. Med. J. *57*:853, 1980.

Beck, R. P., and Hsu, N.: Relationship of urethral length and anterior wall relaxation to urinary stress incontinence. Am. J. Obstet. Gynecol. 89:738, 1964.

Beck, R. P., and Maughan, G. B.: Simultaneous intraurethral and intravesical pressure studied in normal women and those with stress incontinence. Am. J. Obstet. Gynecol. *89*:746, 1964.

Beck, R. P., Arnusch, D., and King, C.: Results in treating 210 patients with detrusor overactivity incontinence of urine. Am. J. Obstet. Gynecol. *125*:593, 1976*a*.

Beck, R. P., Thomas, E. A., and Maughan, G. B.: The detrusor muscle and urinary incontinence. Am. J. Obstet. Gynecol. *94*:483, 1966.

Beck, R. P., Thomas, E. A., and Maughan, G. B.: Surgical results in the treatment of pressure equalization stress incontinence. Am. J. Obstet. Gynecol. *100*:483, 1968.

Beck, R. P., Grove, D., Arnusch, D., et al.: Recurrent urinary stress incontinence treated by the fascia lata sling procedure. Am. J. Obstet. Gynecol. *120*:613, 1974.

Beck, R. P., Daniel, E. E., Fimper, P., et al.: Electromyographic and pressure slides in the canine bladder. Am. J. Obstet. Gynecol. *125*:603, 1976*b*.

Green, T. H.: Development of a plan for the diagnosis and treatment of urinary stress incontinence. Am. J. Obstet. Gynecol. *83*:632, 1962.

Low, J. A.: Management of severe anatomic deficiencies of urethral sphincter function by a combined procedure with a fascia lata sling. Am. J. Obstet. Gynecol. *105*:149, 1969.

MacFarlane, K. T.: Discussion of a sling operation using Marlex polypropylene mesh, for treatment of recurrent stress incontinence. Am. J. Obstet. Gynecol. *106*:376, 1970.

McLaren, H. C.: Fascial slings for stress incontinence. J. Obstet. Gynaecol. Br. Emp. *44*:673, 1957.
Morgan, J. E.: A sling operation using Marlex polypropylene mesh, for treatment of recurrent stress incontinence. Am. J. Obstet. Gynecol. *106*:369, 1970.
Read, C. D.: Stress incontinence of urine with special reference to failure of cure following vaginal operative procedure. Am. J. Obstet. Gynecol. *59*:1260, 1950.
Stallworthy, J.: Personal communication, 1976.
TeLinde, R.: Operative Gynecology. 4th Ed. Philadelphia, J. B. Lippincott, 1970.
The University of Alberta, Bladder Physiology Unit: Unpublished data, 1976.
Zacharin, R. F.: Stress Incontinence of Urine. New York, Harper & Row, 1972.

20

SURGICAL PROCEDURES FOR RECURRENT STRESS INCONTINENCE

R. A. LEE, M.D.

Most frequently, recurrent urinary stress incontinence follows some type of anterior vaginal repair, usually plication of the Kelly-Kennedy type. In some instances, the persistent or recurrent incontinence represents failure of the operative procedure because of poor surgical technique (inadequate plication). In others, it may result from postoperative complications such as infection, hematoma, or catheter trauma. In most instances, the initial result may have been satisfactory for some time, and the recurrent incontinence may be the result of a gradual and progressive postmenopausal (or occupational) deterioration of the musculofascial urethral supports over a period of several years. Just as no single etiologic factor exists in all cases of stress incontinence, there is no single uniformly corrective operative procedure, as attested to by the continual reports of new operations or malfunctions of old procedures.

Most gynecologic surgeons agree that correction of recurrent stress incontinence should be principally surgical — usually by means of a retropubic or combined vaginal-retropubic approach. Although the gynecologic surgeon may have a personal preference, he must be familiar with several basic procedures and their modifications in order to properly select and perform the appropriate operation. In addition, he should be ready to improvise during the operation in order to adapt a technique suitable to the patient's condition.

All successful operations for stress incontinence, whether vaginal plication, suprapubic suspension, or "sling" (or some combination or variation of these), effectively increase the urethral resistance by tightening the musculofascial planes through which the urethra passes, placing the vesical neck in a high retropubic position. In the individual situation it appears that satisfactory surgical results may be obtained by correcting a single facet (functional length, urethrovesical angle, or urethral compliance) of this complex mechanism without affecting other measurable parameters. Possibly this explains the variety of surgical procedures, any one of which gives similar rates of correction (and failure rates) for this distressing problem. Regrettably, *none* of these methods can be 100 per cent effective; the patient who does not have good urethral smooth muscle (quantitatively and qualitatively) will remain incontinent. As emphasized in Chapter 16, regardless of its length, caliber, axis, or angle, a fixed fibrotic, noncontractile urethra will not provide urinary control.

SURGICAL APPROACHES

Sling Operations

FASCIAL SLING

Ridley (1974), Parker and co-workers (1979), and Beck (1976) prefer a sling procedure, for which they favor fascia lata obtained from the lateral aspect of the thigh. Ridley places the patient in the dorsolithotomy position, and the lower abdomen and perineal areas are exposed for a combined approach. At the beginning of the procedure, a Foley urethral catheter is placed to identify any troublesome bleeding and to outline the position of the urethra during the surgical dissection. An 8 to 10 cm. transverse incision is made inferior to the suprapubic catheter, which is situated approximately 4 cm. above the symphysis pubis. Two small incisions are made on each side of the midline through the fascia to enter the space of Retzius.

The vaginal phase is then carried out, separating the vaginal wall from the underlying bladder and urethra. A curved blunt-tipped instrument is passed through one small abdominal incision traversing the space of Retzius alongside the urethra, where it presents vaginally with a gentle thrust. The end of the fascial strip is withdrawn and secured to the anterior abdominal aponeurosis with several 3–0 silk sutures.

A similar procedure is carried out on the other side and the other end of the fascial strip is fixed to the rectus fascia (Figure 20–1). The bladder neck and the proximal one third of the urethra under which the sling will fall are supported but not obstructed. Ridley (1974) noted that one of the most critical aspects of the operation is how tightly the sling is placed beneath the urethra; he suggests that it can scarcely be placed too loosely.

In Ridley's study, from 1948 to 1973, 146 patients underwent this procedure. Of these, 14 patients had this done as primary treatment for urinary incontinence and 132 for recurrent or persistent incontinence. In 127 patients, a fascia lata strip was inserted; no complications occurred that were attributable to this sling material. In three of 17 patients in whom a Mersilene ribbon was used, retropubic infection occurred, and in one patient, erosion into the bladder developed. Other postoperative complications included chronic urinary tract infections in 18 patients and persistent residual urine of 30 ml. or more 6 months after operation in 32 patients. Of the 146 patients, 127 (87 per cent) were considered cured, 11 (8 per cent) were improved, and

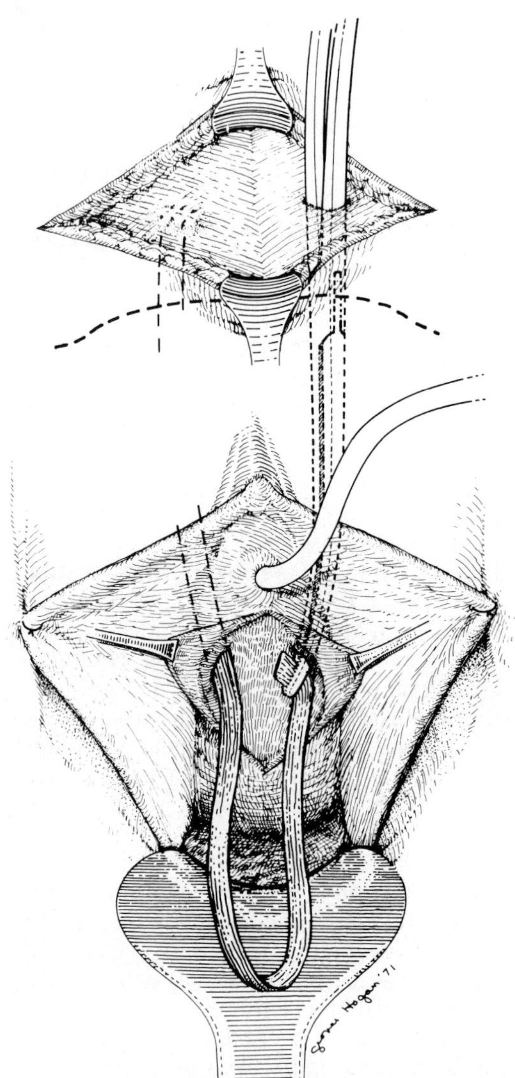

Figure 20–1. Passage of fascia lata strip beneath urethra and retropubically. Strip has been anchored to anterior abdominal fascia on patient's right side and drawn into vagina, and is shown grasped by uterine dressing forceps, to be drawn up on the left side and anchored with proper tension at the other slitlike incision in fascia. Thus, a sling is formed beneath the urethra at the bladder neck. Retention catheter remains in place during the entire sling procedure. (From Ridley, J. H.: Gynecologic Surgery: Errors, Safeguards, and Salvage. © 1974 The Williams & Wilkins Company, Baltimore.)

eight (5 per cent) continued to have urinary stress incontinence.

Similarly, Green (1968) has suggested that the sling procedure may be the most suitable operation for the occasional patient with incontinence after an unsuccessful Marshall-Marchetti-Krantz procedure. He noted that the sling procedure is more complex than the Marshall-Marchetti-Krantz operation and is often followed by significant and prolonged voiding difficulties (Chapter 19). With this approach, however, one can obtain permanent elevation of the urethra and placement of the vesical neck in a high retropubic position. Parker emphasizes that the basic principle of the sling operation is the establishment of a supporting structure beneath the urethrovesical junction, which slightly elevates the urethra in the area with downward movement of the bladder. Unfortunately, synthetic materials, like any foreign body, may provide a nidus for infection, requiring their subsequent removal. Removal may be an arduous task further aggravated by the frequent recurrence of urinary incontinence.

Regardless of the material used for the sling, an appropriate degree of tension is required — tight enough to correct the incontinence and yet loose enough to avoid prolonged urinary retention. Occasionally, because of excessive tension, the narrow band will penetrate the urethra and will present as a ribbonlike wall within the urethral lumen. Parker, while favoring the sling procedure, suggests there are more complications with this operation than with the usual anterior colporrhaphy or Marshall-Marchetti-Krantz procedure. Although Ridley (1974) suggests that the operation is not technically difficult, the excellent results that he has reported may be attributed to his superior clinical judgment and surgical technique based on a very large experience with the fascial sling operations.

The Mersilene Gauze Hammock

Nichols (1979) employed with success a Mersilene gauze hammock as a modification of the Aldridge sling procedure in the treatment of recurrent or severe urinary incontinence. Mersilene gauze, a wide single layer of knitted fabric that does not ravel, permits a gradual permanent infiltration of fibrous connective tissue. This aids in providing future strength to the vesical neck support.

An advantage of this sling procedure, when properly performed, is that it distributes suburethral pressure over a wide area and neither constricts the urethra nor decreases its lumen. Apparently it increases both urethral tone and intraurethral pressure by providing a firm support on which the urethra may rest.

A combined abdominal-vaginal approach is used, and the belly of the Mersilene gauze hammock is sutured to the undersurface of the periurethral connective tissues and to the bladder capsule (Figure 20–2). The ends of the gauze hammock are then sewed without extra tension to the rectus aponeurosis through separate groin incisions. Transvaginal plication of the pubourethral ligament occasionally may be done to support the sling procedure. Because of the risk of infection, all patients are given broad-spectrum antibiotics for 5 days.

In some patients, the vaginal phase of this procedure induced infection around the foreign material (Mersilene), eventually resulting in loss of a portion of the vaginal wall overlying the gauze hammock. In an attempt to avoid this troublesome complication, Nichols (1979) modified his procedure by transplanting a bulbocavernosus fat pad or a separate subepithelial fibromuscular layer of the vagina between the Mersilene hammock and the vaginal wall. If the sling is found to be too loose during the postoperative period, it may be tightened via the groin incision using a urethroscope to visualize the effect on the proximal urethra. This technique, which provides permanent support, is especially appealing in patients with a scarred, fixed vaginal wall that may not lend itself to the retropubic elevation required by a Marshall-Marchetti-Krantz suspension. Recent review of the literature emphasizes that although this surgical option has received international attention, the total reported experience of the results of surgical management is still modest.

Round Ligament Sling

Hodgkinson, in a personal communication, advocates elevation of the urethrovesical junction by means of a suburethral sling fashioned from the two crossed uterine ends of the round ligament. He favors this whenever the anterior vaginal wall has been scarred and shortened from

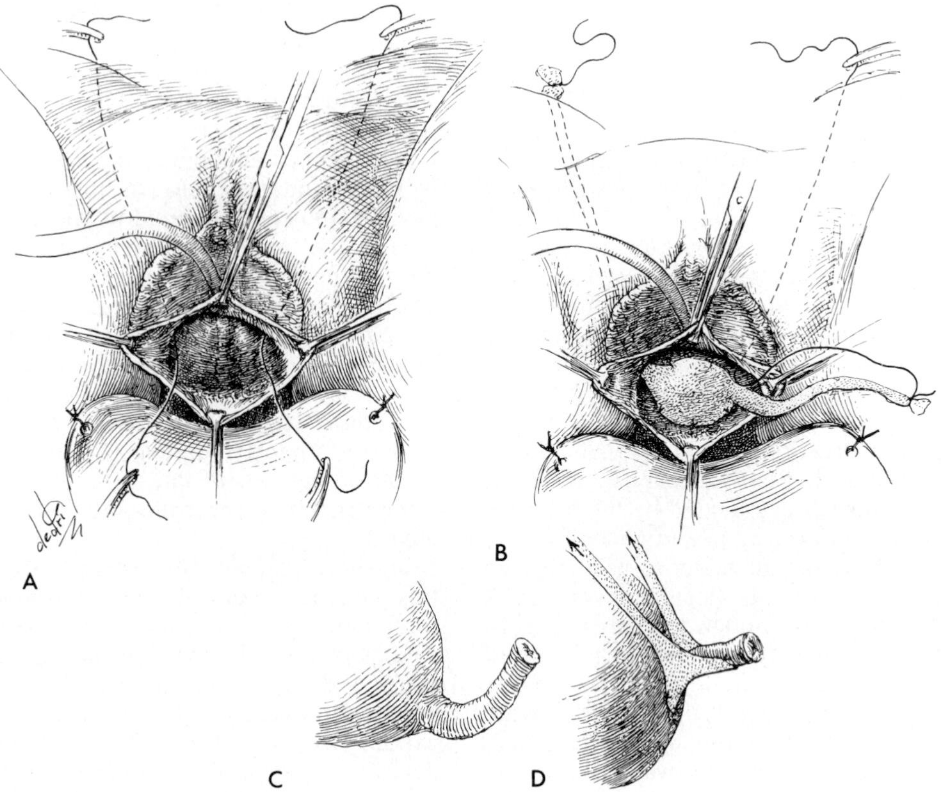

Figure 20–2. Mersilene gauze hammock sling procedure.

A, Short abdominal extraperitoneal incision has been made through each rectus aponeurosis into space of Retzius. Anterior vaginal wall has been opened, and urogenital diaphragm penetrated. Silk pilot suture has been placed through this tunnel on each side.

B, Belly of Mersilene gauze hammock has been tacked in place, and ends tied to vaginal pilot sutures. Traction draws the mesh through each preformed tunnel. After the vagina has been closed, the ends of the gauze hammock are sewn to the rectus aponeurosis.

C, Preoperative deficiency in support of vesicourethral junction is shown, which permits flattening of posterior urethrovesical angle.

D, Diagrammatic representation of effect of Mersilene gauze hammock sling. Vesicourethral junction is elevated over wide area, reducing any tendency toward strangulation and pressure necrosis.

(From Nichols, D. H.: The Mersilene mesh gauze-hammock for severe urinary stress incontinence. Obstet. Gynecol. *41*:88–93, 1973. By permission of Harper & Row, Publishers.)

previous operations. A combined vaginal abdominal approach is used, and the vaginal walls are initially mobilized from the bladder base and proximal three fourths of the urethra.

Lateral to the urethra at the level of the vesical neck, the space of Retzius is entered. A rubber drain is looped around the inferior surface of the urethra, after which the vaginal wall is closed. The space of Retzius is then entered through an abdominal incision, and the ends of the drain, passed through the paraurethral incision, are exposed. One end of the suburethrally placed rubber drain is tied to the ends of two strands of 2-0 catgut suture. The drain is removed by traction, thereby pulling the two sutures to the suburethral location previously occupied by the drain. The ends of the round ligament, which have been mobilized from the uterus, are then tied to the sutures and by traction are displaced to the suburethral location in a parallel side-to-side position (Figure 20–3). The urethra is elevated to a "comfortable-appearing" level and is secured by suturing together the round ligaments.

Each round ligament is secured to the fascia of the ileopectineal line, to provide proper orientation of the sling and to pro-

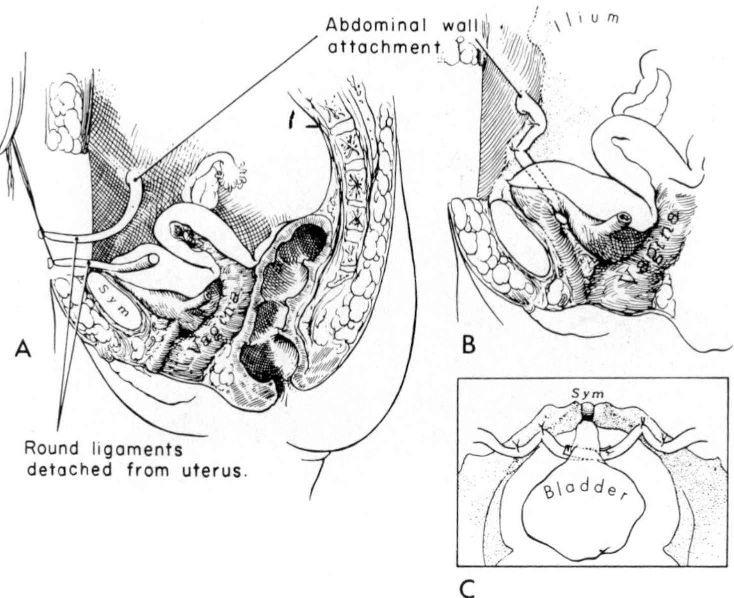

Figure 20–3. *A*, Round ligaments are attached from uterus.

B, Round ligaments are placed beneath vesical neck and sutured to fascia of ileopectineal line to obtain additional security of support.

C, Suburethral position of round ligaments sutured in position. Note additional sutures to fascia of ileopectineal line. (From Hodgkinson, C. P., and Kelly, W. T.: Urinary stress incontinence in the female. III. Round-ligament technic for retropubic suspension of the urethra. Obstet. Gynecol. *10*:493–499, 1957. By permission of Harper & Row, Publishers.)

mote additional security of support. When possible, the anterior vaginal wall is additionally suspended to the retropubic region to further enhance the vesical neck and urethral support.

Hodgkinson, in a personal communication, states he has done over 200 of these procedures, with essentially 95 per cent success rate. He admits that the procedure may result in laceration of the urethra or bladder; however, this is easily recognized and corrected. He continues to be impressed that the round ligament, even in the postmenopausal patient, is quite substantial and of good length. The uniformly excellent results have been obtained except in patients who had previous radiation for pelvic malignancy. This complicating factor also adversely affects any operation for urinary incontinence. Our concern is that with additional time and the "wear and tear of living" the tendency would be for the smooth muscle ligaments to undergo stretch, and attenuation would result in loss of support with recurrent incontinence. This has not been the finding of Hodgkinson. Nonetheless, it should be noted that few have the knowledge and experience of Hodgkinson, who has been a major force in the drive to better understand urinary control.

Suspension Operations

Burch (1961) advocated elevation of the bladdder neck and urethra by suspending the anterior vaginal wall to Cooper's ligament using 2-0 chromic catgut sutures (Figure 20–4). In most cases, hysterectomy was performed, with posterior colpoperineorrhaphy done in selected patients. Enterocele developed in four patients, and vesicovaginal fistula developed in one patient. Burch (1961) has adequately documented that his procedure provides good control of urinary incontinence. The technique is less complex than the sling procedure and does not require the suburethral dissection. It may prove advantageous in patients with a short, scarred urethra in whom only a single pair of Marshall-Marchetti-Krantz su-

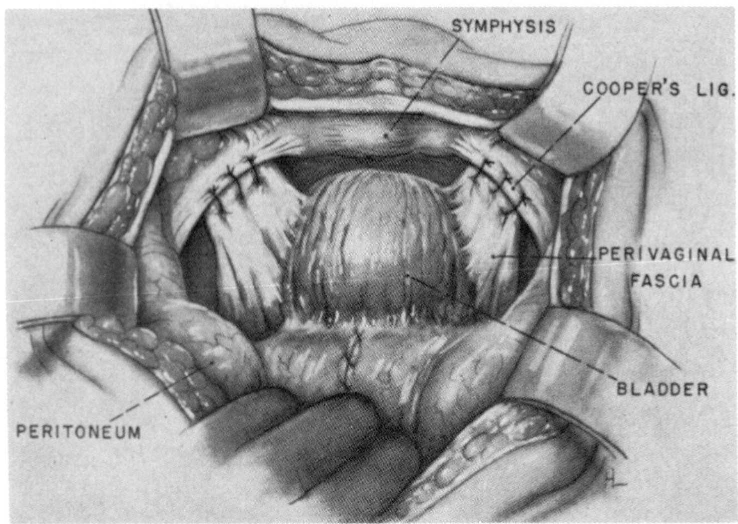

Figure 20–4. Lateral edges of vagina approximated to Cooper's ligament by three interrupted sutures of 2–0 chromic catgut. (From Burch, J. C.: Urethrovaginal fixation to Cooper's ligament for correction of stress incontinence, cystocele, and prolapse. Am. J. Obstet. Gynecol. *81*:281–290, 1961. By permission of C. V. Mosby Company.)

tures can be inserted adjacent to the urethra.

Regrettably, the anterior displacement of the vagina in this procedure encourages the development of posterior enterocele. More recently, the operation has been modified to include cul-de-sac obliteration, which is further enhanced by securing the sigmoid colon to the anterior peritoneum. It should be noted that the placement of absorbable sutures far lateral to the urethra (while forming a vaginal hammock) may not provide sufficient long-term urethral plication and vesical neck support.

Ball and associates (1965) described a combined vaginal-abdominal operation for stress incontinence, which subsequently underwent several modifications. Initially, anterior colporrhaphy was done to lyse any adhesions about the bladder neck, after which an effective plication of the urethra and vesical neck was performed to restore a normal posterior urethrovesical angle. The abdominal phase of the operation consisted of mobilization of the bladder neck and urethra. Plication of the proximal urethra, vesical neck, and 2 cm. of the bladder adjacent to the vesical neck was performed to further increase the functional length of the urethra while decreasing its diameter (Figure 20–5). This also plicated the vesical neck and, at least theoretically, made a portion of the bladder adjacent to this critical area a functional portion of the urethra.

Originally, these workers suspended the anterior vaginal wall of the bladder to the rectus muscle in order to increase the urethrovesical angle. They no longer do this but allow the bladder neck to fall away from the symphysis, where intra-abdominal pressure or stress can be more effectively exerted.

Other variations of the Burch operation suggested by Durfee (1965) and Tanagho and Miller (1970) all essentially accomplish the same support of the proximal urethra with fixation of the anterior vaginal wall to Cooper's ligament or the obturator fascia. Tanagho and Miller did not believe that the free suture (loop) between the vagina and the Cooper's ligament would eventually cut through the vaginal wall. Ball and associates (1965) were particularly vehement in their condemnation of the Marshall-Marchetti-Krantz procedure. They considered that it was unphysiologic and was associated with a high rate of complications and failure. However, in depicting the deficiencies of the operation, they presented what appears to be a rather typical example of an inadequate or "alleged" Marshall-Marchetti-Krantz procedure with only an-

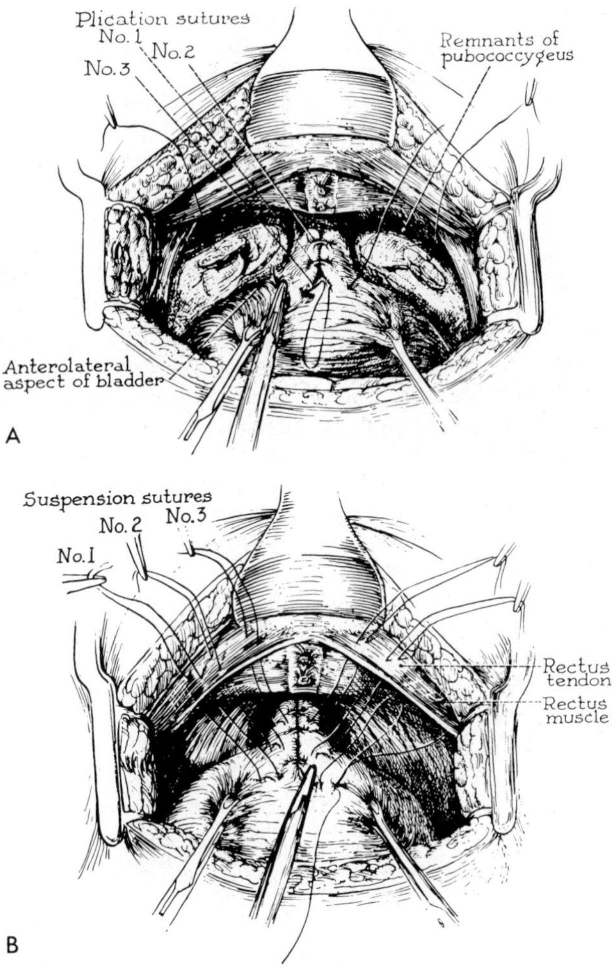

Figure 20–5. *A,* Urethra and bladder neck dissected from their fragile areolar connections to posterior border of symphysis and adjacent descending pubic rami. Three plication sutures are placed in one-end mattress fashion to narrow the urethra and create an anterior urethrovesical angle. *B,* Suspension sutures are placed and passed through rectus tendons on each side. (From Ball, T. L., Natale, R., and Elston, J. H.: Urinary stress incontinence [extension of the indications for the Ball operation and recent modifications in technique]. Nebr. Med. J. *50*:415–423, 1965. By permission of Nebraska Medical Association.)

terior bladder wall suspension to the rectus fascia and little attention directed to support of the urethra and vesical neck.

Marshall-Marchetti-Krantz Procedure

A modified Marshall-Marchetti-Krantz operation (as described in Chapter 16), often combined with a vesical neck plication, has at our institution almost completely replaced other retropubic techniques for the surgical treatment of recurrent urinary incontinence. Infrequently, a preliminary vaginal phase is required to mobilize constricting bands or adhesions, and this permits urethral and anterior vaginal wall elevation during the retropubic phase of the operation. In the absence of previous retropubic surgery, the surgery is carried out as previously described, with accurate placement of the periurethral suspending (hammock) sutures under direct vision with the bladder open. After proper placement of these sutures, the ends are merely tagged and set aside, and the vesical neck and urethra are evaluated for further plication.

In patients who have had multiple operative failures, a remarkable degree of urethral atonicity and loss of resistance can be observed and evidenced by palpation of the vesical neck and proximal urethra through our cystotomy incision. in addition, intraurethral compliance may be measured at 1, 2, and 3 cm. from the vesical neck by means of a water-filled balloon attached to a mobile, two-channel recorder-electromanometer-transducer unit.

In patients who at operation have maximal urethral relaxation with funneling and in whom simple plication or suspension may not sufficiently improve the urethral resistance, a tight plication of the entire length of the urethra is advisable, as suggested by Symmonds (1972). To accomplish this, the anterior cystotomy is extended down through the bladder neck and urethra almost to the level of the external meatus. Contrary to the suggestion of Ball and associates (1965), none of the urethral muscularis is excised; the objective is to preserve and plicate all available smooth muscle so that it may function more effectively on a urethral tube of greater functional length and of smaller caliber, thereby improving urethral resistance.

With the urethra open and under direct observation, it can be tightly plicated on the catheter with interrupted 2-0 chromic catgut sutures, which accurately invert and approximate the epithelial edges without entering the urethral lumen (Figure 20–6). After the suspending Marshall-Marchetti-Krantz sutures have been tied and the urethral catheter has been removed, the urethrovesical junction should appear "tight," with no discernible lumen; that is, it should have the appearance of a normal continent urethra. If further vesical neck plication seems to be advantageous, sutures of 2-0 chromic catgut, one just below the bladder neck and a second just at the level of the bladder neck, may be placed in an endeavor to increase proximal urethral and vesical neck pressure.

If the patient has had a previous retropubic operation, a repeat operation is technically more difficult because of scarring and fixation of the bladder and the urethra to the posterior aspect of the rectus muscle and symphysis pubis. In most of these patients, we have found it expeditious to open the bladder as the initial step, to allow a finger in the bladder. With sharp dissec-

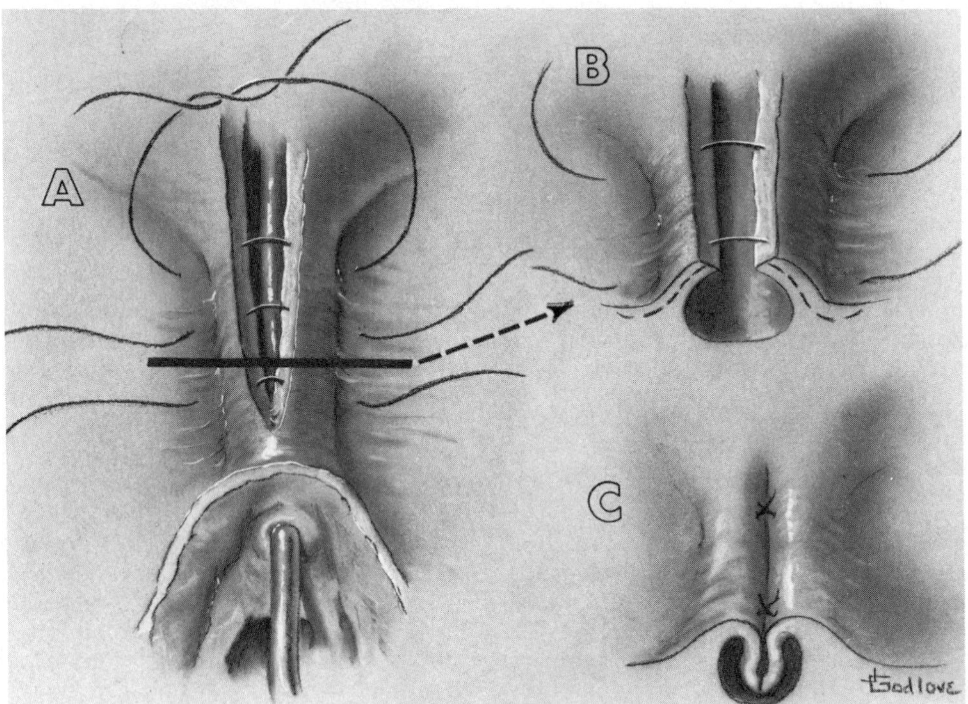

Figure 20–6. *A,* Cystostomy has been extended down through bladder neck and upper two thirds of urethra. (Pubic symphysis not shown for clarity.) *B, C,* Cross-section of urethra, showing method of inserting sutures in urethral smooth muscle (*B*) and diminished caliber of atonic funnel urethra (*C*). (From Symmonds, R. E.: The suprapubic approach to anterior vaginal relaxation and urinary stress incontinence. Clin. Obstet. Gynecol. *15*:1107–1121, 1972. By permission of Harper & Row, Publishers.)

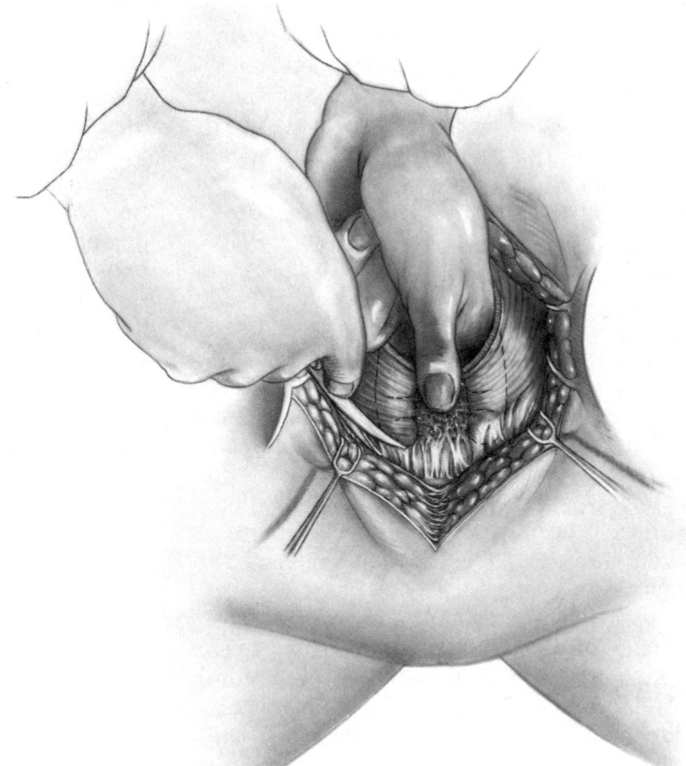

Figure 20–7. Index and middle fingers of surgeon's left hand in bladder, showing sharp dissection of anterior surface of bladder from posterior surface of rectus muscle and back of symphysis.

tion, the bladder wall and urethra can then be mobilized from the back of the rectus muscle and the posterior surface of the symphysis and pubic rami (Figure 20–7).

In many of these patients, observation of the distribution of scarring and fixation revealed that only the upper anterior bladder wall and bladder neck had been suspended at the previous operation. There was no evidence, such as adhesions or scarring, that would indicate placement of the suspending sutures between the symphysis and supporting tissues lateral to the urethra. The lack of such evidence suggests that many of these patients have not had a true urethral and bladder neck suspension but rather merely have had a suture fixation of the anterior bladder wall to the back of the rectus muscle, with little attention to the vesical neck and proximal urethra. Our experience in over 75 patients with previous retropubic operations, at least one of which was a previous Marshall-Marchetti-Krantz, suggests that a repeat procedure properly accomplished will result in correction of urinary incontinence in over 90 per cent of the patients.

POSTOPERATIVE COMPLICATIONS

Postoperative complications with the Marshall-Marchetti-Krantz procedure have been few. Prior to the routine use of cystotomy, two patients had sutures placed inadvertently in the bladder and subsequently required reoperation because of stone formation. Since cystotomy became a regular part of the procedure, our group has not had a complication that can be attributed to this portion of the operation. The suprapubic catheter is generally clamped on the seventh day, and the mean hospital stay is 14 days.

There were no fistulas, nor was repeat

operation required because of urinary retention. Nineteen patients had urinary tract infection. Three patients developed superficial thrombophlebitis with no evidence of pulmonary embolism. Four patients developed ventral hernias, one of which contained the anterior wall of the bladder and required two operative repairs for correction.

Osteitis Pubis

Osteitis pubis, a condition of unknown cause, was noted in six patients. The severity of symptoms and the obvious clinical findings would make this condition difficult to overlook. From 1960 to 1968, over 200 patients underwent a Marshall-Marchetti-Krantz procedure using absorbable suture. From 1968 to 1976, 320 patients had the same procedure done with permanent suture. There was no difference in the frequency of osteitis pubis during the 16 year period. In general, the onset of symptoms was abrupt (at 7 days to 2 months postoperatively). Most patients presented with pain in the pelvic region and extending down the inner or adductor region of one or both thighs. The pain was sharp, aggravated by cough, walking, and especially getting in and out of bed. Usually tenderness over the symphysis was present. Roentgenography demonstrated the characteristic hazy borders of the pubic bone. In five of the six patients, lytic changes were observed 4 to 6 weeks after the onset of symptoms.

In these patients, osteitis pubis was associated with the use of permanent or absorbable sutures and usually not accompanied by any evidence of frank infection. Treatment consisted of bed rest, analgesia, and cortisone acetate. The dosage schedule most often used is 300 mg. of cortisone on the first day, 200 mg. on the second day, and 100 mg. a day for a total of 10 days. There is usually dramatic relief, with disappearance of pain in 24 hours and loss of adductor spasm in 48 hours.

RESULTS

At the Mayo Clinic, from January 1960 through December 1977, 301 patients have undergone a Marshall-Marchetti-Krantz procedure for recurrent urinary stress incontinence. This group of patients had a total of 541 previous operations (an average of 1.8 per patient) specifically for stress incontinence, with a mean follow-up of 7.5 years. Follow-up consisted of reexamination of every patient when possible. If personal interviews and examinations could not be obtained, questionnaires were sent and telephone interviews used.

Two hundred and seventy-three patients (91 per cent) have undergone successful correction of totally disabling stress incontinence. Seven patients in whom recurrent incontinence developed, after having had good urinary control for periods ranging from 8 months to 11 years, subsequently required a "second stage" Kennedy plication of the urethra; this provided complete urinary control in six of the seven patients. Four failures occurred in patients with iatrogenic incontinence: loss of urethra and vesical neck muscle, secondary to transurethral resection of bladder neck, in one; fulguration in one; partial denervation of bladder after radical hysterectomy in one; and distortion of the bladder neck after vaginectomy in one. One of the four patients has undergone correction by a modified sling procedure. These represent some of the more difficult problems in patients with recurrent incontinence.

The Marshall-Marchetti-Krantz operation provides the advantage of a broad suburethral support (a hammock effect), with effective plication of the urethra and high retropubic position of the vesical neck. The technique is relatively simple when compared with other approaches. Whereas the various sling techniques utilizing fascia, Mersilene, or round ligament should provide equally satisfactory elevation of the urethra and bladder neck, there is a distinct hazard that the synthetic materials may provide a nidus for infection or, with time, erode into the bladder or urethra. More commonly, excessive pressure or tension on a relatively short segment of the urethra may produce a persistent mechanical obstruction. This pressure can be unrelenting, and the urinary retention that results can be difficult to correct. Most gynecologic surgeons agree that considerable experience is required to successfully accomplish these more technically demanding procedures if rather serious complications are to be avoided.

Regrettably, the surgical management of these difficult problems has not, and probably will not, become an exact science. Properly performed, each of the retropubic operations can provide urethral support comparable to that achieved with the Marshall-Marchetti-Krantz procedure. With the necessary urethral support, the patient will be cured.

In the proper hands, these same patients probably can be managed with equal success by means of a fascial sling (Ridley, 1974; Parker et al., 1979), a round ligament suspension (Hodgkinson, 1980), a Mersilene sling (Nichols, 1979), a Cooper ligament suspension (Burch, 1961), or perhaps a combined plication (Ball et al., 1965). At any rate, a retropubic operation, whether in the form of a suspension, or a suspension plus plication, or fascial sling or modification thereof, offers the patient with recurrent incontinence the best chance of permanent support of the bladder neck and urethra and good urinary control. Perhaps a few patients will always remain incontinent because of the inherent poor quality and quantity of the contractile smooth muscle in the urethra and vesical neck despite a good anatomic result.

REFERENCES

Ball, T. L., Natale, R., and Elston, J. H.: Urinary stress incontinence (extension of the indications for the Ball operation and recent modifications in technique). Nebr. Med. J. *50*:415, 1965.

Beck, R. P.: Urinary stress incontinence. Ob./Gyn. Digest, pp. 19–35, 1976.

Burch, J. C.: Urethrovaginal fixation to Cooper's ligament for correction of stress incontinence, cystocele, and prolapse. Am. J. Obstet. Gynecol. *81*:281, 1961.

Durfee, R. B.: Anterior vaginal suspension operation for treatment of stress incontinence. Am. J. Obstet. Gynecol. *92*:610, 1965.

Green, T. H., Jr.: The problem of urinary stress incontinence in the female: an appraisal of its current status. Obstet. Gynecol. Surv. *23*:603, 1968.

Hodgkinson, C. P.: Personal communication, 1980.

Nichols, D. H.: The sling operations. In Cantor, E. B. (Ed.): Female Urinary Stress Incontinence. Springfield, Ill., Charles C Thomas, Publisher, 1979.

Nichols, D. H.: Personal communication, 1980.

Parker, R. T., Addision, W. A., and Wilson, C. J.: Fascia lata urethrovesical suspension for recurrent stress urinary incontinence. Am. J. Obstet. Gynecol. *135*:843, 1979.

Ridley, J. H.: Gynecologic Surgery: Errors, Safeguards, and Salvage. Baltimore, Williams & Wilkins Company, 1974, pp. 114–154.

Symmonds, R. E.: The suprapubic approach to anterior vaginal relaxation and urinary stress incontinence. Clin. Obstet. Gynecol. *15*:1107, 1972.

Tanagho, E. A., and Miller, E. A.: Initiation of voiding. Br. J. Urol. 42:175, 1970.

21

VAGINAL REPAIR OF VESICOVAGINAL AND URETHROVAGINAL FISTULAS

WILLIAM C. KEETTEL, M.D.
DOUGLAS W. LAUBE, M.D.

HISTORICAL REVIEW

The problems related to urinary vaginal fistulas date back to antiquity. There are descriptions in the literature of such fistulas found in mummies estimated to be over 4000 years old. Until the seventeenth century there was no cure for these unfortunate patients. However, since that time a number of physicians have made valuable contributions to the development of our present operative knowledge.

In 1672 a Dutchman named H. Van Roonhyse recommended the vaginal approach for fistula repair with proper exposure and wide mobilization of the bladder from surrounding tissues. He recommended that the denuded edges be approximated by means of quills held in place by silk threads. Unfortunately, we do not know whether he was successful with this technique. In 1839, George Hayward at the Massachusetts General Hospital reported a successful repair by dissecting the vaginal mucosa from the bladder prior to closure of the defect.

With the discovery of anesthetic agents, there was increased interest in all types of surgery — including that for vesicovaginal fistula. In 1852, J. Marion Sims, who is generally recognized as having made many of the major contributions to this field, described his technique of repair. In this paper (Sims, 1852) the obstetric causes of fistula were described and preventive measures were recommended. Sims described a vaginal approach, positioning the patient either in the knee-chest or lateral Sims position. He devised the Sims retractor for exposure, facilitating wide mobilization of the fistula, which was closed with silver wire sutures. The silver wire sutures may have been his greatest contribution, since he was the first to attain a consistent success rate in a large number of patients. Sims was a remarkable physician who made equally valuable contributions to other fields of medicine: harelip repairs, repairs of gunshot wounds to the abdomen, and gallbladder surgery. He organized the first Woman's Hospital and late in his career was the first to establish the concept of a cancer hospital.

In 1893 L. Von Dittil described a transperitoneal approach to vesicovaginal fistula. He dissected the bladder from the uterus and the vagina and closed the bladder defect abdominally. The following year, Mackenrodt described a technique of incising the vagina in the midline across the fistula, dissecting the bladder as completely as possible from the vaginal mucosa, and using multilayered closure of the bladder fascia and vaginal mucosa. Latzko (1942) reported his results using a technique suited to the vaginal repair of vesicovaginal fistulas resulting from abdominal tract hysterectomy.

TABLE 21–1. ETIOLOGY OF VESICOVAGINAL AND URETHROVAGINAL FISTULAS REPAIRED AT THE UNIVERSITY OF IOWA, 1926–1980

Etiology	Number of Cases	Per Cent
Gynecologic surgery	145	75.5
Obstetric trauma	28	14.6
Urologic procedures	10	5.2
Trauma from accidents	5	2.6
Radiation complications	4	2.1
Total	192	100.0

ETIOLOGY

Table 21–1 lists the etiologic factors in the 192 vesico- and urethrovaginal fistulas that were repaired at the University of Iowa Hospitals between 1926 and 1980. Three fourths are related to some type of gynecologic surgery. Most of the fistulas caused by obstetric trauma occurred prior to 1940. They resulted from tissue necrosis of the anterior vaginal wall and bladder secondary to prolonged labor, or were sustained at the time of a difficult forceps delivery or podalic version and extraction. With the advent of the antibiotic era and the increased availability of blood, it became relatively safe to perform a low cervical cesarean section, thereby eliminating the need for prolonged labors and traumatic vaginal deliveries. In Third World countries, where hospitals and medical care are still not readily available, obstetric complications remain the leading cause of vesicovaginal fistula.

Today the important etiologic factors in developed nations include: (1) gynecologic surgery, chiefly abdominal hysterectomy, (2) certain urologic procedures, (3) extensive pelvic trauma, and (4) occasional obstetric injury. Fistulas resulting from extension of carcinoma of the cervix or caused by radiation complications represent special problems and will be excluded from this discussion, since they can rarely be repaired vaginally. A fuller discussion is given in Chapters 27 and 28.

Hysterectomy

An increase in the number of operative fistulas has accompanied the greater incidence of hysterectomy. In our series (Table 21–2), 77.5 per cent of the fistulas were related to abdominal total hysterectomy and 20.6 per cent resulted from some type of vaginal operative procedure. It is interesting to note that of the vaginal procedures, only 8.9 per cent of the fistulas resulted from vaginal hysterectomy with anterior wall repair. The major indications for abdominal hysterectomies included small myomas, dysfunctional uterine bleeding, and carcinoma in situ; none of these disease entities should have produced marked anatomic distortion.

The marked difference in incidence of fistulas following abdominal and vaginal surgical procedures may be related to the relative frequency of the procedure. However, it has been my impression that family physicians and general surgeons seldom use the vaginal approach for gynecologic surgery, and family physicians in particular may be overrepresented in abdominal procedures with subsequent fistula formation. Between 1965 and 1980 we identified the specialty of the operator in 52 cases of vesicovaginal fistula. In 40 per cent the surgery was performed by a general practitioner who had surgical privileges, in 4 per cent by a urologist, in 32 per cent by a certified obstetrician and gynecologist, and in 24 per cent by a general surgeon. We do not have accurate information concerning the percentage of all gynecologic surgery done by each of the various groups, but it is our impression that the majority is done by the latter two specialties.

There are many reasons why vesicovaginal fistulas occur following an abdominal total hysterectomy. These include:

1. Distortion of the bladder by large myomas, endometriosis, or previous operative procedures.
2. Lack of experience or care on the part

TABLE 21–2. TYPES OF GYNECOLOGIC SURGERY PRODUCING VESICOVAGINAL FISTULAS

Type of Surgery	Number	Per Cent
Abdominal hysterectomy	111	76.6
Anterior wall repair only	12	8.3
Vaginal hysterectomy with repair	13	8.9
Removal of cervical stump	5	3.4
Radical hysterectomy	4	2.8
Total	145	100.0

of the surgeon in dissecting the bladder from the cervix and upper vagina.

3. Failure to recognize or test for bladder defects or injury at the time of surgery.

4. Failure to recognize the location of the bladder when placing sutures around the vaginal cuff to secure proper hemostasis.

If the surgeon is careful in dissection, tests for bladder defects when indicated, and recognizes the location of the bladder, very few fistulas should result from operative procedures for benign conditions. In our series, the majority of the patients with fistulas were referred to the University of Iowa Hospitals, and only 11 (6 per cent) of this series resulted from complications sustained in our department. This low incidence of fistulas is significant, since the majority of the operations were performed by resident physicians. It is interesting to note that none resulted from obstetric complications, two followed vaginal hysterectomy (0.07 per cent), five resulted from an abdominal hysterectomy (0.08 per cent), and four followed radical hysterectomy for Stage IB cervical cancer. There have been 170 bladder injuries that have been recognized at surgery, and all were successfully repaired.

Urologic Procedures

In the same series (Table 21–1), a variety of urologic procedures accounted for 5.2 per cent of the fistulas. These included extensive urethral dilation, resection of tissue at the vesicourethral junction and "Y-V" plastic repair of the bladder, fulgurations of bladder papillomas, and surgery for urethral diverticulum.

Trauma

There were five cases in which trauma was responsible for the defect, including traumatic perineal injuries with pelvic fractures and vaginal foreign body injuries.

SYMPTOMS AND DIAGNOSIS

Patients with fistulas resulting from obstetric trauma note leakage of urine immediately following delivery. However, patients with fistulas caused by operative trauma often develop their urinary incontinence 5 to 14 days following surgery. The amount of urine lost is directly related to the size and location of the fistula. With a small fistula the urinary leakage may be slight and in some instances dependent upon the position of the patient. These patients may void normal quantities of urine; however, in those with large fistulas, sufficient urine does not collect in the bladder to permit voiding. As long as the urine has free access to the vagina, most vesicovaginal fistulas are painless. It has been our experience that if patients change perineal pads frequently the vaginal leakage of urine does not redden or excoriate the vagina or vulvar tissues, nor does it produce pustules or infection of the vulva. It is true, however, that the odor of the urine may be offensive to the patient and to those in close contact with her. These patients are justifiably uncomfortable and inconvenienced by the continual loss of urine from the vagina.

Often the patients develop considerable hostility toward the responsible surgeon, particularly if he has shown reluctance to investigate the problem and talk to the patient about the cause of the vaginal discharge. Patients are often told that this is the normal discharge seen following surgery of this type and that it will eventually improve. At times, it may be days or even weeks before the correct diagnosis is made and discussed with the patient. During this time the patients are quite certain they are leaking urine from the vagina because of the odor and type of discharge. The importance of early investigation, diagnosis, and patient counseling is emphasized by a recent letter sent to one of us (W.C.K).

"I had a pelvic examination on January 16th because of a vaginal discharge and pelvic pain which was aggravated by sitting and bending. I was told this was caused by a fibroid tumor and infected tubes and that a hysterectomy was necessary. A total abdominal hysterectomy was performed on January 24th and I left the hospital in 7 days, having had no complications. However, soon after leaving the hospital a marked vaginal discharge developed. On February 18th I was re-admitted to the hospital because of vaginal leakage and was seen by a urologist who did a cystoscopic examination. He stated that I either had a (1) kinked ureter following surgery, (2) poisons damaged the bladder before surgery, (3) a doctor missed a stitch at the time of surgery, (4) possible adhesions, or (5) that I had been too active following surgery. My doctor reassured me this was not unusual and the urologist had found nothing wrong. He advised waiting several more months to see how things worked out. I was given prescriptions for estrogen and Tetracycline.

"The leakage continued and I was re-admitted to the hospital one month later and was seen by a second urologist who did another cystoscopic examination and this physician would not talk to me. My physician stated everything looked fine and that this was not uncommon and takes time to heal. In April I was referred to a physician who specializes in female problems and after an hour of testing in his office he stated I had stress incontinence and recommended estrogen injections and an exercise to strengthen my bladder muscles. These recommendations were carried out with no improvement.

"Later in the summer I asked to be referred elsewhere for another opinion. My doctor told me that he would not refer me nor would he send my records but when I threatened to see a lawyer he reluctantly referred me with my records. From July 1948 until my surgery in 1975 I enjoyed a normal marital life. Since my surgery I have given permission to my husband to have sex with other women. Needless to say, this arrangement has created problems and is not satisfactory but I am at 'wits end.' I realize that most doctors are usually run ragged and barely able to breathe but I hope you can help me."

The patient had a small vesicovaginal fistula that was successfully repaired.

As a rule the diagnosis is not difficult. The differential diagnosis includes vesicovaginal fistula, ureterovaginal fistula and severe stress or urge incontinence, vaginitis, and enterovaginal fistula. When the loss of urine is due to weakness of sphincter, urine usually can be seen to spurt from the ureteral meatus with straining. When the fistula is large, it can be palpated through the vagina or seen by careful inspection of the vaginal vault. Smaller fistulas are more difficult to detect. There is usually pooling of urine in the upper vagina, and on inspection one can see a small reddened area at the vaginal apex from which urine escapes. A small flexible wire probe is of help in demonstrating the bladder communication.

Diagnostic Aids

If no fistulous opening can readily be demonstrated, it may be identified by filling the bladder with a dilute solution of methylene blue and then inspecting the upper vagina. If no leakage can be demonstrated, two clean tampons are placed in the vagina, and the patient is asked to drink fluids and walk for a period of time. The tampons are then removed, and the upper one is inspected for the presence of dye. If there is no dye leakage with this test the physician should suspect a ureterovaginal fistula. Indigo carmine should then be given intravenously and the vagina again investigated for the presence of dye. The diagnosis should be confirmed by cystoscopy, which will show the ureteral orifice on the affected side failing to spurt urine. In most cases as a ureteral catheter is passed an obstruction can be felt when the tip reaches the point of ureteral injury.

MANAGEMENT OF VESICOVAGINAL FISTULA

Preparation for Surgery

Once the diagnosis of a vesicovaginal fistula has been established, there is no objection to leaving in a Foley catheter for a short period of time to encourage a spontaneous closure of the fistula. In our experience, however, this rarely occurs; we have seen this happen twice. A number of our patients have had fulguration in an attempt to close the fistula; this again is rarely successful and occasionally may increase rather than decrease the size of the defect.

Preoperative Investigation

All patients with vesicovaginal fistulas should have preoperative cystoscopic examination to determine the size and location of the fistula and particularly the relationship of the ureteral orifices to the fistulous tract. If the ureteral orifices are 0.5 cm. or less from the edge of the fistula or if the fistula is well away from the midline, a ureteral catheter should be placed prior to the surgery.

Intravenous urography should also be a

routine part of the preoperative investigation. Hydroureter or hydronephrosis suggests a ureteral fistula caused by scarring in the region of the ureteral orifice. The preoperative urogram should be a matter of record for the protection of the patient and surgeon.

Management of Incontinence

One of the most distressing problems for the patient awaiting for surgery is the control of the urinary incontinence. There is really no satisfactory method of coping with this problem. The continuous drainage of the bladder with a large Foley catheter may partially reduce the amount of leakage, but is uncomfortable for the patient and may predispose to bladder infections. If there is prolonged administration of antibiotics to prevent recurrent urinary tract infections, the patient is subjected to recurrent candida infections. Some clinicians have advocated the use of a tarsette cup inserted in the upper vagina to collect the urine. In our experience this is seldom successful. In the patients whose preoperative care we have directed, we have not used catheter drainage or antibiotics. If pads are changed frequently, there has been no problem with perineal irritation or urinary tract infections.

Timing of Surgery

The timing of the surgery is most important and must be determined on an individual basis. It may take from 3 to 6 months for the edema and inflammatory changes to subside, and timing is best determined by periodic pelvic examinations. In recent years we have been doing the repair 3 to 4 months following the initial surgery. We have had no experience with the use of large amounts of corticosteroids, as advocated by Collins and associates (1960), to eliminate the inflammatory changes so the the patient may be operated upon within 2 to 3 weeks. This technique has been advocated for a number of years but has not received wide acceptance.

It is well to remember that the physician who performs the initial repair is in the best position to effect a cure.

Surgical Considerations

Choice of Approach

The choice of the approach to repair the vesicovaginal fistula is extremely important and seems to vary with the specialty of the surgeon. Urologists and general surgeons, being more familiar with abdominal surgery, use either a transvesical or transperitoneal approach (Chapter 22). Gynecologists, since the time of Sims, have used the vaginal approach and have achieved the highest cure rates reported. In most instances, the fistula is accessible by the vaginal approach, there is minimal blood loss, the patient has none of the problems of a transabdominal operation, and the morbidity and mortality rates are very low. However, there are a few high-vault fistulas with extensive scarring for which a combined approach (vaginal plus transvesical closure) may be required. There are also combined vesicoureterovaginal or vesicorectovaginal fistulas requiring both a vaginal and abdominal approach. One should not close one's mind to any single technique for the repair, and each case should be considered individually.

In our experience, when the vaginal approach is used, exposure may best be accomplished by placing the patient in the lithotomy position with the buttocks well down on the table. We seldom have had to enlarge the introitus with a Schuchardt's incision to gain access to the fistula. We have not found it necessary to use the knee-chest position or the lateral Sims's position to gain better operative exposure.

Fistula Identification

As mentioned previously, if the ureteral orifices are near the margin of the fistula it is wise to have ureteral catheters placed prior to the surgery. If the fistula is very small it is often helpful to have the urologist pass a small ureteral catheter from the bladder through the tract into the vagina for ease of identification. With a small to moderate-sized fistula, it is wise to place traction sutures above and below the fistula, which may be used for traction and are useful in identifying the opening. If some method of fistula identification is not used, it is surprising how hard it is to find the fistula opening after the dissection has been completed. In some patients we have inserted a small Foley catheter through the fistula and used this for traction.

Technique of Repair

With the patient in the dorsal lithotomy position and using a weighted speculum, the fistula tract is identified using a blunt wire probe. Once the fistula tract is adequately identified, two stay sutures are placed either laterally or in an anteroposterior direction to assist not only in identification of the fistula, but also in tenting the vaginal mucosa during the initial dissection.

The dissection is begun anteriorly, usually 2 to 3 cm. posterior to the urethrovesical angle, much the same as is done in an anterior colporrhaphy (Figure 21–1). As the fistula tract is approached, the dissection is carried laterally around the fistula on either side, continuing to mobilize adequate amounts of pubovesical fascia. This will effect a teardrop configuration when the dissection is completed (Figure 21–2).

There should be wide denudation of the vaginal mucosa, so that the bladder is sufficiently mobilized, permitting a multilayered closure of the bladder defect without undue tension. The mobilization is accomplished by both sharp and blunt dissection, separating the vaginal mucosa from the bladder fascia. Small, long, narrow instruments should be used. For blunt dissection, the use of the knife handle and small pieces of dental roll (Kitners) are of great help. As a rule, excessive blood loss is not a problem. In patients who have had an abdominal hysterectomy, the posterior dissection may be most difficult because of scarring and distortion. One must be careful not to injure the colon, as it may be very close to the margin of dissection. Occasionally, the peritoneal cavity may be entered in this phase of the dissection; after proper identification, the defect is closed. After the

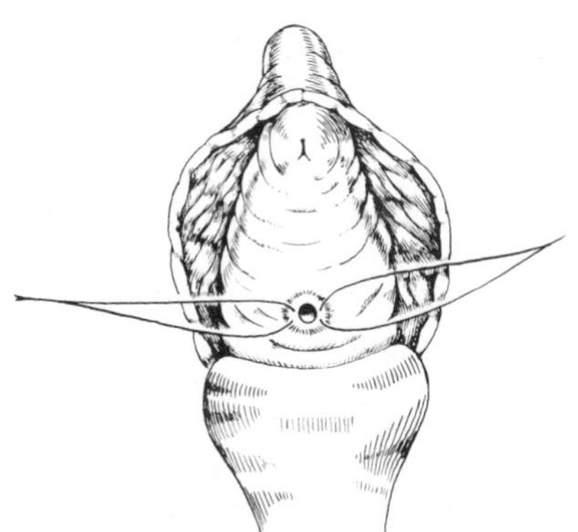

Figure 21–1. Placement of two 2–0 silk identification sutures. These are also used to tent the fistula tract, so that the dissection of the vaginal mucosa can be made more easily.

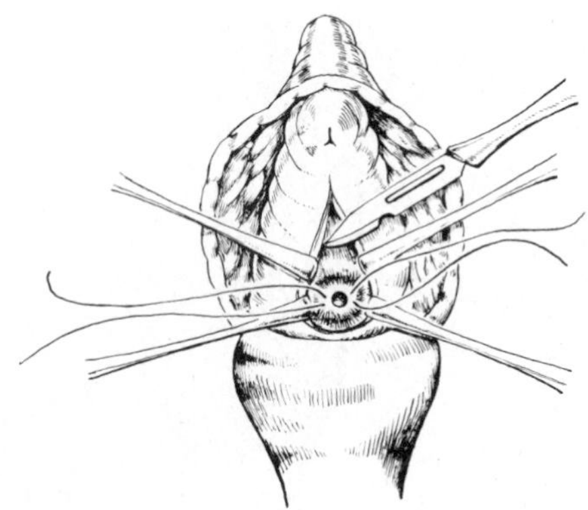

Figure 21–2. Mobilization of the anterior vaginal wall circumferentially around the fistula tract.

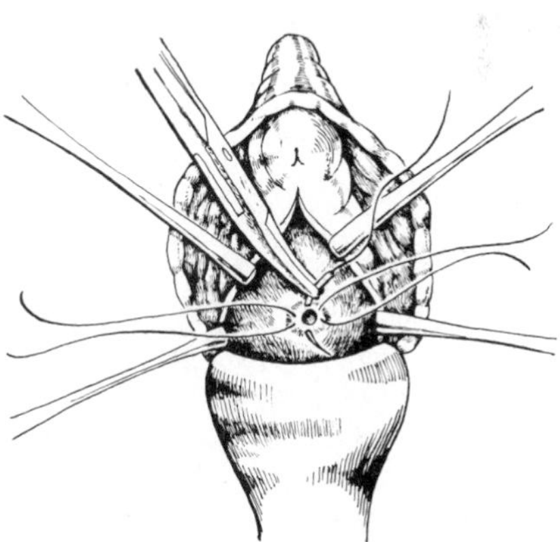

Figure 21–3. Wide mobilization of the tissue surrounding the fistula site is shown. It is imperative to mobilize the pubovesical fascia, not only proximally and laterally, but also distally from the vaginal cuff. After adequate wide mobilization, 3-0 chromic catgut sutures are placed through the fistula tract to effect a watertight first layer closure.

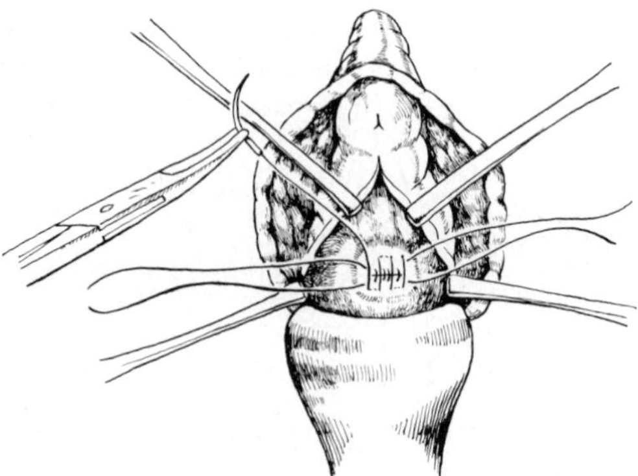

Figure 21–4. The first line of sutures is in place and the second line of imbricating 3-0 chromic catgut sutures is shown. This suture line may be placed either longitudinally or transversely, depending on the direction in which the pubovesical fascia is most adequately dissected.

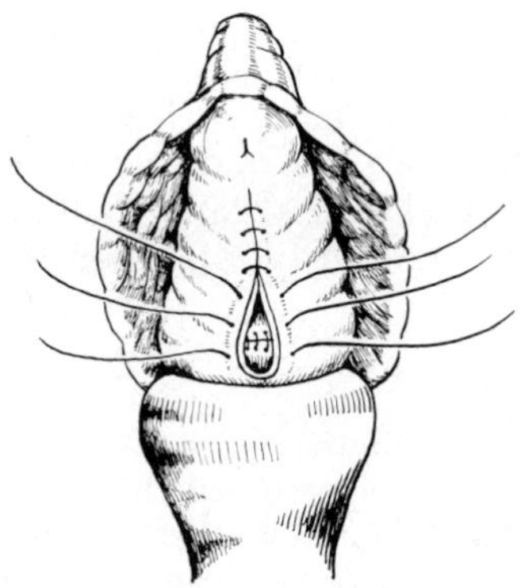

Figure 21–6. Completion of the operation by closure of the vaginal mucosa with interrupted 2-0 chromic catgut sutures over the three-layer closure of this fistula tract.

fistula has been mobilized for a distance of 1.5 to 2 cm., the vaginal epithelium remaining around the fistula opening should be removed. Once adequate wide mobilization has been attained, the first line of suture is placed using 3–0 chromic catgut (Figure 21–3).

Sutures are placed in either corner of the fistula, usually at its lateral extents. Interrupted sutures are used, and the number may range anywhere from as few as three sutures to as many as eight or ten, depending on the size of the fistula. These sutures are then tied, and after this is completed the suture line is checked for watertightness by instilling 200 to 300 ml. of methylene blue into the bladder through a Foley catheter. If the closure is satisfactory, a second imbricating suture line is placed using 3–0 chromic catgut (Figure 21–4).

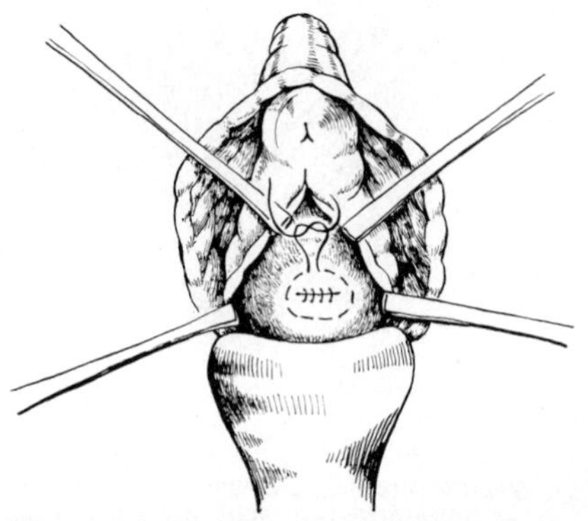

Figure 21–5. Placement of a third suture line. It may be done in either a purse-string fashion, as shown here, or by placing a third imbricating layer of 3-0 chromic catgut in an interrupted fashion.

This may be done in either an anterior or a posterior direction or in a side-to-side direction, depending on where there is adequate mobilization of the pubovesical fascia (Figure 21–5).

A third imbricating layer may be placed, either as a purse-string suture or in an interrupted fashion, usually in an opposite plane from which the second suture line was placed. Occasionally, when there is adequate redundant pubovesical fascia, a fourth suture line may be placed. The repair site is again checked for watertightness, and, if it has been achieved, the vaginal mucosa is then closed over the repair site, and the ureteral catheters are removed (Figure 21–6).

A vaginal pack is not used, as it may cause undue pressure on the closed suture lines.

If the fistula is high in the vault and was not easily mobilized because of scarring and fixation, or if the surgeon is not satisfied with the vaginal closure, a combined transvesical closure will prevent failures. We have used this combined approach on six patients.

As previously mentioned, fistulas due to obstetric trauma are now rarely seen in the United States. Such fistulas, when they occur, are often rather large and frequently involve the entire vaginal wall down to the cervix. These fistulas are readily accessible, and it is relatively easy to dissect the tissues laterally and separate the bladder from the cervix. After such wide mobilization a multilayered closure can be accomplished.

Postoperative Care

The most important aspect of the postoperative care is proper bladder drainage so that the bladder does not become distended. We use a No. 18 French Foley catheter with a 5 ml. bag, which is carefully taped to the inner aspect of the thigh. The catheter is left in place for 12 days; patients void well after its removal and need not be checked for residual urine. In complicated fistulas, where a combined approach has been used, dual drainage (suprapubic and urethral) is used. Prophylactic antibiotics are not employed, and we seldom encounter a urinary tract infection provided that the patient has an adequate fluid intake. With the vaginal approach our morbidity has been below 10 per cent and there has been no mortality.

The patients are encouraged to ambulate the next day, with no restriction on activity. It is advisable to use stool softeners to avoid fecal impactions or excessive straining with a bowel movement. The patients are not examined vaginally at the time of discharge, but a rectal examination should be performed to determine if there is any evidence of operative bed induration. The patients are given careful instructions to refrain from intercourse or douching until after the final examination 6 weeks later.

URETHROVAGINAL FISTULA

A urethrovaginal fistula represents a special problem for many reasons. The causes of these fistulas are slightly different from those of a vesicovaginal fistula. In the 22 patients we have seen with this problem, 10 fistulas were related to obstetric trauma, three resulted from urologic surgery, and two were related to other trauma. The seven that resulted from gynecologic surgery occurred in patients having anterior wall repairs with or without vaginal hysterectomy. One patient developed a fistula 10 years after a Kelly urethral plication with silk sutures. Several sutures had eroded through the urethral mucosa at the vesicourethral junction. This type of fistula may be difficult to diagnose unless direct urethroscopic examination is utilized. It can be difficult to repair because (1) the urethral damage is extensive; (2) the defect may be at the vesicourethral junction, involving both bladder and urethra; (3) there may be extensive scarring, and (4) after the urethral defect has been closed there is often insufficient tissue for a second layer closure. In such cases we have used the bulbocavernosus fat pad from the inner aspect of the large labia as described many years ago by Martius (1956). This has been of great help as a second layer of tissue under the vaginal mucosa. Because of these problems the cure rate is not as high as with vesicovaginal fistula, and some patients have problems with stress incontinence.

WHAT IS THE CURE RATE?

In our clinic we have used the vaginal approach in all patients, except six with high fistulas in whom a combined approach was used, and six in whom an abdominal approach was used. This latter group had unusual combinations of fistulas, such as cecovesicovaginal, sigmoidovesicovaginal, ureterovesicocervical, and ureterovesicovaginal. Between July 1, 1926, and January 1, 1981, we operated upon 192 patients of whom 168 had vesicovaginal fistulas and 24 had urethrovaginal fistulas.

Many of these patients had between one and three previous attempts at closure prior to being referred to the University of Iowa Hospitals. Our initial cure rate was 89.5 per cent, the final cure rate for 168 patients with vesicovaginal fistulas was 94.2 per cent, and the cure rate for the 24 patients with urethrovaginal fistulas 87.5 per cent. One of us (W.C.K.) has personally repaired 75 vesico- and urethrovaginal fistulas with an initial success rate of 91 per cent; six patients required a second operation and one patient had three repairs for a final 100 per cent cure rate. Table 21–3 indicates that our results compare favorably with those of others.

TABLE 21–3. RESULTS IN VARIOUS SERIES OF REPAIRED VESICOVAGINAL FISTULAS

Authors	Year	Cases	%Cured
Sims	1860	261	82.7
Simon	1869	105	89.5
Todd	1909	131	71.5
Bey	1930	300	87.0
Miller	1944	51	84.3
Counsellor	1956	224	87.3
Everett and Mattingly	1956	117	92.2
Moir	1956	133	98.0
Collins and Jones	1957	31	90.9
Keettel and Laube	present series	168	94.2

Delayed Complications

The only late complication which we have noted is that a few patients have had stress or urge incontinence. These problems have tended to occur in the very elderly, in those who have had a radical hysterectomy for cervical cancer, and in those with considerable scarring and bladder fixation. In none of these patients was the problem serious enough to warrant surgery for the stress incontinence.

REFERENCES

Bey, N. M.: Vesicovaginal fistula in women. J. Obstet. Gynaecol. Br. Emp. *37*:566, 1930.

Collins, C. G., and Jones, F. B.: Properative cortisone for vaginal fistulas. Obstet. Gynecol. *9*:533, 1957.

Collins, C. G., Pent, D., and Jones, F. B.: Results of early repair of vesicovaginal fistula with preliminary cortisone treatment. Am. J. Obstet. Gynecol. *80*:1005, 1960.

Counseller, V. S., and Haigler, F. H.: Management of urinary vaginal fistula in 253 cases. Am. J. Obstet. Gynecol. *72*:367, 1956.

Everett, H. S., and Mattingly, R. F.: Urinary tract injuries resulting from pelvic surgery. Am. J. Obstet. Gynecol. *71*:502, 1956.

Kelly, H. A.: The history of vesicovaginal fistula. Trans. Am. Gynecol. Soc. *37*:3, 1912.

Latzko, W.: Postoperative vesicovaginal fistulas. Am. J. Surg. *58*:211, 1942.

Martius, H.: Gynecological Operations. Boston, Little, Brown and Co., 1956.

Miller, N. F.: The surgical treatment and postoperative care of vesicovaginal fistula. Am. J. Obstet. Gynecol. *44*:873, 1942.

Moir, J. C.: Personal experiences in treatment of vesicovaginal fistulas. Am. J. Obstet. Gynecol. *71*:471, 1956.

Sims, J. M.: The treatment of vesicovaginal fistula. Am. J. Med. Sci. *23*:59, 1852.

Todd, J. F.: Instrumental injury of the urinary tract. Women's Med. J. *XIX*:181, 1909.

22

SUPRAPUBIC TRANSVESICAL CLOSURE OF VESICOVAGINAL FISTULA

JOHN B. NANNINGA, M.D.
VINCENT J. O'CONOR, Jr., M.D.

Vesicovaginal fistula results most commonly from pelvic surgical procedures, usually abdominal hysterectomy. Rarely the fistula occurs after prolonged labor or difficult delivery. Surgical procedures on the bladder neck may also contribute to vesicovaginal fistula. In patients who have received radiation therapy, fistulas may occur years later with or without the presence of carcinoma.

The mechanism for fistula formation is either a surgical injury or subsequent necrosis of the bladder wall. The immediate appearance of urine in the vagina after a surgical procedure indicates an injury in the bladder that allows urine to leak out through the vaginal cuff. The development of a urine leak 10 to 20 days postoperatively usually indicates necrosis of tissue on the posterior bladder wall. Contributing to this may be an abscess at the vaginal cuff. In our experience, the average time for the appearance of urine in the vagina following abdominal hysterectomy has been 20 days, with a range of 5 to 120 days. The development of a fistula years after hysterectomy had been performed for carcinoma should be taken as a sign of carcinoma until proved otherwise. If the patient underwent radiation therapy, however, the fistula may be due to necrosis resulting from endarteritis in the involved tissue.

DIAGNOSIS

The diagnosis of vesicovaginal fistula is usually rather obvious. The patient notes the continual leakage of urine from the vagina. The presence of the fistula is confirmed by instilling dye such as methylene blue into the bladder and noting the immediate appearance of the blue color in the vagina. Cystoscopy will aid in locating the site of the fistula in the bladder and in evaluating the condition of the surrounding bladder wall and proximity of the ureteral orifices to the fistula. An excretory urogram will demonstrate any ureteral or renal obstruction. If a ureteral injury is suspected, an intravenous injection of indigo carmine will produce colored urine in the vagina from a ureteral fistula, assuming that the bladder is intact. A retrograde ureterogram usually is required for the diagnosis of a ureteral fistula.

TREATMENT

When a fistula is diagnosed, the patient is placed on indwelling urethral catheter drainage; this in itself may be enough to bring about healing. We have used this successfully in cases of new fistulas as well as in cases of leakage after repair of a

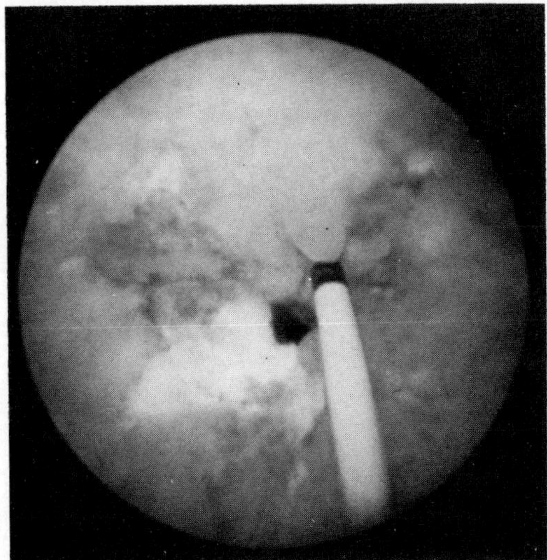

Figure 22–1. A cystoscopic view shows an electrode next to a small vesicovaginal fistula, which is to be fulgurated.

fistula. If the fistula is very small (1 to 2 mm.) and is surrounded by relatively normal tissue, the tract can be coagulated by cystoscopy (Figure 22–1). This has resulted in cure in seven of eight patients in whom it has been performed in the last 10 years. If catheter drainage does not result in healing after several weeks, surgical repair is indicated. During the waiting period for repair, the catheter may or may not be removed, depending on how effectively it keeps the patient dry.

The timing of the closure is quite important in achieving success. A waiting period of about 3 months has been recommended so as to allow the surrounding tissues to regain viability and the scarred, ischemic tissue to delineate. Collins and associates (1971) recommended early closure after a course of steroids, which should decrease inflammation and scarring. As we have not followed this plan, we cannot speak for or against it. Early closure using a peritoneal flap or omental flap to reinforce the repair has also been recommended. The interposed tissue aids in keeping the bladder and vagina separated and in vascularizing the area. In those fistulas that appear immediately after surgery, an early repair may at least be considered because the leak is more likely to be from a surgical injury in the bladder than from necrosis (Persky et al., 1979).

In patients who have undergone radiation treatment, the repair may be delayed up to a year. During this interval, the presence or absence of tumor can be established. The tissue surrounding the fistula may regain some vascularization, although this is unlikely if the fistula occurs many years later. Most fistulas resulting from radiation appear within 2 to 3 years after treatment, although they may occur as long as 20 years later (Graham, 1965).

The choice of operation depends somewhat on the location of the fistula. When the tract is located near the bladder neck or trigone, the vaginal route affords satisfactory exposure for the repair (Chapter 21). Those who employ the vaginal repair have reported excellent results (Keettel et al., 1978).

Our experience has been with the suprapubic transvesical closure of the fistula. This route offers excellent exposure for those fistulas located on the trigone and posterior wall of the bladder. This technique also allows for the reimplantation of the ureter if it is involved in the fistula. Finally, in those fistulas that have recurred

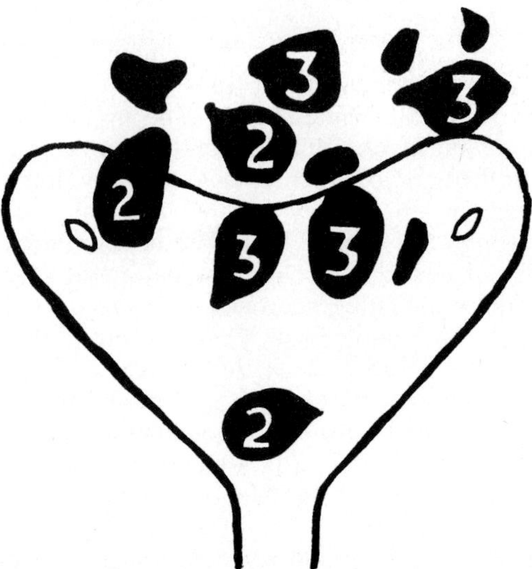

Figure 22–2. The relative sizes and locations of the 23 vesicovaginal fistulas that the authors have repaired during the past 10 years using suprapubic transvesical closure are illustrated.

or are secondary to radiation, omentum or peritoneum can be incorporated in the repair.

Figure 22–2 shows the relative locations and sizes of 23 vesicovaginal fistulas that we have repaired by the suprapubic route during the past 10 years. The fistula resulted from abdominal hysterectomy in 21 patients and from dilatation and curettage in two. Suprapubic transvesical closure was successful on the first attempt in 20 patients; the three patients in whom the first attempt failed each underwent a successful repeat procedure. We attributed the failures of the first attempt to incomplete removal of all of the old scar in the bladder side in two cases and to inadequate mobilization of the apex of the closure, with resultant tension on this part of the suture line, in the third (O'Conor et al., 1973; O'Conor, 1980).

TECHNIQUE

The history and early results of the suprapubic transvesical repair of vesicovaginal fistula have been described by O'Conor (1957). The technique of bisecting the bladder to gain accessibility to the fistula is derived in part from the technique of marsupialization of adherent bladder diverticula and from an intraperitoneal approach, which O'Conor (1957) attributed to Swift-Joly. The procedure will be described as it is now performed.

First, the bladder is exposed through a midline abdominal incision. It may be possible to perform the procedure retroperitoneally, but the peritoneum usually is opened as the bladder is divided down to the fistula. By placement of traction sutures on the bladder wall as it is divided, the fistula is exposed and the bladder can be lifted somewhat to facilitate exposure of the fistula. Figure 22–3*A* shows how the bladder wall is divided and separated from the underlying vagina so that the fistula can be excised. Further dissection then frees the surrounding bladder wall and separates the vagina.

Ureteral catheters aid in identifying the ureter if it is in close proximity to the fistula. When the fistula has been excised and the scarred edges of the vagina trimmed away, the vagina is closed with continuous 2-0 chromic gut and a second layer of 2-0 chromic gut. The bladder is then closed with a continuous 2-0 chromic gut on the muscle layer, the knot being on the outside. There should be no tension on the closure (Figure 22–3*B*). A second layer of sutures, interrupted size 0 chromic gut, is then placed on the seromuscular layer (Figure 22–3*C*). At the end of the closure, a suprapubic catheter is inserted and is left in place for 10 to 14 days.

If the repair was difficult, the catheter is left for several weeks. A urethral catheter may also be used for drainage and irrigation. We do not keep the patient in a prone position or apply suction to the catheter. If there is leakage from the suprapubic site following the removal of the suprapubic tube, a urethral catheter is inserted for several days to allow healing of the suprapubic tract. If a patient has undergone radiation therapy, the catheter drainage is maintained for a minimum of 6 weeks.

For the patient with a large fistula and extensive scarring, the use of a peritoneal flap or pedicle of omentum offers a chance for cure. The idea of using omentum is not new. Walters described its use for vesicovaginal fistula repair in 1937. Subsequently, the use of omentum in the repair of vesicovaginal fistula has been described by others (Turner-Warwick et al., 1967; Kirichuta and Goldstein, 1972; Eisen et al., 1974; Wein et al., 1980).

The omentum, if well mobilized, will extend to the deep pelvis. It is necessary to maintain either of the two gastroepiploic arteries to ensure adequate vascularization. This can be accomplished from either the right or the left side, depending on the location of the bladder defect. The omentum is interposed between the vaginal and bladder suture lines with absorbable sutures. With the omentum between the vagina and the bladder, the bladder is then closed and the omentum is sutured to the posterior aspect of the bladder with 2-0 absorbable sutures. Other anchoring sutures are placed in the omentum and attached to the right or left colic gutter.

We have not used nonabsorbable suture because of the possibility of urine coming into contact with the omental flap. We have

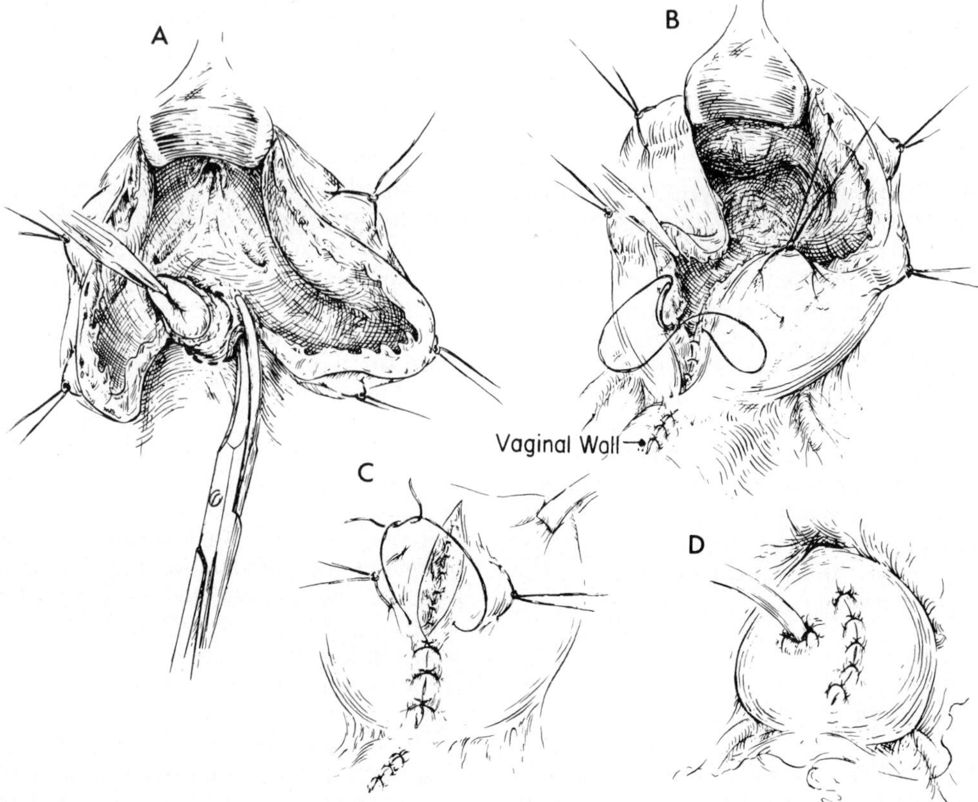

Figure 22–3. Suprapubic transvesical repair of vesicovaginal fistula. *A,* The fistula is being excised after the bladder has been bisected down to the opening. *B,* The vaginal wall has been closed and the first layer of the bladder closure is beginning. *C,* The second layer of the bladder closure is being completed. *D,* The suprapubic catheter is in place. Note that the vaginal closure can be covered with a flap of peritoneum or omentum. (Reproduced with permission from O'Conor, V. J., Jr.: Female urinary incontinence and vesicovaginal fistula. *In* J. F. Glenn [Ed.]: Urologic Surgery. 2nd Ed. Hagerstown, Maryland, Harper & Row, 1975, p. 778.)

noted that in one patient, a small piece of omentum was sloughed from the vagina and urine leaked for about 5 days. The leakage stopped on catheter drainage over a 2 week period, however. Because of the possibility of a urine leak and calcification of nonabsorbable suture, we have used only chromic gut.

Some mention should be made of those patients in whom there is little chance of success in closing the fistula. These include patients who have suffered from recurrent neoplasm, radiation changes, or pelvic trauma, and those in whom multiple attempts at closure have failed. Marshall (1979) has pointed out that in 23 per cent of his cases, no attempt at functional closure was made. Our experience has been that about 30 per cent of patients are ineligible for closure of the fistula for the previously mentioned reasons. In such individuals, the use of some form of urinary diversion usually has been a more realistic means of achieving a dry perineum.

REFERENCES

Collins, C. G., Collins, J. H., Harrison, B. R., Nicholls, R. A., Hoffman, E. S., and Krupp, P. J.: Early repair of vesicovaginal fistula. Am. J. Obstet. Gynecol. *111*:524, 1971.

Eisen, M., Jurkovic, K., Altwein, J., Schreiter, F., and Hohenfellner, R.: Management of vesicovaginal fistulas with peritoneal flap interposition. J. Urol. *112*:195, 1974.

Graham, J. B.: Vaginal fistulas following radiotherapy. Surg. Gynecol. Obstet. *120*:1019, 1965.

Keettel, W. C., Sehring, F. C., deProsse, C. A., and Scott, J. R.: Surgical management of urethrovaginal and vesicovaginal fistulas. Am. J. Obstet. Gynecol. *131*:425, 1978.

Kirichuta, I., and Goldstein, A.: The repair of extensive vesicovaginal fistulas with pedicled omentum: a review of 27 cases. J. Urol. *108*:724, 1972.

Marshall, V. F.: Vesicovaginal fistulas on one urological service. J. Urol. *121*:25, 1979.

O'Conor, V. J.: Suprapubic Closure of Vesicovaginal Fistula. Springfield, Illinois, Charles C Thomas, 1957.

O'Conor, V. J., Jr.: Review of experience with vesicovaginal fistula repair. J. Urol. *123*:367, 1980.

O'Conor, V. J., Jr., Sokol, J. K., Bulkley, G. J., and Nanninga, J. B.: Suprapubic closure of vesicovaginal fistula. J. Urol. *109*:51, 1973.

Persky, L., Herman, G., and Guerrier, K.: Nondelay in vesicovaginal fistula repair. Urology *13*:273, 1979.

Turner-Warwick, R., Wynne, E., and Handley-Ashken, M.: Omental pedicle graft. Br. J. Surg. *54*:849, 1967.

Walters, W.: An omental flap in transperitoneal repair of recurring vesicovaginal fistulas. Surg. Gynecol. Obstet. *64*:74, 1937.

Wein, A. J., Malloy, T. R., Carpiniello, V., Greenburg, S. H., and Murphy, J. J.: Repair of vesicovaginal fistula by a suprapubic transvesical approach. Surg. Gynecol. Obstet. *150*:57, 1980.

23

INCONTINENCE SECONDARY TO NEUROGENIC BLADDER, ANATOMIC DEFECTS, AND URGENCY

STEFAN A. H. LOENING, M.D.
DAVID A. CULP, M.D.

The function of the bladder and urethra is to provide a reservoir and a propelling force for evacuation of urine at appropriate times. Impairment of one or both of these functions may be responsible for urinary incontinence (Herwig, 1974).

TYPES OF INCONTINENCE

In order to choose the most appropriate methods of management, it is important to differentiate clinically between true, overflow (paradoxical), stress, and urge (urgency) incontinence. The type of incontinence can be determined by careful study of the patient's history and symptoms and by thorough physical examination.

True Incontinence

With true incontinence the patient is wet from a constant leakage of urine; there is no sensation of bladder fullness or voiding, and the bladder has lost its capacity to function as a reservoir with appropriate voidings. Trauma to the external sphincter with difficult delivery can result in this type of incontinence.

Overflow Incontinence

Overflow, or paradoxical, incontinence occurs with an overdistended bladder. The intravesical pressure becomes higher than the resistance of the urinary sphincter or the obstruction to bladder outflow, resulting in a constant dribble of urine. On physical examination a distended bladder can be felt suprapubically. The patient with acute overflow incontinence without neurologic deficit is in extreme discomfort. This condition is frequently seen in patients following surgery and demands catheterization. Overflow incontinence may also occur without symptoms, as in urethral stenosis. A gradual buildup of residual urine may go unnoticed by the patient until the urinary incontinence leads to the diagnosis.

Stress Incontinence

Urinary leakage at times of increased intra-abdominal pressure, such as with coughing, laughing, straining, or lifting, is described as stress incontinence. This type of incontinence is often absent or at least milder in the sitting or supine position. With increase of abdominal pressure the urine spurts out involuntarily. The volume evacuated depends on the generated abdominal pressure, the degree of anatomic or neurologic deficit, and the volume of urine present in the bladder. The most frequently found anatomic defects in the female associated with stress incontinence are cystocele and short urethra. Stress incontinence is further described in Chapter 13.

Urge Incontinence

With urge or urgency incontinence the initial sensation of fullness is followed almost immediately by an undeniable urge to void. This type of incontinence can be found in a patient with an irritated bladder secondary to infection or the presence of a stone, tumor, or foreign body, or following x-ray therapy. Uninhibited and reflex neurogenic bladders are also characterized by urge incontinence.

NEUROLOGIC LESIONS PRODUCING INCONTINENCE

Innervation of the Urinary Tract

The frontal lobes anterior to the motor cortex contain the center for the voluntary control of micturition (Chapter 3). From here the first loop of nerves reaches to the pontine mesencephalic reticular formation. At the level of the brain stem this first circuit also receives impulses from the thalamus and cerebellum. The second loop, the reticulospinal circuit, consists of neural pathways from the brain stem to the intermediolateral portion of the sacral spinal cord at the level of S2, S3, and S4, the micturition reflex center. From the sacral cord a third loop innervates the bladder and urethra. These pathways contain parasympathetic motor and somatic nerves. Part of the urethral smooth muscle is supplied by adrenergic fibers and is responsible for some of the tonicity and resistance of the urinary sphincter mechanism. Figure 23–1 shows the innervation of the bladder and the urethra and normal cystometrogram findings.

Tests of Function and Innervation

To determine abnormalities in function and innervation the physician can employ several diagnostic procedures: cystometry, ice water test, electromyography, sphincterometry, and uroflowmetry. Cystometry with air or water is the method most commonly used to evaluate bladder function and sensation. First the patient is asked to urinate. It is important to have a qualified person observe the act of micturition and note the size and force of the urinary stream, as well as hesitancy, straining, or intermittency of urination. After the patient has voided, a urethral catheter is inserted and residual urine measured. During cystometry the volumes at the first desire to void and at the feeling of fullness are recorded. Also noted are uninhibited contractions, which are never seen in the normal bladder. To test sensation, hot and then cold water is instilled. Abnormality in the sensory examination may also be manifested by impaired or absent sensation with bladder filling, bladder pain, or vesical paresthesia. Information gained from sensory examination by cystometry of the bladder mucosa and muscle is of two kinds: (1) exteroceptive, comprising pain, touch, and temperature, and (2) proprioceptive, related to the sensation induced by bladder filling and stretch of the bladder muscle during cystometry (Bradley, 1975). Compared with the characteristic cystometrogram findings of a normal bladder (Figure 23–1), uninhibited and reflex neurogenic bladders, or upper motor neuron bladders, show a "shift to the left" (Figures 23–2, 23–3). Cystometrograms in lower motor neuron bladders show a "shift to the right" (Figures 23–4, 23–5, 23–6).

Other tests of sensory innervation include touch, or pinprick sensation, in the perineal or perianal area. This test yields important clues concerning the intactness of the micturition center located in the sacral cord at S2 to S4, since there dermatomes emanate from the same portion of the cord receiving visceral sensory impulses from the bladder. Another method for determining the intactness of the lower arc is the bulbocavernosus reflex, which clinically evaluates the contractile response in the anal sphincter in response to a stimulation of the bulbocavernosus muscle. If there are normal contractions, the examiner can assume that the reflex arc via the pudendal nerve is intact because the motor innervation of the bladder and urethra

NORMAL BLADDER

RESIDUAL URINE	0 cc
CAPACITY	500 cc
UNINHIBITED CONTRACTIONS	none
URECHOLINE TEST	negative
PROPRIOCEPTIVE SENSATION	
1st. desire	150 cc
fullness	450 cc
EXTEROCEPTIVE SENSATION	
hot	present
cold	present

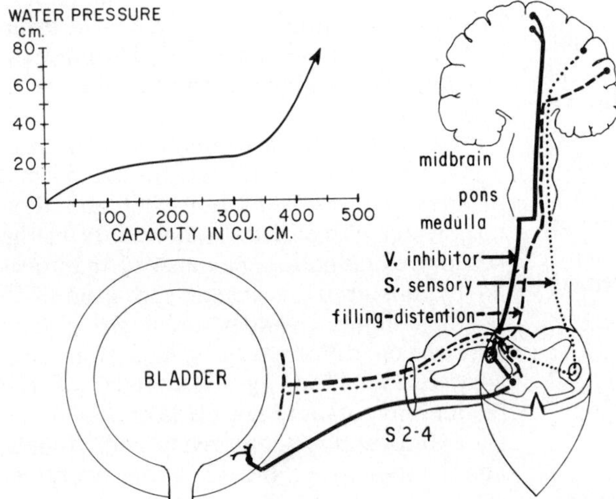

Figure 23–1. Normal bladder innervation and cystometrogram findings.

UNINHIBITED NEUROGENIC BLADDER

RESIDUAL URINE	0 cc
CAPACITY	50–300 cc
UNINHIBITED CONTRACTIONS	present
URECHOLINE TEST	positive
PROPRIOCEPTIVE SENSATION	
1st. desire	50–100 cc
fullness	50–150 cc
EXTEROCEPTIVE SENSATION	
hot	present
cold	present

LESION:
Higher cerebral centers— may be diffuse
a. motor leg
b. internal capsule

s. sensory
v. inhibitor

Figure 23–2. Uninhibited neurogenic bladder: lesions and cystometrogram findings.

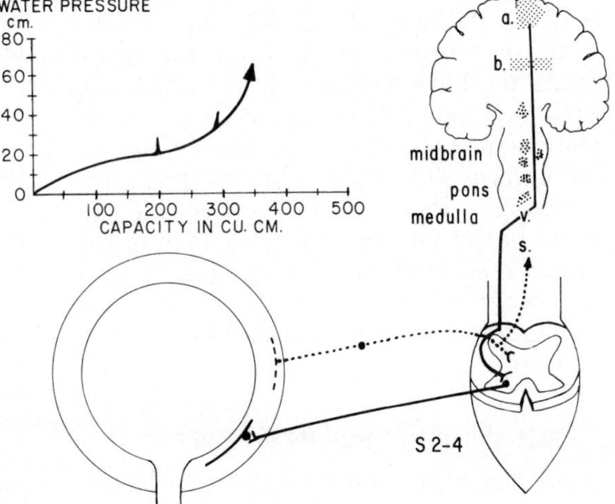

REFLEX NEUROGENIC BLADDER

RESIDUAL URINE __________ increased
CAPACITY __________ decreased
UNINHIBITED CONTRACTIONS __ present
URECHOLINE TEST __________ positive
PROPRIOCEPTIVE SENSATION
1st. desire __________ variable
fullness __________ variable
EXTEROCEPTIVE SENSATION
hot __________ absent
cold __________ absent

LESION:
Transection above sacral segments

s. sensory
v. inhibitor

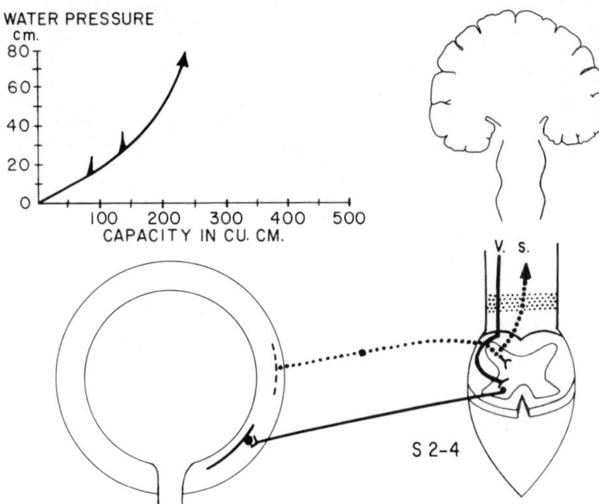

Figure 23–3. Reflex neurogenic bladder: lesions and cystometrogram findings.

MOTOR PARALYTIC BLADDER

RESIDUAL URINE __________ increased
CAPACITY __________ increased
UNINHIBITED CONTRACTIONS __ absent
URECHOLINE TEST __________ positive
PROPRIOCEPTIVE SENSATION
1st. desire ; at high
fullness volumes
EXTEROCEPTIVE SENSATION
hot __________ present
cold __________ present

LESION:
anterior horns and roots

S. sensory
V. inhibitor.

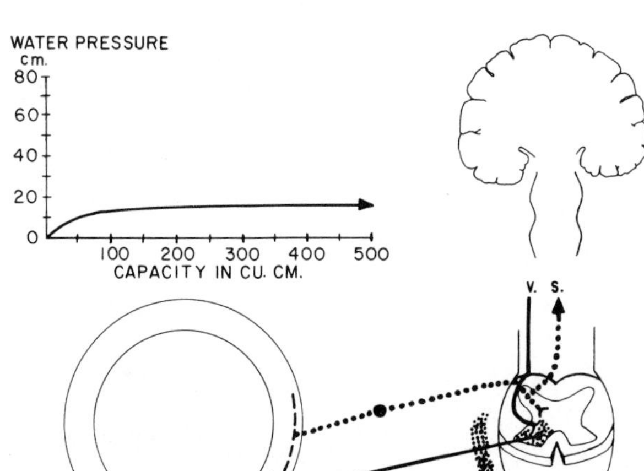

Figure 23–4. Motor paralytic bladder: lesions and cystometrogram findings.

SENSORY NEUROGENIC BLADDER

RESIDUAL URINE ________ increased
CAPACITY ________ increased
UNINHIBITED CONTRACTIONS _ absent
URECHOLINE TEST ________ positive
PROPRIOCEPTIVE SENSATION
  1st. desire ________ absent
  fullness ________ absent
EXTEROCEPTIVE SENSATION
  hot ________ absent
  cold ________ absent

LESION:
sensory pathways _
a. post. roots
b. post. columns

S. sensory
V. inhibitor

WATER PRESSURE
cm.
80
60
40
20
0
100 200 300 400 500
CAPACITY IN CU. CM.
V. S.
a.
b.
S 2-4

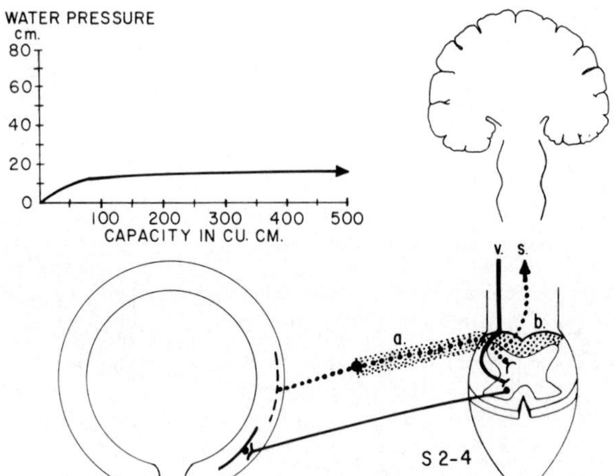

Figure 23–5. Sensory paralytic bladder: lesions and cystometrogram findings.

AUTONOMOUS NEUROGENIC BLADDER

RESIDUAL URINE ________ increased
CAPACITY ________ increased
UNINHIBITED CONTRACTIONS _ absent
URECHOLINE TEST ________ positive
PROPRIOCEPTIVE SENSATION
  1st. desire ________ absent
  fullness ________ absent
EXTEROCEPTIVE SENSATION
  hot ________ absent
  cold ________ absent

LESION:
a. conus
b. cauda equina
c. pelvic nerves

S. sensory
V. inhibitor

WATER PRESSURE
cm.
80
60
40
20
0
100 200 300 400 500
CAPACITY IN CU. CM.
V. S.
a.
b.
c.
S 2-4

Figure 23–6. Autonomous neurogenic bladder: lesions and cystometrogram findings.

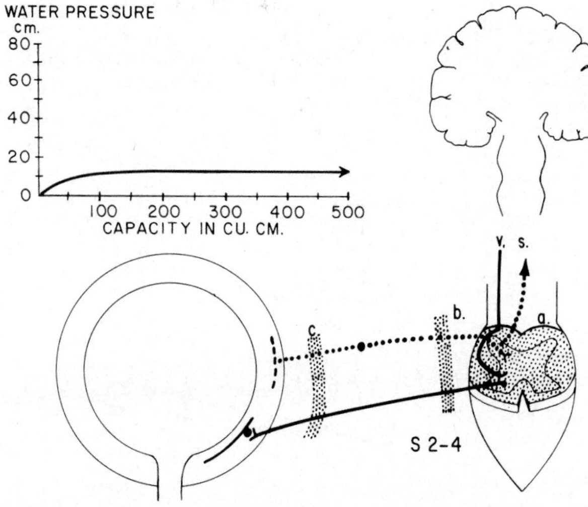

(mostly via the pudendal nerve) is derived from the sacral cord segments S2, S3, and S4, the source of parasympathetic motor and somatic nerves of the bladder (see Figure 23–1).

Contractions of the anal sphincter are characterized by the quick reactions specific for striated muscles. False-positive results may occur if this response is confused with the slow but equally strong, long-lasting contractions of the smooth internal rectal sphincter, which has no neurologic significance but is easily activated by the same type of stimulation. No response of the external anal sphincter is registered when the sphincter is already in contraction prior to the application of the stimulus; this is another source of erroneously negative results.

The denervation sensitivity test as described by Lapides and co-workers (1962) aids in detecting neurologic disease of the sacral spinal cord or reflex arc. The patient is given 2.5 mg. of bethanechol chloride (Urecholine) subcutaneously; after waiting 10 to 20 minutes, a repeat cystometrogram is obtained. The intravesical pressures are then compared to the pressures at comparable volumes on the initial curve. A rise of 15 cm. or more of water after Urecholine administration provides strong evidence in favor of neurologic disease of the sacral spinal cord or the reflex arc. This is due to the fact that the ganglionic synapse and neuromuscular junction are supersensitive to Urecholine, and that impulse transmission is enhanced when neurologic disease is present in the motor nerves (Lapides et al., 1962).

PHARMACOLOGIC CONSIDERATIONS

Sensory, somatic, parasympathetic, and sympathetic nerves play a role in the innervation and function of the bladder. Pharmacologic agents that mimic or counteract the function of acetylcholine and norepinephrine are most commonly used in the treatment of patients with bladder dysfunction, since both serve as neurotransmitters in the bladder and urethra. Other substances — for example, adenosine triphosphate, polypeptides, and prostaglandins — are biologically active neurotransmitters as well but have not found clinical application. Medications in common use, such as tranquilizers, can interfere with voiding and can complicate a patient's problem. A variety of industrial chemicals are neurotoxins, including some heavy metals, organic solvents, n-hexane, n-butylketone, dimethylaminopropionitrile, and organo-phosphorus compounds. Exposure to these chemicals can lead to neurogenic bladder dysfunction (Kreiss et al., 1980).

The neurotransmission of somatic and parasympathetic nerve endings is affected by acetylcholine. Agents that heighten the effects of acetylcholine are termed cholinergic. Competitive inhibitors, on the other hand, block the effect of acetylcholine and are, therefore, anticholinergic. Cholinergic nerve endings are found in the bladder dome and base, as well as in the area of the urethral sphincter. Parasympathomimetic drugs, as well as pelvic nerve stimulation, can excite bladder contraction. In terms of the detrusor muscle, cholinergic drugs encourage whereas anticholinergic drugs inhibit contraction.

Acetylcholine by itself has not been a useful agent. Its actions are diffuse, producing a variety of side effects related to the simultaneous stimulation of cerebral nuclei and the vagus nerve. For this reason, related agents with increased specificity have been developed. There are three main groups: (1) analogues (e.g., bethanechol or Urecholine) and synthetic acetylcholine-like substances (e.g., pilocarpine) affect the same receptor site as acetylcholine; (2) anticholinesterase drugs (e.g., neostigmine and physostigmine) increase the local concentration of acetylcholine by preventing its synaptic breakdown by cholinesterase; (3) competitive inhibitors (e.g., atropine, belladonna, propantheline bromide [Pro-Banthine]) bind the effector cell receptor site and therefore block acetylcholine's effect on the secondary membrane. The action of acetylcholine can be only partially antagonized by atropine.

Adrenergic stimulation via the hypogastric nerves can produce bladder contraction via alpha-receptors and relaxation via beta-receptors in the body of the bladder (Levin and Wein, 1979). On a uropharmacologic basis, one assumes that stimulation of alpha-adrenergic fibers leads to contraction of the sphincteric muscle and a rise in pressure, whereas the inhibitory function of the beta-adrenergic receptors leads to relaxation of the sphincter and drop in closure pressure. Because of overlapping of alpha- and beta-adrenergic endings, no consistent results have been achieved with pharmacologic agents.

Sympathomimetic agents, for example, ephedrine, which by their synaptic stimulation increase outflow resistance, are ganglionic blockers. Those which by their action lead to decreased outflow resistance are isoproterenol (Isuprel), epinephrine, and high-dose norepinephrine. By acting as a blockade of the alpha-synapse, phentolamine (Regitine) and phenoxybenzamine (Dibenzyline) can lead to decreased detrusor contractibility and decreased outflow resistance. Propranolol (Inderal) acts as a sympathetic beta-blocking agent, leading to decreased detrusor relaxation and slight increase of outflow resistance.

Classification of Neurogenic Bladder

Whether the abnormality is a flaccid or a spastic neurogenic bladder depends on the location of the neurologic lesion in the spinal cord; namely, whether it is above or below the micturition center at S2, S3, and S4. This differentiation is used by Bors and Comarr (1971) to classify neurogenic bladders into upper and lower motor neuron bladders. If the conus medullaris and sacral center are undamaged, the reflex patterns via the pelvis (autonomic parasympathetic) and the pudendal (somatic) nerves are intact, resulting in an upper motor neuron bladder, or spastic bladder. Damage to the conus medullaris, the sacral center, or its peripheral nerves leads to an absence of the reflex patterns via the pelvic and pudendal nerves, producing a lower motor neuron bladder, or flaccid bladder.

In the classification proposed by McClellan (1939) and popularized by Lapides (1976), the neurogenic bladder is classified by the response or action of the bladder, not by the type or site of neurologic lesion, as advocated by Bors and Comarr (1971). The five types are as follows:

1. Uninhibited neurogenic bladder.
2. Reflex neurogenic bladder.
3. Motor paralytic bladder.
4. Sensory paralytic bladder.
5. Autonomous neurogenic bladder.

Types of Neurogenic Bladder

A tabulation of findings for the different types of neurogenic bladder is shown in Table 23–1.

Uninhibited Neurogenic Bladder

In the infant and small child the uninhibited neurogenic bladder is a physiologic finding. Inhibitory fibers from higher centers in the cerebral cortex have not matured. Later in life, neurologic diseases, such as cerebrovascular accidents, atherosclerosis, Parkinson's disease, multiple sclerosis, and brain tumors, may damage the inhibitory fibers. Following cerebrovascular accident, the immediate result is usually urinary retention. Often the residual symptoms after the patient's recovery are urgency and urgency incontinence due to loss of inhibitory function. Epileptiform discharges from cortical areas evoke micturition as an initial response of the epileptic attack rather than as a sequela. Sudden uninhibited contractions occurring at lower than normal volumes are seen on the cystometrogram. These occur in the uninhibited as well as the reflex neurogenic bladder and also in an irritable bladder. As a diagnostic test, 15 mg. of propantheline bromide, a parasympatholytic drug, can be used intravenously. This will abolish or markedly diminish the amplitude of bladder contractions of uninhibited or reflex neurogenic bladder, and it will also increase the functional bladder capacity (see Figure 23–2).

Reflex Neurogenic Bladder

In reflex neurogenic bladder, or upper motor neuron type, the spinal lesion is above the sacral cord. The bladder tonus is spastic and the bladder empties reflexly. Figure 23–3 shows the typical cystometrogram findings and the area of anatomic involvement. This type of bladder is most commonly seen after spinal shock has subsided in trauma patients, usually about 8

TABLE 23–1. CHARACTERISTICS OF THE NORMAL AND NEUROGENIC URINARY BLADDERS

	Normal Bladder	Uninhibited Neurogenic Bladder	Reflex Neurogenic Bladder	Autonomous Neurogenic Bladder	Sensory Neurogenic Bladder	Motor Neurogenic Bladder
Residual urine	None	None	Increased	Increased	Increased	Increased
Vesical sensation to hot and cold	Intact	Intact	Absent (except for autonomic hyperreflexia)	Absent	Absent	Intact
Sensation for proprioception (distention)	Intact	Intact	May have autonomic hyperreflexia	Absent	Absent	Intact
Micturition (ability to stop and start)	Intact	Can't stop, may be able to start	Absent	Absent	Intact	Variable
First urge to void	At about 150 ml.	At 50–100 ml. or less	Variable	None	At high volumes	At high volumes
Bladder capacity	About 350–550 ml.	Decreased	Decreased	Increased	Increased	Increased
Uninhibited contractions	None	Present (anticholinergic drugs can abolish contractions)	Present	Absent	Absent	Absent
Bulbocavernosus reflex	Intact	Intact	Highly active	Absent	Variable	Absent
Sensation in saddle area	Intact	Intact	Absent	Absent	Variable	Present
Urecholine test	No exaggerated response	Positive	Positive	Positive	Positive	Positive

weeks after the injury. The patient can initiate the reflex action of the bladder with a variety of stimuli, such as pinching the skin of the thigh.

The external urethral sphincter does not respond to spinal shock in the same flaccid manner as the rest of the lower urinary tract muscle, explaining the high resistance of the external urethral sphincter and the urinary retention characteristic of patients with spinal shock. These patients especially those with high cervical lesions, may perceive bladder fullness through the development of hypertension, severe headaches, sweating, and bradycardia. This array of symptoms is known as autonomic hyperreflexia. Although principally of traumatic origin, the spinal lesion may also occur from tumor, infection, ischemia, or syringomyelia.

Patients with uninhibited contractions and urge incontinence may achieve some control with parasympatholytic drugs such as ProBanthine. Phenoxybenzamine, an oral alpha-adrenergic blocking agent, may improve the voiding pattern in some patients by decreasing urethral resistance (Herwig, 1974). Spasticity of the external sphincter and pelvic floor muscles may necessitate sphincterotomy via, for example, internal urethrotomy to lower urethral resistance. Decreasing urethral resistance improves voiding. This operation may also be indicated for the hypoactive and hypotonic bladder; however, it should be used with caution, as it may result in incontinence. Another mode of relaxing the pelvic floor muscles, with the exception of the levator ani, is section of the pudendal nerve, but this is technically more difficult and often results in only incomplete relaxation.

Following trauma to the spine associated with spinal shock, areflexia and inactivity of the detrusor muscle make catheterization necessary. In this instance, an indwelling urethral catheter may be used over a short period of time when an adequate recording of the patient's input and output is necessary.

Intermittent catheterization has been popularized by Sir Ludwig Guttmann, a neurosurgeon in England (Guttmann and Frankel, 1966). Patients treated by intermittent catheterization tend to develop hydronephrosis, vesicoureteral reflex, kidney and bladder stones, and urinary tract infections *less* often than patients on long-term catheter drainage. When intermittent catheterization is used, the bladder should be emptied at least three or four times during each 24 hour period to avoid overfilling of the bladder. A urinary output between 1.5 and 2 liters per 24 hours must be maintained. Although some advocate catheterization under strict aseptic precautions, Lapides and co-workers (1974) and Rossier (1974) have presented evidence of satisfactory results utilizing unsterile, yet clean, intermittent catheterization. It is crucial to empty the bladder completely, leaving no residual urine; to assure this, manual suprapubic pressure is applied.

A urine culture should be obtained weekly for as long as the patient is on intermittent catheterization in order to uncover and treat urinary tract infections at their inception. It is advisable to use urinary antiseptics (e.g., sulfonamides, nitrofurantoin, methenamine salts, and nalidixic acid). If signs of bladder activity appear, the number of catheterizations may be progressively reduced until the patient can, by initiating the reflex activity of the bladder, achieve a balanced bladder function with residual urine of less than 50 to 100 ml.

Patients with upper motor neuron lesions who develop reflex neurogenic bladder begin, after a variable period of time, to pass urine between catheterizations as a result of reflex activity. This reflex activity may be initiated by gentle tapping of the bladder suprapubically, pinching of the skin, rubbing of the inside of the thigh, or stimulating the perineal area. The trigger area that can initiate the effective emptying contractions of the bladder must be sought in the individual patient.

Motor Paralytic Bladder

Poliomyelitis, polyradiculoneuritis (Guillain-Barré syndrome) multiple sclerosis, trauma, extensive pelvic operations, neoplasms, and herpes zoster infection have all been cited as causes of motor paralytic bladder. The neurologic lesion involves the anterior horn cells of the S2, S3, and S4 parasympathetic motor fibers to the bladder. The supersensitivity test, as described previously, is very helpful in differentiating this type of neurogenic bladder from the hypotonic large capacity bladder secondary to long-standing lower tract obstruction, or from that seen with psychogenic retention, or the habit pattern of infrequent voiding (see Figure 23–4) (Lapides et al., 1972).

The bladder capacity and residual urine in the motor paralytic neurogenic bladder and in the sensory and autonomous neurogenic bladders described later, may be increased markedly. Bladders with large residuals may be stimulated with parasympathomimetic drugs such as Urecholine.

These patients should also be instructed to try to empty their bladders every two to three hours by the clock during the day and several times at night in order to avoid further myogenic decompensation of the bladder.

As has been mentioned before, suprapubic pressure (Credé's maneuver) can also be applied to help evacuate the bladder. Frequently the paraplegic with an autonomous neurogenic bladder is able to effectively use his abdominal muscles augmented with the Credé maneuver. All of these regimens are employed to avoid a chronic overdistention of the bladder muscle, which produces an impairment of blood flow to the bladder, decreasing the resistance to urinary pathogens. As has been mentioned before, these patients also need intermittent catheterizations or continuous catheter drainage. However, one should be aware that the female patient may dribble continuously, although ever larger catheters are used, producing a pressure ulceration of the anterior wall of the urethra.

Urinary diversion may be required to manage a patient with neurogenic bladder disease or to control progressive deterioration of renal function. Persistent reflux with hydronephrosis, failure to relieve outlet obstruction, persistent bladder spasticity with urinary tract obstruction, persistent incontinence, recurrent urinary tract infections with pyelonephritis and sepsis, periurethral abscesses, and urethrocutaneous fistula are the complicating problems that prompt consideration of diverting procedures. The most commonly used methods of urinary diversion are nephrostomy, ureterostomy, ureteroileostomy, vesicostomy, and suprapubic cystostomy. Nephrostomy and suprapubic cystostomy require an indwelling catheter in addition to the use of a collecting device.

The use of various devices with electrical stimulation of the bladder muscle to initiate voiding contractions has been tried repeatedly, but so far consistent results have not been obtained.

Sensory Neurogenic Bladder

Previously tabes dorsalis, the posterior column syndrome, was the principal disease responsible for sensory neurogenic bladder. Today, diabetes mellitus with its segmental demyelinization of the pelvic nerves is the most frequent cause of this disorder (Figure 23–5). Sensory pathways may also be damaged by trauma, surgery, infection, tumor, vascular disease, or other demyelinating diseases.

The urinary incontinence associated with a sensory neurogenic bladder may be of two types: overflow or urgency. The neurological vesical dysfunction appears to be due to the destruction of the afferent limbs in the sacral reflex arc or degeneration of afferent conduction pathways in the spinal cord.

The patient with a sensory neurogenic bladder has no perception of bladder filling, bladder fullness, or voiding and is characteristically in urinary retention with overflow incontinence. The management of this type of neurogenic bladder has been discussed previously (Chapter 3).

Autonomous Neurogenic Bladder

In an autonomous neurogenic (flaccid) bladder or lower motor neuron type, the sacral center, the conus medullaris, or its peripheral nerves, particularly the pudendal nerves, are damaged (Figure 23–6). Trauma, infection, tumor, herniated nucleus pulposus from one or more intervertebral discs, meningomyelocele, and vascular problems may all produce an autonomous bladder. Damage to nerves secondary to extensive operations (e.g., abdominal and perineal resection or radical hysterectomy) may also result in an autonomous neurogenic bladder.

The flaccid bladder may produce a palpable suprapubic mass. Voiding can be initiated and sustained by abdominal straining or the Credé maneuver (suprapubic pressure). However, there is usually a large residual urine volume. Incontinence may be of the overflow or stress type, depending on the resistance of the periurethral striated muscle. The management of the flaccid neurogenic bladder is discussed in Chapter 3.

ENURESIS

Enuresis is the involuntary and unconscious voiding of urine in the absence of congenital or acquired defects of the urogenital and nervous system, persisting after an arbitrary age limit of 3 years. Micturition is usually in a full and steady stream and occurs during sleep (Kuntz, 1965). Involuntary voiding of urine is a normal condition of infancy, and 10 per cent of children between the ages of 5 and 6 years still wet the bed while being otherwise normal. The occurrence of involuntary voiding in association with organic disease, whether in children or adults, is more correctly designated as incontinence of urine. Johnson and Marshall (1954) believe that a subconscious resentment towards parents, a subconscious desire to remain in or return to the irresponsible and protected state of infancy, and the lack of maturity with respect to bladder control are the chief etiologic factors of enuresis.

A certain percentage of enuretic children who do not respond to judicious toilet training or routine medical or psychiatric treatment will, on examination, exhibit organic changes in the urinary tract. Girls with urinary leakage from an ectopic ureteral orifice are often mistakenly treated for enuresis, and this condition may be overlooked even into adulthood. It is estimated that after a thorough examination a urologic abnormality will be found in 1 to 2 per cent of enuretic children. Children with refractory enuresis should therefore have a complete urologic examination. When urologic abnormalities have been excluded, these children may be treated with Tofranil (imipramine hydrochloride), 25 to 75 mg. at bed time. Tofranil's mode of action is unknown, but it is hypothesized to change the sleeping cycle. In enuretic children treated with Tofranil, the most common adverse reactions have been nervousness, sleep disorder, tiredness, and mild gastrointestinal disturbances.

ANATOMIC DEFECTS PRODUCING INCONTINENCE

Congenital or acquired anatomic defects may also produce urinary incontinence. On a congenital basis incontinence is found in patients with ectopic ureteral orifice, epispadias, exstrophy of the bladder, and urethral stenosis.

Ectopic Ureteral Orifice

In females, the location of the ectopic ureteral orifice is beyond sphincter control. In these cases the patient is continuously wet; however, this wetness may show considerable diurnal and nocturnal variation. It is sometimes related to position, with more leakage when the patient is standing. In 75 per cent of the females with ureteral orifice ectopia, normal day and night voiding is usually accompanied by transient urinary dribbling. However, they often have urinary tract infections that independently or together with urinary incontinence lead to urologic examination, diagnosis, and treatment (Harrison et al., 1978). Details regarding the anatomy and pathology of ectopic ureters are presented in Chapter 2.

Bladder Exstrophy and Epispadias

In bladder exstrophy and severe epispadias the bladder has lost its function as a reservoir, resulting in continuous dribbling of urine. This abnormality demands good nursing care to avoid maceration of the surrounding skin. In selected cases, surgical correction of the abnormalities can be attempted immediately. Severe forms require urinary diversion.

Congenital Urethral Stenosis

Congenital urethral stenosis is usually discovered during the first year of life and is occasionally found in females. The stenosis occurs at the external meatus and represents an arrest of the canalization of the urethral epithelium during fetal life. Milder forms of urethral stenosis are found in females of all ages and commonly are discovered with a history of urinary tract infections. Emptying of the bladder is incomplete and dribbling of urine frequently occurs. Incontinence may also result owing to overflow from the overdistended, obstructed bladder (Chapter 29).

Acquired Defects

Acquired defects leading to urinary incontinence may be secondary to interference with sphincter mechanisms, urethral diverticulum, traumatic destruction of the urethra, or the formation of fistulae. The most commonly found abnormality in females that interferes with the urinary sphincter mechanism is a cystocele with stress incontinence as the presenting symptom. Ephedrine sulfate, 25 mg. three or four times a day, can be administered in an attempt to increase the tonicity of the alpha-adrenergic innervated urethral smooth muscle fibers (Chapter 13) (Lapides, 1974).

The most common cause of urethral diverticulum in the female is infection and dilatation of the paraurethral glands. The symptoms are those suggesting chronic or frequently occurring cystitis, namely dysuria, frequency, postvoid dribbling, and urgency incontinence (Harrison et al., 1978). The patient may also complain of dyspareunia with this abnormality (Chapter 13).

Traumatic destruction of the urethra, seen especially after difficult pelvic delivery, may produce urinary incontinence. The formation of fistulae between the urinary tract and surrounding pelvic organs also follows radiation therapy, inflammatory lesions, tumor, or surgery. These topics are covered in detail in Chapters 8, 21, 27, and 28.

OTHER LESIONS PRODUCING URGENCY INCONTINENCE

Disturbances of bladder innervation that produce urgency incontinence are commonly found in the neurogenic bladders with uninhibited contractions. If the involuntary contraction of the bladder cannot be suppressed and urine leaks out, the urgency becomes urge incontinence. The use of parasympatholytic drugs, such as ProBanthine, in these conditions has previously been described.

Along with the well-known symptoms of frequency, dysuria, and suprapubic pain, females also experience urgency and often some urgency incontinence with inflammatory changes of the lower urinary tract, as seen in radiation cystitis and lower urinary tract infections. Urgency incontinence secondary to infection can be handled with appropriate antibiotics, whereas the patient with radiation cystitis may obtain relief of symptoms with the use of parasympatholytic drugs.

Urgency incontinence may be the presenting symptom of vesical and urethral calculi or neoplasms. These conditions require surgical correction, with removal of the stone or tumor, for improvement of the urinary symptoms (see Chapters 26, 27, and 29).

REFERENCES

Bradley, W. E., Timm, G. W., and Scott, F. B.: Cystometry. V. Bladder sensation. Urology *6*:654, 1975.

Bors, E., and Comarr, A. E.: Neurological Urology. Baltimore, University Park Press, 1971.

Guttmann, L., and Frankel, H.: The value of intermittent catheterization in the early management of traumatic paraplegia and tetraplegia. Paraplegia *4*:63, 1966.

Harrison, J. H., Gittes, R. F., Perlmutter, A. D., Stamey, T. A., and Walsh, P. C.: Campbell's Urology. 4th Ed. Philadelphia, W. B. Saunders Co., 1978.

Herwig, K. R.: The history and physical examination in neurogenic bladder disease. Urol. Clin. North Am. *1*:29, 1974.

Johnson, S. H., III, and Marshall, M., Jr.: Enuresis. J. Urol. *71*:554, 1954.

Krane, R. J., and Olsson, C. A.: Phenoxybenzamine in neurogenic bladder dysfunction. II. Clinical considerations. J. Urol. *110*:653, 1973.

Kreiss, K., Wegman, D. H., Niles, C. A., et al.: Neurological dysfunction of the bladder in workers exposed to dimethylaminopropionitrile. J.A.M.A. *243*:741, 1980.

Kuntz, A.: Physiology of Urinary Bladder and Urethra, Normal and Pathological. Encyclopedia of Urology. New York, Springer-Verlag, 1965.

Lapides, J.: Neurogenic bladder. Principles of treatment. Urol. Clin. North Am. *1*:81, 1974.

Lapides, J.: Fundamentals of Urology. Philadelphia, W. B. Saunders Co., 1976.

Lapides, J., Diokno, A., Lowe, B. S., et al.: Followup on unsterile intermittent self-catheterization. J. Urol. *111*:184, 1974.

Lapides, J., Diokno, A., Silber, S. J., et al.: Clean, intermittent self-catheterization in the treatment of urinary tract disease. J. Urol. *107*:458, 1972.

Lapides, J., Friend, C. R., Ajemian, E. P., et al.: Denervation supersensitivity as a test for neurogenic bladder. Surg. Gynecol. Obstet. *114*:241, 1962.

Levin, R. M., and Wein, A. J.: Quantitative analysis of alpha and beta adrenergic receptor densities in the lower urinary tract of the dog and the rabbit. Invest. Urol. *17*:75, 1979.

McClellan, F. C.: The Neurogenic Bladder. Springfield, Ill., Charles C Thomas, 1939.

Rossier, A. B.: Neurogenic bladder in spinal cord injury. Management of patients in Geneva, Switzerland, and West Roxbury, Massachusetts. Urol. Clin. North Am. *1*:125, 1974.

SECTION 4

INFLAMMATORY AND NEOPLASTIC DISEASE; RADIATION INJURY

24

URINARY TRACT INFECTIONS

C. LOWELL PARSONS
SUSHIL S. LACY

INTRODUCTION

Urinary tract infections in women are frequently encountered in the practice of medicine. Patients with these infections are rarely seen initially by the urologist. They are more often seen by the obstetrician-gynecologist, the family physician, or the internist.

Proper management of these patients is often simple and at the same time complex: simple because of the relatively few and well-known causative organisms; complex when the organism involved is resistant to antibiotics, and when the bacterial growth is perpetuated by underlying urinary tract structural defects or underlying systemic disease of the patient. Decreased renal function also makes therapy more complicated. It places the patient at risk not only to the therapy prescribed but also to persistent infection and possibly irreversible renal damage — chronic pyelonephritis.

Over the years, considerable research has helped create a better understanding of the pathogenesis of urinary tract infections in women. An awareness of the possible long-term effects of such infection has aided early diagnosis and treatment. This chapter is a review of these factors and will help define a sound, practical approach in the management of nonpregnant, symptomatic women with urinary tract infections. Urinary tract infections during pregnancy and asymptomatic bacteriuria are discussed elsewhere (Chapter 25).

GENERAL CONSIDERATIONS

Definitions

Terminology related to urinary tract infections can be confusing, since commonly used terms often have different meanings for patients and physicians alike. Hence, a clear concept of generally accepted definitions is essential to better understand the clinicopathologic states, to improve communication among clinicians and with patients, and to formulate rapid patient evaluation and management plans.

Bacteriuria. Bacteriuria, the most commonly used term, literally means the presence of bacteria in the urine. However, the mere presence of organisms does not constitute urinary tract infection. The mucosal surface of the anterior urethra is normally colonized by bacteria, and so are the vaginal vestibule and perineum (Stamey et al., 1965; Elkins et al., 1974). Thus, contamination of voided urine cultures often occurs. Unless critically evaluated, the finding of organisms during a routine urine examination may lead to an incorrect diagnosis and unnecessary treatment.

Significant bacteriuria is generally accepted as indicating bacterial counts of 100,000 or more per milliliter of urine on quantitative cultures in properly collected voided midstream specimens. It appears to correlate well with significant infection as opposed to contamination (Kass, 1956). However, the criteria for significant bacteriuria may vary at times when methods of collection other than the midstream clean-voided route are used. Thus, one may find markedly lower bacterial counts indicating presence of urinary infection in specimens obtained by suprapubic bladder aspiration and by proper urethral catheterization.

Asymptomatic bacteriuria refers to the presence of urinary infection in a patient with no clinical symptoms. By definition, two consecutive positive urine cultures are needed to make the diagnosis.

Pyelonephritis. Pyelonephritis can be broadly defined as renal parenchymal and renal pelvicalyceal system disease caused by bacterial infection. This pathologic process implies vascular, cicatricial, and possibly autoimmune alterations as well as direct effects of inflammation.

Acute pyelonephritis is a clinical syndrome of fever, flank pain, and costovertebral angle tenderness, associated with lower urinary tract irritative symptoms such as urinary frequency and dysuria. Urine culture is diagnostic of causative bacteria.

Chronic pyelonephritis is not synonymous with *chronic urinary tract infection,* which means only prolonged presence of bacteria. Chronic pyelonephritis denotes histologic changes of patchy interstitial nephritis, destruction of tubules, cellular infiltration, and inflammatory changes in the renal pelvicalyceal system. A similar picture may be caused by several underlying diseases of the urinary tract, such as obstruction, vascular disease, phenacetin abuse, hereditary nephritis, and so forth, making it difficult to assess accurately the role of associated symptomatic or asymptomatic bacterial infection. It is now known that progression of this disease does not require presence of demonstrable bacteria.

Cystitis. Cystitis is the term commonly used for infection localized to the urinary bladder, sometimes associated with urethritis. Patients with cystitis usually have symptoms of local irritation such as burning on urination, urgency, urinary incontinence, frequency, nocturia, suprapubic discomfort, and occasionally hematuria. Symptoms such as fever, chills, and flank pain indicate associated pyelonephritis.

Vesicoureteral Reflux. Vesicoureteral reflux is the condition of regurgitation of bladder urine into one or both ureters. Under normal conditions, this is prevented by a competent vesicoureteral junction. Although not all functional implications of reflux are well known, a few factors have been recognized as deleterious to renal function. These include retardation of renal growth in presence of gross, total reflux into the collecting system; increased renal scarring with long-standing reflux; and development of end-stage renal disease secondary to persistent reflux of sterile urine (Hodson, 1967; Salvatierra et al., 1973).

Persistence of Bacteriuria. This persistence indicates the continued presence of the same infecting microorganisms that were isolated at the start of treatment and continue to be isolated while the patient is still on therapy (Figure 24–1). Persistence may be caused by several factors: the organism may be resistant to the antimicrobial drug; the concentration of drug in urine or serum, or both, may be inadequate; the dosage may be inaccurate; or patient compliance with drug therapy may be poor (Kunin, 1963; McCabe and Jackson, 1965).

Superinfection. This refers to the appearance, during treatment of significant bacteriuria, of an organism that is different from the original infecting organism for which therapy was instituted. This new organism may be of a different strain or the same strain as the original but of a different serologic type (see Figure 24–1).

Relapse. Relapse means recurrence of significant bacteriuria with the same species and serologic strain of organism as originally documented. Relapse appears within 2 to 3 weeks of completion of therapy by the patient (Figure 24–1). This may but does not usually signify infection occurring from within the urinary tract, such as the kidneys (Turck et al., 1966). Relapse more likely represents perineal colonization by the infecting organism (Cox et al., 1968; Stamey et al., 1971; Stamey and Sexton, 1975).

Reinfection. On the other hand, reinfection refers to infection occurring after cessation of therapy with a different strain of microorganism or a different serologic type

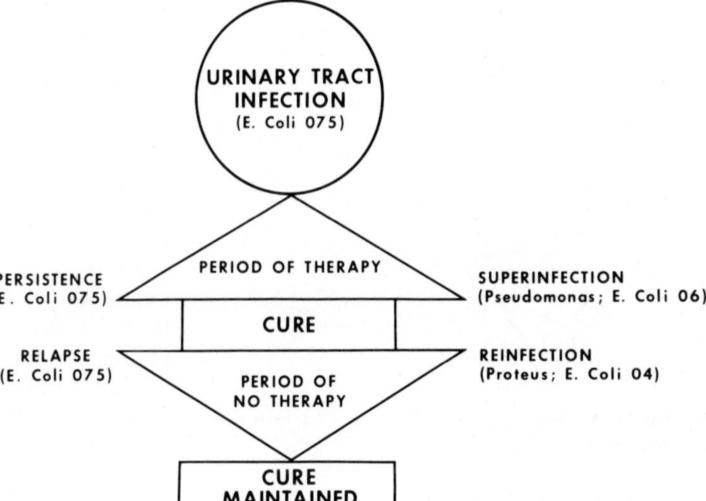

Figure 24–1. Clinical patterns of bacteriuria following therapy in patients with urinary infection.

of the original infecting strain (Figure 24–1). This indicates recurrent bladder bacteriuria, and usually the source of infection is from outside the urinary tract. Typically reinfection occurs some 2 to 12 weeks after a previous episode of infection (Turck et al., 1966).

Prevalence of Bacteriuria

The female is much more susceptible to bacteriuria throughout her lifespan than is the male. This is perhaps because the female urethra is shorter, providing for easier access of bacteria to the bladder. Numerous surveys have helped to define epidemiologic characteristics of urinary tract infection in the female (Kunin, 1970; Asscher et al., 1969).

Two per cent of nonpregnant women in the age group between 15 and 20 years were bacteriuric in one study (Kass et al., 1964). This incidence increased steadily by 1 or 2 per cent per decade to a prevalence rate of 10 per cent between 55 and 64 years of age. Thus, about 4 to 6 per cent of women of childbearing age will have bacteriuria at any one time.

Sexual activity also seems to have a significant role in urinary infection. Only 0.4 to 1.6 per cent of nuns between 15 and 54 years of age were found to have bacteriuria (Kunin and McCormack, 1968). It appears that other factors such as race, marriage, pregnancy, and use of oral contraceptives have no significant effect on the prevalence of bacteriuria except that the condition is twice as common in married women (5.9 per cent) as in single women (2.7 per cent) between 15 and 24 years of age (Kunin and McCormack, 1968).

Long-Term Implications of Bacteriuria

Does bacteriuria lead to progressive renal damage? This question has been asked by many investigators. It appears that the nonpregnant woman with recurrent bacteriuria is probably not at serious risk unless she has an underlying urinary tract obstructive process, vesicoureteral reflux, associated renal disease, or systemic disease (Stamey, 1972). Pyelonephritis is a relatively uncommon cause of end-stage renal disease, accounting for less than 12 per cent of reported cases (Salvatierra, 1979).

PATHOGENESIS

Pathways of Bacterial Entry into the Urinary Tract

Bacteria may gain entry into the urinary tract by three pathways — the ascending route, where the short female urethra is in

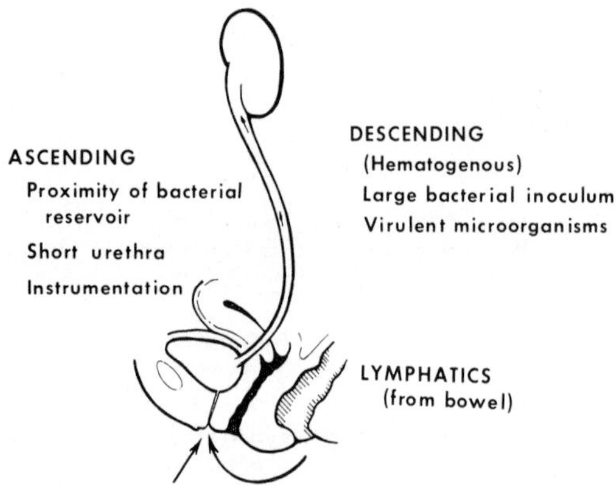

Figure 24–2. Pathways of bacterial entry into the urinary tract.

direct contact with the perineum; the hematogenous route; and the lymphatic route (Figure 24–2).

Ascending Infection

Considerable evidence indicates that, in most instances of urinary tract infection, there is ascending infection through the urethra into the bladder and on occasion through the ureters into the kidneys. Although it is difficult to produce pyelonephritis experimentally by placing microorganisms into the bladder of animals, this can be done by using a large inoculum of bacteria. If one of the ureters of the animal is ligated prior to infection of the bladder, infection occurs only in the unobstructed kidney, which is in direct contact with the bladder (Heptinstall, 1965).

The female is more susceptible to urinary infection not only because of the short urethra but also because of the proximity of the external urethral meatus to a large bacterial reservoir within the intestinal tract (fecal), and along the vaginal vestibule and anterior urethra (introital) (Gruneberg et al., 1968; Cox et al., 1968). This does not explain why some women are more prone to recurrent urinary infections than others, since the presence and distribution of fecal bacteria (mainly *E. coli*) are essentially the same in both groups of women (Gruneberg et al., 1968). Some observers have suggested that the introital bacterial flora of women with no previous history of urinary infections is different from those with recurrent infections. In particular, premenopausal women resistant to urinary infections rarely have introital pathogenic enterobacteria, and when cultured, the organisms (*E. coli*) are very few in number and only transiently present (Stamey, 1972). The question then arises as to the role of introital bacteria in urinary infection. Is the primary determinant of urinary infection host susceptibility — a decrease or lack of natural resistance (Cox et al., 1968) — and not bacterial availability? Or is it possible that changes in urethral flora are directly controlled by changes in the vaginal flora? Well-designed clinical studies indicate that the primary incident in the chain of events leading to bladder bacteriuria is the establishment of pathologic microorganisms (i.e., colonization) on the introitus and their subsequent growth to substantial numbers (Stamey et al., 1971; Schaeffer and Stamey, 1977). Stamey and Timothy (1975) noted that the presence of such bacterial colonization is associated with an elevation of vaginal pH above the normal value of 4.0 (Parsons et al., 1977; Elkins and Cox, 1974; Lang, 1955). Whether or not the vaginal pH is a cause or an effect is unknown. Although not all women with enterobacterial colonization of the perineum develop cystitis, women susceptible to recurrent infection usually have aberrant perineal flora and probably remain at risk for cystitis until their normal flora returns. As discussed below, bladder antibacterial defenses most likely play a role in preventing infection, which may explain why most women do not develop cystitis even when the perineum contains potential pathogens. Normal vaginal antibacterial mechanisms appear to be an important first line of defense against cystitis. These mechanisms have not yet been defined but may involve pH, antibodies, or normal flora interfering with and supervening as the predominant microorganisms.

Descending Infection

Descending infection through the hematogenous route occurs only under special circumstances. Experimentally, an obstructed kidney appears to be more susceptible to an inoculum of intravenously injected bacteria than is an unobstructed one. Clinically, however, it is difficult to ascertain the exact importance of this, since significant clinical bacteremia prior to an episode of urinary infection is uncommon. The kidney may be involved in high-grade staphylococcal bacteremia or endocarditis with multiple cortical abscesses. Also, occasionally a patient develops bacteremia following urethral instrumentation. In such cases the urethral organisms are most likely forced into the circulatory system and could produce pyelonephritis if there were preexisting obstructive disease. Renal tuberculosis almost always is acquired via the hematogenous route.

Lymphatic Spread. Experimental evidence to date suggests the possible spread of bacterial infections along *lymphatic channels* connecting the bowel and the urinary tract. Carbon particles have been demonstrated to migrate through lymphatics into the kidneys in an animal model when intravesical pressure is increased to extremely high levels. In spite of these studies, the clinical implication remains unclear regarding lymphatic spread of urinary infection.

Host Defense Mechanisms

Normally there is a state of balance between the host and the bacterial population. Entrance of bacteria into the urinary tract does not necessarily result in infection. It has been shown that women have had bacterial contamination following pelvic examination. More vigorous urethral trauma, such as during sexual intercourse, may force bacteria into the bladder. However, not all women undergoing pelvic examinations develop significant bacteriuria (Bran et al., 1972). It becomes apparent, then, that any abnormality underlying the patient's defense mechanism or an alteration in the virulence or size of bacterial inoculum might set the stage for urinary infection.

Normal periodic voiding is one of the most important *"extrinsic"* bladder defense mechanisms. In a classic clinical study, the introduction of 10 million bacteria into normal male volunteers failed to establish infection. They rapidly cleared the organisms by voiding, dilution with fresh urine, and voiding again (Cox and Hinman, 1961). Since even after complete bladder emptying there is a small amount of urine left in the bladder, it would appear that mechanical factors alone would not adequately provide normal defense, and perhaps other associated defense mechanisms exist. Attempts to accurately define these *"intrinsic"* defense factors have not determined whether the mechanism resides in the bladder wall (mucosal) and is of a cellular nature, as in active phagocytosis, or whether it is immunologic in nature, e.g., bacterial antigens eliciting specific antibody production (Norden et al., 1968). One important intrinsic bladder antibacterial defense mechanism has been better defined, however. Parsons and associates (1980) have shown that the bladder is lined by a layer of one or more sulfonated glycosaminoglycans that acts as an anti-adherence factor, preventing bacteria from adhering to the transitional cells and thereby allowing them to be washed to the exterior.

The renal medulla is much less resistant to infection than is the renal cortex. This seems related to the high osmolality and ammonia content of the medulla, which inhibits activity of complement, which together with antibody is bactericidal to gram-negative bacteria. The normal high osmolality of the medulla also prevents rapid mobilization of leukocytes and phagocytosis of bacteria. Cell wall-deficient bacteria (L-forms) could possibly persist in the hypertonic renal medullary environment and may explain the mechanism of relapse in some cases (Guze and Kalmanson, 1964).

Urine itself, though a good growth medium for bacteria, has its own potentially inhibitory factors that prevent continued, rapid bacterial multiplication. Urine of women is often of a more suitable pH and osmolality to support bacterial growth than is urine of men. The inhibiting activity is most active under pH 5.5 and tends to decrease with urinary dilution. The urine of pregnant women usually supports bacterial growth better than does urine of nonpregnant women (Roberts and Beard, 1965). Besides pH, other factors such as urine osmolality, urea content, ammonium, and organic acid concentration also have effects on bacterial growth. Of these, urea content appears to be the most important antibacterial factor (Kaye, 1975). The gram-positive urethral bacteria rarely are uropathogens, most likely because they grow poorly in urine (Stamey and Mihara, 1980).

Factors Encouraging and Perpetuating Urinary Tract Infections

Any abnormality in the host, particularly within the urinary tract, can predispose the patient to infection. Establishment of infection in turn can produce abnormalities resulting in perpetuation. In the host, the abnormality may be transient or permanent, and the alteration or reduction in resistance may be local or systemic. Infection may be related to obstruction, neurologic disease, and calculi in the urinary tract. Often genetic factors and underlying renal disease are the perpetuating factors.

Stasis and Obstruction

Structural abnormalities of the urinary tract causing obstruction may be congenital or acquired and can occur at any level of the system. Essentially, obstruction causes ineffective drainage, and the stasis encourages bacterial growth. Ureteropelvic junction obstruction, ureteral strictures, urethral stenosis, and vesicoureteral reflux are the more common abnormal clinical findings in patients with recurrent or chronic urinary tract infection. Calculi not only cause urinary obstruction but may also initiate and perpetuate infection. When antimicrobial therapy is discontinued, the nidus of bacteria in the stone produces a relapse of infection. Vesicoureteral reflux carries organisms freely into the renal pelvis and calyces, creating a predisposition to renal infection. Urinary infection itself may induce reflux, especially in patients with recurrent or chronic cystitis, by producing an incompetent vesicoureteral junction. In addition to anatomic reasons for susceptibility to urinary tract infection, placement of an indwelling catheter totally bypasses all bladder defenses and leads to bacteriuria no matter what chemical or mechanical therapy is instituted (Andriole, 1975).

Functional Abnormalities

These are usually neurologic deficits that produce ineffectual bladder emptying or increased urethral resistance. Women may have occult or subclinical neurogenic bladder disease specific to the detrusor muscle. Some women develop the habit of inefficient and incomplete voiding. These "infrequent voiders" over a period of time may develop an atonic bladder and provide a continuous pool of infected residual urine. Pregnancy also produces transient functional ureteral obstruction mechanically and by hormonal changes. Subsequent to these changes, the smooth muscle of the ureter becomes relatively atonic, and urinary stasis occurs within the upper urinary tract, predisposing the women to infection. Dynamic distention may itself open the lumen and produce transitory reflux. Microorganisms, particularly *Escherichia coli* and its endotoxin (pharmacologic concentrations), directly suppress ureteral smooth muscle by producing temporary hydroureteronephrosis (Teague and Boyarsky, 1968).

Systemic Factors

Diabetics have asymptomatic bacteriuria no more frequently than the general population; however, diabetics do show greater incidence of chronic pyelonephritis at postmortem examination. And, in one study, the prevalence of bacteriuria was 18.8 per cent among diabetic women, compared with only 7.9 per cent in nondiabetic women (Vejlsgaard, 1965). Diabetics are prone to develop neurogenic bladder dysfunction and severe vascular disease, both of which predispose to infection. Other genetic problems associated with urinary infection are gouty nephropathy, sickle cell trait, and cystic renal disease. Metabolic disorders, such as nephrocalcinosis, chronic potassium deficiency, and renal tubular defects, appear to increase susceptibility to pyelonephritis as seen under experimental and clinical conditions (Rocha, 1972). It is essential that the clinician be aware of all factors predisposing to and perpetuating infection when evaluating a female with recurrent or chronic urinary tract infection.

SIGNS AND SYMPTOMS

The clinical manifestations of urinary tract infection can be diverse, but usually certain signs and symptoms are associated with specific anatomic areas of involvement. It is helpful to distinguish lower urinary tract infection (cystitis) from upper urinary tract infection (pyelonephritis), not only to decide on the proper antimicrobial therapy but also to plan proper evaluation and follow-up.

Lower Tract Infection

Cystitis and associated urethral irritation are manifested by lower urinary tract irritative symptoms that may be mild to severe. Usually symptoms are dysuria, frequency with small amounts of voided urine, and urgency, occasionally to the point of mild incontinence. Nocturia, suprapubic tenderness, and low backache and flank pain are often present. Occasionally there is hematuria at the end of voiding, or the urine may be grossly bloody. Systemic symptoms are usually not seen with lower urinary tract infections.

Upper Tract Infection

Women with infection involving the renal pelvis, calyces, renal parenchyma, and ureters usually present with fever, chills, general malaise, and occasionally anorexia, nausea, and vomiting. Flank or costovertebral angle pain and tenderness is a common finding. Lower urinary tract irritative symptoms may precede the onset of other symptoms by a few days. Severe flank pain or renal colic suggests coexistent urinary obstructive disease and on occasion may be due to necrotizing papillitis with a sloughed papilla secondary to diabetic or analgesic nephropathy.

CLINICAL CLASSIFICATION OF NONPREGNANT, SYMPTOMATIC WOMEN WITH URINARY TRACT INFECTION

In clinical practice, management of patients becomes easier with rapid and accurate categorization in broad groups, if it is at all possible. This is certainly true for patients with urinary tract infection (Table 24–1). Differentiation of patients by the severity of clinical symptoms when first seen, their history relative to urinary infections, and the type of microorganism isolated on culture supplies the best guidelines

TABLE 24–1. CLINICAL CLASSIFICATION OF NONPREGNANT, SYMPTOMATIC WOMEN WITH URINARY TRACT INFECTION

Clinical Classification	History of Urinary Tract Infection	Severity of Symptoms	Causative Organisms	Associated Conditions
ACUTE UNCOMPLICATED	First episode of infection or infrequent reinfection or relapse	Usually mild (cystitis) to moderate (pyelonephritis); rarely severe (bacteremia)	*Escherichia coli*	Usually none Perineal colonization by uropathogen (most common)
ACUTE COMPLICATED	Frequent reinfection; persistence or relapse (*chronic bacteriuria*)	May be mild; usually moderate to severe	*Escherichia coli* (occasionally resistant) *Klebsiella-Enterobacter* *Proteus, Enterococcus* *Pseudomonas* (rare)	Structural and functional disorders of urinary tract; calculi; diabetes mellitus

for instituting therapy and estimating the prognosis.

Acute Uncomplicated Urinary Infections

Patients most often seen in the office practice are those with mild uncomplicated urinary tract infection. These have typical symptoms of cystitis, such as dysuria, urgency, frequency, hesitancy, and suprapubic pain. They are seen with either their first episode of infection or an episode far removed in time from a previous urinary infection (infrequent relapse or reinfection). The causative organism is usually *E. coli* from the patient's enteric pool which is sensitive to all antimicrobials effective against gram-negative organisms including sulfonamides and nitrofurantoin. Bacteriuria is eradicated in more than 90 per cent of these women, and it is uncommon to find any underlying disease.

With moderate infection, patients often have associated signs and symptoms of upper urinary tract involvement (pyelonephritis) secondary to ascending infection. It is extremely rare to see a patient with a severe degree of clinical symptoms, e.g., bacteremia, in this group.

Acute Complicated Urinary Infections

Clinically, these infections may be designated as being of mild, moderate, or severe degree. The patient's urologic history often indicates frequent reinfections or relapse. Overall, this occurs in 15 to 20 per cent of all females who develop cystitis. The typical relapse usually develops within 2 weeks of cessation of therapy, the typical reinfection after 2 to 12 weeks. (Reinfection and relapse are arbitrary terms originally meant to help differentiate patients with pyelonephritis from those whose recurrent bacteriuria comes from a source outside the genitourinary tract [Turck et al., 1966].) Between clinical episodes of infection, some of these women continue to have bacteriuria — asymptomatic and chronic bacteriuria. Evaluation of these patients is warranted, since they have a slightly higher incidence of underlying primary or secondary anatomic defects and functional disorders. The majority, however, will have none of these abnormalities. Some have concomitant systemic disease or metabolic disorders. Although *E. coli* is predominant, other organisms frequently isolated are *Proteus, Klebsiella-Enterobacter,* and *Enterococcus*.

The response to therapy in this group depends on the efficacy of antimicrobial therapy and the correction of any underlying perpetuating factor. The most common source of the recurrent bacteriuria is colonization of the urethra and vagina as a unit by a uropathogen (Cox et al., 1968; Stamey et al., 1971; Stamey and Sexton, 1975), as discussed earlier. It may be a transient phenomenon, but usually it persists for several months before spontaneously reverting to normal. The problem is much more common in postmenopausal women and seems to account for their greater susceptibility to lower urinary tract infection. Severe cases of acute complicated urinary infection characterized by bacteremia and septicemia are seen most often in older, debilitated women undergoing gynecologic surgery and requiring ureteral or bladder catheterizations.

DIAGNOSTIC STUDIES

Urine Culture

A quantitative urine culture is the most important laboratory test in the diagnosis and immediate management of urinary tract infection. Various clinical criteria, such as history, physical findings, and microscopic examination of urine for pyuria and bacteria, may suggest the presence of infection but are not adequate for proper documentation of urinary infection. In the busy office practice, the quantitative urine culture is often neglected in the interest of time or in an effort to reduce expense to the patient. Unfortunately, this frequently results in unnecessary treatment with antimicrobials for symptoms mimicking urinary tract infection. In cases in which infection is present, the patient may be subjected to prolonged morbidity and further expense for reevaluation if the organism happens to be resistant to the initial therapy. Hence, the need for the quantitative culture in women suspected of having urinary tract infection cannot be overemphasized. Isolation of the organism followed by antibiotic sensitivity tests allows determination of appropriate therapy.

Pour-Plate Dilution Technique

In most major hospital laboratories, the quantitative culture is done by the pour-plate dilution technique. Although this method is extremely accurate (it is used as a standard of comparison for other methods), it is time consuming.

Calibrated Bacteriologic Loop Technique

The calibrated bacteriologic loop technique is now more common in the busy microbiologic laboratories and does save considerable time. The correlation between the two techniques is high, and under controlled standard conditions false-positive and false-negative results with the loop technique average approximately 5 per cent.

Office Urine Culture Kits

Recently, numerous simple quantitative urine culture kits have been developed for routine office diagnostic studies. They are inexpensive and easy to work with, and they provide a high degree of sensitivity (few false negatives) and specificity (few false positives) for initial identification of the microorganism. Subculture and antibiotic sensitivity testing can then be easily

TABLE 24–2. PARTIAL LIST OF COMMERCIALLY AVAILABLE OFFICE URINE CULTURE KITS

Name	Source	Principle	Remarks
Testuria	Ayerst Laboratories, New York, N.Y.	Filter paper method	Use of only one culture medium Initial identification and assessment of contaminating organisms is poor
Uricult	Bristol Laboratories, Syracuse, N.Y.	Dip slide method	Use of two culture media Contamination detected by growth of mixed colonies on nonselective media
Oxoid	Flow Laboratories, Rodeville, Maryland	Dip slide method	
Dipinoc	Stayne Diagnostics, East Rutherford, N.J.	Dip slide method	
Clinicult	Smith, Kline & French Laboratories, Philadelphia, Pa.	Dip slide method	
Speci-test	Ross Laboratories, Columbus, Ohio	Cup method	Limited by use of only one culture medium
Bacturcult	Wampole Diagnostics, Stamford, Connecticut	Cup method	
UTI-tect	Abbott Laboratories, North Chicago, Ill.	Cup method	Use of four culture media provides selective growth and identification of organisms
Culture-Pette	Scott Laboratories, Inc., New York, N.Y.	Pipet method	Limited by use of one culture medium
Microstix	Ames Company, Div. of Miles Laboratories, Inc., Elkhart, Indiana	Pad culture method	Selective growth by use of two culture media Incorporates nitrites test

done. Some of these kits have incorporated chemical tests that simply screen the urine for presence of bacteria. The most commonly used is the nitrites test (Griess's test), based on the principle that nitrate normally present in the urine is reduced to nitrite by bacteria. This change can be detected by change of color on a reagent pad, indicating bacteriuria. In our laboratories, both the filter paper method kit (Testuria) and the pad culture method kit (Microstix) have given satisfactory results. The Microstix kit has the advantage of having a nitrite test chemical reagent pad besides two pads containing culture media. Though it will detect both gram-positive and gram-negative bacteria, it does not detect *Candida*. The kit has a reported sensitivity of 90.7 per cent and specificity of 99.1 per cent in detecting colony counts of 10^5 or more per milliliter of urine (Kunin, 1974).

Table 24–2 provides a partial list of commercially available office culture kits for easy reference. The choice depends on the ease of handling and of interpretation of results by the physician and office staff.

Vaginal Studies

Vaginal Culture

For women with repetitive infection, a culture obtained by swirling a cotton swab, in a circular fashion, around the vaginal introitus often will yield the source of the recurrent infection. A woman with enteric colonization often will need to be placed on suppressive therapy (see later discussion). Cultures can be repeated at 2 month intervals, and when they show that vaginal flora has reverted to normal, therapy can be terminated.

Vaginal pH

Vaginal pH may be used as an index for monitoring the efficacy of suppressive antimicrobial therapy. One can stop medications when the pH returns to normal, since in our experience the vaginal flora reverts to normal (pH 4.0 to 4.5) in over 90 to 95 per cent of cases when pathogenic bacterial growth disappears. The only accurate way to measure vaginal pH is to employ a pH meter and to place the probe into the vaginal introitus. Various pH indicator papers are too inaccurate to give meaningful information.

Urinalysis

Microscopic examination of the urine for bacteria is an excellent *presumptive* test for presence of urinary infection, that can be done easily and rapidly. It is to be emphasized that for diagnosis of urinary tract infection, one must also have a culture of the urine. With a little experience one can consistently estimate the number of bacteria seen on microscopic examination with quantitative cultures. Urinalysis also allows initial determination of the bacterial morphology, which becomes easier with examination of a stained urine specimen. Depending on personal preference and confidence, either uncentrifuged or centrifuged specimens of urine may be examined. I prefer to examine the unstained, uncentrifuged specimen (a drop of urine on the slide covered with a cover slip) with the phase contrast microscope. This method provides better than 90 per cent accuracy in detecting significant bacteriuria when one or more bacteria are seen per high power ($\times$ 400) field. A methylene blue or Gram stain helps detect bacteria with greater ease, especially the cocci.

The presence of white blood cells (pyuria) and red blood cells suggests infection but is not a reliable index without documented presence of bacteria. Pyuria without significant bacteria may indicate nonbacterial inflammation or a urinary tract foreign body or tumor and is a classic finding in urinary tuberculosis. Approximately 15 to 20 per cent of women with pyuria do not have urinary tract infection. Casts are rare, but when present they indicate renal parenchymal disease. Since diabetics are more susceptible to urinary tract infection, and since infection often produces an alkaline urine, the specimen should be tested for glycosuria and pH. These parameters are easily determined by the plastic urine examination dip sticks available commercially.

ORGANISMS CAUSING BACTERIURIA

Urinary tract infection in the nonpregnant, symptomatic female is usually due to enteric strains of gram-negative aerobic organisms. Of these, *Escherichia coli* is the predominant causative organism in 80 to 85 per cent of patients. The remaining less common organisms are *Klebsiella-Enterobacter, Proteus* species, *Enterococcus, Staphylococcus* and group D *Streptococcus* (Figure 24–3). *Pseudomonas* rarely causes urinary tract infection, except in the presence of significant urinary tract pathology, because it is not part of the bowel flora. In hospitalized females undergoing instrumentation or requiring indwelling catheters, one may see *Serratia marcescens* as the etiologic agent, usually representing nosocomial infection. Anaerobic fecal bacteria do not grow well in urine and are rarely seen in urinary infections. Yeasts such as *Candida albicans* rarely occur except in such abnormal cases as individuals with diabetes or patients receiving immunosuppressive therapy. Candiduria may be difficult to treat and is best handled by intravesical chemotherapy with amphotericin B. In the presence of indwelling catheters and foreign bodies, yeasts are difficult to eradicate and may on occasion cause systemic infection.

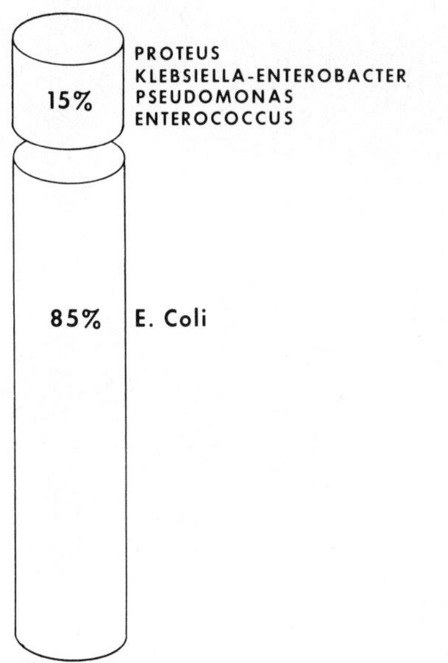

Figure 24–3. Organisms usually causing urinary tract infection.

URINE SPECIMEN COLLECTION METHODS

Accuracy and reliability are of utmost importance in the documentation of significant bacteriuria. Unreliability creates physician frustration, poor patient response, morbidity, and often unnecessary, expensive, and improper antimicrobial therapy. Accurate interpretation of the results of urine examination (culture and urinalysis) depends largely upon the proper collection of the specimen, the timing of specimen analysis, and the individual examiner's experience and interpretative skills (confidence level). Confidence is acquired by practice and an understanding of basic principles involved. The timing of the examination is important, because rapid growth of organisms in urine left standing for more than 30 minutes at room temperature will invalidate the results of both microscopic examination and culture, giving a false-positive result. The false-positive culture presents a major obstacle to consistently accurate diagnosis of urinary tract infection. On the other hand, error in diagnosing significant bacteriuria (false negative) with colony counts below 10,000 (10^4) is extremely rare (less than 2 per cent). Urine specimens that cannot be immediately examined should be refrigerated and studied within 3 to 4 hours.

Suprapubic Aspiration

Suprapubic aspiration of urine directly from the bladder allows the most accurate specimen. It is rarely used in an adult female since midstream voided specimens and catheterized specimens are more rapidly and easily obtained and are reliable.

Midstream Clean-Catch Method

The midstream clean-catch voided specimen is quite acceptable for documentation of true bacteriuria when correctly obtained by the patient or nurse. It has an 80 per cent reliability, which increases to 95 per cent if two consecutive specimens show a colony count of 100,000 or more of the same organism per milliliter of urine. In routine cases of uncomplicated infection, presence of two or more species of organisms normally suggests contamination. Various commercial firms market midstream collection kits with cleansing agents, collecting bottles, and complete instructions.

Urethral Catheterization

Urethral catheterization to obtain the urine specimen is often advisable to avoid contamination from vaginal flora or from splattering of the female urinary stream, ineffective cleansing in obese patients, or the patient's failure to follow instructions precisely.

This method should not be used routinely even though it has been shown to cause bladder bacteriuria in only 1 per cent of nonhospitalized young women without any medical illness or lower urinary tract abnormalities (Turck et al., 1962). However, the risk is somewhat higher in hospitalized women and those with abnormal underlying host defense mechanisms. A positive urine culture (100,000 or more bacteria per milliliter of urine) of a catheterized patient has a 95 per cent accuracy, and false-positive cultures are rare.

EVALUATION OF WOMEN WITH URINARY TRACT INFECTION

Clinical Evaluation

Somewhat controversial is the *extent of evaluation* that a physician should perform on a woman with mild uncomplicated acute urinary infection. Some clinicians are prone to do nothing more than a urinalysis prior to prescribing therapy, whereas others go to extremes of subjecting patients to a complete workup including radiologic and endoscopic studies. I have found that a careful history taken at the initial visit often helps to uncover the pattern of urinary tract infections. If the history clearly indicates a first episode of infection or extremely infrequent reinfection — episodes spaced over a period of years rather than months or weeks — evaluation may be limited to physical examination, urinalysis, and initial as well as follow-up urine cultures. However, if the history indicates recurrent episodes of urinary tract infection (frequent reinfections or relapse), every effort should be made to rule out any underlying host factors that may encourage or perpetuate infection. This evaluation should be undertaken after completion of initial therapy, following the second documented episode of infection.

A thorough physical examination, particularly of the external genitalia and vagina, is most helpful in the *differential diagnosis* of acute uncomplicated urinary tract infection. Vaginitis and senile urethritis are common conditions that may cause burning on urination, frequency, and local periurethral irritation that the patient is unable to clearly define. When vaginitis and urethritis occur concomitantly with urinary infection, they should also be treated appropriately, since they may encourage urinary infection by

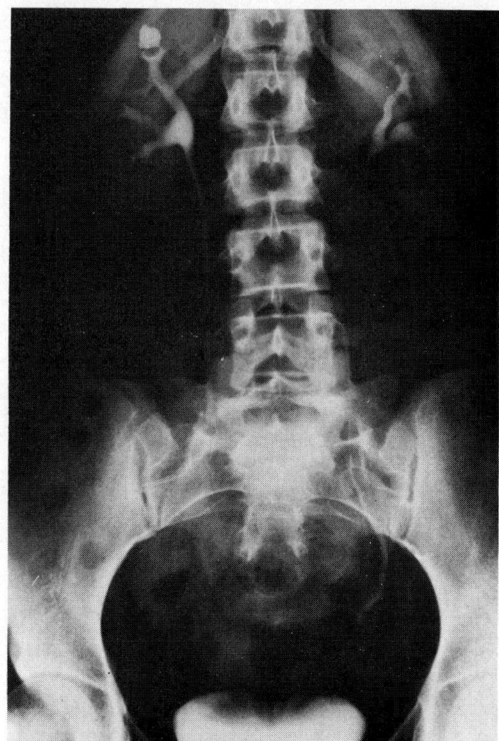

Figure 24–4. Excretory urogram. Right upper pole renal calyceal diverticulum in a 25-year-old female with history of recurrent urinary infections. A calyceal diverticulum is often a site of calculus formation and a possible predisposing factor in relapse.

altering local defense mechanisms. Young women may forget and leave foreign bodies in the vagina, causing lower urinary tract irritative symptoms. I have on several occasions removed an old tampon and in one instance the remains of a decaying black olive! Courses of antimicrobial therapy with poor clinical results may be avoided in these cases.

Roentgenographic Studies

Intravenous Excretory Urography

An intravenous excretory urogram, with its acceptable minimal morbidity and ease of performance, should be the first study obtained. Women with infrequent infections do not need this evaluation since they almost never have an underlying pathologic condition (Fair et al., 1979). In women with rapidly recurring urinary tract infections or infections caused by unusual species of bacteria (e.g., *Proteus)* one might wish to perform an intravenous urogram. It provides in most instances maximal information about the urinary tract anatomy (Figure 24–4), any gross changes in renal function, and the presence of calculi (Figure 24–5, *A* and *B*). Classic radiographic changes suggestive of bacterial inflammation involving the upper urinary tract include irregularity of calyceal outline with blunting or clubbing, cortical scarring with loss of the normal smooth renal outline, and, in severe cases, marked reduction in size of a renal segment or the entire kidney. On rare occasion the pelvicalyceal system may be outlined by intraluminal gas, since bacterial strains other than the clostridial group have been known to produce gas under certain conditions (Figure 24–6). Excretory urography is not contraindicated in acute renal infections; in fact, it should be performed whenever acute pyelonephritis is suspected. This examination is an important diagnostic aid, since one often is uncertain of the exact diagnosis. The intravenous pyelogram should be obtained before therapy (or immediately thereafter), since it will show poor function in the affected tissue, which quickly will revert to normal (Davidson and Talner, 1973), often by 48 hours after initiation of treatment.

Cystography and Voiding Urethrocystography

Cystograms and voiding urethrocystograms delineate the lower urinary tract better than the excretory urogram and provide information about bladder capacity, residual bladder urine, and vesicoureteral reflux. They occasionally suggest neurogenic detrusor dysfunction. These studes are indicated when follow-up cultures are negative and the patient is asymptomatic, since acute cystitis may produce transient reflux and since the risk of developing bacteremia during catheterization and the study itself is higher. A urethral diverticulum may be detected only on the postvoid film because the contrast-filled bladder is usually superimposed on the cystogram films (Figure 24–7, *A*, *B*, and *C*). The intravenous (excretory) urogram often appears to be grossly within normal limits even in the presence of severe vesicoureteral reflux (Figure 24–8, *A* and *B*). Hence, cystography and voiding urethrocystography are a necessary part of patient evaluation.

Retrograde Pyeloureterography

Retrograde pyeloureterography is used less frequently with the advent of improved contrast media for excretory urography, newer radiologic techniques, and tomography. Retrograde studies should be done when the patient is sensitive to the contrast medium or has marked renal insufficiency, or when the initial excretory urogram is inadequate. The risk of introducing bacteria into the urinary tract and possibly causing bacteriuria in the presence of infection makes this study less attractive for routine use.

Endoscopic Studies

Cystoscopy and Urethroscopy

Cystoscopy and urethroscopy in the adult female are easy to do under local anesthesia and are often part of an office examination. There is little indication for these procedures in the patient with acute uncomplicated urinary tract infection. Besides providing visual confirmation of lower urinary tract disease or abnormalities,

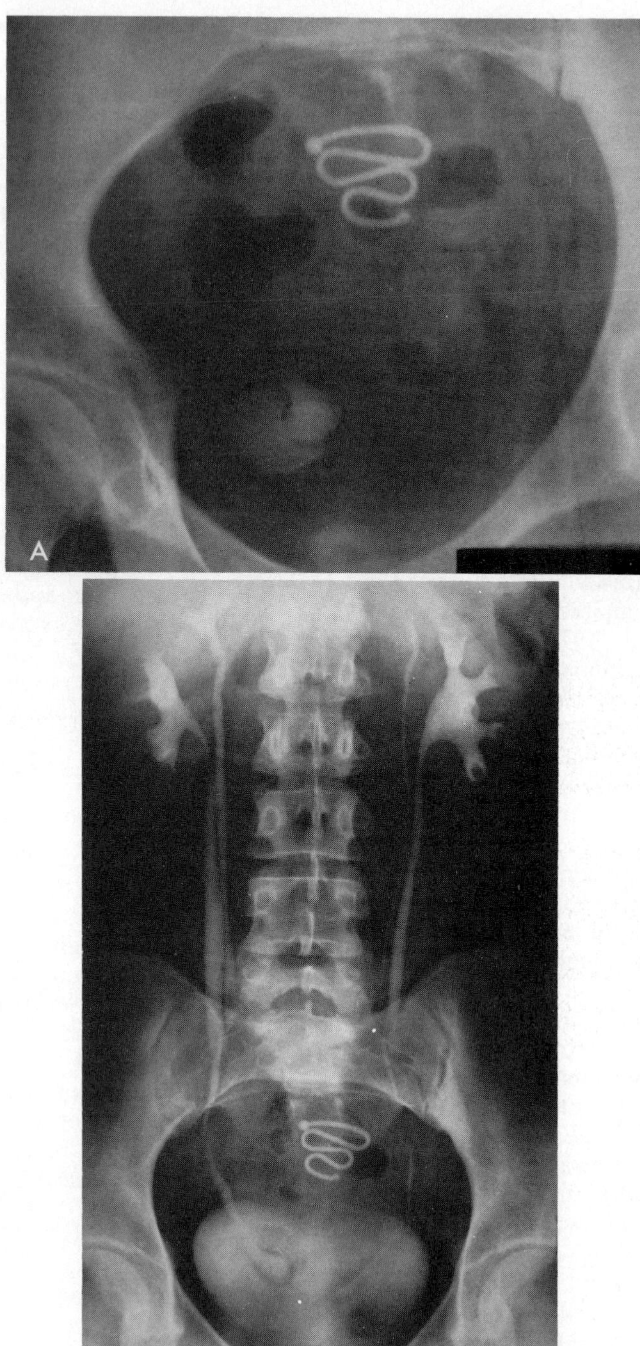

Figure 24–5. Right ureterocele with calculus in a female 36 years of age with a history of recurring urinary infection. *A*, Plain film of pelvis. A large calcific shadow is visible in area of the bladder. *B*, Excretory urogram showing bilateral duplication of upper urinary collecting system and the calculus within the ureterocele. (Intrauterine device is seen in uterus.)

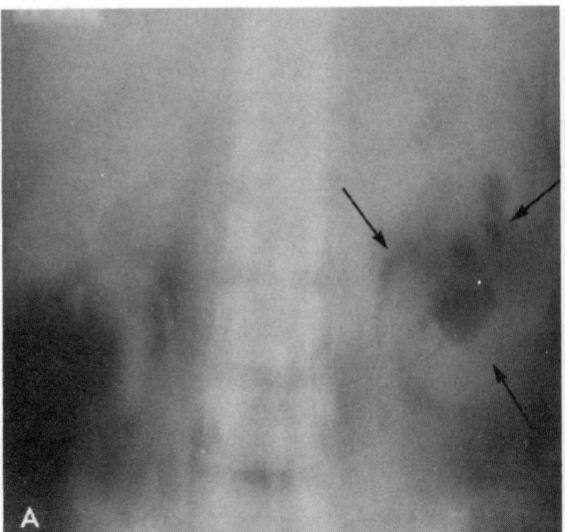

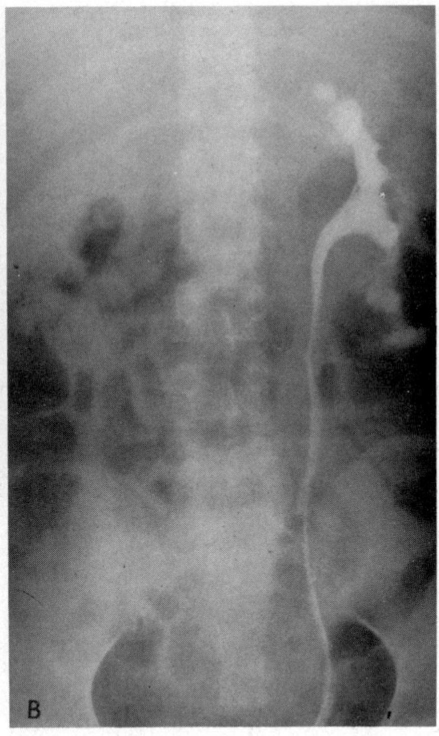

Figure 24–6. Pyelonephritis, left kidney. A 32-year-old female seen initially with severe colicky left flank pain suggestive of ureteropelvic obstruction by calculus. She had minimal systemic symptoms. *A*, Excretory urogram showing delayed function of left kidney. Pelvicalyceal system outlined by intraluminal gas. Urine culture isolated *Escherichia coli*. *B*, Left retrograde pyelogram done at a later date when the patient was asymptomatic reveals extensive blunting of calyces and papillary necrosis.

urethrocystoscopy may be combined with retrograde ureteral catheterization to obtain urine samples from the kidneys in patients with suspected upper tract infection and it may be combined with urethral calibration to detect significant urethral stenosis. The spectrum of cystoscopic findings in patients with recurrent urinary tract infection includes chronic trigonitis, cystitis cystica, ureteroceles, abnormal ureteral orifices with lateral displacement on the bladder wall suggesting presence of reflux, foreign bodies within the bladder, bladder and urethral diverticulum, bladder wall thickening with trabeculation, and, on occasion, gross changes that suggest neurogenic bladder disease. Vaginoscopy, as mentioned earlier, is indicated if not previously done as part of the initial physical examination.

Renal Function Studies

Baseline renal function studies early in evaluation may indicate preexistent renal insufficiency and help in the selection and dosage formulation of the antimicrobial therapy. Studies such as blood urea nitrogen and serum creatinine, though gross parameters of renal function, are usually adequate to monitor antimicrobial drug therapy. Creatinine clearance is often necessary, especially in hospitalized patients and in cases of marked renal insufficiency. Ordinarily, none of these studies is required in women with acute uncomplicated urinary infection, but they are essential when using a potentially nephrotoxic antibiotic (e.g., the aminoglycosides).

Urodynamic Studies

These studies include gas cystometry combined with electronically integrated sphincter electromyography, urethral pressure profile recording, urinary flow rates, and intravesical pressure tracings. There is no place for routine use of any of these, except in a female with some indication of micturition dysfunction or underlying neu-

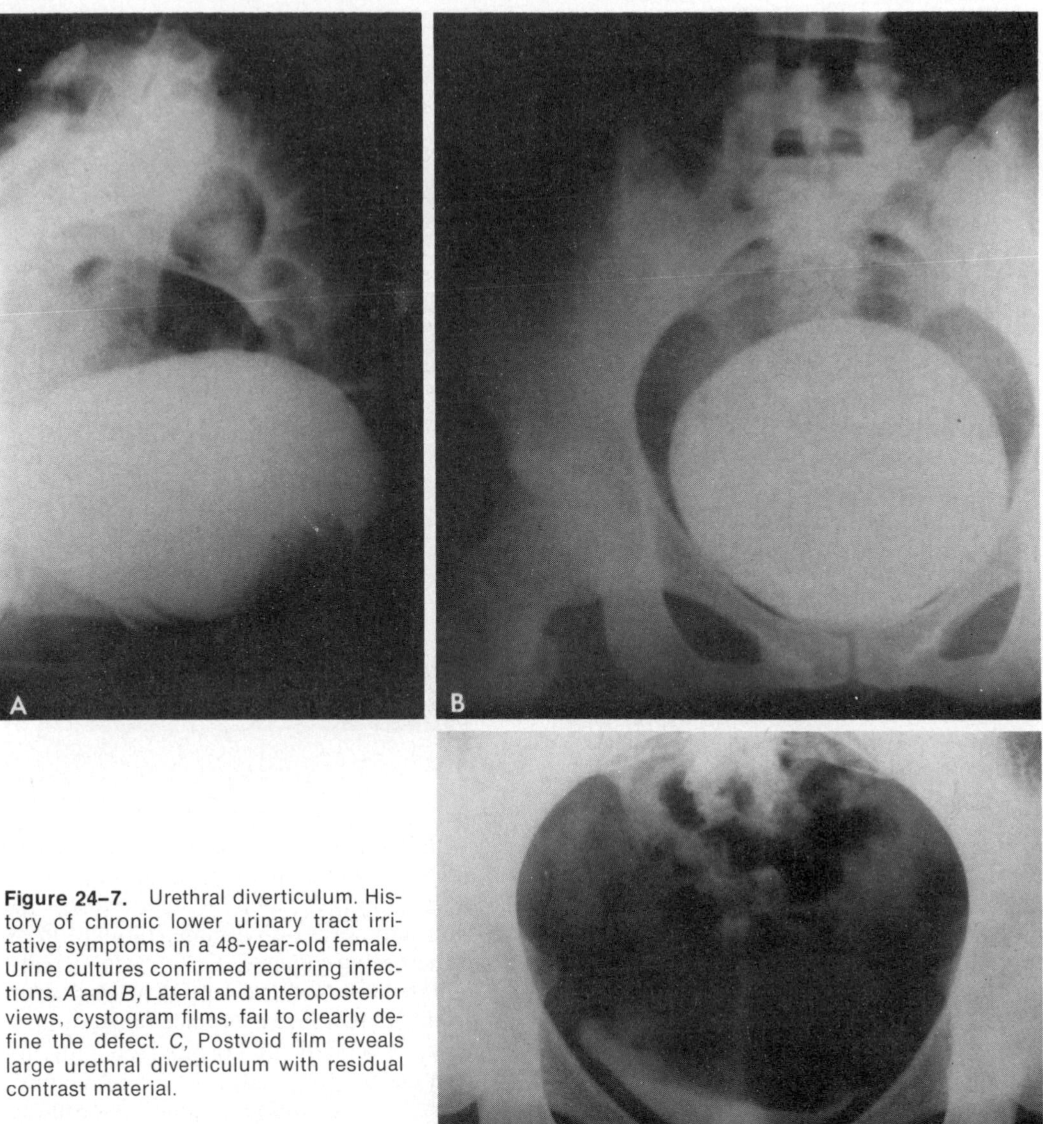

Figure 24–7. Urethral diverticulum. History of chronic lower urinary tract irritative symptoms in a 48-year-old female. Urine cultures confirmed recurring infections. *A* and *B*, Lateral and anteroposterior views, cystogram films, fail to clearly define the defect. *C*, Postvoid film reveals large urethral diverticulum with residual contrast material.

rogenic bladder disease producing a functional obstruction and large residual urine.

Urinary Tract Infection Localization Studies

Since the urinary tract is essentially a contiguous, open system from the urethral meatus up to the kidneys, a positive urine culture simply denotes the presence of infection within the system. In patients with history of frequent reinfection or relapse, it is helpful to differentiate bladder bacteriuria from renal bacteriuria. Many of these women have periods of asymptomatic bacteriuria; this also justifies efforts to exclude a locus for recurrent bacteriuria from within one or both kidneys. The clinical usefulness lies in planning patient manage-

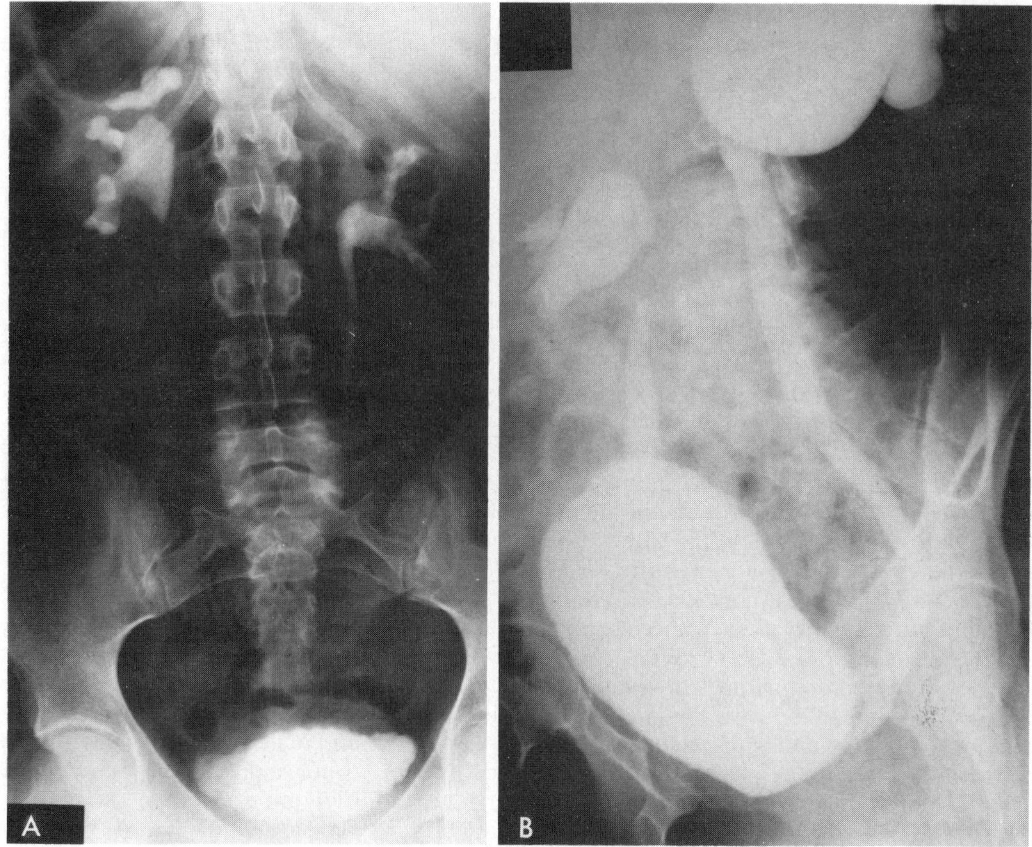

Figure 24–8. Chronic pyelonephritis of right kidney and bilateral total vesicoureteral reflux in a 19-year-old female with past history of numerous episodes of urinary infection. *A*, Excretory urogram. Except for blunting of calyces, especially the right upper pole calyx, the study is relatively unimpressive. *B*, Cystogram revealing underlying gross reflux with dilatation of ureters, pelves, and calyces.

ment, since the presence of renal infection might suggest a more vigorous and extended therapeutic approach than does the presence of lower urinary tract infection alone.

Indirect Methods

Indirect methods of localizing urinary tract infection, being noninvasive, appear attractive at first glance. Unfortunately none of these has found acceptance in clinical practice. They include: (1) special staining of urinary sediment to detect polymorphonuclear leukocytes originating in the kidney (''glitter cell'' stain); (2) examination of urinary sediment after intravenous injection of bacterial pyrogen or adrenocorticoids; (3) measurements of various urinary enzyme excretion; (4) tests of maximal urinary concentrating ability; and (5) determination of the immunologic response by estimating serum antibody titers against type-specific organisms in the urine (Cobbs, 1972).

Another useful method is to examine the urine for bacteria that are ''antibody-coated'' (Thomas et al., 1974). This is based on the observation that unlike bladder bacteriuria, renal infection produces a systemic antibody response. The urine sample is collected by catheterization. A 15 ml. aliquot is centrifuged immediately and the sediment placed on a slide, air dried, and fixed with acetone. The sample is then treated with the fluorescein-labeled antihuman IgG and examined for fluorescent bacteria. A positive test suggests that the upper urinary tract is the source of bacteriuria. The principal source of error is from the perineal flora, which may be antibody coated. For this reason, a voided specimen should never be used.

Direct Methods

Direct methods of localizing urinary infection are more accurate but invasive. Examination of renal tissue for bacteria or bacterial antigen by the *fluorescent antibody technique* has not been reliable and appears to be rather drastic for routine use. Fortunately, when properly performed, *selective ureteral catheterization* via cystoscopy and urine sampling for culture provides accurate localization of renal infection with little if any morbidity (Stamey et al., 1965). This is the method I use when necessary.

Another technique of ureteral urine sampling is the *bladder wash-out technique,* which requires only bladder catheterization (Fairley et al., 1967). The bladder urine is sent for culture; then neomycin solution is instilled and left within the bladder for an hour. The neomycin kills the bladder bacteria but not those in the ureters or kidneys. The bladder is then thoroughly washed out with approximately 2 liters of sterile water. Urine samples are then collected every 10 minutes for half an hour. These samples, representing ureteric and renal urine, are sent for culture. The bladder wash-out method is somewhat time consuming and does not designate the side of renal involvement. It may also be inaccurate if vesicoureteral reflux exists.

Patterns of Response to Antimicrobial Therapy

Perhaps the most feasible approach in a majority of patients with chronic bacteriuria is to study their pattern of response to prescribed antimicrobial therapy. Patients with bladder bacteriuria differ from those with renal bacteriuria in the results of treatment and in the pattern of recurrence of infection after seemingly effective antimicrobial therapy. In 80 per cent of patients with recurrences of upper urinary tract infection, the recurrences involved the same organisms as the original infection; i.e., the recurrences were relapses. On the other hand, in 71 per cent of the patients with recurrences of bladder bacteriuria, the recurrences were actually reinfections with new organisms (Turck et al., 1968). The patient's pattern of response should be defined in light of this information, and therapy modified as necessary.

MANAGEMENT OF URINARY TRACT INFECTIONS

The chief goals in the treatment of women with urinary tract infection are to decrease morbidity due to the accompanying symptoms, eradicate the causative bacteria, and prevent recurrences to deter secondary changes of renal functional abnormalities and structural damage to the urinary tract.

In the practice of ambulatory medicine, the majority of women seen have symptoms suggestive of mild (cystitis) to moderate (pyelonephritis) degrees of urinary tract infection. Unless physical examination and urinalysis (bacteriuria) clearly indicate urinary infection, it is advisable to withhold definitive antimicrobial therapy until diagnostic cultures are available. Symptoms along with pyuria are not enough to diagnose urinary infection in the absence of bacteria. And as a general rule, one should treat bacteriuria and not pyuria.

General Measures

Rest and *adequate hydration* are important for all patients. Hydration helps to bring about more frequent bladder emptying and dilution of bacterial counts, and also decreases renal medullary osmolality, to assist phagocytosis and perhaps destroy cell wall-deficient bacterial strains. Hydration may also help to decrease the concentration of bacterial growth factors such as glucose and organic acids. *Acidification* of urine has been employed to increase the antibacterial property of urine and inhibit bacterial multiplication (Table 24–3). We have found, however, that urinary acidification has little effect in "in vitro" testing of bacterial growth as well as little clinical effect. Consequently, acidification generally is not indicated, especially since the patient is being treated with a course of

TABLE 24–3. URINARY ACIDIFIERS: Listed in order of preference

Agent	Usual Dose	Remarks
Ascorbic acid	500 mg. twice daily May be increased if necessary	Patient acceptance excellent. Very large doses may cause urate and oxalate stones.
Cranberry juice	Large amounts at frequent intervals	Patient acceptance fair to good.
Ammonium chloride	12 gm. a day in divided doses	Patient acceptance poor. Contraindicated in renal and hepatic failure.
Methionine	12 gm. a day in divided doses	Patient acceptance poor. Contraindicated in renal failure.
Sodium acid phosphate (NaH_2PO_4)	1 gm. four times a day orally	Patient acceptance poor. Contraindicated in renal and cardiac failure.

antimicrobial drug that is much more effective. However, it is helpful in patients with recurrent urinary infections and patients taking methenamine compounds, since the antibacterial activity of these agents is maximal at a pH of 5.5 or less. I find that having the patient frequently check the urinary pH with nitrazine paper is the most effective means of maintaining low urinary pH over a period of time. *Urinary analgesic agents* such as phenazopyridine hydrochloride (Pyridium) help relieve pain and burning on urination. If prescribed they should be used for only 2 to 3 days along with a specific antibacterial agent. I use these agents frequently in managing women with lower urinary tract irritative symptoms but without any indication of infection.

Basic Principles of Antimicrobial Therapy

Choice of Agent

Because as many as 10 to 20 per cent of women will have relapsing infections, the choice of which of the many antimicrobial agents to employ should be based on certain important considerations. These are discussed in detail here.

Host Factors. Known hypersensitivity reaction to a drug obviously would contraindicate its use in an individual patient. In addition, presence of underlying structural defects of the urinary tract or presence of calculi and catheters, or other foreign bodies, may alter the expected response to a therapeutic agent. In patients with infected foreign bodies, one can never hope to sterilize the urinary tract but at best only to suppress the growth of bacteria. Such cases make up a small part of those seen in routine practice, however, and their management will not be discussed in detail.

With the relapse rate after urinary tract infection being 10 to 20 per cent, it is important that the antibiotic therapy will not alter the rectal flora, which is the reservoir of microorganisms in these individuals and which intermittently or continually colonizes the perineum. The principal way in which the reservoir is altered is by unabsorbed drug that passes into the fecal stream and is capable of rapidly selecting for resistant organisms. The two principal compounds that act in this way are the tetracyclines and ampicillin, neither of which should be a first-line drug for treatment of simple cystitis.

With the vaginal vault and periurethral area being the source of pathogenic bacteria in recurrent urinary tract infection, it would be best to use an antibiotic that does not destroy the normal flora, which could potentially prevent the growth of the uropathogens by acting in a bacterial interference fashion. The compounds most likely to destroy the normal vaginal flora and set up a vaginitis are the penicillins, particularly ampicillin, and tetracycline.

Another criterion in the selection of antibiotics for treating cystitis should be low cost. Since many antimicrobial compounds are relatively inexpensive there are many from which to choose, even in the presence of sensitivity reactions.

Finally, one would want a compound that

concentrates well in the urine since this is where the infection is. Invariably the oral antibiotics all develop very high urinary levels; in fact, the urine levels are often well in excess of the sensitivity assays that are reported by most laboratories.

Serum Levels. A high serum level of an antibiotic is undesirable in treatment of acute cystitis, since the goal is to achieve a urine level of the antibiotic sufficient to kill the pathogenic bacteria without altering the normal flora anywhere in the body. Preservation of normal flora prevents vaginitis, which might lead to a vicious circle of vaginitis-cystitis. A high serum level of antibiotic also can alter the bowel flora, which is the ultimate reservoir of pathogenic microorganisms in the urinary tract. Most of the oral preparations attain reasonably significant serum levels that can alter the bowel and vaginal flora. The penicillins and tetracyclines significantly affect the vaginal flora. Trimethoprim/sulfamethoxazole (Septra, Bactrim) has a significant effect on the bowel flora, due most likely to its serum level. The compounds that have an extremely low serum level, with a half-life of only 19 minutes, are the nitrofurantoins. These are excellent compounds to use because the only antibacterial level obtained in the body is in the urine. This may explain why there has been no selection or change in the resistance pattern to this compound in the 25 years that it has been on the market. Macrodantin, the macrocrystalline form of nitrofurantoin, should be used because the gastrointestinal side effects of the generic compound are so marked that the patient compliance is poor.

Bacteriologic Data. The bacteriologic data are largely dependent on the urine culture and disc sensitivity patterns. These studies are particularly important for systemic infections, such as pyelonephritis, where one would wish to obtain an adequate serum level to treat the infection. Although one may employ these disc sensitivity patterns for lower urinary tract infections, many of the bacterial species are susceptible to the very high levels of antibiotic obtained in the urine. For example, *E. coli* and *Proteus* species are susceptible to greater than 60 μg of penicillin G, a level easily obtained in the urine (Kulers and Bennett, 1975). *Pseudomonas* species are 80 per cent susceptible to urine levels of tetracycline. This drug can also be used empirically to treat *Pseudomonas* infections, although they rarely are found in female outpatients with cystitis.

Table 24–4 summarizes the usual sensi-

TABLE 24–4. USUAL SPECTRUM OF ANTIMICROBIAL SENSITIVITY OF ORGANISMS CAUSING URINARY TRACT INFECTION

Organisms	Trimethoprim-sulfamethoxazole	Nitrofurantoin	Nalidixic acid	Ampicillin	Cephalothin	Tetracyclines	Kanamycin	Gentamicin	Polymyxins	Carbenicillin
Escherichia coli	+	+	+	+	+	±	+	+	+	+
Kiebsiella	+	±	+	−	+	±	+	+	+	−
Enterobacter	+	−	+	−	−	−	+	+	+	+
Proteus mirabilis	+	−	+	+	+	−	+	+	−	+
Indole-positive *Proteus; vulgaris, morganii* and *rettgeri*	±	±	±	−	−	±	+	+	−	+
Pseudomonas	−	−	−	−	−	−	−	+	+	+
Enterococcus	−	±	−	+	±	+	−	−	−	−
Staphylococcus	−	+	−	+	+	+	+	+	−	+
Serratia marcescens	+	−	−	−	−	−	−	+	−	−

\+ Effective — Not effective ± Occasionally effective

tivity patterns of most species of gram-negative bacteria to antibiotics (Cox, 1974; Appel, 1977a, b, c).

Systemic Urinary Tract Infection. For patients who have systemic infection — that is, principally pyelonephritis — the physician should select an antibiotic that will attain a significant serum level, since the badly infected renal unit is poorly perfused. The agent selected should be based on the sensitivity data when they become available. Prior to that, one may initiate the broad-spectrum coverage necessary to treat the organisms expected to be causing the infection. Although an in-depth review of the principles of management of pyelonephritis is not within the scope of this chapter, it is a general rule that compounds such as ampicillin should be used to cover enterococci, in combination with the aminoglycoside of choice. When sensitivity data become available, one may then use the least toxic drug to which the organism is susceptible. In the presence of positive blood cultures, the treatment should continue for a minimum of 10 days by the intravenous route.

Lower Urinary Tract Infections. Since patients with lower urinary tract infection make up the majority of individuals who are treated for infections, the bulk of the following discussion will concern their management.

Precautions

The kidney is the major route for excretion of most of the antimicrobial agents. In cases of decreased renal function, toxicity may be caused by accumulation and prolonged exposure to increased levels of the drug or its metabolite. Many antibiotics have direct nephrotoxicity, making it more important to reduce the dose of antibiotic (Whelton, 1974). Continual monitoring of renal function is advisable when these potentially toxic agents are used in patients with azotemia. There are two ways to adjust dosage in these patients: (1) by giving the dose of the drug in the usual manner but increasing the interval between subsequent doses, depending on serum creatinine or creatinine clearance values (variable frequency regimen; dosage intervals should not be greater than 24 hours, however) or (2) by administering smaller doses after the initial loading dose while maintaining a constant interval between doses (variable dosage regimen).

In cases of lower urinary tract infections in individuals with impaired renal function, antibiotic therapy should be selected with prevention of toxicity in mind (Table 24–5). In general, one should select an antibiotic that is both filtered and secreted by the kidneys in order to obtain maximum urine levels to treat the infection, e.g., penicillin, cephalosporins, or sulfonamides. One should avoid compounds such as nalidixic acid, which is rapidly inactivated by the liver and therefore attains less than adequate urine levels. Tetracycline also should be avoided in patients with significantly impaired renal function, since the tetracyclines tend to be catabolic and perhaps increase the degree of renal failure. Most importantly, nitrofurantoin compounds should be avoided, since they are very rapidly metabolized, having a serum half-life of only 19 minutes, and attain inadequate urine levels while their toxic metabolites accumulate in the serum.

Clinical Management of Women with Urinary Tract Infection

First Episode or Infrequent Reinfection

In a first episode of lower urinary tract infection or a rare reinfection, the organism involved usually is *E. coli,* which is sensitive to almost all of the standard oral antimicrobials. In 80 per cent of women, a short course of therapy results in bacteriologic cure. The principal compounds available and guidelines for management and follow-up are listed in Table 24–6. The length of therapy can be extremely short; in fact, one dose is sufficient to eradicate the infection in 80 per cent of women (Rubin et al., 1980; Ronald et al., 1976). As a general rule, an effective and inexpensive therapeutic course should consist of approximately 3 days of full-dose antibiotic therapy followed by suppression for 4 more days with one dose at bedtime.

TABLE 24–5. SERUM AND URINARY LEVELS OF ANTIMICROBIAL DRUGS, THEIR POTENTIAL TOXICITY, AND DOSAGE MODIFICATION IN PRESENCE OF RENAL INSUFFICIENCY

Antimicrobial Drug	Serum Level	Urinary Level	Major Toxic Properties	Dosage Change in Renal Failure
Trimethoprim-sulfamethoxazole	±	++	Allergic reactions; blood dyscrasias	Reduce dose
Nitrofurantoin	−	++	Peripheral neuropathy; pneumonitis	Avoid use
Nalidixic acid	+	++	Central nervous system	Avoid use
Ampicillin	+	++	Allergic reactions; pseudomembranous colitis	No change
Cephalothin, Cephalexin, Cephazolin	++	++	Allergic reactions; hepatic dysfunction	No change or slight
Cephaloridine	++	++	Nephrotoxic	Avoid use
Tetracyclines*	±	± to +	Hepatic dysfunction; nephrotoxic	Avoid all preparations except doxycycline
Kanamycin	++	++	Ototoxic (auditory); nephrotoxic	Major dose reduction
Gentamicin	++	++	Ototoxic (vestibular); nephrotoxic	Major dose reduction
Polymyxins	++	± to +	Peripheral neuropathy; nephrotoxic	Major dose reduction
Carbenicillin	++	++	Allergic reactions	No change or slight
Indanyl ester of carbenicillin	±	++	Bleeding diathesis	No change or slight

++ Good + Adequate ± Borderline − Negligible

*Serum and urinary concentrations vary with different tetracycline preparations.

Frequent Reinfection or Recurrence

Women who are highly susceptible to frequent reinfections that are not adequately controlled by short-course therapy may be placed on long-term suppressive antimicrobial therapy (Stamey et al., 1977). This is performed by selecting from the list in Table 24–6 the highest compound on the list to which the patient has no sensitivity. The patient should first receive low-dose therapy for 3 days to clear her urine, and then the dose should be reduced to one tablet at bedtime. If she remains infection-free on this regimen, she may then be placed on a dosage of one tablet every other night. Monitoring the patient is best done by culturing the vaginal introitus, the source of the recurrent bacteriuria, at 4 to 6 month intervals. When the uropathogens causing the infections have disappeared according to vaginal introital cultures, suppressive therapy may be stopped.

Relapsing or Persistent Infection

In a small percentage of women, relapsing or persistent urinary tract infection is caused by surgically correctable abnormalities. For this reason, women with relapsing infection should have complete evaluation, including radiologic examinations, to uncover any such factors. In some of the patients, however, relapse occurs despite surgical correction of the underlying fac-

TABLE 24–6. MANAGEMENT OF SYMPTOMATIC URINARY TRACT INFECTION

Women with first episode of urinary infection or with an infrequent episode of reinfection

Severity of Clinical Illness	Antimicrobial Agents	Duration of Therapy	Follow-up Schedule for Urine Cultures
Mild (cystitis)	Sulfonamides Nitrofurantoin Nalidixic acid Trimethoprim-sulfamethoxazole	10 to 14 days	(a) 42 to 72 hours after start of therapy, especially if no symptomatic response (b) 7 to 10 days post therapy, then (c) Once a month for 3 months, then (d) Once every 3 months for one year, then (e) Once every 6 months for one year
Moderate (pyelonephritis)	Ampicillin Cephalosporins: Cephalexin Cephradine Tetracyclines	As above	As above

tors, and in others no abnormalities may be found. If one suspects that the renal units are the source of the recurrent infection in such patients, therapy may be extended to 6 weeks of full-course oral medication (Turck et al., 1966). If relapse still occurs, further prolongation of therapy may be necessary. Since patients in this group often represent cases of acute complicated urinary tract infection, the pathogenic organisms often are resistant to multiple drugs and systemic antibiotic therapy may be necessary. Many patients, however, will have a fixed renal reservoir of organisms and will respond successfully to long-term oral antibiotic therapy.

Prophylactic Therapy after Sexual Intercourse

Some women who are susceptible to urinary tract infection can relate the onset of their cystitis to recent sexual intercourse. After the acute infection has been treated, reinfection can be prevented by a single dose of antibiotic (see Table 24–6) after intercourse (Stamey, 1972; Vosti, 1975).

Antimicrobial Drugs

The number of microbial agents increases every year with the introduction of new drugs. Many of these represent small molecular structural alteration of older, well-established drugs. Usually they offer no significant advantage and are often more expensive than the older standard preparations. No attempt will be made to discuss at any length the various groups of antibacterial agents. However, we would like to mention a few significant aspects of some of the relatively newer agents.

Among the penicillins, *amoxicillin* does have the pharmacokinetic advantage of being better absorbed (80 per cent) and has a longer half-life. Therefore, the dose required is lower and less frequently given than ampicillin and has far less effect on the bowel flora. Except that amoxicillin causes less diarrhea, the two drugs are essentially identical in their side-effects and antibacterial activity. Carbenicillin is the first of the semisynthetic penicillins to inhibit *Pseudomonas* and indole-positive *Proteus*. The sodium salt of the *indanyl ester of carbenicillin* (Geocillin) is the only oral preparation available today for treatment of urinary tract infection due to *Pseudomonas* organisms in ambulatory patients.

Ticarcillin is a more recently introduced semisynthetic penicillin with antipseudomonal activity. It is at least twice as active in vitro as is carbenicillin against *Pseudomonas* and equally active against *E. coli* and *Proteus* species. It produces adequate serum and urine levels even with marked renal insufficiency and can be used in much lower dosage than can those recommended for carbenicillin. Ticarcillin may be useful in serious infections due to susceptible gram-negative organisms in patients not allergic to penicillin.

The original cephalosporin group consisted of cephalothin, cephaloridine, and cephalexin for intravenous, intramuscular and oral use respectively. *Cephazolin* produces higher and more prolonged serum levels than cephalothin and cephaloridine. It also lacks the potential of renal toxicity and hence has replaced cephaloridine as an intramuscular agent. *Cephapirin* also gives good blood levels and causes less incidence of phlebitis on intravenous use. *Cephradine* is a new oral cephalosporin that offers no significant advantage over cephalexin. The antibacterial activity of all cephalosporin preparations is the same.

The group of aminoglycoside antibiotics was recently joined by tobramycin and amikacin. *Tobramycin* and gentamicin have similar antibacterial activity; however, tobramycin has one significant advantage over gentamicin in that it is less toxic to the kidneys, as proved by animal studies and more recently by human studies (Kumin, 1980). However, in vitro susceptibility studies have consistently shown *Pseudomonas aeruginosa* to be two to four times more sensitive to tobramycin than to the other two drugs. Tobramycin is less active against *Serratia marcescens* and *Enterobacter*. *Amikacin* has the advantage of having an accepted safe dose at least three times greater than that of gentamicin or tobramycin. It provides reliable serum levels that do not require frequent monitoring except in renal failure. This may be an advantage in community practice where aminoglycoside levels cannot be easily determined. The most important role of amikacin appears to be in the treatment of infections due to gentamicin- and tobramycin-resistant organisms (Yu et al., 1977). Where such resistance does not exist or is very low, amikacin should be withheld to delay emergence of amikacin-resistant organisms.

REFERENCES

Andriole, G.: Urinary tract infections. Urol. Clin. North Am. *2*:451, 1975.

Appel, G. B., and Neu, H. C.: The nephrotoxicity of antimicrobial agents. N. Engl. J. Med. *296*:663, 1977a.

Appel, G. B., and Neu, H. C.: The nephrotoxocity of antimicrobial agents. N. Engl. J. Med. *296*:722, 1977b.

Appel, G. B., and Neu, H. C.: The nephrotoxicity of antimicrobial agents. N. Engl. J. Med. *296*:784, 1977c.

Asscher, A. W., Sussman, M., Waters, W. E., et al.: The clinical significance of asymptomatic bacteriuria in the nonpregnant woman. J. Infect. Dis. *120*:17, 1969.

Bran, J. L., Levison, M. E., and Kaye, D.: Entrance of bacteria into the female urinary bladder. N. Engl. J. Med. *286*:626, 1972.

Cobbs, C. G.: Localization of urinary tract infection. *In* Kaye, D. (ed.): Urinary Tract Infection and Its Management. St. Louis, C. V. Mosby Co., 1972, p. 52.

Cox, C. E.: Urinary infection and renal lithiasis. Urol. Clin. N. Amer. *1*:279, 1974.

Cox, C. E., and Hinman, F., Jr.: Experiments with induced bacteriuria, vesical emptying and bacterial growth on the mechanism of bladder defense to infection. J. Urol. *86*:739, 1961.

Cox, C. E., Lacy, S. S., and Hinman, F., Jr.: The urethra and its relationship to urinary tract infection. II. The urethral flora of the female with recurrent urinary tract infection. J. Urol. *99*:632, 1968.

Davidson, A. J., and Talner, L. B.: Urographic and angiographic abnormalities in adult onset acute bacterial nephritis. Radiology *106*:249, 1973.

Elkins, I. B., and Cox, C. E.: Perineal, vaginal and urethral bacteriology of young women. I. Incidence of gram-negative colonization. J. Urol. *3*:88, 1974.

Fair, W. R., McClennan, B. L., and Jost, R. G.: Are excretory urograms necessary in evaluating women with urinary tract infection? J. Urol. *121*:313, 1979.

Fairley, K. F., Bond, A. G., Brown, R. B., et al.: Simple test to determine the site of urinary tract infection. Lancet *2*:427, 1967.

Gruneberg, R. N., Leigh, D. A., and Brumfitt, W.: *Escherichia coli* serotypes in urinary tract infection: Studies in domiciliary antenatal and hospital practice. *In* O'Grady, F., and Brumfitt, W. (eds.): Urinary Tract Infection. London, Oxford University Press, 1968, p. 68.

Guze, L. B., and Kalmanson, G. M.: Persistence of bacteria in "protoplast" form after apparent cure of pyelonephritis in rats. Science *143*:1340, 1964.
Heptinstall, R. H.: Experimental pyelonephritis: A comparison of blood-borne and ascending patterns of infection. J. Pathol. *89*:71, 1965.
Hodson, C. J.: The radiological contribution toward the diagnosis of chronic pyelonephritis. Radiology *88*:857, 1967.
Kass, E. H.: Asymptomatic infections of the urinary tract. Trans. Assoc. Amer. Physicians *69*:56, 1956.
Kass, E. H., Savage, W. D., and Santamarina, B. A. G.: The significance of bacteriuria in preventive medicine. *In* Kass, E. H. (ed.): Progress in Pyelonephritis. Philadelphia, F. A. Davis Co., 1964, p. 3.
Kaye, D.: Host defense mechanisms in the urinary tract. Urol. Clin. N. Amer. *2*:407, 1975.
Kulers, A., and Bennett, N. M.: The Use of Antibiotics. Philadelphia, J. B. Lippincott Company, 1975, p. 212.
Kumin, G. D.: Clinical nephrotoxicity of Tobramycin and Gentamicin. A prospective study. J.A.M.A. *244*:1808, 1980.
Kunin, C. M.: Microbial persistence versus reinfection in recurrent urinary tract infections. Antimicrobial Agents and Chemotherapy 1962, 1963, p. 21 (American Society for Microbiology, Ann Arbor).
Kunin, C. M.: A ten-year study of bacteriuria in school girls: Final report of bacteriologic, urologic and epidemiologic findings. J. Infect. Dis. *122*:382, 1970.
Kunin, C. M.: Detection, Prevention and Management of Urinary Tract Infections. Philadelphia, Lea and Febiger, 1974, p. 92.
Kunin, C. M., and McCormack, R. C.: An epidemiologic study of bacteriuria and blood pressure among nuns and working women. N. Engl. J. Med. *278*:635, 1968.
Lang, W. R.: Vaginal acidity and pH. A review. Obstet. Gynecol. Surv. *10*:546, 1955.
Levison, M. E., and Kaye, D.: Management of urinary tract infection. *In* Kaye, D. (ed.): Urinary Tract Infection and Its Management. St. Louis, C. V. Mosby Co., 1972, p. 188.
McCabe, W. R., and Jackson, G. R.: Treatment of pyelonephritis: bacterial, drug and host factors in success or failure among 252 patients. N. Engl. J. Med. *272*:1037, 1965.
Norden, C. W., Green, G. M., and Kass, E. H.: Antibacterial mechanisms of the urinary bladder. J. Clin. Invest. *47*:2689, 1968.
Parsons, C. L., Lofland, S., and Mulholland, S. G.: The effect of trichomonal vaginitis on vaginal pH. J. Urol. *118*:621, 1977.
Parsons, C. L., Stauffer, C., and Schmidt, J. D.: Bladder surface glycosaminoglycans: An efficient mechanism of environmental adaptation. Science *208*:605, 1980.
Roberts, A. P., and Beard, R. W.: Some factors affecting bacterial invasion of bladder during pregnancy. Lancet *1*:1133, 1965.
Rocha, H.: Epidemiology of urinary tract infection in adults. *In* Kaye, D. (ed.): Urinary Tract Infection and Its Management. St. Louis, C. V. Mosby Co., 1972, p. 148.
Ronald, A. R., Boutros, P., and Mourtada, H.: Bacteria localization and response to single-dose therapy in women. J.A.M.A. *235*:1854, 1976.
Rubin, R. H., Fang, L. S. T., Jones, S. R., et al.: Single-dose amoxicillin therapy for urinary tract infection. Multicenter trial using antibody-coated bacteria localization technique. J.A.M.A. *244*:561, 1980.
Salvatierra, O., Jr.: Renal transplantation. J. Continuing Education Urol. *18*:13, 1979.
Salvatierra, O., Kountz, S. L., and Belzer, F. O.: Primary vesicoureteral reflux and end-stage renal disease. J.A.M.A. *226*:1454, 1973.
Schaeffer, A. J., and Stamey, T. A.: Studies of introital colonization in women with recurrent urinary infections. X. The role of antimicrobial therapy. J. Urol. *118*:221, 1977.
Stamey, T. A.: Urinary Infections. Baltimore, Williams & Wilkins Co., 1972, pp. 80 and 269.
Stamey, T. A., Condy, M., and Mihara, G.: Prophylactic efficacy of nitrofurantoin macrocrystals and trimethoprim-sulphamethoxazole in urinary infections. Biologic effects on the vaginal and rectal flora. N. Engl. J. Med. *296*:780, 1977.
Stamey, T. A., Govan, D. E., and Palmer, J. M.: The localization and treatment of urinary tract infections: The role of bactericidal urine levels as opposed to serum levels. Medicine *44*:1, 1965.
Stamey, T. A., and Mihara, G.: Observations on the growth of urethral and vaginal bacteria in sterile urine. J. Urol. *124*:461, 1980.
Stamey, T. A., and Sexton, C. C.: The role of vaginal colonization with Enterobacteriaceae in recurrent urinary infections. J. Urol. *113*:214, 1975.
Stamey, T. A., Timothy, M., Millar, M., et al.: Recurrent urinary infections in adult women. The role of introital enterobacteria. Calif. Med. *115*:1, 1971.
Stamey, T. A., and Timothy, M. M.: Studies of introital colonization in women with recurrent urinary infections. I. The role of vaginal pH. J. Urol. *114*:261, 1975.
Teague, N., and Boyarsky, S.: Further effects of coliform bacteria on ureteral peristalsis. J. Urol. *99*:720, 1968.

Thomas, V., Shelokov, A., and Forland, M.: Antibody-coated bacteria in the urine and the site of urinary tract infection. N. Engl. J. Med. *290*:588, 1974.

Turck, M., Anderson, K. N., and Petersdorf, R. G.: Relapse and reinfection in chronic bacteriuria. N. Engl. J. Med. *275*:70, 1966.

Turck, M., Goffe, B., and Petersdorf, R. G.: The urethral catheter and urinary tract infection. J. Urol. *88*:834, 1962.

Turck, M., Ronald, A. R., and Petersdorf, R. G.: Relapse and reinfection in chronic bacteriuria. II. The correlation between site of infection and pattern of recurrence in chronic bateriuria. N. Engl. J. Med. *278*:422, 1968.

Vejlsgaard, R.: Bacteriuria in patients with diabetes mellitus. *In* Kass, E. H. (ed.): Progress in Pyelonephritis. Philadelphia, F. A. Davis Co., 1965, p. 478.

Vosti, K. L.: Recurrent urinary tract infections: Prevention by prophylactic antibiotics after sexual intercourse. J.A.M.A. *231*:934, 1975.

Whelton, A.: Antibacterial chemotherapy in renal insufficiency: A review. Antibiot. Chemother. *18*:1, 1974.

Yu, V. L., Rhame, F. S., Pesanti, E. L., et al.: Amikacin therapy. Use against infections caused by gentamicin- and tobramycin-resistant organisms. J.A.M.A. *238*:943, 1977.

25

AGE-SPECIFIC URINARY TRACT PROBLEMS

PART 1 PEDIATRIC

GEORGE W. KAPLAN, M.D.
WILLIAM A. BROCK, M.D.

PART 2 ADOLESCENT/SEXUALLY ACTIVE

ALVIN L. BREKKEN, M.D.

PART 3 POSTMENOPAUSAL

ROBERT CORLETT, M.D.

PART 1

PEDIATRIC

INTRODUCTION

In the broad spectrum of gynecologic and urologic disorders, the problems of the infant and prepubertal girl deserve separate consideration. In this age group, congenital abnormalities of anatomic or hormonal genitourinary development are more likely to be encountered than are the acquired lesions seen in the pubertal or adult female. This is an area of interest that has been at the periphery of the practicing urologist or gynecologist and often falls in between their areas of expertise. By virtue of a primary interest in congenital genitourinary disorders, the pediatric urologist has inherited the care of many young girls with primary gynecologic complaints — if not by active pursuit then frequently by default. This section will deal with those developmental and acquired disorders of the genitourinary tract that are most likely to present at birth or during childhood. Pubertal and adolescent urinary tract problems will be discussed later in this chapter.

A proper understanding of the pathogenesis and management of most childhood urologic-gynecologic disorders is based on a thorough working knowledge of the embryologic development of the urogenital system. This has been reviewed in Chapter 1. Development of the entire urinary tract is closely tied to development of the fallopian tubes, uterus, and vagina in the female. As will be seen later, disorders of development of either system may affect not only those structures of the other system in close anatomic proximity but distant urogenital structures as well.

PROBLEMS PRESENTING AT BIRTH

Mode of Examination of the Newborn or Infant Female

The gynecologic-urologic examination of a newborn female requires more than a cursory glance at the external genitalia and anus. A checklist of specific features should be completed before the infant's genitourinary tract is pronounced normal.

The need for inspection of the abdomen for obvious abdominal wall defects and palpation of the abdomen for masses applies to both sexes. The inguinal areas of the female should be palpated for the presence of gonadal tissue and a search made for any signs of virilization of the external genitalia. The presence and relative size of the labia majora and minora should be noted. In a newborn the effect of maternal and placental hormones renders these tissues more turgid and plump than in the older child; they may even appear edematous. Any labial fusion or rugation should be noted. The presence, shape, and relative size of the clitoris should be determined; it is proportionally larger in the normal newborn than it will be later. The introitus should be exposed by grasping the labia majora and drawing them down and toward the examiner. This should allow localization of the urethral meatus and establish both the patency of the hymen and the presence of the vagina. Vulvar examination of the infant is aided by abducting and flexing the hips of the child onto the abdomen. Frequently the turgid state of the vulvar tissues necessitates gentle probing with a lubricated catheter tip, probe, or moist cotton-tipped applicator to prove the presence and normality of these structures; it is essential that this be determined at birth. Introital masses can be noted and their location defined in relation to the urethra, vagina, and anus.

The position and patency of the anus should be noted. In the child with an abdominal mass or a genital abnormality, a digital rectal examination, usually with the fifth finger, should be performed. The cervix is usually palpable upon rectal examination in the neonate up to a few weeks of age. Abdominal masses can be localized as either anterior or posterior to the rectum by digital and bimanual abdominal-rectal examination. Anal tone and perineal sensation can be ascertained in the child with suspected myelodysplasia. The back should be examined for evidence of myelodysplastic disorders. If vaginoscopy of the infant is indicated, it usually will necessitate anesthesia; an infant cystoscope has proved to be the most efficacious tool for visualizing the vaginal vault in this age group.

Ambiguous Genitalia

The most obvious problem that may be encountered in the newborn is the inability to assign the sex of the child because of genital ambiguity. The entire spectrum of intersex is complex and includes many disorders that present only in adolescence or in later life. Neonatal ambiguous genitalia, however, most commonly fall into one of four definable categories: (1) female pseudohermaphroditism, (2) mixed gonadal dysgenesis, (3) male pseudohermaphroditism, and (4) true hermaphroditism. There is a continuum of virilization of the indifferent female genitalia from normal female through ambiguity to normal male. A complete discussion of normal and abnormal sexual differentiation is contained in Chapter 7.

Duplication of the external genitalia is an exceedingly rare disorder. It may be complete or incomplete. If duplication is complete there usually is a side-by-side double vagina, cervix, and uterus as well as a duplicated urethra, two bladders, two ani, and a bifid sacrum (Figure 25–1). Each bladder drains a single ipsilateral ureter and kidney, and the lower bowel usually unites proximally. This anomaly may be due to partial twinning. Treatment must be individualized in each instance. There have been reports of successful pregnancy in

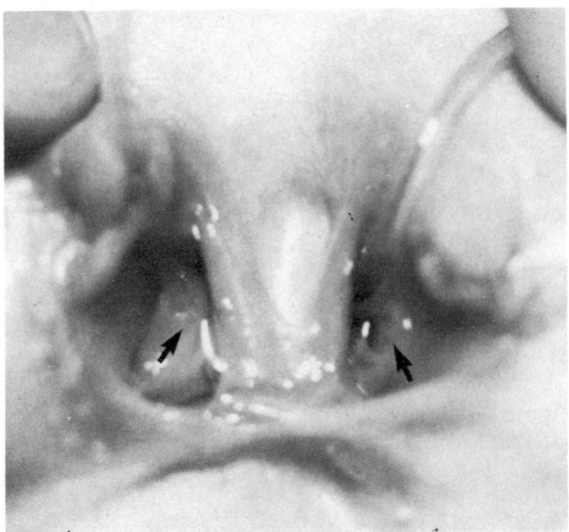

Figure 25–1. Vaginal and urethral duplication. Note catheters in the two urethras (arrows). The bladder itself was single, that is, it was not duplicated. (From Belman, A. B., and Kaplan, G. W.: Genitourinary Problems in Pediatrics. Philadelphia, W. B. Saunders Company, 1981.)

patients with duplicated external genitalia (Jones and Heller, 1966).

VAGINAL CYSTS

Cysts of the vagina are not uncommon in newborn girls. The etiology of these cysts varies; they may arise from müllerian remnants, vestigial wolffian duct structures, Skene's paraurethral glands, or urothelial inclusion cysts. In adult females, epithelial inclusion cysts after episiotomy or perineal trauma are most common; in infants, the etiology is more often exaggerated response of müllerian duct remnants to maternal hormonal stimulation (Deppisch, 1975; Gottesman and Sparkuhl, 1979; Cohen et al., 1957). Most introital cysts in newborns are located at the distal extent of the urethrovaginal septum, posterior to the urethra and anterior to the hymen (Figure 25–2). They appear to contain pearly, cream-colored material. Occasionally it is difficult to determine the precise site of origin of an introital cyst. Gentle probing usually will permit visualization of both the urethral and hymenal orifices.

Vaginal introital cysts usually are noted at the time of the newborn examination. Their primary significance lies in the need to differentiate them from a prolapsed ectopic ureterocele. As maternal hormone levels subside in the infant, introital cysts regress and an expectant course of treatment can be taken. If the cysts do not regress or if they cause obstruction of the urethral or vaginal outlet, they should be marsupialized into the introitus rather than excised, to avoid urethral injury. They do not tend to recur (Cohen et al., 1957). Differentiation of the cysts from an ectopic ureterocele can be made by intravenous pyelography if regression does not occur or if the child has urinary symptoms. There has been a report of ipsilateral renal agenesis associated with a Gartner's duct cyst (Gadbois and Duckett, 1974). Determination of the exact origin of the cyst (e.g., Skene's versus Gartner's duct, and so forth) is not necessary.

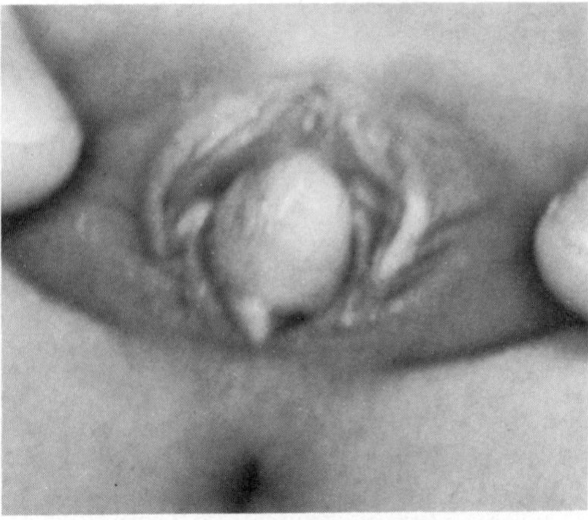

Figure 25–2. Neonatal vaginal introital cyst.

Exstrophy/Epispadias

The exstrophy/epispadias complex of anomalies is of uncertain etiology but appears to be due to an abnormal overdevelopment of the cloacal membrane, preventing medial ingrowth of the mesenchymal tissue of the lower abdominal wall. The classic form of exstrophy, in which the urinary tract is open and everted from the urethral meatus to the umbilicus, is the most common form encountered. It occurs in from 1 in 35,000 to 1 in 50,000 births (Figure 25–3). When classic exstrophy occurs the diagnosis is obvious in the delivery room. Babies with this anomaly

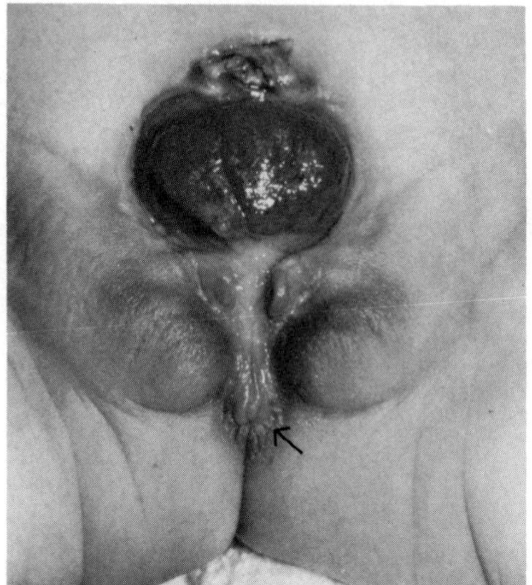

Figure 25–3. Classic form of exstrophy in newborn female. Note bifid clitoris and anteriorly placed anus (arrow).

otherwise are quite healthy, and the success of reconstruction may depend on the adequacy of the initial care by the primary physician. The exstrophic bladder should be protected from external irritants, such as diapers, gauze, and so forth, and should be kept moist with a fine, warm saline mist until a decision regarding reconstruction has been made.

We favor early attempts at reconstruction during the first week of life if the bladder appears large enough to close. Delays in reconstruction lead to significant thickening and contraction of the bladder wall as well as to polypoid hyperplasia of the mucosa that may render closure impossible. We have utilized bilateral iliac osteotomies — even in the newborn — as an effective aid to closure. The majority of children will require second-stage bladder neck reconstruction and ureteral reimplantation to attain continence and to correct the vesicoureteral reflux that is present in all of these patients. Up to 43 per cent of females with exstrophy may have associated gynecologic anomalies that require later treatment (Stanton, 1974). Most are fertile and capable of successful pregnancy.

Alternative treatment consists of delayed cystectomy and urinary diversion, usually by means of a primary or staged ureterosigmoidostomy (Hendren, 1976). Arap and co-workers (1980) recently described an

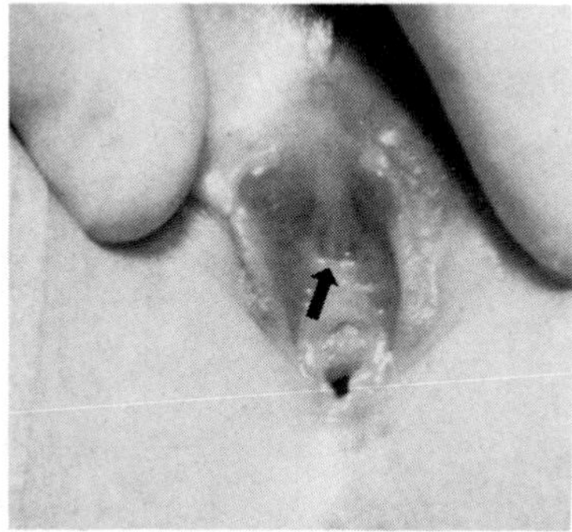

Figure 25–4. Bifid clitoris and epispadiac urethral meatus (arrow) in a girl with urinary incontinence.

interesting alternative method of staged reconstruction that may be useful in the smaller bladder. Exstrophic bladders, if not closed, have a tendency toward adenomatous metaplasia and possible development of adenocarcinoma, a factor that must be remembered during the long-term follow-up of these children.

The less common, milder forms of epispadias, in which the bladder is intact but the urethra remains unformed, may go unrecognized at birth unless a careful examination is performed and attention paid to the associated findings that suggest the presence of the condition (for example, bifid clitoris) (Figure 25–4). Treatment depends on the degree of urinary continence. Bladder neck reconstruction may be required.

Urogenital Sinus and Cloacal Abnormalities

COMMON UROGENITAL SINUS (FEMALE HYPOSPADIAS)

If the urethrovaginal septum fails to form completely, varied degrees of foreshortening of the female urethra may occur. The exact pathogenesis of the problem is unknown. Mild degrees of insignificant foreshortening of the urethra occur in many girls and may be noted only at the time of attempted urethral catheterization. The more proximal degrees of female hypospadias in which the urethral meatus lies deep in the vagina are rare; they may lead to urinary incontinence if the internal vesical sphincter mechanism is deficient. Treatment must be individualized and may include construction of a neourethra from vaginal, thigh, or labial flaps coupled with bladder neck revision (Hendren, 1980*a*). If incontinence or significant vaginal pooling of urine are problems, urethroplasty is indicated (Antolak et al., 1969).

PERSISTENT CLOACA

The failure of complete development of the urorectal septum in the female fetus leads to abnormal termination of the urinary, genital, and gastrointestinal tracts into a single common passage or cloaca. On physical examination the hallmark of this rare condition is the female with a single perineal orifice (Cheng et al., 1974). Various patterns of this anomaly have been described and include the entire spectrum of imperforate anus and anorectal agenesis (Raffensperger, 1976; Stephens, 1963). Classification has been based on the level of opening and the extent of communication of the three involved tracts as well as on the length of the common chamber (Figure 25–5).

Affected children are at serious risk (up to 86 per cent) for the intestinal and urinary tract obstruction that can result from this anomaly as well as from a high incidence of anomalies in other organ systems (Raffensperger, 1976). Children with imperforate anus also have an unusually high incidence of associated neurogenic bladder.

On physical examination, in addition to the single perineal orifice, there may be apparent posterior labial fusion or absence of the labia; an anal dimple may be visible. Abdominal distention often is present secondary to obstruction of the colonic outlet or from hydrometrocolpos with or without secondary bladder outlet obstruction. The child may pass meconium-stained urine.

Evaluation includes careful, sterile perineal examination followed by a sterile radiograph of the cloaca. This is performed by injecting a contrast agent retrogradely into the common perineal orifice. An intravenous pyelogram is mandatory and often will reveal hydronephrosis or nonobstructive renal anomalies. Significant vesicoureteral reflux is a common finding at the time of cystography. Careful endoscopic evaluation should allow visualization of the urinary, genital, and colonic outlets and help in planning either temporizing or definitive surgical intervention. These children usually require urgent decompression and diversion of the gastrointestinal tract by loop colostomy and often will need drainage of the hydrocolpos to relieve the secondary urinary outlet obstruction. This can be done by dilatation of the urogenital sinus or by tube vaginostomy. Vesicostomy may be required in some. The question of when to do definitive repair has not been answered. Raffensperger (1976) has proposed early definitive separation of the three involved systems but others believe that definitive repair is best done when the child is older and has a better grasp on life (Hendren, 1980*b*; Cheng et al., 1974). Because of the complexity of this anomaly, treatment must be individualized for each patient, and definitive repair should be performed by a surgeon or a team of surgeons experienced with these complexities.

Genital Prolapse

Procidentia, or genital prolapse, occurs rarely during the first week or two of life and almost always is associated with pelvic floor paralysis secondary to myelodysplasia. Bilateral ureteral obstruction results and requires urgent attention to the prolapse. Manual reduction of the prolapse, maintained by binding the infant's legs together, coupled with catheter drainage of the bladder, usually suffices as treatment. This treatment should be maintained for a few weeks. This condition does not usually recur (Johnston, 1968).

PROBLEMS PRESENTING IN INFANCY AND CHILDHOOD

After the neonatal age period, congenital anomalies present clinically far less commonly than do acquired problems and tumors. Presumably most of the congenital anomalies of the genital tract either were manifest at birth or will not become mani-

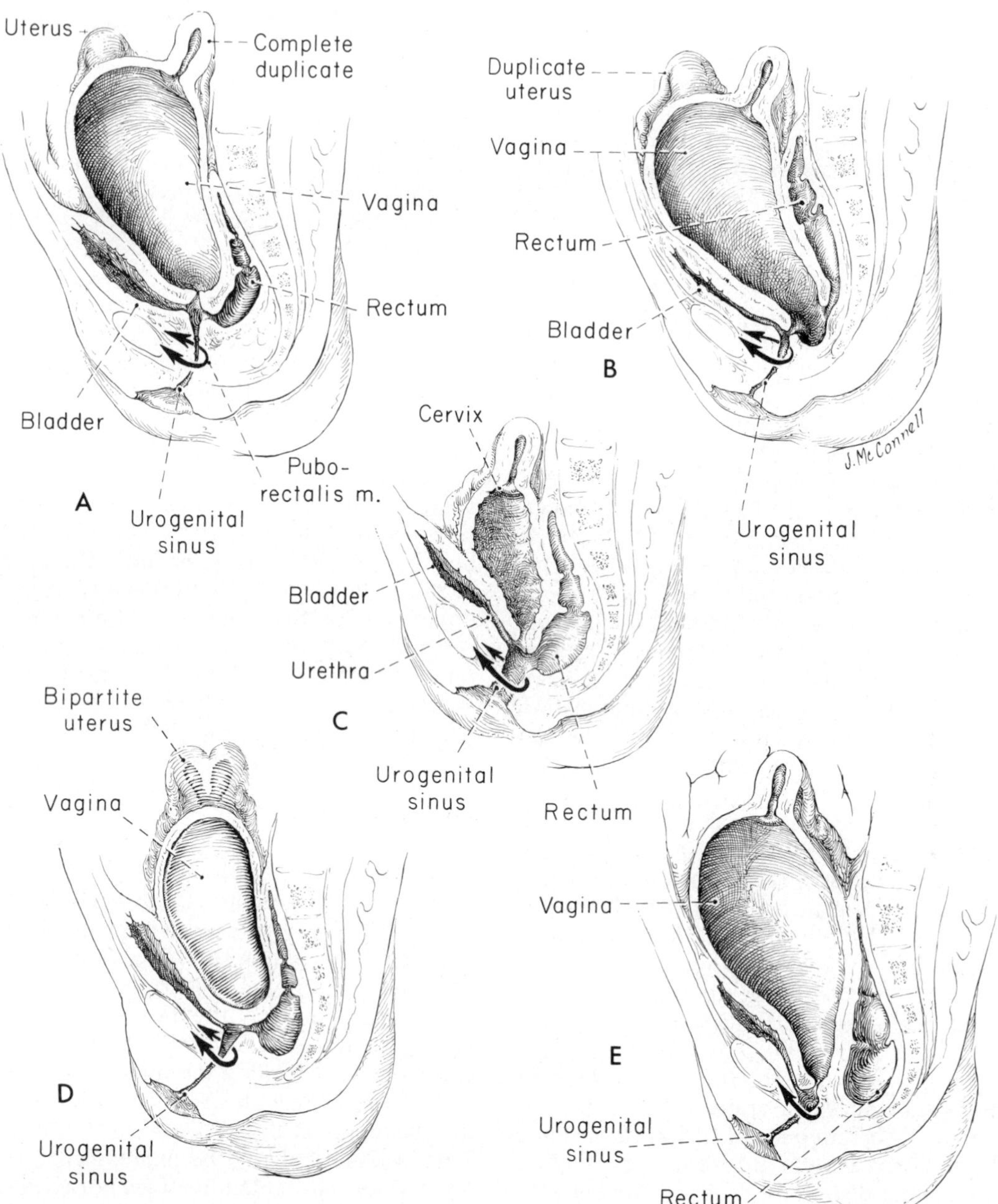

Figure 25–5. Varieties of cloacal anomalies. The double arrow indicates the position of the puborectalis muscle, which is essential to the development of fecal continence after operation. (From Raffensperger, J. G.: Anomalies of the Female Genitalia. *In* Kelalis, P. P., and King, L. R.: Clinical Pediatric Urology. Vol. 2. Philadelphia, W. B. Saunders Company, 1976.)

fest until after puberty. Congenital anomalies of the urinary tract, on the other hand, often become manifest between infancy and puberty, especially after the age of 2 years, because it is not until after the child is toilet-trained that many such defects are recognized.

Mode of Examination of the Older Child

Prepubertal children usually are quite cooperative during perineal examination if one approaches them in a confident and reassuring manner. The examination itself should be relatively free of discomfort; hence, one should have no hesitation about necessary examinations of the female genitalia in children. Initial inspection usually is performed with the child supine on the examining table with knees flexed and the hips abducted. As an alternative, especially in younger children, the same examination can be performed while the child is in the mother's lap. A penlight usually will provide adequate illumination. Attention should be paid to the anatomy of the external genitalia as well as to the character of the skin immediately surrounding the genitalia. Hernias usually are readily apparent as a bulge in the inguinal area, especially if the child is crying. If no hernia is present, palpation of the labia majora for the presence of gonads or lesions usually is unrewarding.

One should note the position of both the urethral and hymenal orifices, but in most instances it is unecessary to inspect the vaginal vault itself. If inspection of the vaginal vault is required, this often can be accomplished using an otoscope with or without a veterinary otoscope speculum (Billmire et al., 1980). Placing the child in the knee-chest position often allows even better visualization of the interior of the vaginal vault (Emans and Goldstein, 1980). Rectal examination is an important adjunct to examination of the girl's perineum. Special attention should be paid to the character of the anal tone, large boluses of firm stool in the rectal ampulla, and any extraluminal palpable masses either anteriorly or posteriorly.

Vulvovaginitis

Vulvovaginitis occurs rather frequently in girls before puberty. It most often is manifest as dysuria or hesitancy but occasionally may present as a frank vaginal discharge. Nonspecific vulvovaginitis is, without question, the most common type of vulvovaginitis in childhood (Gray and Kotcher, 1961) and is part of the "tight bottom" syndrome to be discussed later. Girls with nonspecific vulvovaginitis usually present with urinary symptoms such as dysuria, frequency, urgency, or incontinence. Physical examination will reveal mild erythema of the vulvar tissues and the vaginal vault. Vaginal discharge usually is not present. Because the child has dysuria she may not empty her bladder completely, so that there may be residual urine on a more or less voluntary basis. Cultures of the vaginal secretions reveal only normal flora.

Nonspecific vulvovaginitis often will respond, at least temporarily, to warm sitz baths containing either sodium bicarbonate or colloidal oatmeal. Bland ointments to protect the perineal skin also are sometimes of value. Recurrences of nonspecific vulvovaginitis are common.

Urinary Tract Infection

It is important to differentiate girls with nonspecific vulvovaginitis from those presenting with true urinary infections. This is accomplished by culturing a carefully collected specimen of urine (Stephens, 1963). Because the vulva is inflamed and because many girls fill the vagina in the act of voiding, with consequent mixing of vaginal epithelial cells and leukocytes, reliance on a urinalysis alone for diagnosis is fraught with danger.

The peak incidence of symptomatic urinary tract infection in girls occurs between the ages of 2 and 5 years (Kunin, 1971). Many of these infections are lower tract in origin but mixed in this group are a significant minority of upper tract problems as well (Smellie and Normand, 1975). Because the first symptom or sign of upper tract anomalies may be a urinary infection, it is important to accurately identify those children with true urinary infections and then to proceed to evaluation. The key to accurate identification of a urinary infection is a urine culture obtained from a properly collected urine specimen. In a toilet-trained girl a voided specimen is totally reliable only if it is negative. Hence, if there is any doubt about the diagnosis of urinary infection, urine should be collected either by catheterization or by suprapubic aspiration before institution of therapy so that one may ascertain the presence or absence of urinary infection. If urinary infection is identified, the child should then be evaluated with an intravenous urogram and a voiding cystourethrogram to rule out any significant anomalies of the urinary tract (Kunin, 1971).

"Tight Bottom" Syndrome

There is a group of girls who present with lower urinary tract symptoms, with or without perineal discomfort, in whom neither a frank vulvovaginitis nor a definite urinary infection can be identified. We have, for lack of a better term, labeled this problem as the "tight bottom" syndrome (Kaplan and Brock, 1980). Girls with this syndrome usually have frequency, urgency, and dysuria. They often have both day and night urinary incontinence. Additionally, they often have a typical posturing that has been called the "curtsy sign," in which they attempt to forestall an imminent detrusor contraction by squatting and forcing the heel of one foot into the perineum (Vincent, 1966). Many seem to have problems with constipation or encopresis as well. Often upon rectal examination one will find the child's rectal ampulla filled with a mass of relatively hard stool.

To conceptualize this problem, it would seem that some painful event or series of events (such as recurrent detergent vulvovaginitis, recurrent anal fissure, or even urinary infection) produces a childhood response: "That hurts. I don't want to do that any more." The child then attempts to avoid passing urine or stool. Voiding and defecating without complete perineal relaxation frequently are painful and this consequently reinforces the child's thinking. A repetitive pattern in which voiding and defecating are delayed and are associated with pain is reinforced and the above-mentioned symptom complex results. Therapy for these children is somewhat prolonged and involves the use of stool softeners, bulk-producing laxatives, sitz baths, reassurance, and time. Hypnosis and biofeedback also have been used to effect a behavioral change in these patients (Hinman, 1974).

Urethral Prolapse

Urethral prolapse presents during childhood as a relatively asymptomatic reddish mass surrounding the entire circumference of the urethra (Figure 25–6). The prolapsed urethra may bleed easily so that some children may present with a bloody vaginal discharge. There usually are no urinary symptoms associated with the lesion. Urethral prolapse is much more common in black children than in whites (Klaus and Stein, 1973). The etiology of the lesion is unknown. The treatment is surgical and consists of excision of the prolapsed mucosa with reanastomosis of the remaining urethral mucosa to the vulvar epithelium (Belman and Kaplan, 1981). Recurrences are uncommon.

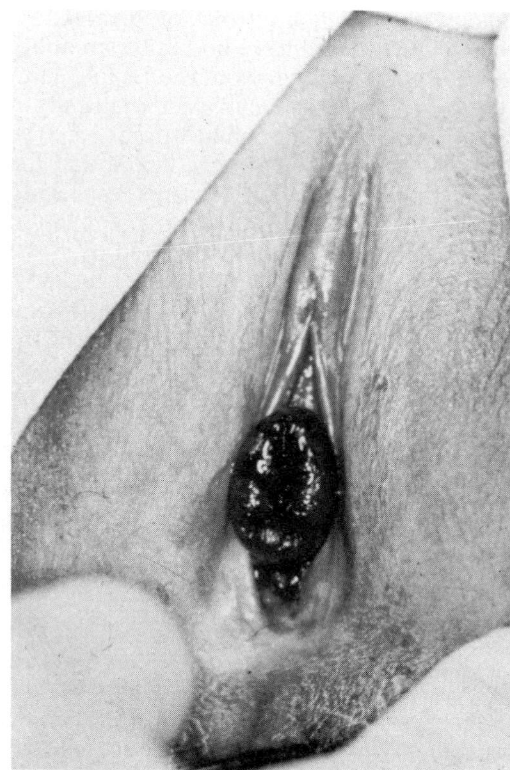

Figure 25–6. Urethral prolapse in a 7-year-old girl. (From Belman, A. B., and Kaplan, G. W.: Genitourinary Problems in Pediatrics. Philadelphia, W. B. Saunders Company, 1981.)

Genital Trauma

Many little girls inadvertently fall and injure the perineum. Such injuries often are emotionally traumatic as well, but fortunately usually are of little medical consequence. There may be a laceration of the

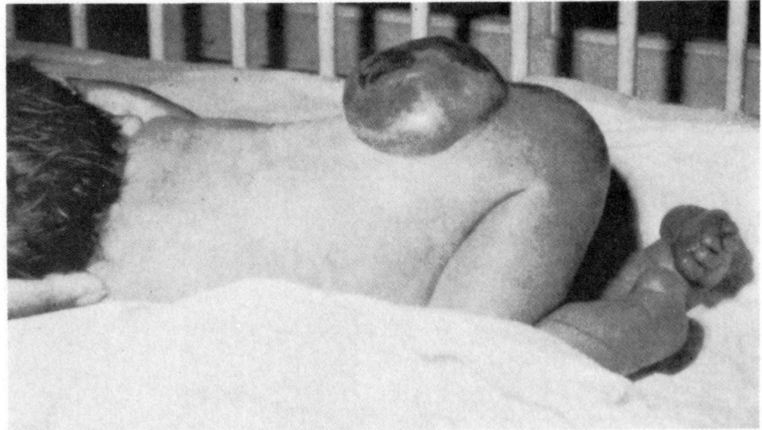

Figure 25–7. Newborn with an intact myelomeningocele. (From Kaplan, G. W.: Myelomeningocele. *In* Harrison, J. H., et al.: Campbell's Urology, 4th Edition. Philadelphia, W. B. Saunders Company, 1979.)

vulva, which initially bleeds profusely but stops promptly. General anesthesia may be required for an adequate examination. A rather common sequel to such an injury, however, is a fear of voiding, which may last anywhere from a few hours to several days. During this period it is best to avoid urethral catheterization if possible. Often the child can be coaxed to void either in a tub of warm water or following the judicious use of bethanechol (Urecholine), but, failing this, suprapubic aspiration or the percutaneous placement of a suprapubic catheter may be warranted.

Urinary Incontinence

Urinary incontinence is a very frequent presenting complaint in early childhood. Many such episodes are caused by voiding dysfunctions, such as the "tight bottom" syndrome, as well as by urinary tract infection. A carefully obtained history is paramount to diagnosis. Pure nocturnal enuresis, a very common problem in children, almost never is associated with structural abnormalities (McKendry and Stewart, 1974). Intermittent daytime incontinence most often is associated with voiding dysfunction or with true urinary infection. The history of the girl who voids normally and yet is wet continually is almost pathognomonic of a child with an ectopic ureter. Physical examination will reveal obvious problems such as exstrophy, epispadias (Figures 25–3 and 25–4), or neurogenic dysfunction (Figure 25–7) (most often caused by myelodysplasia or other spinal dysrhaphic problems). Careful inspection of the perineum may lead to observation of a jet of urine from an ectopic ureter (Figure 25–8).

Intravenous urography is of importance in the examination of the incontinent child (excluding pure nocturnal enuresis). Patients with ectopic ureters often have subtle findings on intravenous urography, which must be pursued for an accurate diagnosis. The most common of these is the presence of ureteral duplication, with the ectopic

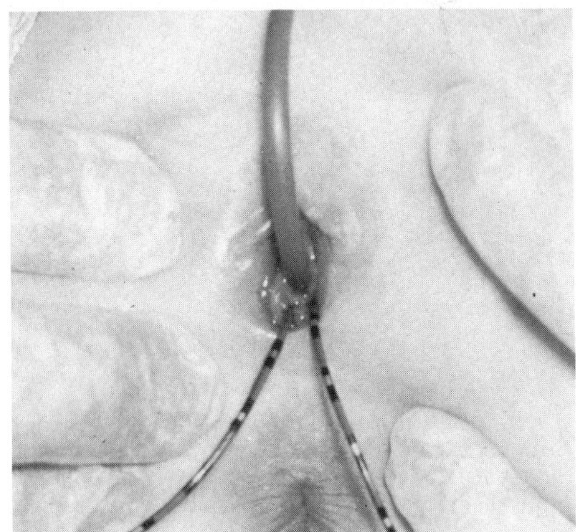

Figure 25–8. Bilateral ectopic ureters. (From Kelalis, P. P.: Anomalies of the urinary tract. B. Renal pelvis and ureters. *In* Kelalis, P. P., and King, L. R.: Clinical Pediatric Urology. Vol. 1. Philadelphia, W. B. Saunders Company, 1976.)

ureter arising from a poorly functioning upper pole moiety of the duplication (Figure 25–9). The embryologic basis of this anomaly has been detailed in Chapter 1. Obstructive lesions as a cause of urinary incontinence in girls are most uncommon, but such problems as an ectopic ureterocele ball-valving into the bladder neck rarely may present with incontinence. (Figure 25–10). The surgical management of major anomalies of the urinary tract in children is beyond the scope of this presentation, and the interested reader is referred to standard textbooks of pediatric urology.

Tumors

Tumors of the female pelvis are uncommon, but when they are present they may affect the urinary tract of children. Ovarian teratomas are among the more common tumors of the female pelvis in childhood and most often are discovered as an asymptomatic mass (Siegel et al., 1978). Occasionally such a tumor may twist on its pedicle and present as an ovarian torsion with the acute onset of lower abdominal pain. Rarely ovarian tumors may become so large that they fill the entire true pelvis and by mechanical means obstruct the urinary tract (Figure 25–11). Surgical resection of the ovarian tumor in such instances effects a cure, but in those few individuals with obstructive uropathy secondary to the presence of the tumor one must watch for a postobstructive diuresis when the tumor has been removed.

Girls with pelvic neuroblastoma may present with an asymptomatic mass, but on many occasions the mass, by virtue of its size, impinges on the lower urinary tract

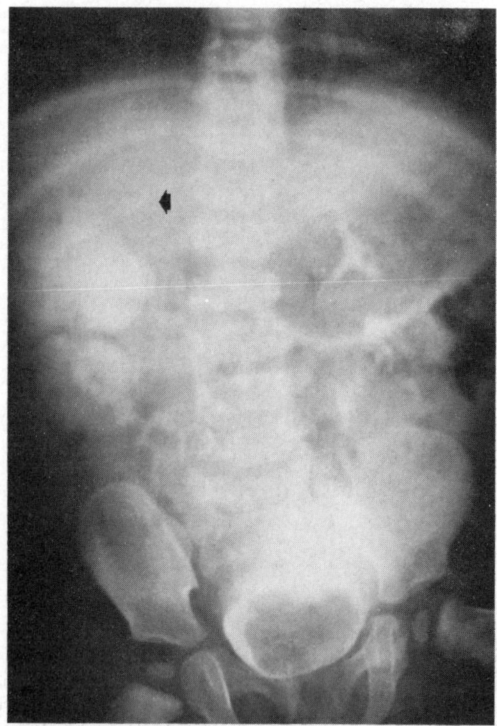

Figure 25–10. Intravenous pyelogram from a child with bilateral ureteral duplication and ectopic ureterocele arising from poorly visualized right upper pole segment (arrow). There is dilatation of the lower collecting system on the right. The lucency within the bladder is the ureterocele. (Reproduced with permission from Kaplan, G. W., and Brock, W. A.: Voiding dysfunction in children. *In* Gluck, L., et al. [Eds.]: Current Problems in Pediatrics. Copyright © 1980 by Year Book Medical Publishers, Inc., Chicago.)

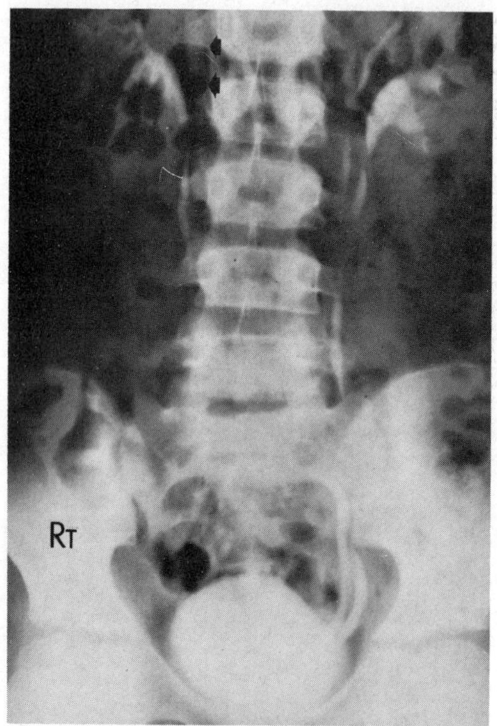

Figure 25–9. Intravenous pyelogram from a girl with bilateral ureteral duplication and urinary incontinence. Right upper pole collecting system (arrows) is dilated and only faintly visualized; it opened into an ectopic vaginal location, causing incontinence. (Reproduced with permission from Kaplan, G. W., and Brock, W. A.: Voiding dysfunction in children. *In* Gluck, L., et al. [Eds.]: Current Problems in Pediatrics. Copyright © 1980 by Year Book Medical Publishers, Inc., Chicago.)

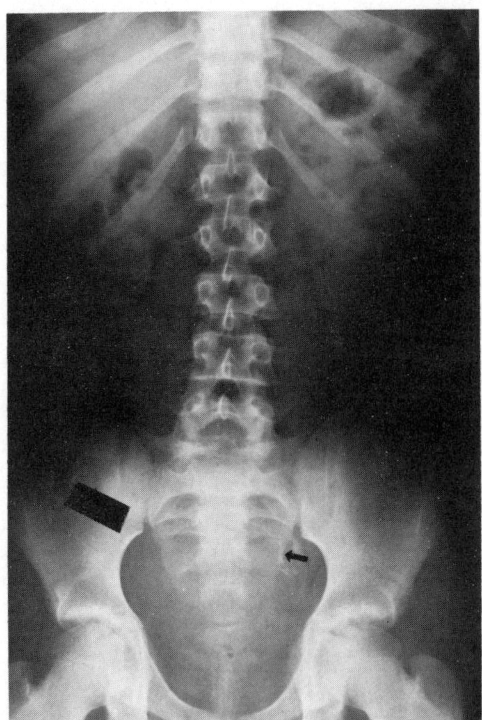

Figure 25–11. Intravenous urogram from an 11-year-old girl with an ovarian dermoid filling the bony pelvis and producing bilateral hydronephrosis. Arrow indicates calcification in the tumor in this 30-minute film of the urogram, also showing faint visualization of a bilaterally dilated collecting system.

and causes symptoms of obstructive uropathy. Because the pelvic ganglia are involved, excision of a pelvic neuroblastoma does carry the risk for the subsequent development of neurogenic bladder dysfunction. The latter must be carefully sought in patients who have undergone excision of such tumors. Additionally, in patients with pelvic neuroblastoma the bladder itself may be invaded by the tumor, so that marked hematuria may result and pose a management problem. In rare instances, cystectomy may be necessary as a therapeutic adjunct for these patients.

Rhabdomyosarcoma is a relatively uncommon childhood tumor that may arise in the pelvis, either in the bladder or in the vagina. These tumors often achieve rather massive dimensions before they are recognized. Those that involve the cavity of the bladder or the vagina may present by the passage of small bits of grape-like tissue (sarcoma botryoides), with signs and symptoms of obstructive uropathy, or with vaginal bleeding. Formerly radical extirpative surgery was believed essential for cure, and the prognosis seemed very bleak (Tefft and Jaffe, 1973). In recent years, however, it has been shown that many affected patients will respond to chemotherapy and radiation therapy without extirpative surgery (Ghaumi et al., 1975). Consequently the current recommended approach to treatment of these tumors includes biopsy and intense chemotherapy with vincristine, actinomycin, and cyclophosphamide. If the tumor does not respond, radiation therapy is added; only if the tumor is not eradicated by these means is extirpative surgery utilized. The current 2-year survival rates observed in children with rhabdomyosarcoma treated by this approach approximate 50 per cent.

REFERENCES

Antolak, S. J., Jr., Smith, J. R., and Doolittle, K. H.: Female hypospadias. J. Urol. *102*:640, 1969.

Arap, S., Giron, A. M., and Menezes de Goes, G.: Initial results of the complete reconstruction of bladder exstrophy. Urol. Clin. North Am. *7*:477, 1980.

Belman, A. B., and Kaplan, G. W.: Genitourinary Problems in Pediatrics. Philadelphia, W. B. Saunders Company, 1981.

Billmire, M. E., Farrell, M. K., and Dine, M. S.: A simplified procedure for pediatric vaginal examination: use of veterinary otoscope specula. Pediatrics *65*:823, 1980.

Cheng, G. K., Fisher, J. H., O'Hare, K. H., et al.: Anomaly of the persistent cloaca in female infants. Am. J. Roentgenol. *120*:413, 1974.

Cohen, H. J., Klein, M. D., and Laver, M. B.: Cysts of the vagina in a newborn infant. Am. J. Dis. Child. *94*:322, 1957.

Deppisch, L. M.: Cysts of the vagina: classification and clinical correlations. Obstet. Gynecol. *45*:632, 1975.

Emans, S. J., and Goldstein, D. P.: The gynecologic examination of the prepubertal child with vulvovaginitis: use of the knee-chest position. Pediatrics *65*:758, 1980.

Gadbois, W. F., and Duckett, J. W., Jr.: Gartner's duct cyst and ipsilateral renal agenesis. Urology *4*:720, 1974.

Ghaumi, F., Exelby, P. R., D'Angio, G. J., et al.: Multidisciplinary treatment of embryonal rhabdomyosarcoma in children. Cancer *35*:677, 1975.
Gottesman, J. E., and Sparkuhl, A.: Bilateral Skene duct cysts. J. Pediatr. *94*:945, 1979.
Gray, L. H., and Kotcher, E.: Vulvovaginitis in childhood. Am. J. Obstet. Gynecol. *82*:530, 1961.
Hendren, W. H.: Exstrophy of the bladder. An alternative method of management. J. Urol., *115*:195, 1976.
Hendren, W. H.: Construction of female urethra from vaginal wall and a perineal flap. J. Urol. *123*:657, 1980*a*.
Hendren, W. H.: Urogenital sinus and anorectal malformation: Experience with 22 cases. J. Pediatr. Surg. *15*:628, 1980*b*.
Hinman, F.: Urinary tract damage in children who wet. Pediatrics *54*:142, 1974.
Johnston, J. H.: The female genital tract. *In* Williams, D. I. (Ed.): Pediatric Urology. New York, Appleton-Century-Crofts, 1968, pp. 475–485.
Jones, H. W., and Heller, R. H.: Pediatric and Adolescent Gynecology. Baltimore, Williams & Wilkins Company, 1966.
Kaplan, G. W., and Brock, W. A.: Voiding dysfunction in children. Curr. Probl. Pediatr. *10*:1, 1980.
Klaus, H., and Stein, R. T.: Urethral prolapse in young girls. Pediatrics *52*:645, 1973.
Kunin, C. M.: Epidemiology and natural history of urinary tract infection in school age children. Pediatr. Clin. North Am. *18*:509, 1971.
McKendry, J. B. J., and Stewart, D. A.: Enuresis. Pediatr. Clin. North Am. *21*:1019, 1974.
Raffensperger, J. G.: Anomalies of the female genitalia. *In* Kelalis, P. P., King, L. R., and Belman, A. B. (Eds.): Clinical Pediatric Urology. Vol. 1. Philadelphia, W. B. Saunders Company, 1976.
Siegel, M. J., McAlister, W. H., and Shackelford, G. D.: Radiographic findings in ovarian teratomas in children. Am. J. Roentgenol. *131*:613, 1978.
Smellie, J. M., and Normand, I. C. S.: Bacteriuria, reflux, and renal scarring. Arch. Dis. Child. *50*:581, 1975.
Stanton, S. L.: Gynecologic complications of epispadias and bladder exstrophy. Am. J. Obstet. Gynecol. *119*:749, 1974.
Stephens, F. D.: Congenital malformations of the rectum and anus in female children. *In* Congenital Malformation of Rectum, Anus and Genito-Urinary Tracts. Edinburgh, E. & S. Livingstone, 1963.
Tefft, M., and Jaffe, N.: Sarcoma of the bladder and prostate in children. Cancer *32*:1161, 1973.
Vincent, S. A.: Postural control of urinary incontinence: The curtsy sign. Lancet *2*:631, 1966.

PART 2

ADOLESCENT/SEXUALLY ACTIVE

INTRODUCTION

Sexual activity appears to increase a woman's risk of developing urinary tract infections. Urinary tract infections occur with greater frequency in married women than in nuns (Kunin and McCormack, 1968). Bran and co-workers (1972) demonstrated that milking the urethra can introduce bacteria into the bladder. The thrusting motion of intercourse is associated with the entry of bacteria into the bladder. Furthermore, oral-genital contact allows for exposure of the urethra to the flora of the mouth. Urinary symptoms in sexually active women may occur without clinical evidence of infection.

PATHOPHYSIOLOGY

The pathophysiology of urinary tract infection is related to the existence of bacteria, the body's intrinsic defense mechanisms, and the presence of obstruction or stasis.

It is commonly believed that bacteria enter the bladder from the perineum and anus. The organism recovered by culture in 80 per cent of instances is *Escherichia coli*. There is ample evidence, however, that a host of organisms may gain entry to the bladder through the urethra. These include normal inhabitants of the oral and genital tracts plus Chlamydiae, *Neisseria meningitidis*, Mycoplasma organisms, *Mycobacterium tuberculosis*, and Blastomyces. Descending infection from the kidney and spread of infection via the vascular tree may occur. The shortness of the female urethra and its close proximity to the vagina and rectum contribute to the incidence of infection (Lapides, 1973).

Several intrinsic urinary tract antibacterial mechanisms have been suggested. Urine itself may be bacteriostatic; Kaye (1973) reports that bacterial growth is greater in trypticase soy broth than in urine. Urea, low pH, and urine hyperosmolality tend to inhibit bacterial growth. Bacteria may be entrapped by the mucosa with subsequent phagocytosis by leukocytes. Immune defense mechanisms in the bladder have not been clearly demonstrated. It is reasonable to postulate, however, that immune defense mechanisms exist in the bladder as well as elsewhere in the body.

There is ample evidence that obstruction or stasis is associated with increased infections related to urinary calculi, stenosis, infrequent voiding and distention, or neurogenic bladder. Adatto and co-workers (1979) state that women who void frequently will have a much lower incidence of urinary tract infections. Voluntary retention of urine for more than 1 hour after the urge to urinate was first experienced was present in 61 per cent of patients with infections and in only 11 per cent of controls. Mehrotra (1953) presents experimental evidence that overdistention of the bladder interferes with vascularity. This causes sludging and vascular stasis, with subsequent ecchymosis. Chronic urinary tract infection in the hypotonic neurogenic bladder is well known.

The use of oral contraceptives and intrauterine devices has been shown to be associated with increased urinary tract infections. The increased incidence of infection is thought to be correlated with sexual activity per se rather than with any particular method of contraception.

SPECIFIC SYMPTOM COMPLEXES

Cystitis

Frequency, urgency, dysuria, pelvic pressure, and fullness characterize cystitis. Abdominal examination may disclose lower abdominal tenderness. Findings on pelvic examination include urethral tenderness, anterior pelvic discomfort, and nontender adnexae. The patient often is afebrile but may have mild temperature elevation. The diagnosis is confirmed by examination of the urinary sediment. Leukocytes, erythrocytes, and bacteria will be visible on microscopic examination. In significant disease, 10 or more leukocytes and 20 or more bacteria per high power field are found when a spun specimen is examined.

Escherichia coli is the most common pathogen in cystitis. Frequent recurrences with the same organism should arouse suspicion of the presence of urinary calculi, obstruction, or inadequate emptying. Treatment of cystitis should include a liberal amount of oral fluids, which will provide a mechanical "washing out" of the bladder. The patient should be encouraged to void and not to "hold her urine."

Antimicrobial therapy includes the use of sulfonamides, nitrofurantoins, and trimethoprim. A dosage of sulfisoxazole, 4 gm. initially followed by 1 gm. four times daily for 10 days, is widely used. Nitrofurantoin, 50 to 100 mg. three times daily for 10 days, is also commonly employed. It is inappropriate to utilize bactericidal antimicrobials in the treatment of simple cystitis. Phenazopyridine hydrochloride (Pyridium) has long been utilized, as it is excreted in the urine, where it exerts a topical analgesic effect. It should be emphasized that it is a purely analgesic and not an antimicrobial agent. Therapy with Pyridium should be short-term; it is important to warn patients that a reddish-orange discoloration of the urine will occur.

A thorough evaluation of the urinary tract should be undertaken in patients with frequent and recurrent bacterial cystitis. This examination should include an intravenous pyelogram, cystoscopy, and renal function tests, such as serum creatinine, creatinine clearance, and blood urea nitrogen (BUN) determinations.

Honeymoon Cystitis

The symptom complex of honeymoon cystitis is identical to that of cystitis. Temporally it is related to increased sexual activity. Therapy should include precoital and postcoital voiding, liberal fluid intake, and administration of urinary antimicrobials and urinary analgesics.

O'Donnell (1968), Hirschhorn (1965), and

Reed (1970) have described surgical techniques performed to minimize urinary symptoms. Basically these are designed to increase the diameter of the vagina at the introitus. O'Donnell's method is to incise the hymenal ring vertically and to close it transversely. Hirschhorn and Reed describe advancement of the urethra by a transverse incision between the urethra and the introitus. The incision is then closed vertically, which advances the urethral orifice up and away from the vaginal orifice and minimizes the intravaginal advancement of the urethra with coitus. The surgical approach for treatment of urinary symptoms exemplifies the range of therapies available. In most cases, however, lower urinary tract symptoms can be treated with more conservative measures.

Urethral Syndrome

The "urethral syndrome," or abacterial cystitis, is characterized by frequency and dysuria with sterile urine cultures. Its etiology remains obscure. Theoretic explanations variously attribute the urethral syndrome to urethral trauma from sexual activity, urethral glandular infection, trigonitis, drug therapy, and excessive consumption of coffee and tea (see Chapter 20).

The urethral syndrome in women may be related to a low-grade indolent infection with *Chlamydia trachomatis*. Genital chlamydial infections are becoming widely recognized; excellent reviews by Eschenbach (1980) and Johannisson and co-workers (1980) point out the clinical implications of such infections. Chlamydiae attach to columnar or transitional cells and most commonly do not invade tissues deeply. In the male, nonspecific urethritis or nongonococcal urethritis is most often attributed to chlamydiae. Tissue culture methods are necessary to demonstrate the presence of a chlamydial infection.

Other suggested causes of the urethral syndrome include bacterial pathogens with culture growth below 100,000 organisms per milliliter of urine, coitus, menopause, defective immune mechanisms, menses, instrumentation of the urethra, emotional stress, and changes in the weather. The cause of the urethral syndrome remains an enigma, yet it continues to trouble many women (Brooks and Maudar, 1972; Maskell et al., 1979).

Approaches to the treatment of urethral syndrome have included surgery and multiple drug regimens. The most common surgical approach is urethral dilatation. Gentle and careful urethral dilatations performed periodically will relieve urinary symptoms in some cases. The mechanism by which this salutary effect is achieved is obscure. The progressive dilatation of the urethra may well cause a traumatic rupture of the periurethral glands, which then for a period of time allows egress of the glandular secretions.

A persistent urethral syndrome demands evaluation. A careful history should include documentation of previous surgery, voiding patterns, sexual practices, drug therapy, and medical problems such as diabetes and multiple sclerosis. During the examination a search should be made for urethral drainage or a mass. Skenitis or urethral diverticulum may be evident. Urinalysis and urine culture should be done. Cystoscopic examination of the urethra and bladder may be of significant value. Robertson (1976) reports significant advantages to the use of the carbon dioxide urethroscope in visualization of the urethra. Urethral diverticula, urethritis, ectopic ureteral openings, scarring from previous surgery, and a hypoestrogenic state may be noted. In addition, cystometric examination will provide information regarding bladder function and may lead one to suspect neuropathy secondary to diabetes, multiple sclerosis, spinal cord tumor, or syphilis.

SUMMARY

Urinary tract problems are more common in the sexually active woman. Potential pathogens frequently are found in the distal urethra (Stamey et al., 1965). During coitus the urethra is compressed and driven inward; the subsequent milking action results in the deposition of bacteria in the bladder. The presence of bacteria in the bladder and proximal urethra may result in urinary infection. Natural defense mechanisms generally prevent disease; when these mechanisms fail as a result of obstruction, stasis, or calculi, chronic and recurring infections occur. Careful evaluation, including urinalysis, culture, cystoscopy, serum creatinine and BUN determinations, and intravenous pyelography, should be performed to rule out the presence of life-threatening disease and to provide a rational basis for therapy. Treatment should include education of the patient in proper voiding habits, for infrequent voiding clearly is associated with a greater incidence of lower urinary tract disease. Hygiene is important; adequate fluid intake is necessary. Appropriate antimicrobial therapy, including sulfonamides, nitrofurantoins, and trimethoprim, should be given. To date, no evidence is available to incriminate the use of any specific method of contraception in causation of urinary tract infections in the sexually active woman.

REFERENCES

Adatto, K., Doebele, K. G., Galland, L., et al.: Behavioral factors and urinary tract infections. J.A.M.A. *241*:2525, 1979.

Bran, J. L., Levison, M. E., and Kaye, D.: Entrance of bacteria into the female urinary bladder. N. Engl. J. Med. *286*:626, 1972.

Brooks, D., and Maudar, A.: Pathogenesis of the urethral syndrome in women and its diagnosis in general practice. Lancet *2*:893, 1972.

Eschenbach, D.: Recognizing chlamydial infections. Contemp. Obstet. Gynecol. *16*:15, 1980.

Hirschhorn, R. C.: Urethral-hymenal fusion: A surgically correctable cause of recurrent cystitis. Obstet. Gynecol. *26*:903, 1965.

Johannisson, G., Löwhagen, G. B., and Lycke, E.: Genital Chlamydia trachomatis. Infection in women. Obstet. Gynecol. *56*:671, 1980.

Kaye, D.: Host defense mechanisms in the urine and urinary bladder. Bacteriuria and urinary tract infections. Proceedings of the International Symposium of the National Kidney Foundation. Section III. Chapter 1. 1973.

Kunin, C. M., and McCormack, R. C.: An epidemiologic study of bacteriuria and blood pressure among nuns and working women. N. Engl. J. Med. *278*:636, 1968.

Lapides, J.: Pathophysiology of urinary tract infections. Bacteriuria and urinary tract infections. Proceedings of the International Symposium of the National Kidney Foundation. Section IV. Chapter 3. 1973.

Maskell, R., Pead, L., and Allen, J.: The puzzle of "urethral syndrome": A possible answer. Lancet *1*:1058, 1979.

Mehrotra, R. M. L.: An experimental study of the vesical circulation during distention and in cystitis. J. Pathol. Bacteriol. *66*:79, 1953.

O'Donnell, R. P.: An intrapartum surgical technique for the prevention of chronic honeymoon urethritis. Int. Surg. *50*:428, 1968.

Reed, J. F.: Urethral-hymenal fusion: A cause of chronic adult female cystitis. J. Urol. *103*:441, 1970.

Robertson, J. R.: Urethroscopy — the neglected gynecologic procedure. Clin. Obstet. Gynecol. *19*:315, 1976.

Stamey, T. A., Govan, D. E., and Palmer, J. M.: The localization and treatment of urinary tract infections. The role of bactericidal urine levels as opposed to serum levels. Medicine *44*:1, 1965.

PART 3
POSTMENOPAUSAL

It is important to appreciate the complexity of the integral reflexes of continence and micturition to understand the changes that occur in the genitourinary system of the postmenopausal female. Much of this change is inevitable and not satisfactorily treated. Although the discovery of estrogen receptors in the urethra is relatively new, it has been known for several decades that the urethra is hormone sensitive and therefore is responsive to estrogen treatment in the menopause. Recent research, however, has suggested an even greater role for estrogens in the process of aging than is appreciated at present. Gerontologists have for many years considered the aging process as involving changes in both the endocrine and neurologic systems.

Dysfunction of the lower urinary tract is a common problem of the aging female and cannot always be approached in the usual fashion. The presenting symptom complex is variable, and similar symptoms may result from different pathophysiologic processes. Adequate hormone replacement therapy, a pubococcygeal exercise program, and enlargement of the outflow tract with dilatation or urethrotomy may be indicated in the therapy of menopausal problems. Parasympathomimetic agents and anticholinergic drugs may also have a role, but their use must be tempered by recognition of the increased drug sensitivity found in the elderly.

As with other organ systems, the lower urinary tract is more often a target for disease or for symptomatic expression of an alteration in normal physiologic activity in the elderly than in the younger individual. Changes in vesical function with age are not limited to women, but this discussion is restricted to women in the postmenopausal age group.

The appearance of new problems (or the exacerbation of preexisting ones) may be broadly considered to be secondary to one of two separate factors: (1) the process of aging itself and (2) the diminished estrogen levels associated with cessation of ovarian function. The symptom complex caused by either of these two processes, i.e., aging or estrogen deficiency, may be identical (incontinence, nocturia, frequency, and so forth). The pathophysiology, the clinical and urodynamic findings, and the therapy may be different, however. For ease of discussion the negative influence of these two inexorable developments will be discussed separately, although they can, and usually do, occur together.

AGING

To better understand the changes that affect the genitourinary system of the menopausal woman, the reader is referred to a full discussion of the normal neurophysiology of micturition and continence included in Chapters 3 to 5.

An irrefutable decline in the integrity of the neuromuscular system is a normal accompaniment of age. Various age-related degenerative changes in the sensory and autonomic ganglia have been described. The deep tendon reflexes (DTRs) become increasingly sluggish with age and ultimately may disappear. The loss of DTRs begins around the age of 50 years; by age 80 few people have intact ankle jerk reflexes (Johnson, 1960). The blunting of abdominocutaneous reflexes, prolongation of pupillary reaction time, diminution of olfactory, gustatory, and auditory sensation, and a progressive loss of vibratory sensation (approximately half of those over 80 years old will have lost these sensations in the lower extremities) are some of the neurologic changes that are a direct result of the aging process.

The range of ocular motion is frequently limited in all directions, and a generalized age-related weakness of striated musculature is widely recognized. In all muscles studied there is an increase in interstitial connective tissue (Johnson, 1960). In general, the conditioned and unconditioned responses are of much lesser magnitude in the elderly than in the normal young adult (Welford and Birren, 1965).

Continence

Considering first the neurophysiology of storage (or continence), one can appreciate that a decline in either the sympathetic, parasympathetic, or somatic (pudendal nerves) nervous system can upset the delicate homeostasis between continence and incontinence. For example, a "slowdown" of the sympathetic stabilizing reflexes permits development of detrusor irritability (or loss of accommodation) and causes loss of the appropriate increase in urethral resistance in response to an increasing intravesical volume. Would this type of incontinence be considered neurogenic or anatomic? Would the therapy be medical or surgical? Tanagho and co-workers (1966) have shown that in the normal continent individual an increase in the urethral pressure profile accompanies an increasing vesical volume. The incontinent woman, however, does not demonstrate this compensatory change. Another normal reflex relies on an intact pelvic floor for activation of detrusor inhibitory fibers. What happens in the elderly woman with no pubococcygeal tone whatever? Similarly, normal reflexes are ineffective in the absence of normal pelvic floor striated muscles.

Micturition

At the other end of the spectrum are disorders of voiding associated with impairment in the finely coordinated integral reflexes. Partial failure of urethral or pelvic floor relaxation during micturition may cause inefficient voiding, with subsequent development of increased intravesical pressure, increased residual urine, recurrent bacteriuria, and overflow incontinence. These may be manifested by a myriad of symptom complexes, including hesitancy, frequency, nocturia, a feeling of incomplete voiding, and postvoid dribbling. These changes can, of course, occur in the woman who has suffered a neurologic accident but may also occur in the patient whose urinary tract appears neurologically intact. Thus, with prolongation in latency periods, degenerative changes in autonomic ganglia, and so forth, a situation that clinically mimics bladder instability or true stress incontinence can exist.

ESTROGEN DEFICIENCY

The distinction made empirically in this chapter between postmenopausal changes due to senescence or aging and those due to estrogen deprivation may be more apparent than real. The human female is somewhat unique among mammals in that much of her total life span exists after cessation of reproductive life. One third of her life follows the menopause, whereas in the mouse, monkey, and rat, only 10 to 15 per cent of the total life span occurs in the menopausal period (Eskin, 1980).

In the woman reproduction may serve as a biologic model for aging. Decreasing steroid production by the ovaries results in the senescent changes of the secondary sexual organs. The decline in production of these sex steroids, principally 17β-estradiol, which begins several years before menopause, is responsible for subtle changes that cannot readily be separated from the sequences resulting from aging.

The clinical symptoms are varied and not limited to the genital system. In the brain, estrogens provide certain enzymes necessary for proper transmission of nerve impulses. In addition, estrogen receptor concentrations in the brain diminish with aging (Eskin, 1980).

The lower urinary tract and the reproductive tract are of similar embryologic origin (Chapter 1). Estrogen receptors have been demonstrated in the urethra (Sjogren, et al., 1980). Although no receptors have yet been demonstrated in the bladder, some evidence exists that suggests a steroid responsiveness by the bladder.

Studies of urethral pressures reveal this to be an age-related phenomenon. Edwards and Malvern (1974) found an inverse relationship between age and urethral pressure profile and developed a formula that expresses this relationship:

Amplitude = 92 − patient's age in years
(in cm. of water)

Plante and Susset (1980) found the maximum urethral pressure to be significantly lower in women over 70 years old compared to younger women. They believed that a loss of urethral compliance occurs, resulting in loss of urethral elasticity. This loss of compliance was aggravated if there had been prior "significant urogynecological operations" (Susset and Plante, 1980). Tanagho and Miller (1973) concur: "In women, vaginal urethral dissection inevitably damages the striated external sphincter." This may occur as a consequence of urethral or periurethral fibrosis, which probably develops in varying degrees with dissection of the anterior vaginal wall.

As one might expect, an organ that demonstrates estrogen receptors and changes associated with menopause should respond to the administration of estrogens. Faber and Heidenreich (1977), treating stress incontinence, and Smith (1976), treating atrophic urethritis, achieved excellent results using estrogen replacement. A significant

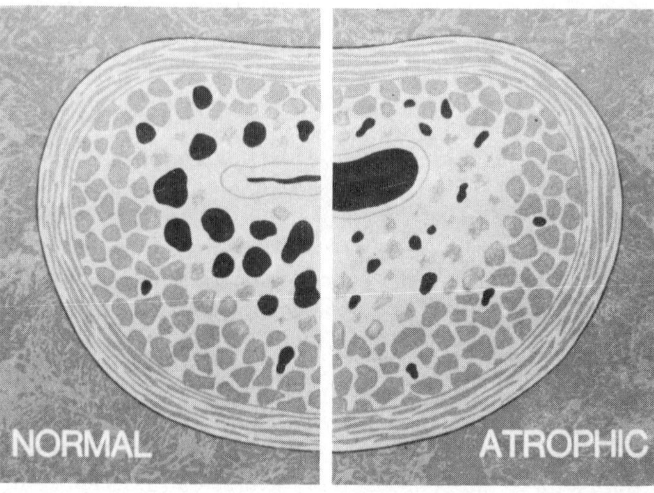

Figure 25–12. The rich venous network that lies between the mucosa and the muscularis of the urethra becomes atrophic in the postmenopausal woman. The washer-like effect of this erectile tissue may be restored by hormone replacement therapy.

rise in the urethral pressure profile was demonstrated by Faber and Heidenreich (1977) in 95 per cent of patients after estrogen treatment for 2 to 4 months. Estrogen treatment causes a proliferation of the atrophic urethral epithelium that can be demonstrated by cytologic methods. Lack of maturation of the squamous epithelium from estrogen deficiency can convert the entire distal urethra to a rigid, inelastic tube. Eventually, the thin, friable epithelium may take on the same inflamed, ulcerative appearance as is seen in the vagina in the more commonly recognized senile vaginitis. With time, strictures develop. In addition to its proliferating effect on the urothelium, estrogen increases the vascularity of the urethra and thus enhances the vascular sleeve surrounding the urethra (Figure 25–12).

CLINICAL PRESENTATION

The 1980 census claimed 30,000,000 women past the age of 50 years. The incidence of incontinence in geriatric patients in hospitals ranges from 25 to 40 per cent. A similar survey in outpatients reveals a slightly lower incidence (13 to 42 per cent) (Brocklehurst, 1978).

Incontinence is not the most common symptom in postmenopausal women. Nocturia was reported in 61 to 67 per cent in three different series reported by Brocklehurst (1978). Other symptoms included daytime frequency (23 to 35 per cent), "scalding" (13 per cent), and difficulty in voiding (3 to 7 per cent). Bacteriuria is age related and may be as high as 10 per cent in the menopausal woman (Corlett, 1979).

Incontinence is, of course, a symptom and may be a result of a number of different pathologic processes. It may be due to the process of aging itself, as a result of weakened compensatory neurologic reflexes with or without associated urethral and pelvic floor atrophy. Probably the most common cause of significant urinary incontinence, especially in the elderly menopausal woman, is an unstable bladder. Brocklehurst and Dillane (1966), using cystometrography, demonstrated a high incidence of uninhibited neurogenic bladder in elderly continent women. Nearly all women with known neurologic lesions had abnormal cystometrograms, and of the neurologically intact group, 15 of 24 women demonstrated an abnormal cystometrogram (uninhibited detrusor contractions, reduced capacity, or elevated residual urine). They state that "it appears that a poorly functioning bladder is a common accompaniment of old age even among those who are not suffering from incontinence." It is obvious that these functional changes may cause, in addition to urinary incontinence, nocturia, enuresis, daytime frequency, and urgency.

Stress urinary incontinence in the menopausal female is another common problem. With clinical and urodynamic findings supporting the diagnosis and no other findings of depressed bladder function, the problem

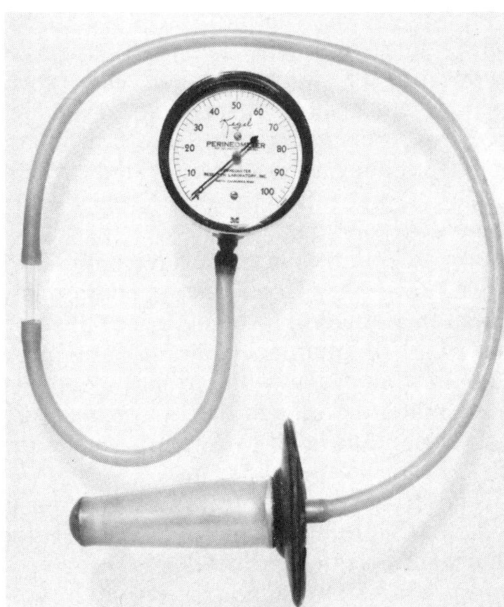

Figure 25–13. The perineometer consists of a pneumatic vaginal chamber connected by rubber tubing to a manometer calibrated in millimeters of mercury. The tubing is long enough to allow the patient to hold the manometer for observation during an exercise period. (Reproduced with permission from Current Problems in Obstetrics and Gynecology II *1*:4, 1978. Copyright © 1978 by Year Book Medical Publishers, Inc., Chicago.)

may be approached in the usual fashion. Pubococcygeal exercise has been reported effective in the management of stress incontinence (Kegel, 1956), but in my experience this modality is curative only in the milder cases. To be most efficacious these exercises should be started in the reproductive years, before a clinical problem has developed. The clinician may diagnose pubococcygeal atrophy and instruct the patients by means of a digital examination of the vagina. To quantify the findings, however, the perineometer may be used (Figure 25–13). This may be given to the patient so that she, too, can measure her efforts. The patient is instructed to exercise twice daily and to progress to at least 100 contractions per session.

Surgery for stress incontinence in the elderly woman must be selective. Since problems with impaired voiding and urinary retention are more common in this group, adequate evaluation is required (Fig. 25–14). The extent of correction of the anatomic defect should take into consideration the patient's degree of activity. Unlike the 40-year-old jogger or tennis player, the 68-year-old woman may require less elevation of the bladder neck for comparable results. Otherwise, as with the patient illustrated in Figure 25–14, outflow obstruction may develop. Overcorrection may respond incompletely to internal urethrotomy or urethral dilatation. Thus, the clinical picture and the patient's age and activity should dictate the type of surgical procedure selected.

As a rule, estrogen replacement and Kegel's exercises should be utilized before surgery. Either oral estrogen or vaginal estrogen cream is helpful. Because of the dangers of estrogen replacement treatment in postmenopausal women, many patients

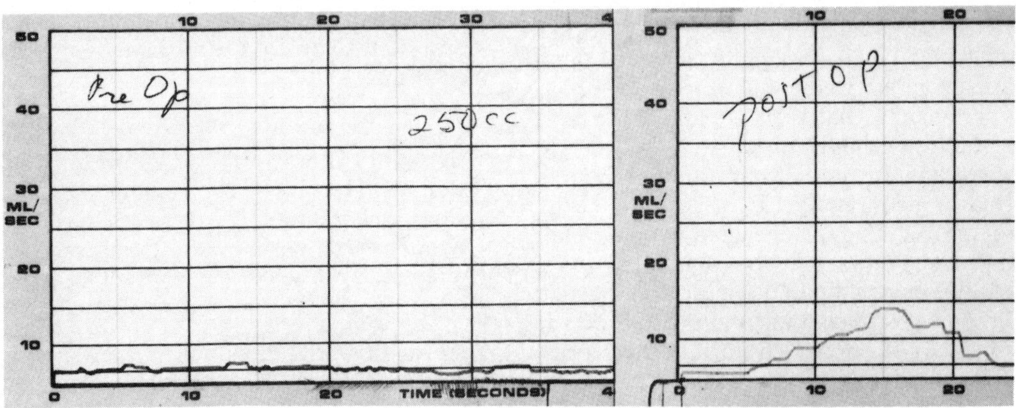

Figure 25–14. The flow rate on the graph on the left was obtained from a menopausal woman 1 year following a Marshall-Marchetti-Krantz procedure. The graph on the right was obtained in the same patient following an internal urethrotomy. (Reproduced with permission of PW Communications, Inc., The Female Patient *4*:30, 1979.)

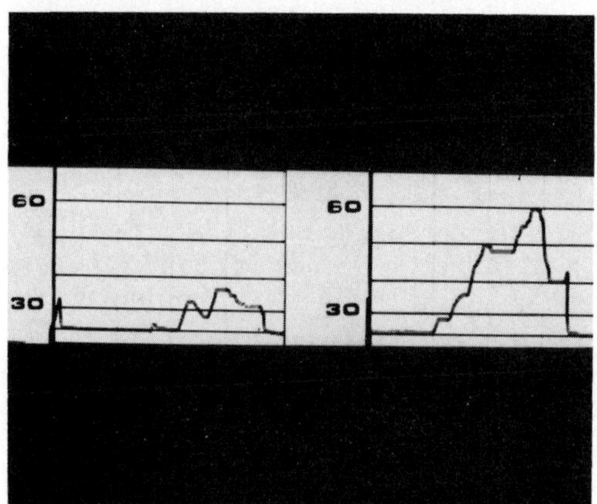

Figure 25–15. The graph on the left is the urethral pressure profile from a menopausal patient before vaginal estrogen treatment and the graph on the right following treatment. Note the significant improvement in maximal pressure as well as functional length. (Reproduced with permission of PW Communications, Inc., The Female Patient *4*:30, 1979.)

prefer vaginal cream to oral estrogen. A significant amount of estrogen is absorbed through the vaginal mucosa, a fact the clinician should realize (Schief et al., 1977; Rigg et al., 1978). The improvement can be dramatic at times (Figure 25–15) and is a result of better apposition of the urethral walls and the increased urethral tone associated with improved vascularity (Figure 25–12).

Other medications with α-adrenergic effects may be utilized to improve urethral pressure. Such drugs as phenylpropanolamine (Ornade), ephedrine, and imipramine (Tofranil) can be used for this purpose, but in the author's experience they have not proved very helpful in the patient with a stable bladder. Additionally, many of these patients have medical problems, such as hypertension, that would make the use of these drugs inadvisable.

Overflow incontinence is another form of urinary incontinence that is found with greater frequency in the aged woman. Outflow obstruction may be functional (as a result of uncoordinated micturition) or anatomic, but either type can result in the sequence of increased intravesical pressure, bladder decompensation, increased residual urine, bacteriuria, and trabeculation. Brocklehurst (1978) studied the bladders from 25 autopsies on patients 74 to 102 years old. The majority showed trabeculation, which was due partly to hypertrophy of the detrusor bundles and partly to loss of supporting elastic tissue. The elderly patient is much more susceptible to adverse drug reactions; therefore, if overflow incontinence, poor flow rate, or elevated residual urine is present, a careful drug history should be obtained to rule out the use of any medication that might have anticholinergic properties. Dopamine, phenylpropanolamine (Ornade), promethazine (Phenergan) and imipramine (Tofranil) are but a few of the drugs with strong secondary anticholinergic effects that may cause urinary retention in the susceptible individual.

The urethral syndrome is a condition in which symptoms of disturbed micturition (burning, frequency, hesitancy, nocturia, and urgency) are found in association with sterile urine cultures. In reality this is not a single entity, but probably has several different causes with similar presentation. Lipsky (1977) performed a urodynamic evaluation on a group of 43 women with the urethral syndrome. He demonstrated outflow obstruction in over half the patients. Two types of obstruction were noted: the first, found mainly in menopausal women, was a narrowing of the distal segment of the urethra. The second type of obstruction was seen in younger women and was a result of incomplete relaxation of the external sphincter. The main criterion for obstruction was the peak flow rate; rates less than 15 ml./second are considered compatible with obstruction. The flow rate varies inversely with age, and this must be kept in mind when evaluating specific values. Abrams and Torrens (1979) gave the following norms:

Men $<$ 40 years	$>$ 22 ml./second
Men 40–60 years	$>$ 18 ml./second
Men $>$ 60 years	$>$ 13 ml./second
Women $<$ 50 years	$>$ 25 ml./second
Women $>$ 50 years	$>$ 18 ml./second

In recording flow rates, we found that voided volumes as small as 200 ml. were acceptable, but the coefficient of variation was least when the volume was in excess of 300 ml. (Corlett and Roy, 1979). In addition to peak flow, the curve should demonstrate a rapid acceleration so that the maximum rate is reached within the first one third of the total voiding time.

The postmenopausal women with obstruction were treated satisfactorily with oral estrogen and either external urethroplasty or urethral dilatation. Schleyer-Saunders (1976) treated 300 women who had mixed urinary symptoms, including dysuria and incontinence, using only hormone implants and reported overall improvement in 70 per cent: good results in 30 per cent and fair results in 40 per cent. Smith (1976), who has written extensively on the subject, observed that when symptoms were present for less than 12 months, treatment with conjugated estrogens (Premarin) alone, 0.6 mg. daily for three weeks per month for a total of three months, was often successful. But if symptoms were present for longer than 1 year, urethral dilatation added to hormone replacement improved results (Smith, 1976). Internal urethrotomy may be utilized in place of urethral dilatation. It is believed by some to have a more prolonged effect than dilatation. Stanton and associates (1980) achieved good success in menopausal patients with obstruction using the Otis urethrotome. They noted, however, greater improvement in those patients with bladder instability, demonstrated by uroflowmetry, in addition to obstruction.

In those patients responding to estrogen treatment alone, improvement was noted as early as 1 week following institution of therapy. The patients remained symptom-free for 6 to 24 weeks after stopping treatment, but then symptoms returned with progressive severity. In view of the temporary nature of recovery following temporary treatment, it would seem reasonable to treat indefinitely. It may well be that lower doses given less frequently will suffice for the prevention of the atrophic changes discussed earlier. Once the estrogen deficiency has proceeded unchecked to the point of causing anatomic changes in the lower urinary tract, a higher dose, more frequently administered, is required.

Given the controversy regarding estrogen replacement therapy, the reader is referred to Greenblatt and associates (1980) for a discussion of estrogen dose and the relative risks of developing endometrial carcinoma.

REFERENCES

Abrams, P., and Torrens, M.: Clinical urodynamics. Urol. Clin. North Am. *6*:71, 1979.

Brocklehurst, J. C.: The bladder. *In* Brocklehurst, J. C. (ed.): Textbook of Geriatric Medicine and Gerontology. London, Churchill Livingstone, 1978.

Brocklehurst, J. C., and Dillane, J. B.: Studies of the female bladder in old age. I. Cystometrograms in non-incontinent women. Geront. Clin. *8*:285, 1966.

Corlett, R. C.: Urologic problems in menopause. Female Patient *4*:30, 1979.

Corlett, R., and Roy, S.: Carbon dioxide uroflowmetry. J. Urol. *122*:512, 1979.

Edwards, L., and Malvern, J.: The urethral pressure profile: theoretical considerations and clinical application. Br. J. Urol. *46*:325, 1974.

Eskin, B. A.: Aging and the menopause. *In* Eskin, B. A. (Ed.): The Menopause. Comprehensive Management. New York, Masson Publishing, 1980.

Faber, P., and Heidenreich, J.: Treatment of stress incontinence and estrogen in postmenopausal women. Urol. Int. *32*:223, 1977.

Greenblatt, R., Nezhat, C., and Karpas, A.: The menopausal syndrome hormone replacement therapy. *In* Eskin, B. A. (Ed.): The Menopause, Comprehensive Management. New York, Masson Publishing, 1980.

Johnson, W.: The Older Patient. New York, Paul Hoeber, Inc., 1960.

Kegel, A.: Stress incontinence of urine in women: physiologic treatment. J. Int. Coll. Surg. *25*:487, 1956.

Lipsky, H.: Urodynamic assessment of women with urethral syndrome. Eur. Urol. *3*:202, 1977.

Plante, P., and Susset, J.: Studies of female urethral pressure profile. Part I. The normal urethral pressure profile. J. Urol. *123*:64, 1980.

Rigg, L., Hermann, H., and Yen, S. C.: Absorption of estrogen from vaginal creams. N. Engl. J. Med. *298*:195, 1978.

Schief, I., Tulchinsky, D., and Ryan, K.: Vaginal absorption of estrone and 17β-estradiol. Fertil. Steril. *28*:1063, 1977.

Schleyer-Saunders, E.: Hormone implants for urinary disorders in postmenopausal women. J. Am. Geriatr. Soc. *24*:337, 1976.

Sjogren, C., Lindskog, M., Ulmsten, U., et al.: Estrogen binding sites in nuclear fractions from the rat urogenital tract. Presented at 10th Meeting of the International Continence Society, Los Angeles, California, October 9, 1980.

Smith, P.: Postmenopausal urinary symptoms and hormonal replacement therapy. Br. Med. J. *2*:941, 1976.

Stanton, S., Hilton, P., Cardoza, L., and Annan, H.: Internal urethrotomy in the management of impaired voiding in the female. Presented at 10th Meeting of the International Continence Society, Los Angeles, California, October 9, 1980.

Susset, J., and Plante, P.: Studies of female urethral pressure profile. Part II. Pressure profile in female incontinence. J. Urol. *123*:70, 1980.

Tanagho, E., and Miller, E.: Functional consideration of urethral sphincteric dynamics. J. Urol. *109*:273, 1973.

Tanagho, E., Miller, E., Meyers, F., et al.: Observation on the dynamics of the bladder neck. Br. J. Urol. *38*:72, 1966.

Welford, A. T., and Birren, J. E.: Behavior, Aging and the Nervous System. Springfield, Illinois, Charles C Thomas, 1965.

26

URINARY TRACT INVOLVEMENT BY BENIGN AND MALIGNANT GYNECOLOGIC DISEASE

S. LIFSHITZ, M.D.
H. J. BUCHSBAUM, M.D.

Diseases of the female genital tract can cause functional and morphologic alterations in the urinary tract. The close anatomic and physiologic relationship of the gynecologic and urologic systems, developed in embryonic life, makes one organ system responsive to alterations in the other. Most striking in its effect on the urinary tract is cervical carcinoma (see Chapter 27). Other benign neoplastic or inflammatory conditions of the female genital tract can also affect the urinary tract. Everett and Sturgis (1940) found bladder symptoms in 46 per cent of patients with common gynecologic disorders. Solomons and co-workers (1960) and Kokkonen and associates (1971) reported a 20 to 32 per cent incidence of unsuspected ureteral involvement in patients with benign gynecologic disease. The disease processes that cause urinary symptoms can arise at any site in the genital tract: ovary, parovarium, fallopian tube, uterine corpus, cervix, or vagina.

We will discuss urinary tract involvement by the more frequently encountered benign and malignant uterine and adnexal diseases, by endometriosis, and by the ovarian remnant syndrome.

I. Uterine corpus disease
  - Leiomyomata uteri
  - Endometrial carcinoma
  - Uterine sarcoma

II. Adnexal disease
  - Pelvic inflammatory disease
  - Ovarian neoplasms, benign and malignant
  - Embryonic rest tumors (parovarian cysts, Gartner's duct cysts)

III. Endometriosis

IV. Ovarian remnant syndrome

The obstetrician-gynecologist must recognize that gynecologic disease can often involve the urinary tract and that treatment, particularly surgery, can result in injury. When involvement of the urinary tract is suspected, evaluation not only will document distortion and displacement but will identify measurable changes by which appropriateness of therapy can be assessed. The urologist must also be aware of the effect of gynecologic disease on the urinary tract, because he may be the first physician consulted and may often be asked to participate in medical management.

UTERINE CORPUS DISEASE

Leiomyomata Uteri

Leiomyomata uteri (fibroids), benign tumors of the uterine musculature, are

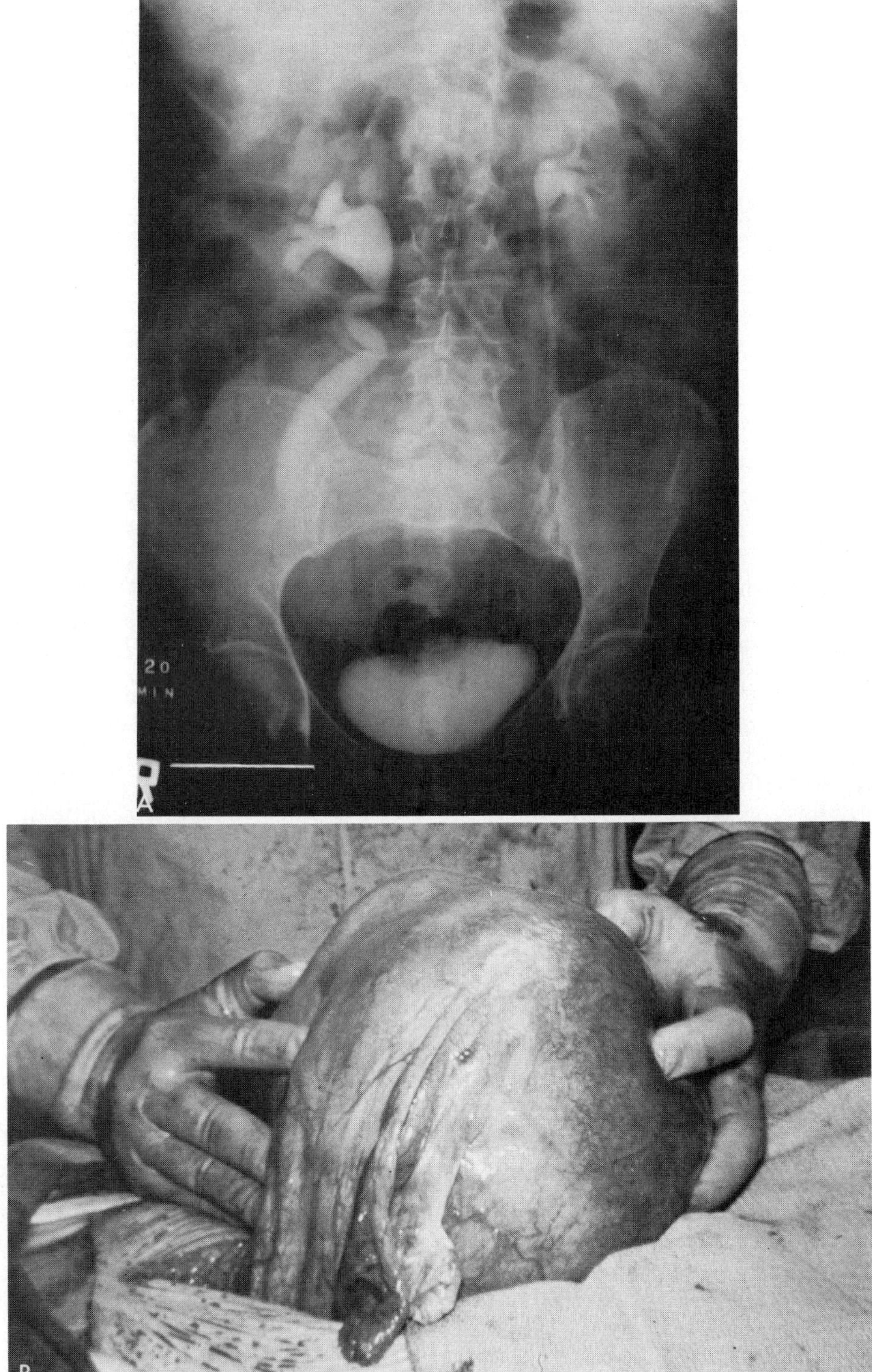

Figure 26–1. Uterine myomas. *A*, Pyelogram in patient with large uterine myoma causing right ureteral obstruction at the pelvic brim. *B*, Large myomatous uterus delivered through abdominal incision at time of hysterectomy.

among the most common tumors of the female pelvis. Myomas are found in approximately 25 per cent of uteri of women during the reproductive years (Hall, 1963).

Although most myomas are asymptomatic, they may grow to considerable size. Myomas can remain intramural, become submucous, protruding into and distorting the endometrial cavity, or become subserous and pedunculated (Figure 26–1). In most cases they are firm with a smooth surface and mobile, but they can become adherent to other pelvic or abdominal viscera when pelvic inflammatory disease or endometriosis is present. Symptoms and findings in the urinary tract relate to the size and location of the myomas, and to the presence of inflammatory disease or endometriosis.

Bladder

When the myomas are small, they are generally asymptomatic. As they enlarge, they may encroach on other organs and cause pressure symptoms. The proximity of the urinary bladder to the uterus, in the funnel-shaped rigid pelvis, makes the bladder most susceptible to the increasing size of uterine myomas. The most common urinary symptom produced by myomas is frequency, resulting from external pressure on the bladder. Rarely, cervical or lower corpus myomas, arising below the bladder flap, can cause urethral obstruction. They elevate the bladder base so that it presses against the region of the internal sphincter, causing ureteral displacement and blockage.

Ureters

Significant ureteral obstruction from myomas is far less frequent than one might anticipate. In the absence of an inflammatory process or endometriosis, even an enlarged uterus is mobile. Furthermore, myomas are firm and do not mold to or comply with the shape of the upper pelvis. The ureters in their extraperitoneal location avoid the pressure of an intraperitoneal tumor.

The frequency with which partial ureteral obstruction occurs is difficult to assess. Ureteral changes relate to the *size* and *location* of myomas and to the presence of concomitant inflammatory disease. Exceptionally large myomas may cause ureteral obstruction at the pelvic brim (Figure 26–1). Morrison (1960) reported some degree of ureteral obstruction in 11 of 61 patients (18 per cent) with myomas. Ureteral obstruction was present in nine of 32 patients (28.1 per cent) with myomas that filled the pelvis or were palpable above the symphysis and in only 6.9 per cent (two of 29 patients) with small fibroids. Both patients with small myomas had underlying disease that accounted for the hydroureteronephrosis.

Kretschmer and Kanter (1937) noted some degree of ureteral obstruction in 70.8 per cent of patients with myomas above the pelvic brim and in 54.5 per cent of patients with smaller tumors, but they did not identify other conditions that might have been present. Chamberlin and Payne (1944) also suggested a correlation between tumor size and ureteral obstruction and reported an overall incidence of upper tract dilatation secondary to myomas in 72.5 per cent of patients. None of these reports notes the degree of obstruction. Consequently it is of interest that Long and Montgomery (1950) found only a slight degree of distention in 31 of 66 patients with upper urinary tract dilatation. Many of these reports emanated from urology services, suggesting some degree of selection. It is interesting to note that at the University of Iowa in a 5-year period ending December 1975, significant ureteral obstruction was found in only nine of 598 patients with myomas of all sizes.

Fixed and intraligamentous tumors, as expected, are more likely to affect the ureters. The incidence of ureteral displacement and obstruction in fixed and intraligamentous tumors is nearly double that of freely movable myomas (Chamberlin and Payne, 1944). Intraligamentous tumors are most likely to displace the ureters laterally and posteriorly and to cause obstruction by compressing them against the bony pelvis (Figure 26–2). Chamberlin and Payne (1944) reported ureteral obstruction in 48 per cent and displacement in 20 per cent of 25 patients with intraligamentous tumors. A combination of obstruction and displacement was present in 16 per cent of patients studied.

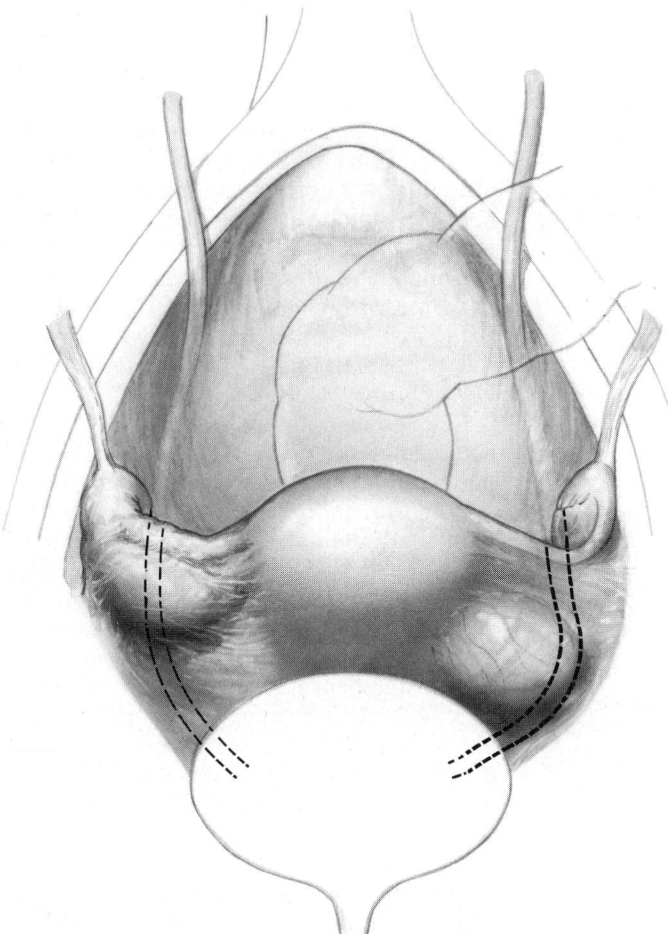

Figure 26–2. Tubo-ovarian abscess involving right adnexa. Inflammatory mass is fixed and can obstruct the ureter. An intraligamentous myoma is shown in the left broad ligament. Tumors at this site cause deviation and occasionally obstruction of the ureter.

The presence of pelvic inflammatory disease is another factor that alters the effect of myomas on the urinary tract. Fixation of myomas can also result from endometriosis or diverticulitis of the bowel. Long and Montgomery (1950) found some degree of ureteral obstruction in 39.4 per cent of patients with myomas. The incidence of ureteral obstruction increased to 84 per cent when pelvic inflammatory disease was present with the myomas.

In almost all of the reports, the right ureter is more frequently displaced or obstructed by myomas. The frequency of right ureteral involvement may be three to four times as great as that of left ureteral involvement. Right-sided predominance has been postulated to be due to the anatomic difference between the course of the ureter as it crosses the left and right iliac arteries. The left ureter is protected in its course by the sigmoid colon, which overlies it, making it less exposed to pressure than is the right.

Dilatation of the ureters produced by myomas does not generally alter renal function as measured by BUN and creatinine tests. When the offending uterus is removed, these changes quickly regress and normal appearance is restored. When removing the myomatous uterus care should be taken not to injure the urinary bladder, which may be greatly distorted by the tumor. The uterovesical fold should be divided and dissected downward from the anterior surface of the uterus before the uterine vessels are clamped. Adequate exposure is imperative at all times to avoid damage to the urinary tract. Myomectomy for low-lying myomas may be helpful.

Intraligamentous tumors should be removed by dividing the round ligament near the uterus and by creating a plane of cleavage between the anterior leaf of the broad ligament and the tumor. The infundibulopelvic ligament with the ovarian vessels should then be clamped, divided, and ligated with the ureter under direct vision. This plane of dissection, once developed, can be continued posteriorly, and with careful blunt dissection the mass can be delivered from between the leaves of the broad ligament. The remainder of the operative procedure can be completed in a routine fashion. When dissecting intraligamentary masses, the surgeon must be cognizant of possible displacement of the ureter from its normal location (Figure 26–2). Preoperative intravenous pyelography or ureteral catheterization, or both, can be selectively used by the surgeon unfamiliar with the course of the ureter.

Endometrial Carcinoma

Adenocarcinoma of the endometrium involves the urinary tract less frequently than does malignancy of the uterine cervix. In the later stages of endometrial carcinoma, after endocervical involvement has occurred (Stage II), the malignancy spreads laterally along tissue planes toward the pelvic sidewall. This spread is in the base of the broad ligament, the cardinal ligaments and the paracervical tissues. The cancer can break through the serosa of the uterus and involve the parametrium.

As the disease progresses to the lateral wall it can cause obstruction of the ureter, commonly by compression or rarely by invasion. The incidence of pelvic and para-aortic lymph node involvement is directly related to the degree of tumor differentiation and depth of myometrial invasion (Creasman, 1976). With pelvic lymph node involvement comes the possibility of ureteral obstruction or medial displacement of the distal ureter (Figure 26–3). Not only must distal ureteral obstruction secondary to pelvic lymph involvement be considered, but in addition nearly 60 per cent of patients with pelvic node disease secondary to endometrial carcinoma will have para-aortic nodal involvement as well (Boronow, 1976). Extensive involvement of the para-aortic lymph nodes can cause lateral displacement of the proximal ureter.

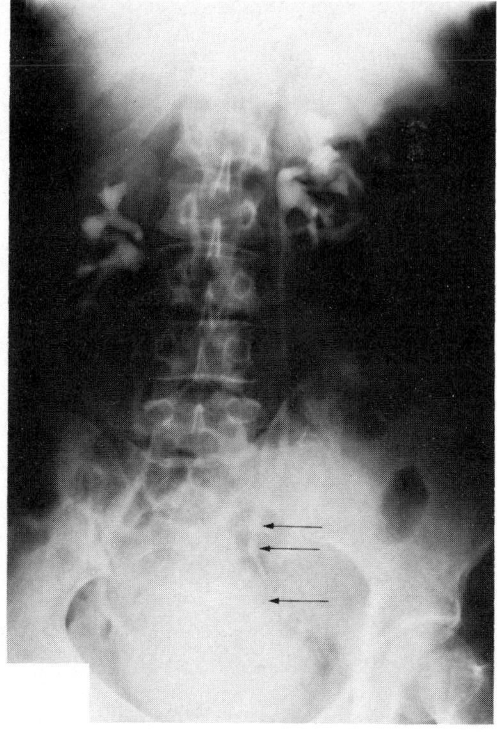

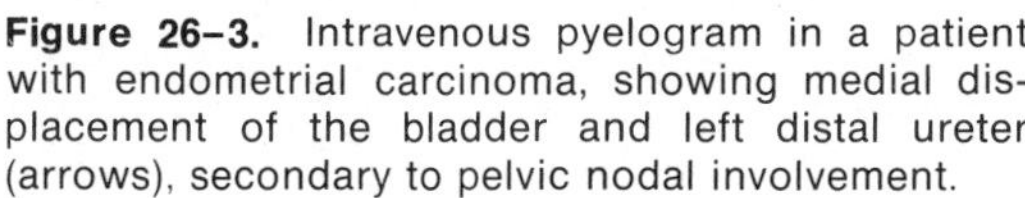

Figure 26–3. Intravenous pyelogram in a patient with endometrial carcinoma, showing medial displacement of the bladder and left distal ureter (arrows), secondary to pelvic nodal involvement.

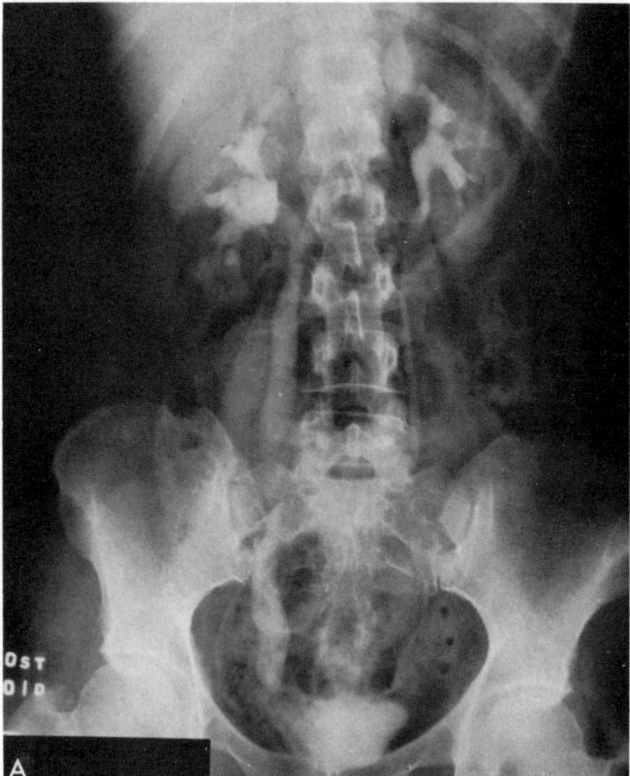

Figure 26–4. Patient with endometrial stromal sarcoma.

A, Intravenous pyelogram showing deformity of the right side of the bladder and obstruction of the right ureterovesical junction.

B, Photomicrograph showing endometrial stromal sarcoma (T) involving bladder musculature (M) and submucosa (S). (Hematoxylin-eosin stain, ×50.)

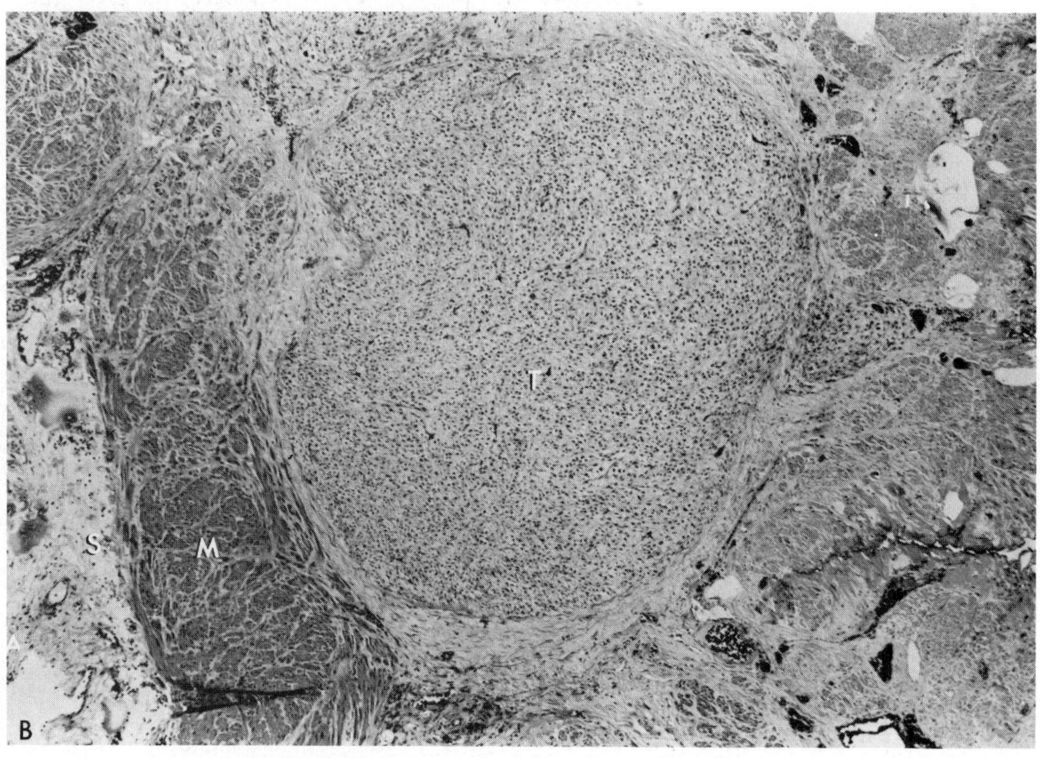

The bladder is generally spared by endometrial carcinoma, and direct invasion is rarely encountered. Ureteral and urethral involvement are more common. Metastasis to the anterior vaginal wall, probably by retrograde vascular or lymphatic routes, occurs in 10 to 15 per cent of patients following primary treatment (Finn, 1950; Dede et al., 1968; Ingersoll, 1971). It is not uncommon to see patients with distal urethral obstruction secondary to metastatic adenocarcinoma of the endometrium. When tumor invades the myometrium, more often in poorly differentiated tumors (Cheon, 1969; DiSaia et al., 1975), extension through the lower anterior uterine wall may continue directly into the bladder.

Uterine Sarcoma

Uterine sarcomas spread primarily via the bloodstream; the lung is the most common site of metastatic disease. Endometrial stromal sarcoma, a pure homologous tumor, recurs more commonly in the pelvis and can involve the bladder via external compression or by direct invasion. Because of the proximity of the bladder base to the anterior aspect of the uterus, direct extension of the malignant process can involve the urethra, the ureters, or both (Figure 26–4*A*).

When the bladder musculature is involved (Figure 26–4*B*) and the tumor has not broken through the bladder mucosa, the cystoscopic picture is one of bullous edema. With mucosal involvement the lesion can appear as an ulcer or as an exophytic tumor projecting into the bladder. The most frequent manifestation of bladder mucosal involvement is hematuria. This may be gross but most often is microscopic and may be intermittent. Other clinical urinary symptoms in order of occurrence are frequency, dysuria, and pyuria.

ADNEXAL DISEASE

Pelvic Inflammatory Disease

Pelvic inflammatory disease (PID) is rapidly reaching epidemic proportions. The acute episode, precipitated by a gonococcal infection, involves the lower genital and urinary tracts. Affected are the urethra, urethral glands, Bartholin's glands, and cervix. Dysuria and vaginal discharge are the usual early complaints (Cuman et al., 1975). Without treatment or with delayed or inadequate treatment, the disease progresses and ascends through the endometrial cavity to involve the fallopian tubes.

The early upper gynecologic tract disease involves first the endosalpinx and later the full thickness of the fallopian tube. Inflammatory exudate can leak out the distal end of the fallopian tube, causing acute pelvic peritonitis. In untreated or reinfected cases, the disease process destroys the tubal mucosa, distending the fallopian tube with pus (a pyosalpinx). Several cycles of the disease may occur with episodes of acute exacerbation. When the disease process involves the ovary, a fixed and firm inflammatory mass, a tubo-ovarian abscess, results. (See Figure 26–2.)

Nongonococcal pelvic infection, secondary to pregnancy termination or the intrauterine device, can also result in tubo-ovarian abscess (Taylor et al., 1975). When pelvic abscess formation is associated with recent major gynecologic surgery or malignancy, occasionally fistula formation to the vagina or other pelvic viscera may develop. London and Burkman (1979) reported two patients with tubo-ovarian abscess secondary to the intrauterine device who developed fistula formation into the urinary bladder. With drainage of the pelvic abscess and adequate antibiotic treatment, the fistulas healed spontaneously. Unlike myomas and benign ovarian neoplasms, a tubo-ovarian abscess is fixed to the pelvic peritoneum overlying the ureter. Prior to the advent of antibiotic therapy, patients with chronic pelvic inflammatory disease commonly showed upper urinary tract dilatation. Everett and Sturgis (1940) reported hydroureter and hydronephrosis in 44.4 per cent of patients with chronic salpingitis. When inflammatory masses were present this was increased to 58.5 per cent. Long and Montgomery (1950) cite similar figures: 23 of 47 patients (48 per cent) with extensive pelvic inflammatory disease had dilatation of the upper urinary tract with delayed drainage. Ten of the 23 patients had urinary tract symptoms. With *acute* pelvic inflam-

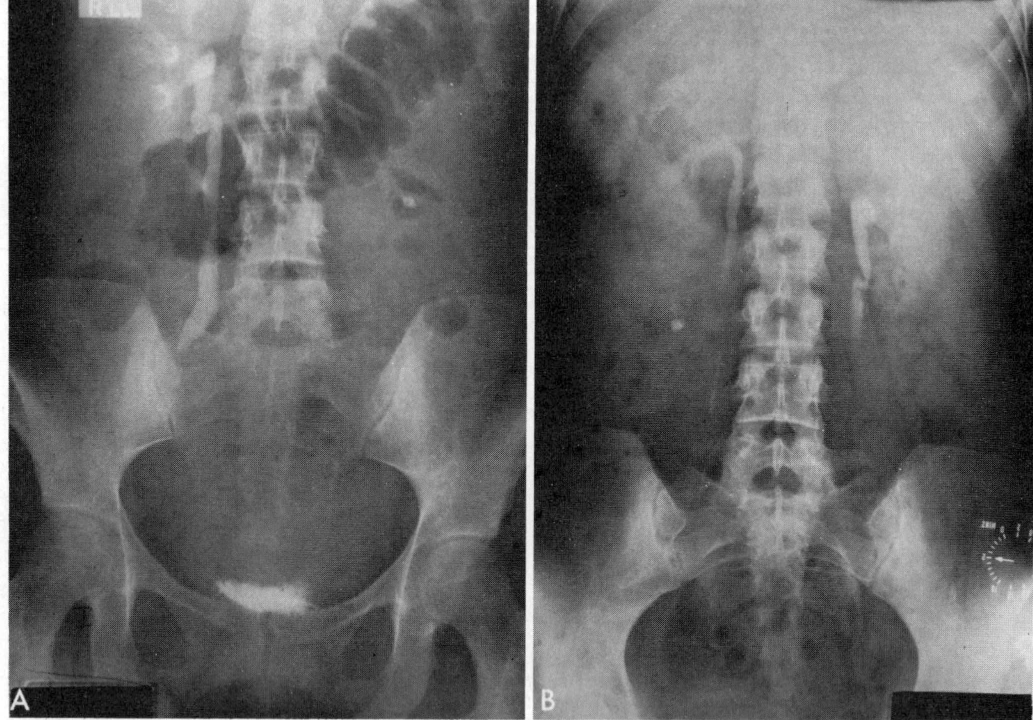

Figure 26–5. Patient with pelvic inflammatory disease.
A, Preoperative intravenous pyelography demonstrating moderate right hydroureter.
B, Postoperative study after total abdominal hysterectomy and bilateral salpingo-oophorectomy, showing resolution of ureteral obstruction.

matory disease nine of 28, or 31.1 per cent, had some degree of upper urinary tract involvement. With *chronic* PID four of eight patients (50 per cent) had upper urinary tract changes, whereas these abnormalities were present in nine of 10 patients with pelvic abscess. Kretschmer and Kanter (1937) examined a single patient with a tubo-ovarian abscess (side and size not given) and found no alterations on pyelography, and this report is frequently cited when urinary tract alterations secondary to PID are discussed.

With the apparent increase in the incidence of pelvic inflammatory disease, we are seeing more patients with obstructed upper urinary tracts. Figure 26–5*A* is a preoperative film showing chronic pelvic inflammatory disease in a young woman. After definitive surgery, total abdominal hysterectomy and bilateral salpingo-oophorectomy, the changes are reversed (Fig. 26–5*B*). However, the regression is not as rapid or complete as it is with myomas or benign adnexal cysts.

Ovarian Neoplasms, Benign and Malignant

Benign ovarian tumors can affect the urinary tract in a fashion similar to that of myomas. Like myomas, they can cause extrinsic pressure on the bladder, leading to frequency and the urge to void. They are generally more mobile than myomas and located higher in the pelvis. Ovarian neoplasms can compress the superior aspect of the bladder, particularly if they are anterior to the uterus. Occasionally a rapidly growing ovarian tumor lying posterior to the uterus in the cul-de-sac can displace the uterus and bladder anteriorly. Under extreme conditions this can result in urethral obstruction with urinary retention due to impingement of the urethra or vesical neck against the symphysis pubis (Figure 26–6).

Cystic and even solid ovarian tumors are softer than myomas and can mold or form to the irregular shape of the lateral pelvis. In this way they can compress the ureter. But benign cysts confined to the true pelvis

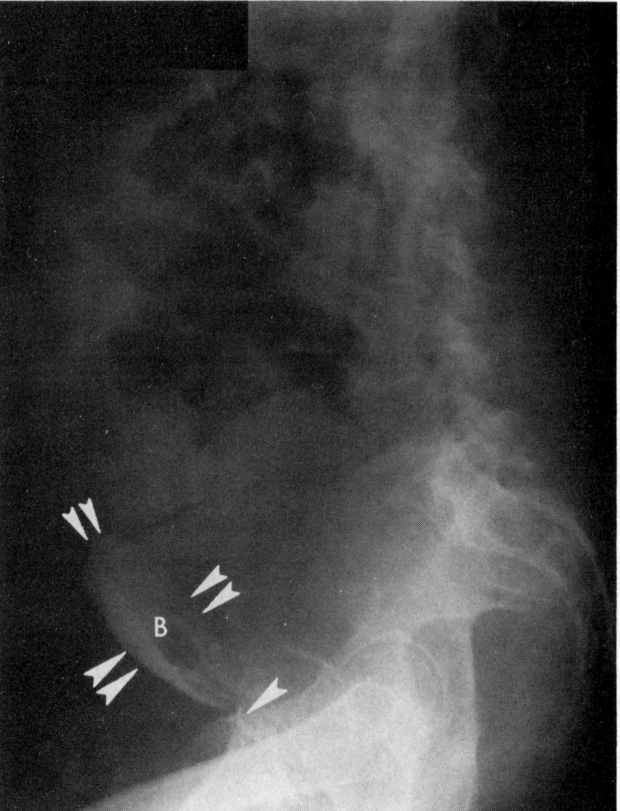

Figure 26–6. Cystogram in a patient with ovarian carcinoma presenting with acute urinary retention. The bladder (double arrows) is displaced superiorly and anteriorly by large tumor causing impingement of the urethra against the symphysis pubis (arrow). Note Foley catheter in bladder.

rarely obstruct the ureter. Pyelography often shows bilateral deviation with bowing of the pelvic ureter. Tumors reaching above the pelvic brim are more likely to cause ureteral obstruction by compression at the inlet (Figure 26–7). The incidence of ureteral obstruction secondary to large ovarian neoplasms has been variously reported as 40 to 81 per cent (Everett and Sturgis, 1940; Kretschmer and Kanter, 1937). Chamberlin and Payne (1944) found ureteral obstruction in three, displacement in one, and both obstruction and displacement in two of 14 patients with ovarian cysts. Forty-three per cent of patients with ovarian cysts had some preoperative changes on pyelography. In all instances the roentgenographic findings reverted to normal after operation. Morrison (1960) reported upper urinary tract changes in six of 14 patients (43 per cent) with ovarian tumors. Once again, no sequelae were found in patients operated upon.

The likelihood of ureteral obstruction in ovarian neoplasms is directly related to the size and histologic characteristics of the tumor. Long and Montgomery (1950) reported ureteral obstruction in 57.8 per cent of patients with benign ovarian tumors (larger than a uterus of 4 months' gestation) and in 69.2 per cent (nine of 13) with malignant tumors. These authors also noted that most changes regressed following surgery.

In addition to bladder compression and ureteral pressure, ovarian carcinoma can involve the pelvic and para-aortic lymph nodes (Bergman, 1966). While intraperitoneal tumors are likely to displace the ureters laterally, retroperitoneal lymph node masses secondary to ovarian carcinoma will displace the ureters medially. The bladder is rarely involved by ovarian carcinoma (Bernstein, 1936). We have seen two cases of ovarian carcinoma with bladder invasion (Figure 26–8) in over 350 cases of ovarian carcinoma in 7 years. The ureters may become obstructed by the primary intraperitoneal tumor or as a result of retroperitoneal pelvic nodal involvement. Me-

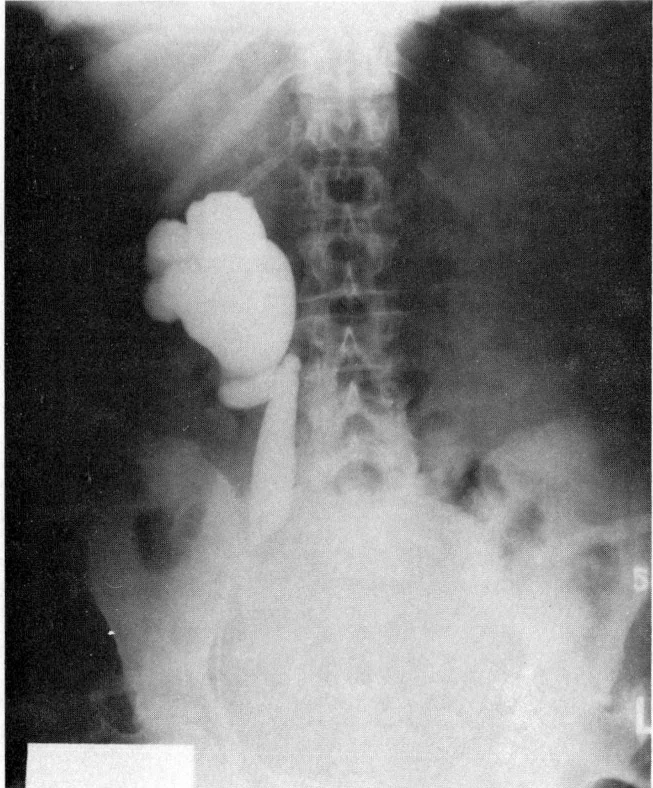

Figure 26–7. Right retrograde pyelogram in a patient with a large benign ovarian cyst, demonstrating marked hydroureteronephrosis. Obstruction is at the pelvic brim.

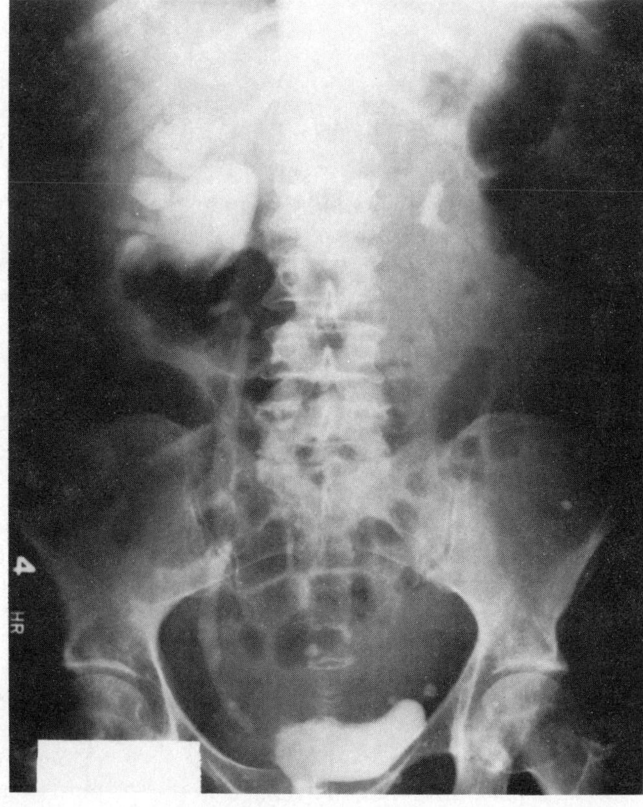

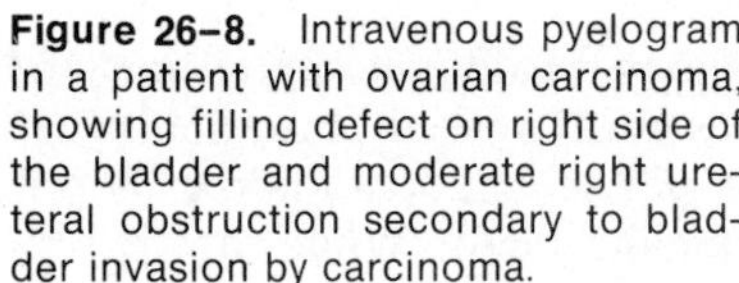

Figure 26–8. Intravenous pyelogram in a patient with ovarian carcinoma, showing filling defect on right side of the bladder and moderate right ureteral obstruction secondary to bladder invasion by carcinoma.

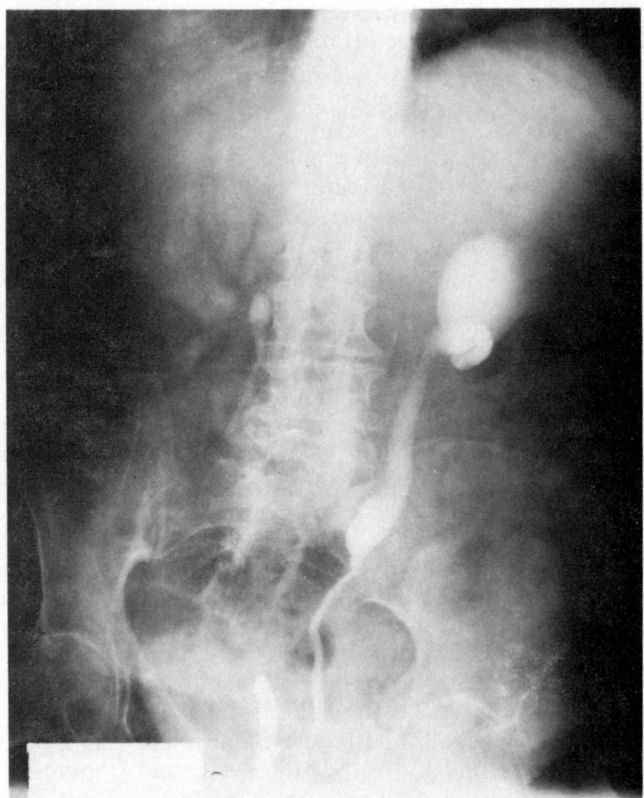

Figure 26–9. Left retrograde pyelogram in a patient with ovarian carcinoma, demonstrating moderate hydroureteronephrosis secondary to histologically proved metastases in the left common iliac lymph nodes. (Right oblique view.)

tastases in the common iliac nodes are especially likely to place the ureter in jeopardy. Figure 26–9 shows a patient with retroperitoneal metastatic spread of ovarian carcinoma with left ureteral obstruction.

Surgery for ovarian neoplasms and that for pelvic inflammatory disease present similar problems. Adnexal masses adherent to the lateral pelvic wall or broad ligament present considerable technical problems in their removal. The infundibulopelvic ligament often is shortened, and the tumor or abscess wall may lie against both the ureter and the iliac vessels. In dissecting these masses, the posterior parietal peritoneum lateral to the pelvic vessels should be incised and the position of the ureter determined before clamping the ovarian vessels. Care should be taken not to tear any collateral vessels that may have developed to supply the tumor. If the adnexal mass is large and interferes with good exposure, it can be removed separately from the uterus.

Embryonic Rest Tumors

In the mesosalpinx, between the tube and the ovary, is situated the parovarium (epoophoron), a vestigial remnant of the wolffian body. Its main excretory duct, the wolffian or mesonephric duct, extends from the caudal pole of the ovary downward along the lateral margin of the uterine corpus and cervix and the lateral wall of the vagina (see Chapter 1).

Parovarian Cysts

From the parovarium, cysts of various sizes can develop. These parovarian cysts can be recognized by their position between the tube and the ovary, the latter being intact while the tube is greatly elongated and stretched over the upper border of the tumor. The effect of these cysts on the urinary tract is similar to that produced by the more common ovarian cysts. The likelihood of ureteral obstruction is related to the size; those cysts reaching above the true pelvis can cause ureteral obstruction by compression at the brim.

Gartner's Duct Cysts

The lower portion of the mesonephric duct is known as Gartner's duct. Cystic dilatation of this duct may occur at any point in its course; when it occurs in the portion located between the folds of the broad ligament, pathologic changes in the urinary tract may be produced by a mechanism similar to that of intraligamentous myomas. These cysts are likely to displace the ureters laterally and cause obstruction by compression against the pelvic sidewalls. (See earlier discussion).

ENDOMETRIOSIS

Next to myoma uteri, endometriosis may be the most common pathologic condition found in the female pelvis. The histologic picture is that of ectopic endometrium, stroma, and glands. Although Sampson's theory of spread by retrograde menstruation is the most widely held, hematogenous, lymphatic, and direct extension, as in adenomyosis, have also been considered as possible mechanisms. Endometriosis has been reported at laparotomy in 1.04 to 32 per cent of women (Meigs, 1938; Brzezinski et al., 1962).

Any portion of the pelvic peritoneum may be involved by endometriosis. Urinary tract involvement is rare. Kerr (1966) estimated the incidence of involvement of the urinary tract by endometriosis at 1.2 per cent. The bladder is most frequently involved, followed by ureters and kidneys. Urethral involvement is extremely rare. If endometrial tissue is present at the urethral meatus, the lesion will be painful and seen to enlarge at the time of menstruation.

Bladder

Over 150 cases of bladder endometriosis have been reported. Careful history and physical examination will aid the physician in arriving at a diagnosis. Whereas small lesions may be asymptomatic, larger lesions will cause dysuria, frequency, and urgency. These symptoms are usually aggravated prior to and during menstruation. Cyclic hematuria (20 to 25 per cent of cases) may give a clue as to the cause (Kerr, 1966). The most common involvement of the bladder is a mucosal lesion that results from a serosal focus involving the full thickness of the bladder wall. Although early lesions may be small, endometriomas of the bladder can exceed 8 cm.

Findings on cytoscopic examination vary with the site and size of the tumor. If the lesion is submucosal, only bullous edema may be apparent. With mucosal involvement bluish lesions are visible; these may appear as cysts or as ulcerative lesions. Moore and co-workers (1943) in a literature review found that in 21 of 46 patients with endometriosis of the bladder the lesion was palpable on vaginal examination. After menstruation the symptoms tend to regress as the lesion shrinks and the edema of the surrounding tissue subsides. History and physical examination may aid in establishing a diagnosis of bladder endometriosis, but rarely is the bladder the only site of involvement. The cul-de-sac and uterosacral ligaments are accessible to bimanual and rectovaginal examination, and the laparoscope can be very effective in establishing a diagnosis. On cytoscopic examination, bladder biopsy may be necessary to rule out bladder carcinoma.

Symptomatic lesions of the bladder can be treated by transurethral resection. Since the bladder is rarely the only involved site, a systemic form of treatment should also be used.

Ureter

Involvement of the ureter by endometriosis has been classified as (1) intrinsic, when the ureter is compressed by periureteral endometriotic tissue or by direct invasion of the wall of the ureter, and (2) extrinsic, when ureteral compression results from external pressure from an endometriotic site in the parietal peritoneum, ovary, or broad ligament. The first type, intrinsic involvement, is rare (Figure 26–10). Kerr (1966) in a complete review of the literature reported 43 cases of ureteral involvement by endometriosis, 9 intrinsic and 34 extrinsic.

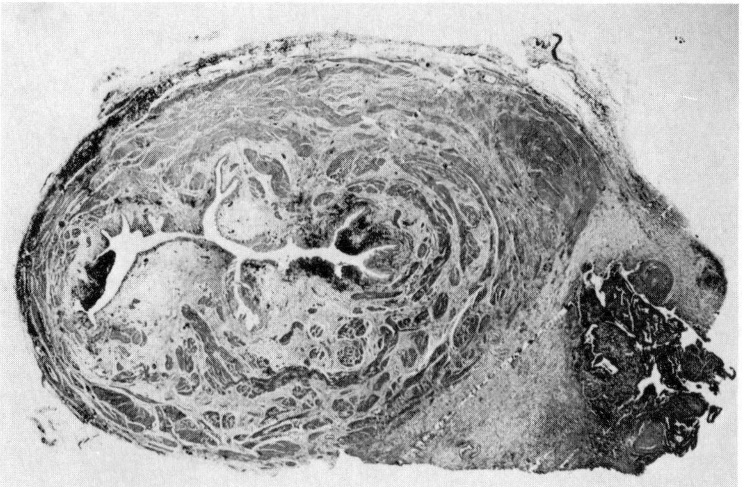

Figure 26–10. Extrinsic endometriosis. Low power photomicrograph showing area of endometriosis beside collapsed ureter. (From Moore, J. G., et al.: Urinary tract endometriosis: Enigmas in diagnosis and management. Am. J. Obstet. Gynecol. *134*:162, 1979. By permission of C. V. Mosby Company.)

Ureteral endometriosis usually is located 2 to 5 cm. from the ureterovesical junction. The disease has a predilection for the segment of the ureter corresponding to the approximate site of the posterior attachment of the ureterosacral ligaments (Pollack and Wills, 1978).

The roentgenographic findings in ureteral involvement by endometriosis are nonspecific (Figure 26–11).

When ureteral obstruction is present, flank or abdominal pain is the most common symptom. This was present in 49 per cent of the 43 patients surveyed by Kerr (1966). The pain is not cyclic, suggesting that it is secondary to ureteral obstruction and hydroureteronephrosis. In only three patients was the pain cyclic, becoming more severe during menstruation. Gross hematuria occurred in six patients, microscopic hematuria in six. Five of the six patients with gross hematuria had intrinsic involvement of the ureter by endometriosis. There is a rather poor outcome in this reported group of 43 patients, with nephrectomy in 10 patients and intentional ureteral ligation in two; in addition, two patients had nonfunctioning kidneys. The total complication rate was 32.5 per cent. Stanley and co-workers (1965) and Moore and associates (1979) have also indicated that approximately 25 per cent of the kidneys are lost when endometriosis obstructs the ureter.

Treatment of histologically proved endometriosis with extensive urinary tract involvement consists of extirpative surgery, including a total abdominal hysterectomy and bilateral salpino-oophorectomy. Endometriotic implants should be treated by resection or fulguration (Langmade, 1975). Ureteral obstruction secondary to endometriosis should be treated early in order to protect renal function. This can be accomplished by lysing periureteral adhesions, or with partial ureteral resection with reanastomosis or ureteroneocystostomy. Occasionally a temporary nephrostomy will be required to obviate renal damage, while the disease is brought into remission by castration or hormonal therapy. In these cases, return of ureteral patency can be documented with antegrade pyelographic studies, at which time the nephrostomy tube can be removed and normal urine flow reestablished.

Less extensive urinary tract involvement can be treated with conservative surgery and hormonal therapy.

OVARIAN REMNANT SYNDROME

The ovarian remnant syndrome is a rare complication of difficult oophorectomy in patients in whom the ovaries are encased in dense fibrous adhesions. The syndrome is

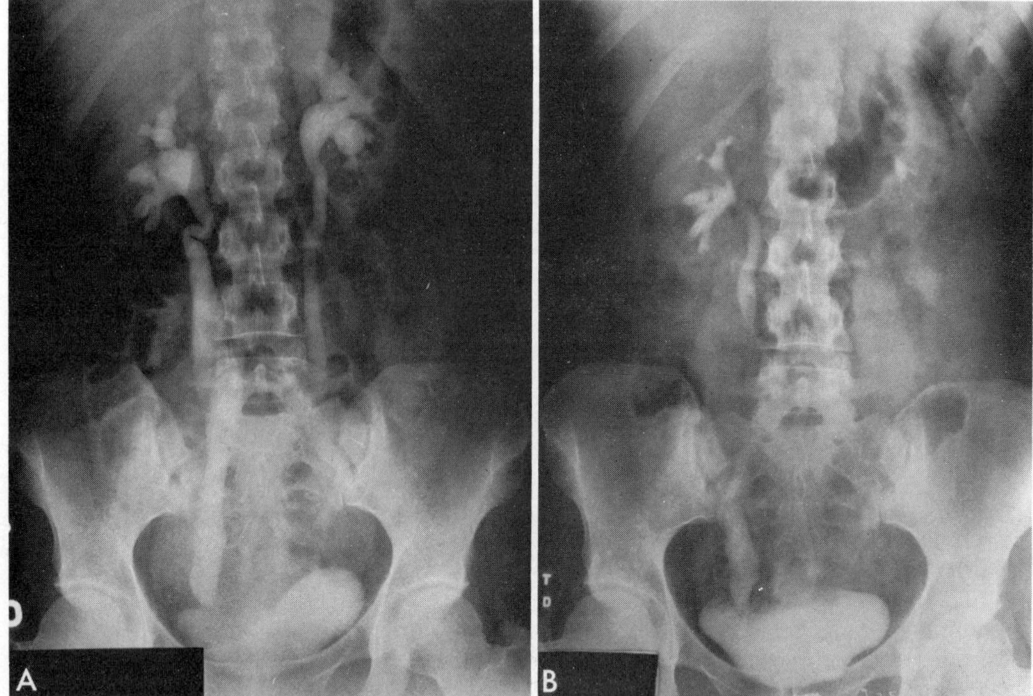

Figure 26–11. Patient with endometriosis.
A, Preoperative intravenous pyelogram demonstrating bilateral hydroureteronephrosis.
B, Study 3 months after total abdominal hysterectomy, bilateral salpingo-oophorectomy and lysis of periureteral adhesions. Moderate improvement is seen in hydroureteronephrosis.

characterized by lower abdominal pain with or without a palpable mass or a palpable cystic pelvic mass without symptoms. Surgery and pathologic studies confirm the presence of ovarian tissue where there should be none (Symmonds and Pettit, 1979).

The frequency with which ovarian tissue is inadvertently left behind after pelvic surgery is unknown, but several reports in the literature indicate that such remnants can form cysts or masses that lead to serious clinical problems.

Unilateral ureteral obstruction due to the ovarian remnant syndrome has been documented in eight patients in the recent English literature (Scully et al., 1979). Three of the patients reported had originally undergone surgery for pelvic inflammatory disease, three for endometriosis, and one for an ectopic pregnancy. In the eighth case no diagnosis was documented, but adhesions were noted at the time of primary pelvic surgery. All the patients presented with acute or chronic pain, and a pelvic mass was palpable in three. At operation, the cysts were found to range from 1 to 7 cm. in diameter, and all of them were said to be corpus luteum cysts.

Treatment of the ovarian remnant syndrome consists of surgical excision of the remnants and contiguous adherent structures. Serious urologic sequelae are avoided by identification and mobilization of the ureter at the time of operation (Berek et al., 1979).

REFERENCES

Berek, J. S., Darney, P. D., Lopkin, C., et al.: Avoiding ureteral damage in pelvic surgery for ovarian remnant syndrome. Am. J. Obstet. Gynecol. *133*:221, 1979.

Bergman, F.: Carcinoma of the ovary, a clinical pathological study of 86 autopsied patients with special reference to mode of spread. Acta Obstet. Gynecol. Scand. *45*:211, 1966.

Bernstein, P.: Tumors of the ovary. A study of 1101 cases of operations for ovarian tumor. Am. J. Obstet. Gynecol. *32*:1023, 1936.
Boronow, R. C.: Endometrial cancer. Not a benign disease. Obstet. Gynecol. *47*:360, 1976.
Brzezinski, A., Koren, A., and Kedar, S.: Contribution to the problem of the etiology of endometriosis. Isr. Med. J. *21*:111, 1962.
Chamberlin, G. W., and Payne, F. L.: Urinary tract changes with benign pelvic tumors. Radiology *42*:117, 1944.
Cheon, H. K.: Prognosis of endometrial carcinoma. Obstet. Gynecol. *34*:680, 1969.
Creasman, W. T., Boronow, R. C., Morrow, C. P., DiSaia, P. J., and Blessing, J.: Adenocarcinoma of the endometrium: Its metastatic lymph node potential. Gynecol. Oncol. *4*:239, 1976.
Cuman, J. W., Rendtorff, R. C., Chandler, R. W., et al.: Female gonorrhea: Its relation to abnormal uterine bleeding, urinary tract symptoms and cervicitis. Obstet. Gynecol. *45*:195, 1975.
Dede, J. A., Plentl, A. A., and Moore, J. G.: Recurrent endometrial carcinoma. Surg. Gynecol. Obstet. *126*:533, 1968.
DiSaia, P. J., Morrow, C. P., and Townsend, D. E.: Synopsis of Gynecologic Oncology. New York, John Wiley & Sons, 1975, p. 113.
Everett, H. S., and Sturgis, W. J.: The effect of some common gynecological disorders upon the urinary tract. Urol. Cutan. Rev. *44*:638, 1940.
Finn, W. F.: Time, site and treatment of recurrences of endometrial carcinoma. Am. J. Obstet. Gynecol. *60*:773, 1950.
Hall, J. E.: Applied Gynecologic Pathology. New York, Appleton-Century-Crofts, 1963, p. 161.
Ingersoll, F. M.: Vaginal recurrence of carcinoma of the corpus. Management and prevention. Am. J. Surg. *121*:473, 1971.
Kerr, W. S.: Endometriosis involving the urinary tract. Clin. Obstet. Gynecol. *9*:331, 1966.
Kokkonen, J., Koskela, O., and Vahala, J.: Benign gynaecological tumours and radioisotope renography. Acta Obstet. Gynec. Scand. *50*:275, 1971.
Kretschmer, H. L., and Kanter, A. E.: Effect of certain gynecologic lesions on the upper urinary tract. J.A.M.A. *14*:1097, 1937.
Langmade, C. F.: Pelvic endometriosis and ureteral obstruction. Am. J. Obstet. Gynecol. *122*:463, 1975.
London, A. M., and Burkman, R. T.: Tuboovarian abscess with associated rupture and fistula formation into the urinary bladder: Report of two cases. Am. J. Obstet. Gynecol. *135*:1113, 1979.
Long, J. P., and Montgomery, J. B.: The incidence of ureteral obstruction in benign and malignant gynecologic lesions. Am. J. Obstet. Gynecol. *59*:552, 1950.
Meigs, J. V.: Endometriosis — a possible etiological factor. Surg. Gynecol. Obstet. *67*:253, 1938.
Moore, J. G., Hibbard, L. T., Growdon, W. A., et al.: Urinary tract endometriosis: Enigmas in diagnosis and management. Am. J. Obstet. Gynecol. *134*:162, 1979.
Moore, T. D., Herring, A. L., and McCannel, D. A.: Some urologic aspects of endometriosis. J. Urol. *49*:171, 1943.
Morrison, J. K.: The ureter and hysterectomy. Including the effects of certain gynaecological conditions on the urinary tract. J. Obstet. Gynaecol. Br. Emp. *67*:66, 1960.
Pollack, H. M., and Wills, J. S.: Radiographic features of ureteral endometriosis. Am. J. Roentgenol. *131*:627, 1978.
Scully, R. E., Galdabini, J. J., and McNeely, B. V.: Case records of the Massachusetts General Hospital. Case 48–1979. N. Engl. J. Med. *301*:1228, 1979.
Solomons, E., Levin, E. J., Bauman, J., and Baron, J.: A pyelographic study of ureteric injuries sustained during hysterectomy for benign conditions. Surg. Gynecol. Obstet. *111*:41, 1960.
Stanley, K. E., Utz, D. C., and Dockerty, M. B.: Clinically significant endometriosis of the urinary tract. Surg. Gynecol. Obstet. *120*:491, 1965.
Symmonds, R. E., and Pettit, P. D. M.: Ovarian remnant syndrome. Obstet. Gynecol. *54*:174, 1979.
Taylor, E. S., McMillan, J. H., Greer, B. E., et al.: The intrauterine device and tubo-ovarian abscess. Am. J. Obstet. Gynecol. *123*:338, 1975.

27

URINARY TRACT INVOLVEMENT BY INVASIVE CERVICAL CANCER

J. R. Van NAGELL, Jr., M.D.
E. S. DONALDSON, M.D.
E. C. GAY

ANATOMIC RELATIONSHIPS OF THE FEMALE UROLOGIC AND INTERNAL GENITAL SYSTEMS

The lower urinary tract is in direct apposition to the cervix and pericervical and perivaginal lymphatics. Since the ureters and bladder are often compromised by enlarging tumor masses of the cervix, it is pertinent to review the anatomic relationship between the female urologic and internal genital organs.

The distal ureter enters the pelvis crossing over the common iliac artery just medial to its bifurcation. It descends along the lateral pelvic wall retroperitoneally beside the hypogastric vessels and, starting at the level of the ischial spine, follows a medial and anterior course to enter the base of the broad ligament. At the vaginal fornix approximately 2 cm. lateral to the cervix, the ureter lies just beneath the uterine artery and above the vaginal artery (Figure 27–1). Here, it continues through the vascular web in the uterovaginal fascia crossing the upper anterior vagina to enter the bladder at the trigone. The lymphatics of the pelvic portion of the ureter usually join those from the posterior surface of the bladder and empty into the common and internal iliac lymph nodes.

The bladder lies anterior to the vagina and lower uterine segment, and posterior to the symphysis pubis. The bladder base and the urethra lie against the anterior vaginal wall, separated by a thin layer of endopelvic fascia. Bladder lymphatics originate from two plexuses — one on the anterior and one on the posterior bladder surface. The lymphatic efferents from the anterior surface drain into the anterior vesical and external iliac nodes. Those lymphatics from the posterior surface anastomose with lymphatics from the cervix and upper vagina, and empty into the internal iliac nodes.

CERVICAL LYMPHATIC DRAINAGE

Small lymphatic vessels originate from three distinct systems that coincide with the three cervical anatomic layers — the endocervical mucosa, the cervical stroma, and the uterine serosa. These three systems empty into a broad subserosal network that gives rise to the final collecting trunks. Within the stromal layers, there is communication between the lymphatics of the lower uterine segment and the cervix. This is clinically significant in that early anatomic studies have shown that some cervical cancers spread superiorly into the lower uterine wall (Seelig, 1894).

The efferent collecting trunks draining the cervix share pathways parallel to the

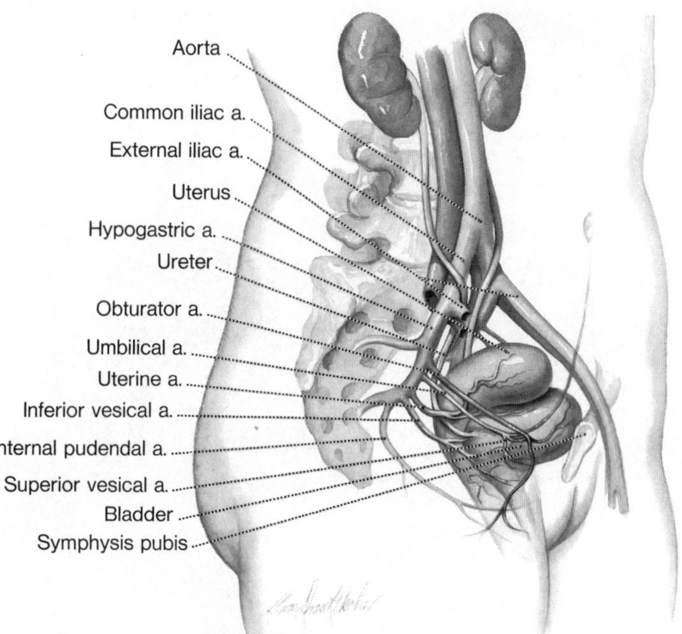

Figure 27–1. The anatomic relationship of the female urologic and internal genital organs.

uterine corpus and vagina. Valves preventing the retrograde flow of lymph are present below a cervical stromal depth of 5 mm.

The lymphatic efferents from the cervix and supravaginal region can be divided into anterior, posterior, and lateral main trunks. The anterior lymphatic trunk (Figure 27–2, inset) originates from the anterior surface of the upper portion of the cervix and crosses the vesicouterine plica to insert on the posterior bladder surface. It then follows a lateral course toward the superior vesical artery and drains into the internal iliac nodes. The posterior lymphatic trunk originates on the posterior aspect of the cervix at the insertion of the uterosacral ligament and follows this structure to the rectal fascia, where it divides into medial and lateral branches. The medial branch follows the retrorectal space to the superior rectal and subaortic nodes. The lateral branch travels through the pararectal space in the ureteric sheath to terminate in the common iliac and subaortic nodes.

The lateral main trunk, which is clinically the most significant, drains directly through the cardinal ligament to the periureteral, obturator, and internal iliac nodes (Figure 27–2).

PATHS OF DIRECT AND LYMPH NODAL SPREAD IN CERVICAL CANCER

Cervical cancer spreads by local invasion and by embolization into lymphatic channels, resulting in regional lymph nodal metastases. Vascular spread of cervical cancer does occur, but this is the pathway in less than 5 per cent of cases (Corscaden, 1962).

Paths of Direct Invasion

There are three major paths of direct invasion of cervical cancer (Figure 27–3):

1. Superiorly, cervical cancer cells spread in the stroma and stromal lymphatics to invade the uterine wall. The International Federation of Gynecology and Obstetrics Staging System (Table 27–1) ignores this type of extension; therefore, the incidence and significance of this finding have not been thoroughly investigated. Uterine involvement by cervical cancer has been reported in 4 to 17 per cent of patients (Wentz and Jaffe, 1966; Perez et al., 1975). Gusberg and co-workers (1953), for exam-

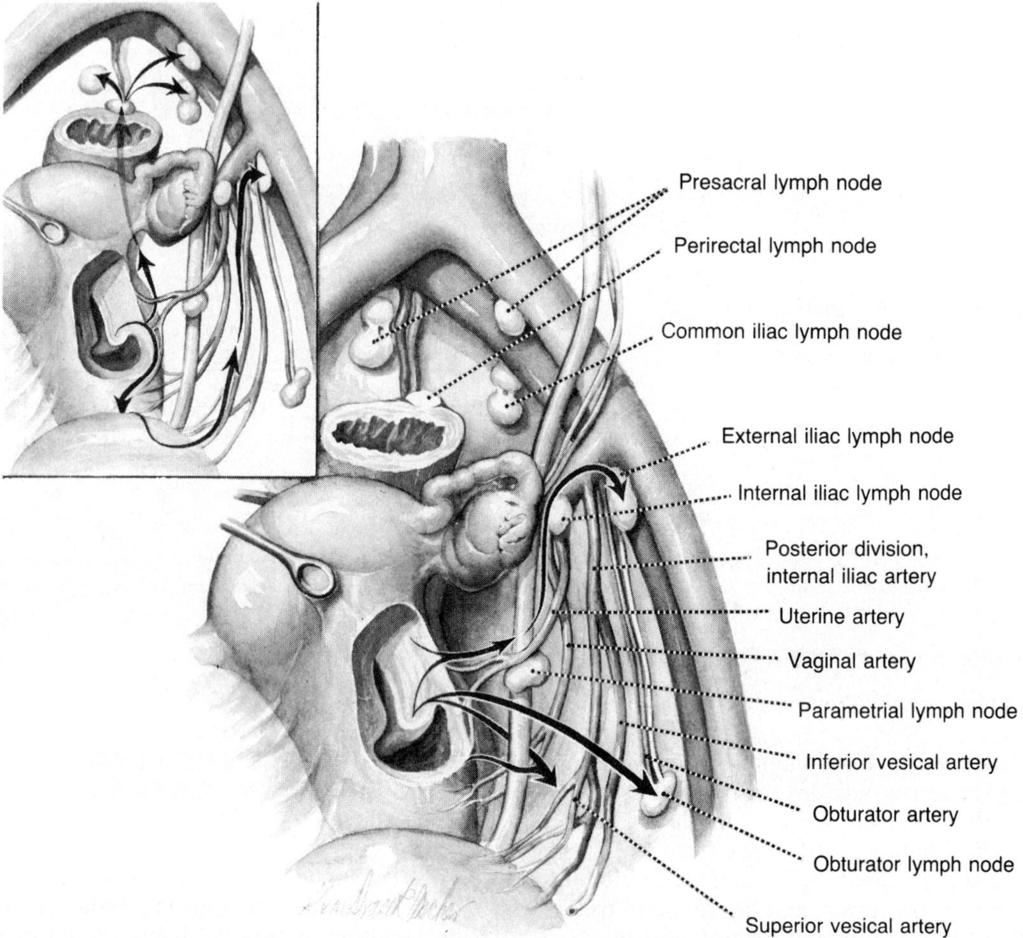

Figure 27–2. Major pathways of lymph nodal spread by invasive cervical cancer.

ple, studied the pathways of direct extension of cervical cancer and noted a 10 per cent incidence of endometrial spread. The incidence of endometrial and myometrial spread correlated directly with the size of the lesion.

2. Inferiorly, cervical cancer invades the stroma beneath the vaginal mucosa. When the lesion in this type of spread is clinically palpable and confirmed by vaginal biopsy, the patient is placed into Stage IIa or IIIa, depending upon whether or not tumor has invaded the lower one third of the vagina (Table 27–1).

3. Lateral paracervical and parametrial invasion is the most common pathway of spread of cervical cancer. Parametrial lymphatics carry tumor emboli directly to the regional pelvic lymph nodes, which in turn drain superiorly to the para-aortic nodes.

Lymph Nodal Metastases: Incidence and Distribution

The incidence of lymph nodal metastases in cervical cancer is directly related to the size and extent of the lesion. In a summary of over 2000 patients with cervical cancer, Plentl and Friedman (1971) reported lymph nodal metastases in 15 per cent of patients with Stage I disease, 29 per cent of patients with Stage II disease, and 47 per cent of patients with Stage III disease. External iliac nodes were most commonly involved, followed in order by obturator, internal iliac, common iliac, and parametrial lymph node groups.

The distribution of lymph nodal metastases in early cervical cancer has recently been studied at the University of Kentucky Medical Center. Sixty-two patients with

TABLE 27–1. INTERNATIONAL CLASSIFICATION OF CANCER OF THE CERVIX

Stage 0	Carcinoma in situ, intraepithelial carcinoma
	(Cases of Stage 0 should not be included in any therapeutic statistics)
	Invasive Carcinoma
Stage I	Carcinoma strictly confined to the cervix (extension to the corpus should be disregarded)
Stage Ia	Microinvasive carcinoma (early stromal invasion)
Stage Ib	All other cases of Stage I. Occult cancer should be marked "occ."
Stage II	The carcinoma extends beyond the cervix but has not extended onto the pelvic wall. The carcinoma involves the vagina, but not the lower third
Stage IIa	No obvious parametrial involvement
Stage IIb	Obvious parametrial involvement
Stage III	The carcinoma has extended onto the pelvic wall. On rectal examination there is no cancer-free space between the tumor and the pelvic wall. The tumor involves the lower third of the vagina. All cases with a hydronephrosis or nonfunctioning kidney
Stage IIIa	No extension onto the pelvic wall
Stage IIIb	Extension onto the pelvic wall and/or hydronephrosis or nonfunctioning kidney
Stage IV	The carcinoma has extended beyond the true pelvis or has clinically involved the mucosa of the bladder or rectum
Stage IVa	Spread of the growth to adacent organs
Stage IVb	Spread to distant organs

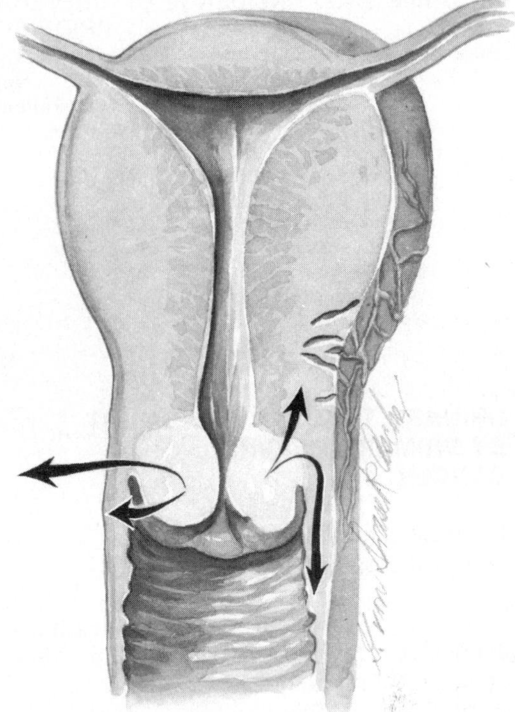

Figure 27–3. Sites of direct invasion by invasive cervical cancer.

clinical Stage Ib squamous cell carcinoma of the cervix were treated with radical hysterectomy, pelvic lymphadenectomy, and upper vaginectomy. Of these patients, 16 (26 per cent) had histologic spread of disease beyond the cervix. Three had extension into the parametrium without nodal involvement. In 13 patients (20 per cent), pelvic lymph nodes contained foci of cervical cancer. Metastases occurred most frequently in the obturator and internal iliac lymph node groups.

Piver and Chung (1975) have recently reported a direct correlation between tumor size and the incidence of lymph nodal metastases. Patients with Stage Ib cervical cancers less than 3 cm. in diameter had a 21 per cent incidence of spread to pelvic nodes, whereas those with lesions greater than 3 cm. in diameter had a 35 per cent incidence of pelvic lymph nodal metastases.

In patients dying of cervical cancer, lymph nodal distribution of tumor is somewhat different. Hendrikson (1949) and Holzaepfel and Ezell (1955) noted paracervical or parametrial spread in over 70 per cent of the cases, and metastases to the internal iliac chain were present in 25 per cent of patients. Unarrested tumor growth in the parametrium often resulted in hydroureter, hydronephrosis, complete ureteral obstruction, and finally death due to renal failure.

TABLE 27–2. INCIDENCE OF URETERAL OBSTRUCTION BY CERVICAL CANCER PRIOR TO THERAPY

Investigator	Number of Patients in Series	Number of Patients with Ureteral Obstruction
Aldridge and Mason (1950)	333	115 (34.5%)
Burns et al. (1960)	365	118 (32.3%)
Rhamy and Stander (1962)	305	43 (14.1%)
Barber et al. (1963)	503	105 (20.9%)
Kottmeier (1964)	1402	268 (19.1%)
Midboe et al. (1969)	541	92 (17.0%)
Waggoner and Spratt (1969)	945	215 (22.8%)
Bosch et al. (1973)	990	143 (14.4%)

URINARY TRACT INVOLVEMENT BY PRIMARY CERVICAL CANCER

Incidence and Significance of Ureteral Obstruction

The most common cause of death in cervical cancer remains renal failure secondary to ureteral obstruction by tumor. Hendrikson (1949) noted that 78 per cent of patients who died following treatment for cervical cancer had evidence of ureteral compression and kidney damage at autopsy. Also, ureteral obstruction by tumor is associated with a high incidence of pelvic lymph nodal metastases. Symmonds and co-workers (1968) reported that 43 per cent of patients with ureteral obstruction had pelvic lymph nodes involved with tumor. For these reasons, involvement of the urinary tract by cervical cancer is of prognostic significance.

The reported incidence of ureteral obstruction by cervical cancer prior to therapy is summarized in Table 27–2. The frequency of unilateral or bilateral ureteral compression by tumor in over 4000 patients studied varied from 14 to 34 per cent at the time of initial staging.

The prognostic significance of ureteral obstruction in patients with invasive cervical cancer is illustrated in Table 27–3. The 5-year survival rate of patients with ureteral obstruction varied from 8 to 33 per cent (average 18 per cent). In contrast, the 5-year survival rate in patients without ureteral obstruction was 22 to 59 per cent (average 50 per cent). Ureteral obstruction was therefore associated with a decrease in the overall survival rate of 32 per cent. Previous staging systems for cervical cancer disregarded the importance of ureteral obstruction. Because of its prognostic significance, however, the most recent Cancer Committee of the International Federation of Gynecology and Obstetrics has recommended that all patients with ureteral obstruction be placed in Stage IIIb (Table 27–1).

It is important to note that certain patients with no palpable evidence of parame-

TABLE 27–3. FIVE-YEAR SURVIVAL RATES OF PATIENTS WITH AND WITHOUT URETERAL OBSTRUCTION BY CERVICAL CANCER

Investigator	Number of Patients in Series	Five-Year Survival Rate	
		Patients Without Ureteral Obstruction	*Patients With Ureteral Obstruction*
Aldridge and Mason (1950)	333	59%	16 %
Burns et al. (1960)	365	62%	24 %
Barber et al. (1963)	503	22%	7 %
Kottmeier (1964)	1402	56%	8.8%
Bosch et al. (1973)	990	51%	33 %
	3593 (Total)	50% (Average)	18% (Average)

TABLE 27–4. FINDINGS ON INTRAVENOUS PYELOGRAPHY IN PATIENTS WITH CERVICAL CANCER

		Patients with Abnormalities				
Initial Stage	**Total Patients**	*Ureteral Obstruction*	*Pelvic Mass*	*Renal Calculus*	*Double Collecting System*	**Patients with Normal Findings**
I	181	4	3	2	0	172
IIa	40	0	3	1	0	36
IIb	159	12	10	2	2	133
IIIa	9	2	1	0	0	6
IIIb	115	38	6	0	0	71
IV	79	30	6	0	0	43
Total	583	86	29	5	2	461

trial extension will have ureteral obstruction by tumor. Van Nagell and colleagues (1975) reported that 4 of 181 patients (2.8 per cent) with palpable evidence of Stage I disease actually had obstructive uropathy on intravenous pyelography (Table 27–4). Ureteral obstruction occurred at the ureterovesical junction (Figure 27–4) or in the distal one third of the ureter (Figure 27–5) in over 90 per cent of the cases, as compared with only 1 per cent in the proximal ureter (Table 27–5). The incidence of obstructive uropathy increased to 38 per cent in patients with clinical Stage IV disease

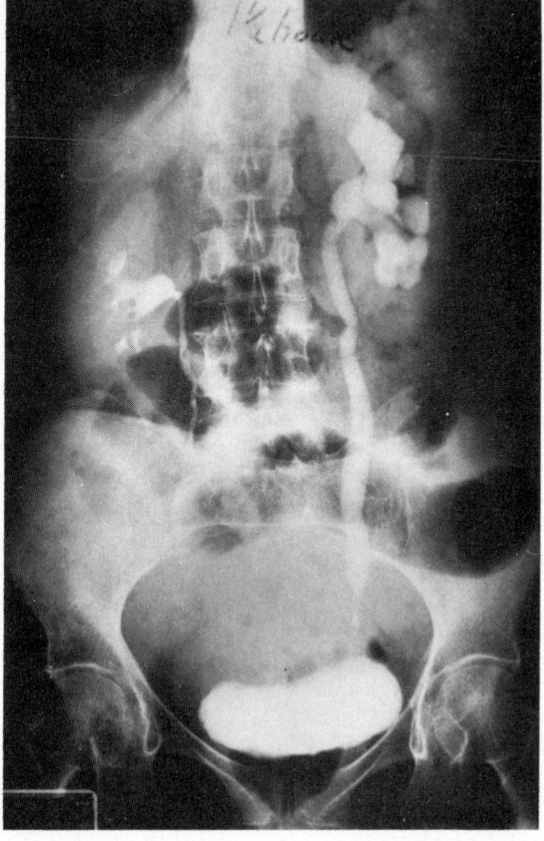

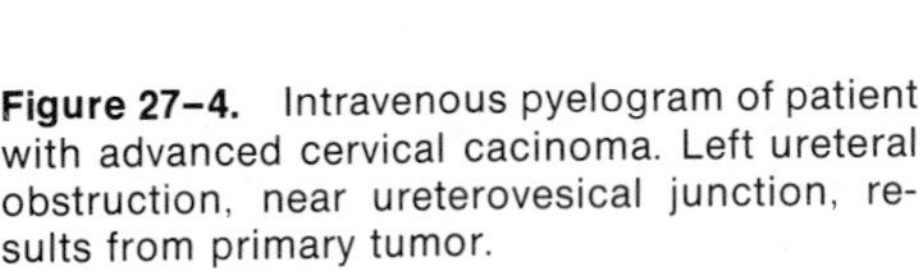

Figure 27–4. Intravenous pyelogram of patient with advanced cervical cacinoma. Left ureteral obstruction, near ureterovesical junction, results from primary tumor.

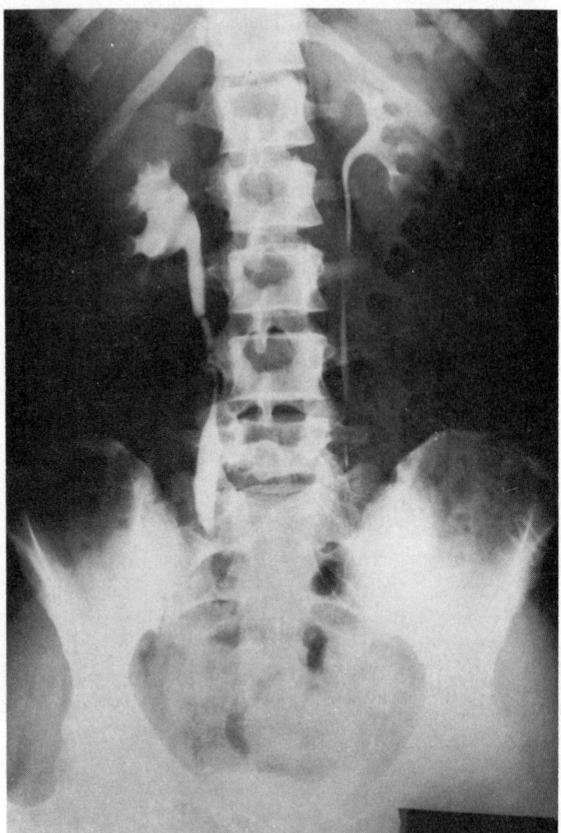

Figure 27–5. Intravenous pyelogram of patient with advanced cervical carcinoma, demonstrating obstruction at the middle third of the right ureter. Obstruction at this site is by metastatic tumor in common iliac lymph nodes.

(Table 27–6). No patient with early stage disease had bilateral ureteral obstruction. However, bilateral ureteral obstruction occurred in 6 per cent of those patients with advanced (Stages III and IV) disease.

Mechanism of Obstruction

The mechanism of ureteral obstruction appears to be extrinsic compression by tumor in the periureteral lymphatics rather than direct involvement of the ureteral wall. In 42 patients with cervical cancer and ureteral obstruction who were explored surgically at the University of Kentucky Medical Center, 33 had metastases in the pelvic lymph nodes and 18 had tumor involving the para-aortic lymph nodes. Tumor was fixed to lateral pelvic wall structures in 27 patients and involved the bladder in 14 patients. Eight patients with ureteral obstruction and central pelvic tumor underwent total pelvic exenteration. Examination of the surgical specimens failed to show direct involvement of the ureteral wall by tumor in any case. Ureteral obstruction was uniformly caused by extrinsic pressure of a tumor mass.

TABLE 27–5. LOCATION OF URETERAL OBSTRUCTION

Ureterovesical junction	33
Distal one third of ureter	36
Middle one third of ureter	2
Proximal one third of ureter	1
Nonfunctioning kidney	14
Total	86

Diagnostic Aids

Cytologic Techniques

The diagnosis of bladder involvement by cervical cancer has traditionally been made by cystoscopically directed biopsy. However, certain cytologic techniques have

TABLE 27–6. URETERAL OBSTRUCTION RELATED TO STAGE IN CERVICAL CANCER

Stage Prior to Intravenous Pyelography	Patients	Patients with Obstruction on Intravenous Pyelography	
		Unilateral	*Bilateral*
I	181	4 (2.2%)	0
IIa	40	0	0
IIb	159	12 (7.5%)	0
IIIa	9	1 (11.1%)	1 (11.1%)
IIIb	115	32 (27.8%)	6 (5.2%)
IV	79	24 (30.4%)	6 (7.6%)

been effective in the diagnosis of transitional cell carcinoma of the bladder and could be applied to metastatic bladder lesions as well. Reichborn and co-workers (1972) reported that bladder cytology was accurate in the diagnosis of recurrent transitional cell carcinoma of the bladder in 90 per cent of the cases. Other investigators (e.g., Trott and Edwards, 1973) have reported increased accuracy of bladder washings compared with conventional urine samples in the diagnosis of bladder carcinoma.

Urinary CEA Determination

The recent findings of elevated carcinoembryonic antigen (CEA) levels in the urine of patients with transitional cell carcinoma of the bladder (Pugh, 1973; Hall, 1973) are of theoretical importance. Several investigators (Khoo and Mackay, 1973; van Nagell et al., 1975; DiSaia et al., 1976) have shown that CEA level is elevated in the plasma and tumors of patients with carcinoma of the cervix. In addition, Goldenberg and associates (1976), using the immunoperoxidase technique, reported the localization of CEA on the cell membrane in squamous cell carcinoma of the cervix. It now appears that approximately 50 per cent of cervical cancers have detectable CEA present in the cytoplasm or on the cell membrane of tumor cells (van Nagell et al., 1979). Urinary CEA determination may therefore be a useful adjunct to exfoliative cytologic examination in the detection of early spread of cervical cancer to the bladder.

Cystoscopy

Although biopsy-proved involvement of the bladder by tumor is a necessary prerequisite for inclusion into Stage IVa (Table 27–1), indications for cystoscopy in patients with cervical cancer have not been clearly defined. Some investigators have favored examining all patients under anesthesia and performing cystoscopy at that time, whereas others have felt that cystoscopy is indicated only in the presence of palpable or visible extension of cervical cancer anteriorly. Furthermore, the question as to whether cystoscopy used in evaluating the spread of cervical cancer should best be performed under general or local anesthesia has not been answered.

Other Prognostic Implications

Cystoscopic findings in 583 previously untreated patients with cervical cancer have recently been reported (van Nagell et al., 1975), and are represented in Table 27–7. Bladder biopsies were performed in 120 patients, and invasion of the bladder mucosa by cervical cancer was confirmed in 45 patients. It is of interest that no patient with palpable evidence of Stage I or II disease had extension of invasive cervical cancer to the bladder mucosa. The incidence of biopsy-proved cervical cancer in the bladder was 20 per cent in patients with clinical findings of Stage IIIb disease and 23 per cent in patients with evidence of Stage IV disease (Table 27–8).

The significance of a tumor mass elevating the bladder, but not involving the bladder mucosa, has not been properly evaluated. It has been estimated that this finding may be present in up to one third of patients with advanced cervical cancer. However, no long-term follow-up studies to evaluate the prognostic implications of bladder elevation by tumor are available.

TABLE 27–7. CYSTOSCOPIC FINDINGS IN PATIENTS WITH CERVICAL CANCER

Stage Prior to Cystoscopy	Patients	Patients with Abnormalities				
		Invasive Cancer	*Mass Elevating Bladder*	*Bullous Edema*	*Bladder Inflammation*	*Vesico-vaginal Fistula*
I	177	0	0	1	4	0
IIa	40	0	2	0	0	0
IIb	147	0	6	5	3	0
IIIa	7	0	1	0	0	0
IIIb	133	27	41	6	0	0
IV	79	18	5	1	0	2
Total	583	45	55	13	7	2

Metastatic spread of primary cervical cancer to the kidneys is rare. Extrapelvic metastases occur in approximately 35 per cent of patients treated for invasive cervical cancer (Hendrikson, 1949; Halpin et al., 1972). In a review of 202 patients with distant metastases from cervical cancer, Hendrikson (1949) noted that only three patients had renal involvement with tumor. This confirms numerous studies showing that cervical cancer spreads primarily to lower urinary tract structures rather than to the kidney or proximal ureters.

The futility of trying to prolong life in patients with primary cervical cancer by palliative urinary diversion is illustrated by the report of Chua and colleagues (1967). These authors found no statistically significant difference in the survival of cervical cancer patients with ureteral obstruction who received urinary diversion prior to therapy and those that did not. It is evident, therefore, that palliative urinary diversion is contraindicated in patients with cervical cancer.

Summary

It is apparent that urinary tract involvement by cervical cancer is of both therapeutic and prognostic significance. All patients with primary cervical cancer should, therefore, have extensive evaluation of the urinary tract prior to therapy. Intravenous pyelography should be performed in all patients, and cystoscopy should be carried out in those patients whose cancer has palpably extended beyond the cervix.

URINARY TRACT INVOLVEMENT BY RECURRENT CERVICAL CANCER

Diagnostic Considerations

In the United States there are approximately 20,000 cases of invasive cancer of the cervix diagnosed per year, and in approximately 40 per cent of these the patient will have recurrent or persistent disease following therapy. The diagnosis of recurrent cervical cancer is often quite difficult to establish. Most patients have been treated for the primary cancer by irradiation, and cervical cytologic samples are difficult to interpret. In addition, tumor may recur in a site which is not readily palpable and cannot be biopsied.

Several adjunctive diagnostic methods including lymphangiography and needle biopsy have been recommended in order to increase diagnostic accuracy. Lehman and co-workers (1975) and Piver and Barlow (1973) have reported greater than 90 per

TABLE 27–8. BIOPSY-PROVED BLADDER INVASION RELATED TO STAGE IN PATIENTS WITH CERVICAL CANCER

Stage Prior to Cystoscopy	Total Patients	Patients with Bladder Invasion
I	177	0
IIa	40	0
IIb	147	0
IIIa	7	0
IIIb	133	27 (20.3%)
IV	79	18 (22.8%)

cent correlation between positive findings on lymphangiography and bulky metastatic involvement of pelvic and aortic lymph nodes. However, both investigators note that this technique may not be accurate in the diagnosis of small lymphatic metastases. Gary and colleagues (1964) advocated the use of parametrial needle biopsy to diagnose recurrent cervical carcinoma of the pelvis, but this procedure is associated with a 10 per cent false-negative rate (El-Minawa and Perez-Mesa, 1974) and is often ineffective in diagnosing upper pelvic recurrence. Consequently, many patients must undergo exploratory laparotomy and selected biopsies simply to establish the diagnosis of recurrent cervical cancer.

Involvement of the urinary tract, specifically ureteral obstruction, is one of the few objective signs of tumor recurrence. Ureteral stricture and subsequent obstruction caused by radiation are relatively rare, occurring in approximately 2 to 3 per cent of patients experiencing obstructive uropathy (Slater and Fletcher, 1971; Villasanta, 1972). Any patient, therefore, who develops ureteral obstruction following radiation therapy for primary cervical cancer should be suspected of having recurrence, and appropriate measures should be undertaken to confirm the presence of tumor histologically.

Evaluation of Patients for Radical Surgery

Intravenous pyelography should be performed on all patients suspected of having recurrent tumor in order to determine the lateral extent of the disease. Since the majority of patients with cervical cancer have been treated with radiation therapy to the limit of normal tissue tolerance, radical surgery is the method of choice in the treatment of pelvic recurrence. This type of surgery is quite extensive, often requiring bowel or urinary tract diversion, and is associated with a significant incidence of major postoperative complications (Rutledge and Burns, 1965; Symmonds et al., 1968).

Although the overall 5-year survival rate after exenterative surgery has been 20 to 30 per cent, higher survival rates are possible with careful patient selection. In an effort to define the group of patients most suited for radical surgery, several authors (Creasman and Rutledge, 1972; Barber, 1969) have proposed a uniform evaluation system for all patients with recurrent disease prior to operation. The factors for this evaluation include (1) location of tumor; (2) presence and duration of symptoms; and (3) intravenous pyelographic findings. Centrally located recurrence, whether involving the bladder or not, is often surgically resectable with a high percentage of cure.

Tumor involving the lateral pelvic wall structures is not curable. Creasman and Rutledge (1972), for example, reported that 82 per cent of patients with central pelvic recurrence had resectable lesions, and 51 per cent survived at least 2 years following surgery. More lateral lesions were resectable in only 38 per cent of cases, and the 2-year survival rate fell to 20 per cent.

Prognostic Implications

Ureteral Obstruction by Recurrent Tumor

The prognostic implication of ureteral obstruction by recurrent tumor has been studied by a number of investigators. Van Dyke and van Nagell (1975) reported that 78 per cent of patients whose recurrent tumor was resectable had normal intravenous pyelograms, whereas the majority of patients with unresectable disease had either unilateral or bilateral ureteral obstruction. Radical surgery was performed on 40 of 110 patients with recurrent cervical cancer. Fifty-eight per cent of patients with normal intravenous pyelograms survived 2 to 10 years (mean, 50 months) following surgery. However, all patients undergoing pelvic exenteration who had ureteral obstruction died within 2 years of operation from recurrent carcinoma.

Similarly, Halpin and co-workers (1972), in a review of 134 patients with recurrent cervical carcinoma, noted no 5-year survivors among patients with obstructive uropathy. In the largest series, Barber and co-workers (1963) reported a 5-year survival rate of 10 per cent following pelvic exenteration in patients with unilateral ureteral obstruction. There were no 5-year survivors with ureteral obstruction deep in the posterolateral aspect of the pelvis.

There is no doubt that all patients with recurrent cervical cancer who are able to tolerate pelvic exenteration physically and psychologically should be surgically explored. However, when recurrent carcinoma produces total ureteral obstruction, the possibility of patient survival is so limited that ultra-radical surgery is an impractical therapeutic method.

Palliative urinary diversion in patients with ureteral obstruction due to recurrent cervical cancer is generally not favored by the authors. These patients have usually had a complete course of pelvic irradiation, and the high incidence of operative complications as well as the minimal duration of survival outweighs any advantages of the procedure. In a recent study, Meyer and co-workers (1980) reported that 44 cervical cancer patients who underwent urinary diversion because of impending renal failure had a mean survival of 3.8 months. The most common method of urinary diversion was unilateral nephrostomy, and this procedure was associated with only minimal complications. These investigators concluded that urinary diversion could be of benefit to selected patients particularly if there was no histologic evidence of tumor recurrence.

Bladder Involvement by Recurrent Tumor

Bladder involvement by recurrent cervical cancer is associated with a poor prognosis both because of the extent of local spread and because it is often accompanied by lateral pelvic wall or nodal disease. Spratt and colleagues (1973), for example, reported that extension of cervical cancer into the bladder was associated with a significant decrease in survival following pelvic exenteration. It is pertinent to note that the incidence of lymph nodal spread is directly related to the depth of bladder wall invasion by cervical cancer. Perez-Mesa and Spjut (1963), in a study of 83 patients undergoing pelvic exenteration, reported that the incidence of pelvic lymph nodal metastases increased from 16 to 32 per cent when the depth of invasion by cervical cancer progressed from the serosal to the mucosal layer of the bladder. Patient survival was more directly related to the incidence of lymph nodal spread than to extension of tumor into the bladder. The 5-year survival rate following pelvic exenteration of patients with bladder involvement by cervical cancer was 33 per cent, whereas for those with pelvic lymph nodal spread it was less than 10 per cent.

In summary, the anatomic relationship of the urinary tract to the internal female genital system makes it a common site of involvement of both primary and recurrent cervical cancer. It is only by a thorough evaluation of urinary tract structure and function that the oncologist can obtain the knowledge necessary to plan optimal therapy for each patient with cervical cancer.

REFERENCES

Aldridge, C. W., and Mason, J. T.: Ureteral obstruction in carcinoma of the cervix. Am. J. Obstet. Gynecol. *60*:1272, 1972.

Barber, H. R. K.: Relative prognostic significance of preoperative and operative findings in pelvic exenteration. Surg. Clin. North Am. *49*:431, 1969.

Barber, H. R. K., Roberts, S., and Brunschwig, A.: Prognostic significance of preoperative non-visualizing kidney in patients receiving pelvic exenteration. Cancer *16*:1614, 1963.

Bosch, A., Frias, Z., and de Valda, G. C.: Prognostic significance of ureteral obstruction in carcinoma of the cervix uteri. Acta Radiol. *12*:47, 1973.

Burns, B. C., Everett, H. S., and Brack, C. B.: Value of urologic study in the management of carcinoma of the cervix. Am. J. Obstet. Gynecol. *80*:997, 1960.

Chua, D. T., Fawzi, I. A., O'Leary, J. A., et al.: Palliative urinary diversion in patients with advanced carcinoma of the cervix. Cancer *20*:93, 1967.

Corscaden, J. A.: Gynecologic Cancer. Baltimore, The Williams & Wilkins Co., 1962, p. 147.

Creasman, W. T., and Rutledge, F.: Preoperative evaluation of patients with recurrent carcinoma of the cervix. Gynecol. Oncol. *1*:111, 1972.

DiSaia, P. J., Morrow, C. P., Haverback, B. J., et al.: Carcinoembryonic antigen in cervical and vulvar cancer patients — serum levels and disease progress. Obstet. Gynecol. *47*:95, 1976.

El-Minawa, M. F., and Perez-Mesa, C. M.: Parametrial needle biopsy follow-up of cervical cancer. Int. J. Obstet. Gynecol. *12*:1, 1974.

Gary, R. K., Sala, J. M., and Spratt, J. S.: The detection and treatment of post-irradiationally recidivated cancers of the cervix uteri. Radiology *83*:203, 1964.

Goldenberg, D. M., Pletsch, Q., and van Nagell, J. R., Jr.: Immunoperoxidase localization of carcinoembryonic antigen in squamous cell carcinoma of the cervix. Gynecol. Oncol. *4*:204, 1976.

Gusberg, S. B., Fish, S. A., and Wang, Y. Y.: The growth pattern of cervical cancer. Obstet. Gynecol. *2*:557, 1953.

Hall, R. R.: Carcinoembryonic antigen and urothelial carcinoma. Br. J. Urol. *45*:88, 1973.

Halpin, T. F., Frick, H. C., III, and Munnell, E. W.: Critical points of failure in the therapy of cancer of the cervix; a reappraisal. Am. J. Obstet. Gynecol. *114*:755, 1972.

Hendrikson, E.: The lymphatic spread of carcinoma of the cervix and body of the uterus. Am. J. Obstet. Gynecol. *58*:924, 1949.

Holzaepfel, J. H., and Ezell, H. E.: Sites of metastases of uterine carcinoma. Am. J. Obstet. Gynecol. *69*:1027, 1955.

Khoo, S. K., and Mackay, E. V.: Carcinoembryonic antigen in cancer of the female reproductive system — sequential levels and effects of treatment. Aust. N.Z. J. Obstet. Gynecol. *13*:1, 1973.

Kottmeier, H. L.: Surgical and radiation treatment of carcinoma of the uterine cervix. Acta Obstet. Gynecol. Scand., *43*(Suppl. 12):1, 1964.

Kroemer, P.: Die Lymphorgane der weiblichen Genitalien und ihre Veranderungen bei malignen Erkankungen des Uterus. Arch. Gynaekol. *73*:57, 1904.

Lehman, M. H., Park, R. C., Barham, E. D., et al.: Pretreatment lymphangiography in carcinoma of the uterine cervix. Gynecol. Oncol. *3*:354, 1975.

Meyer, J. E., Yatsuhashi, M., and Green, T.: Palliative urinary diversion in patients with advanced pelvic malignancy. Cancer *45*:2698, 1980.

Midboe, D. K., Roddick, J. W., Jr., and Catron, F. H.: Prognostic significance of urinary tract involvement by cervical cancer. Cancer *24*:84, 1969.

Perez, C. A., Zivnuska, F., Askin, F., et al.: Prognostic significance of endometrial extension from primary carcinoma of the uterine cervix. Cancer *35*:1493, 1975.

Perez-Mesa, C., and Spjut, H. L.: Persistent postradiation carcinoma of the cervix uteri; a pathologic study of 83 pelvic exenteration specimens. Arch. Pathol. *75*:462, 1963.

Piver, M. S., and Barlow, J. J.: Paraaortic lymphadenectomy, aortic node biopsy, and aortic lymphangiography in staging patients with advanced cervical cancer. Cancer *32*:367, 1973.

Piver, M. S., and Chung, W. S.: Prognostic significance of cervical lesion size and pelvic lymph node metastasis in cervical carcinoma. Obstet. Gynecol. *46*:507, 1975.

Plentl, A., and Friedman, E. A.: Lymphatic System of the Female Genitalia. Philadelphia, W. B. Saunders Co., 1971, p. 91.

Pugh, R. C.: Pathology of cancer of the bladder. Cancer *32*:1267, 1973.

Reichborn, R., Kjennerud, S., and Hoeg, K.: The value of urine cytology in the diagnosis of recurrent bladder tumors. Acta Cytol. *16*:269, 1972.

Rhamy, R. K., and Stander, R. W.: Pyelographic analysis of radiation therapy in carcinoma of the cervix. Am. J. Roentgenol. Radium Ther. Nucl. Med. *87*:41, 1962.

Rutledge, F. N., and Burns, B. C.: Pelvic exenteration. Am. J. Obstet. Gynecol. *91*:692, 1965.

Seelig, A.: Pathologisch-anatomische Untersuchungen über die Ausbreitungswege des Gebärmutterkrebses. Strassburg, A. Volkmann, 1894, p. 10.

Slater, J. M., and Fletcher, G. H.: Ureteral strictures after radiation therapy for carcinoma of the uterine cervix. Am. J. Radiol. *61*:269, 1971.

Spratt, J. S., Jr., Butcher, H. R., Jr., and Bricker, E. M.: Exenterative Surgery of the Pelvis. Philadelphia, W. B. Saunders Co., 1973, p. 49.

Symmonds, R. E., Pratt, J. H., and Welch, J. S.: Exenterative operations. Am. J. Obstet. Gynecol. *101*:66, 1968.

Trott, P. A., and Edwards, L.: Comparison of bladder washings and urine cytology in the diagnosis of bladder cancer. J. Urol. *110*:664, 1973.

Van Dyke, A. H., and van Nagell, J. R., Jr.: The prognostic significance of ureteral obstruction in patients with recurrent carcinoma of the cervix uteri. Surg. Gynecol. Obstet. *141*:371, 1975.

Van Nagell, J. R., Jr., Meeker, W. R., Parker, J. C., et al.: Carcinoembryonic antigen in patients with gynecologic malignancy. Cancer *35*:1372, 1975.

Van Nagell, J. R., Jr., Sprague, A. D., and Roddick, J. W., Jr.: The effect of intravenous pyelography and cystoscopy on the staging of cervical cancer. Gynecol. Oncol. *3*:87, 1975.

Van Nagell, J. R., Donaldson, E. S., Gay, E. C., Hudson, S., Sharkey, R. M., Primus, F. J., Powell, D. F., and Goldenberg, D. M.: Carcinoembryonic antigen in carcinoma of the uterine cervix. II. Tissue localization and correlation with plasma antigen concentration. Cancer *44*:944, 1979.

Villasanta, U.: Complications of radiotherapy for carcinoma of the cervix. Am. J. Obstet. Gynecol. *114*:717, 1972.

Waggoner, C. M., and Spratt, J. S. Jr.: Prognostic significance of radiography ureteropathy before and after irradiation therapy for carcinoma of the cervix uteri. Am. J. Obstet. Gynecol. *105*:1197, 1969.

Wentz, W. B., and Jaffé, R. M.: Squamous cell carcinoma of the cervix with higher uterine involvement. Obstet. Gynecol. *28*:271, 1966.

28

RADIATION CYSTITIS, FISTULA, AND FIBROSIS

H. J. BUCHSBAUM, M.D.
J. D. SCHMIDT, M.D.
C. PLATZ, M.D.
A. J. WHITE, M.D.

RADIATION THERAPY — RISKS VERSUS BENEFITS

Radiation therapy in gynecologic practice is currently restricted to the treatment of pelvic malignancy, although in the past it was used in the treatment of infertility and dysfunctional uterine bleeding and for ovarian ablation. Alone or in combination with surgery, radiation therapy is widely used in the treatment of gynecologic malignancies (Table 28–1). For many diseases, particularly in advanced stages of uterine carcinoma, radiation therapy is the preferred form of treatment.

Because of the close proximity of the female genitalia and the lower urinary tract, a malignancy in the former can invade or obstruct the latter. It is important, therefore, to determine the extent of urinary tract involvement prior to the start of radiation therapy. This is particularly true when recurrent carcinoma is suspected, since the clinical signs and symptoms of radiation injury, as well as the radiographic findings, mimic recurrent cancer.

TABLE 28–1. RADIATION THERAPY OF GYNECOLOGIC MALIGNANCIES

Site	Therapeutic Mode		
	Radium	*Teletherapy*	*Isotopes*
Cervix	+	+	+(1)
Endometrium	+	+	
Ovary		+	+
Vulva	+(2)	+	
Vagina	+	+	
Fallopian tube		+	+

(1) No longer used.
(2) Mold or needles.

The kidney, the most radiation-sensitive of the urinary tract structures, is spared exposure to the ionizing radiation in the standard treatment fields for gynecologic cancer; however, the lower ureters and bladder receive almost the same total dose as does the malignancy. These urinary tract structures cannot be shielded from the external beam and are in close proximity to the tandem and colpostats used in the treatment of uterine cancer (Figure 28–1). The uterus (corpus and cervix) can tolerate high doses of irradiation, as much as 20,000 to 30,000 rads in 2 to 3 weeks. When irradiated, this organ becomes nonfunctional and is unaffected by postirradiation fibrosis.

The administered doses are calculated to effectively control disease at the lowest complication rate. Bloomer and Hellman (1975) discussed the risk-benefit problem of radiation therapy and presented theoretical curves showing the probability of tumor control and the risks of radiation complications plotted as a function of radiation dose

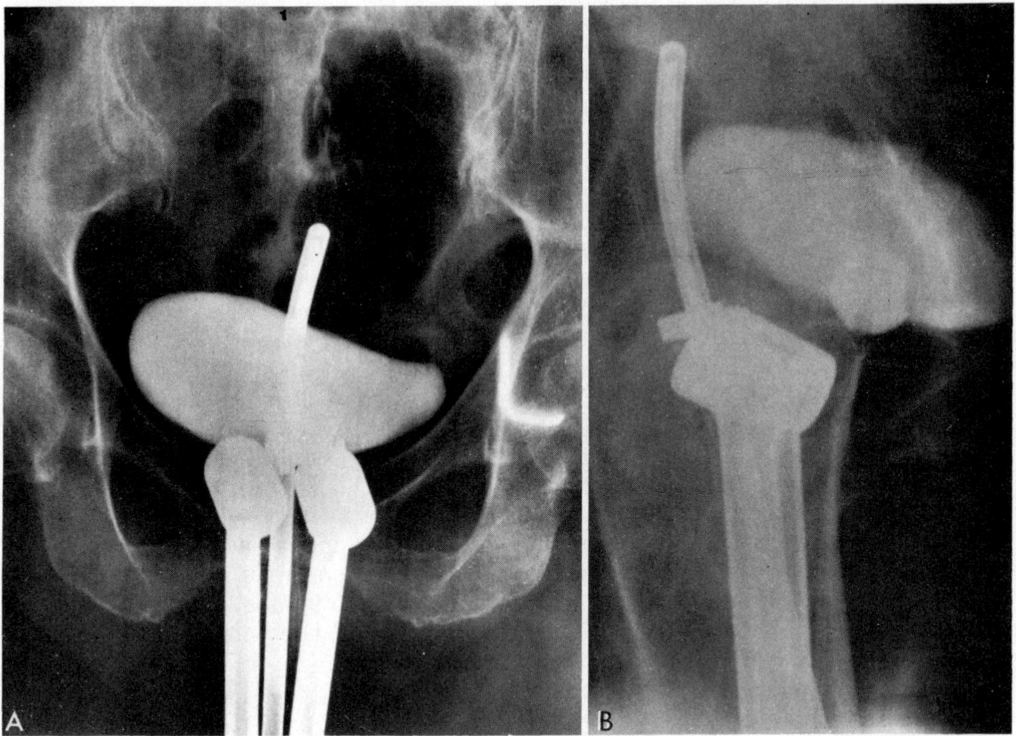

Figure 28–1. Cystogram with radium applicator used in the treatment of cervical carcinoma. Note proximity of bladder to radium sources. *A,* Anteroposterior view. *B,* Lateral view.

(Figure 28–2). The distance between the curves represents the therapeutic gain. The tumoricidal dose for epithelial tumors of the genital tract and the sensitivity of the bladder and ureters make it impossible to separate the two curves for a significant therapeutic gain. The therapist can choose two doses, A or B, as shown in Figure 28–2. With the lower dose (A), major complications are kept to a minimum, but the tumor control is not as good as with the slightly higher dose (B). Greater tumor control at

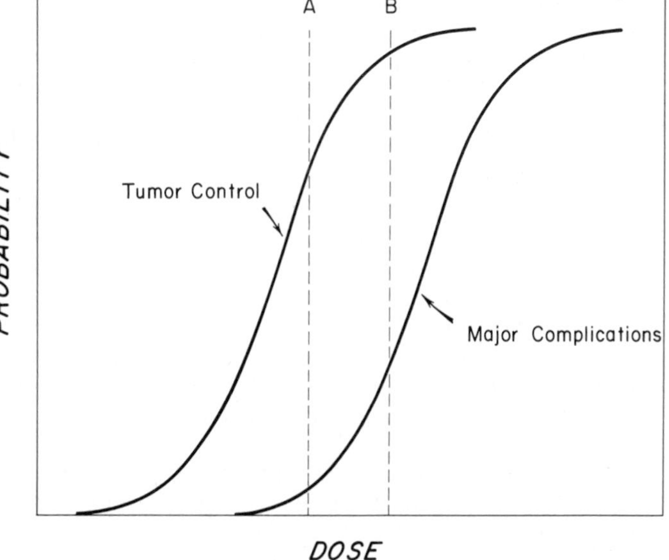

Figure 28–2. Theoretical curves describing probability of achieving tumor control and the development of major complications as a function of the radiation dose. *A* and *B* represent two different programs. (Reprinted by permission from Bloomer, W. D., and Hellman, S.: Normal tissue responses to radiation therapy. N. Engl. J. Med. *293*:80, 1975.)

level B is achieved at the cost of a higher complication rate.

In spite of the individualization of radiation therapy resulting from computerized dosimetry, the application of dosimetry probes, and fractionation of treatment, radiation injuries still occur. Such injuries may be an unavoidable complication of therapy in a small number of patients, and not the result of poor technique or technical error. The physician is therefore likely to continue seeing patients with urinary tract problems following radiation therapy of gynecologic malignancies.

The likelihood of urinary injury is related to the amount of radiation delivered and the time over which it is administered (time/dose relationship). Higher doses, larger fields, and treatment with higher energy beams increase the chances of injury. The most common urinary problems following radiation therapy of gynecologic malignancies are radiation cystitis, vesicovaginal fistula, and ureteral fibrosis. Surgery following radiation therapy, as well as re-irradiation, significantly increases the complication rate.

BLADDER INJURY (RADIATION CYSTITIS)

Bladder injury following radiation can be mild and transitory, moderate, or severe. Factors that alter the susceptibility of the bladder to radiation injury are oxygenation of the tissue, invasion by tumor, infection, systemic diseases, and prior or concomitant administration of cytotoxic drugs. Mild reactions may be evident after 3000 rads and present minimal objective findings and mild symptoms that abate. It is rare to find significant changes in the bladder even after 5000 rads delivered over 5 weeks; the bladder can easily tolerate 6500 to 7000 rads of teletherapy at the usual rate. Morphologic changes begin to appear at about 8000 rads as mucosal ulceration, and the patient may complain of pain and hematuria. Severe reactions are irreversible and present as contracted bladder or vesicovaginal fistula.

Serious bladder injury has been reported in 3 to 5 per cent of patients receiving radiation therapy for treatment of cervical carcinoma (Calame and Wallach, 1967; Stockbine et al., 1970; Buchler et al., 1971; Boronow and Rutledge, 1971; Villa Santa, 1972; van Nagell et al., 1974; Bosch and Frias, 1977). Most authorities agree that intracavitary and vaginal radium is the major contributor to bladder injuries. A greater degree of uniformity can be achieved with the external beam than with radium therapy. The individual anatomic configuration can cause variations in the geometry of the radium application. The loading adds another variable to the system. Attempts to reduce injury by measuring bladder dose with probes have generally been unsuccessful. There appears to be no correlation between measured dose and subsequent bladder injury (Peckham et al., 1969). Lee and co-workers (1976) found that in radium treatment the dose rate, rather than treatment time, is the critical parameter in modifying the risk of normal tissue injury.

Histopathology

The urinary bladder responds to irradiation in much the same fashion as do other mucosa-lined structures. Dean (1933) described three types of bladder reaction to irradiation: acute, subacute, and chronic, dependent on the onset of symptoms. The early histologic changes are those reflecting cellular damage, largely due to direct cellular injury; those occurring later are the result of the repair process, primarily as it affects connective tissue and blood vessels.

Early Changes

Little descriptive material is available concerning the histology of the earliest changes, most descriptions being drawn from observations on irradiated skin. The earliest response of the canine bladder (Hueper et al., 1942) is congestion and dilatation of the submucosal capillaries with edema of the submucosa. This is followed by the development of degenerative changes in the epithelium, characterized by cytoplasmic vacuolization and nuclear pyknosis. A perivascular lymphocytic infiltration surrounds dilated capillaries, and mucosal hemorrhages are seen. As degenerative changes progress in the epithelium, microcyst formation occurs, with accompanying infiltration of polymorphonuclear leukocytes and lymphocytes, and subsequent appearance of syncytial epithelial clusters. Desquamation of the epithelium may occur, resulting in superficial ulceration with a covering of fibrin and leukocytes. Endothelial proliferation may be noted at this time, although it is generally not obliterative. Focal vacuolar and hyaline changes in the muscularis are also seen (Hueper et al., 1942; Gowing, 1960).

Ulcers that occur early are often due to the destruction of neoplasm that has replaced portions of the bladder wall. These ulcers tend to be deeper than those resulting from radiation therapy, since tumor invasion may involve the full thickness of bladder wall.

Late Changes

Following cessation of radiation, many of these changes regress. Hueper and coworkers (1942) noted the persistence of the cellular reaction in the submucosa. Capillary proliferation may follow, with the formation of ectatic vessels, while other capillaries show narrowing of their lumina due to endothelial proliferation and subendothelial fibrosis. As fibrosis occurs in the submucosa, hyalinization of the connective tissue is seen. This fibrotic reaction also involves the muscularis, displacing damaged muscle fibers (Figure 28–3). Large, often bizarre fibroblasts ("radiation fibroblasts") may be found in the fibrous reaction and may prove to be a source of error in the search for recurrent tumor (Figure 28–4). The epithelium may return to normal, or it may exhibit varying degrees of atrophy (see Figure 28–3) or ulceration, depending largely on the response of the fine vasculature and connective tissue. The extent and rapidity of healing are also dependent on the presence or absence of associated infection, the urinary bladder being more prone to infection under these circumstances (Watson et al., 1947).

The remote responses of the bladder,

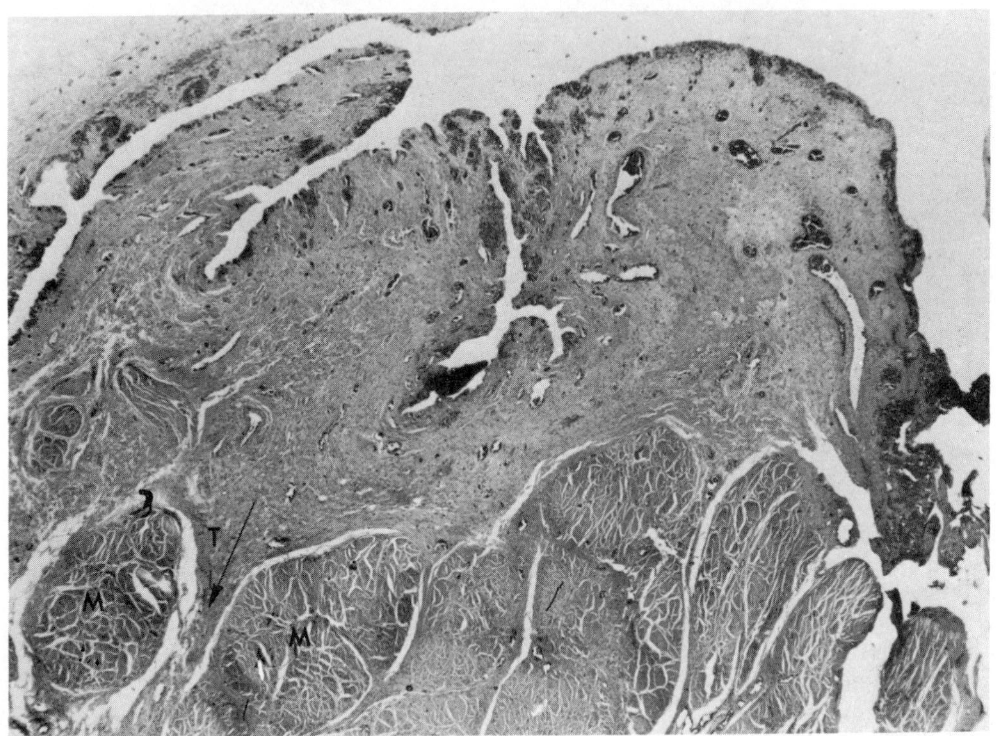

Figure 28–3. Microscopic appearance of radiation cystitis. The submucosa is widened and fibrotic, with extension of fibrosis (arrow) into the muscularis, separating bundles of smooth muscle (M). Ectatic capillaries are also evident beneath an atropic epithelium. (Hematoxylin-eosin stain, ×12.5.)

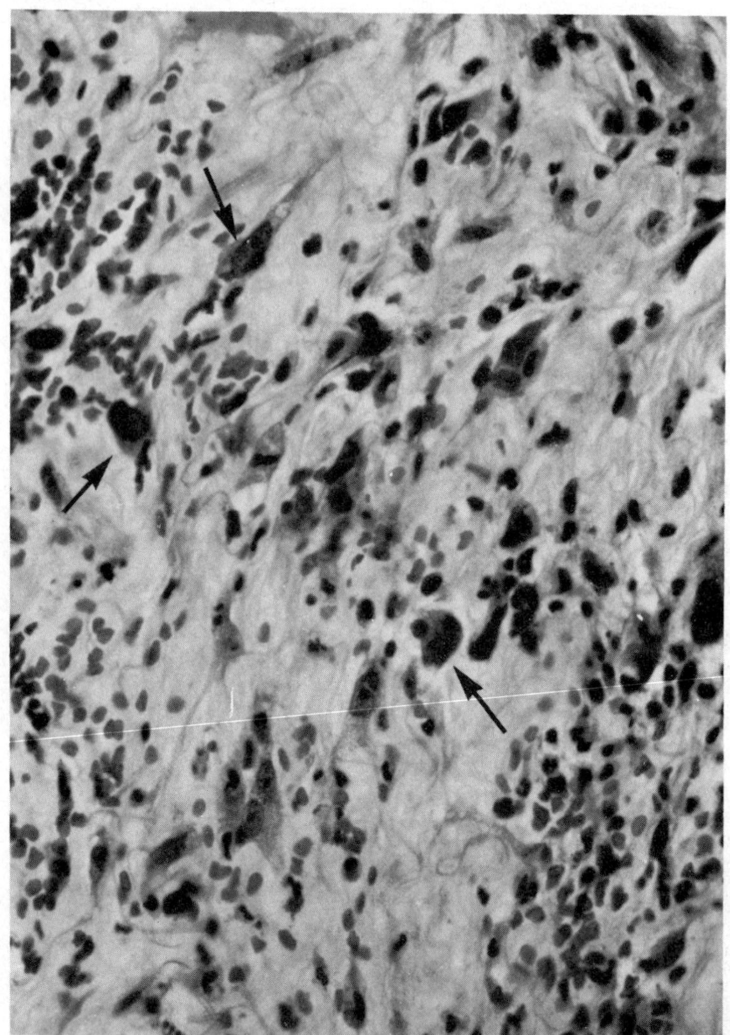

Figure 28–4. Microscopic picture of bladder submucosa following radiation therapy. Large, bizarre fibroblasts ("radiation fibroblasts") are seen in submucosa (arrows). Inflammatory cells, lymphocytes, and plasma cells are also present. (Hematoxylin-eosin stain, ×300.)

i.e., those occurring after apparent healing or resolution has taken place, are largely the result of slow but progressive changes in the vessels and connective tissue (Watson et al., 1947; Rubin and Casarett, 1968). An obliterative arteritis can be observed in medium-sized and small vessels, which may be so severe as to completely occlude the lumen (Figure 28–5 *A, B*). There is increasing fibrosis in the submucosal tissue, which may limit distensibility of the bladder.

The vascular changes are presumed to interfere with the blood supply to the epithelium and adjacent tissues, resulting in atrophy or necrosis of the epithelium, with ulceration and formation of fissures or fistulas. Because of the slow progression of the vascular changes, this process may take years to develop. Following the establishment of an ulcer or fistula, an accompanying inflammatory reaction and granulation tissue proliferation can occur. Often the tissue is sufficiently ischemic so that little reaction occurs, leaving the margins of the ulcer or fistula with a wall of dense connective tissue (Figure 28–6) (Gowing, 1960). The surface of the ulcer may be covered with necrotic debris in which calcification takes place (Figure 28–7).

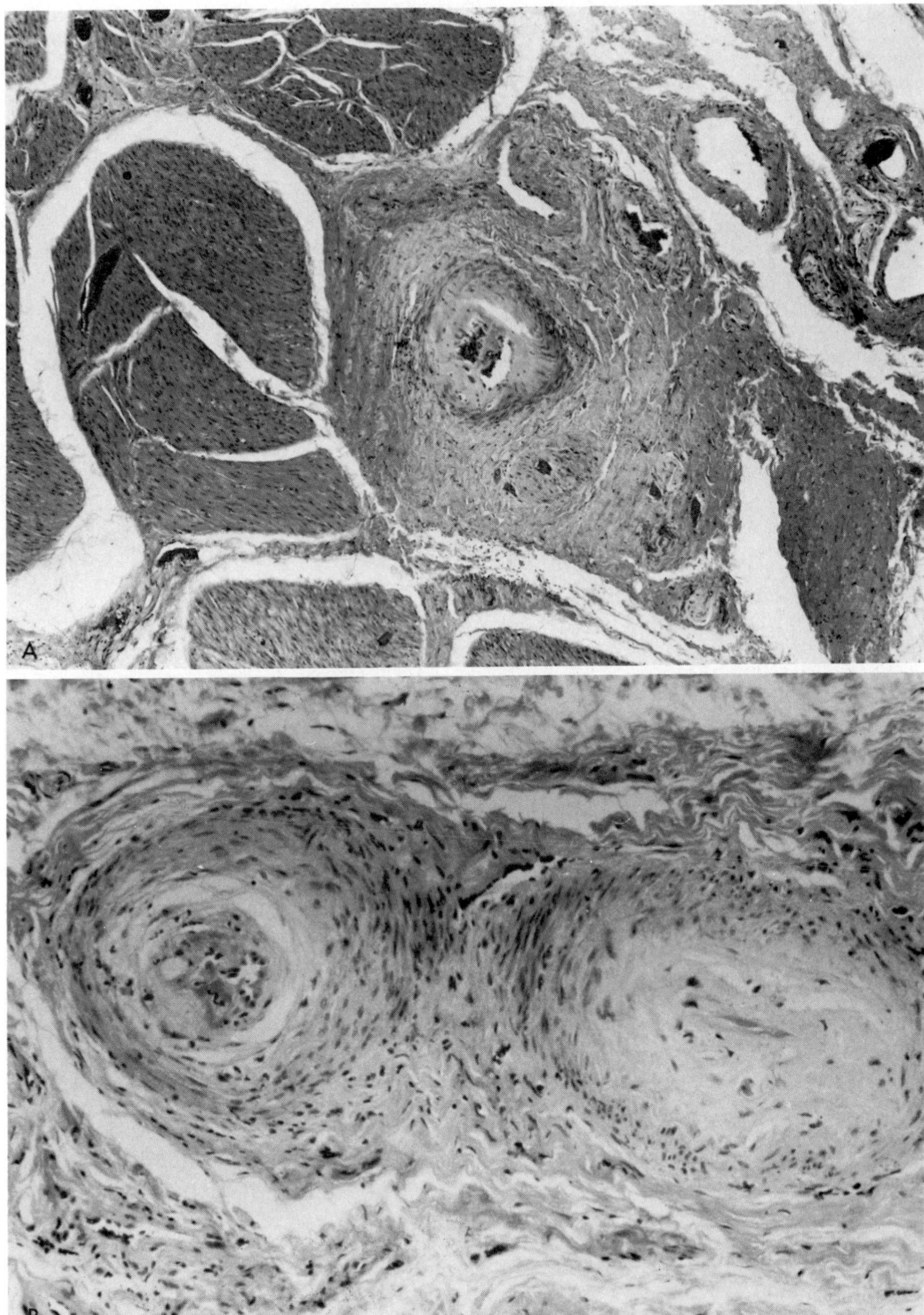

Figure 28–5. Vascular changes following radiation therapy.

A, Bladder. Artery in the muscularis of the bladder shows intimal thickening and perivascular fibrosis. The vessels in the upper right show little or no alteration. This variation in degree of obstruction is typical for radiation reaction. (Hematoxylin-eosin stain, ×50.)

B, Ureter. The lumen of this artery from the adventitia of the distal ureter is nearly obliterated by intimal proliferation. (Hematoxylin-eosin stain, ×125.)

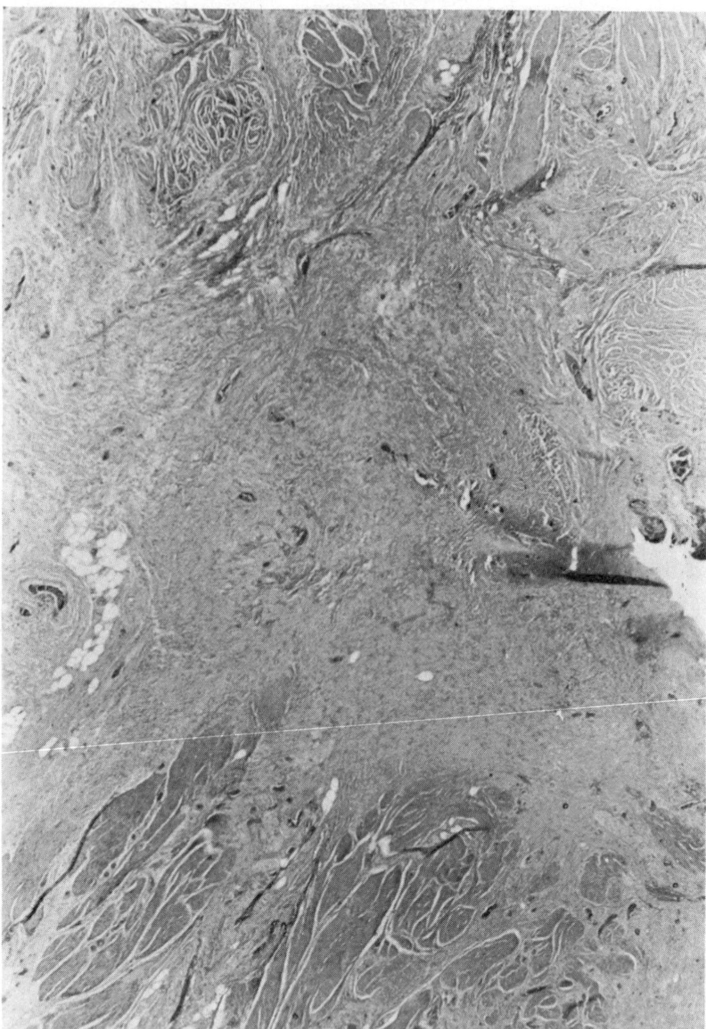

Figure 28–6. The fibrosis in the base of this ulcer extends through the entire muscular wall of the bladder. The surface is largely devoid of inflammatory reaction or vascular proliferation, a finding common in late post-irradiation ulcers. (Hematoxylin-eosin stain, ×12.5.)

Until recently, there has been no serious attempt to grade the severity of injury following radiation therapy. Kagan and associates (1979) proposed a staging system for gastrointestinal and urinary tract injuries following radiation therapy for cervical carcinoma. The criteria that apply to the urinary tract are the following:

R_1: Complete recovery following symptoms such as urinary burning and bleeding and hydroureter.

R_2: Incomplete recovery from urinary bleeding, edematous bladder mucosa, persistent hydroureter. Continuous medication required.

S_1: Requires surgical intervention for a single organ injury: total cystectomy, urinary diversion, or ureteral implantation.

S_2: Requires extensive surgery for injury to two organs.

Such a grading system would help in objectively evaluating radiation injury, but the proposed system could be improved by having parallel grades for subjective complaints and for objective findings.

Clinical Findings

The acute phase of radiation cystitis can begin 3 to 6 weeks after the start of radiation therapy, with symptoms of cystitis that may be indistinguishable from the more common acute hemorrhagic cystitis of bacterial origin. The acute changes may subside after completion of radiation therapy. The subacute changes start 6 months to 2

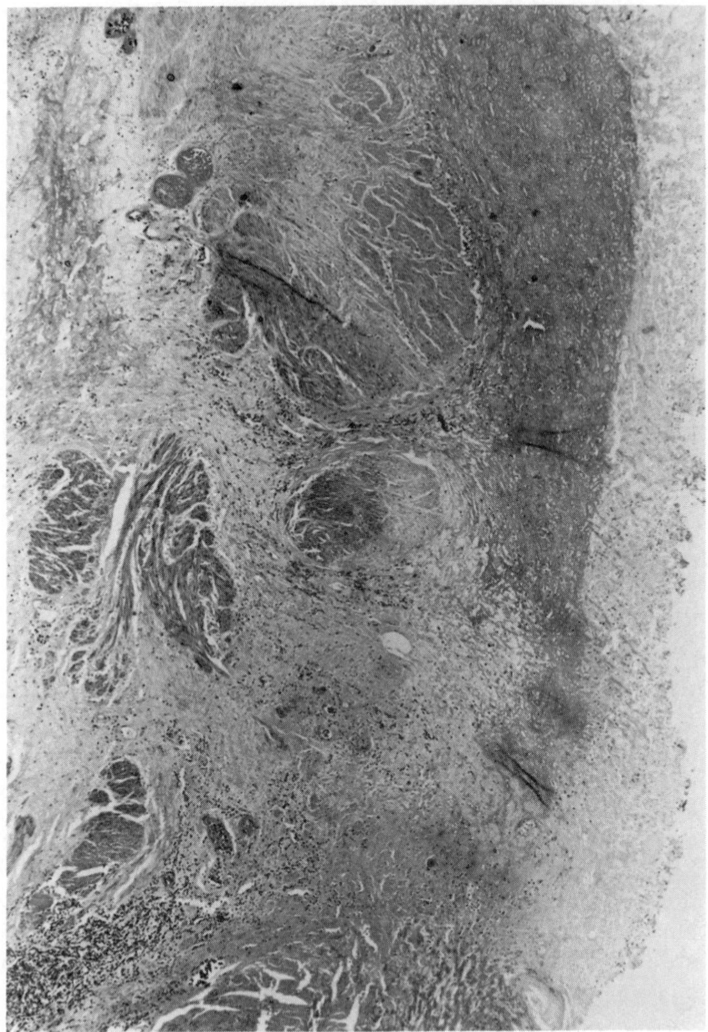

Figure 28-7. Necrotic debris covers base of a radiation ulcer, with underlying fibrosis of the muscularis. Vascular proliferation (granulation tissue) is minimal, and the inflammatory reaction is scanty. (Hematoxylin-eosin stain, ×300.)

years after therapy and result in more significant objective and subjective findings. Chronic changes generally result in a very-low-capacity bladder with mucosal ulceration or fistula.

Acute Cystitis

The symptoms of acute radiation cystitis are those of bladder irritation, including frequency, urgency, suprapubic pain, burning or pressure sensation on urination, and urge incontinence. Gross hematuria may occur with or without pain and may be noted initially, throughout the act of voiding, or at its termination. Women who are particularly aware of their voiding habits may even note the passage of small particles of tissue, which represent necrotic bladder debris. Flecks of calcium, "sand," or stones may also be voided.

A woman may be aware not only of persistent bladder irritation with increased diurnal and nocturnal frequency but also of a definite decrease in bladder capacity. In Kottmeier's series (1964) of 3484 patients treated for cervical carcinoma, 8 per cent had some bladder complaints. Minimal bladder symptoms were present in 229 of 279, the symptoms and findings disappearing several weeks after completion of therapy. Nineteen patients had extensive bladder necrosis with hemorrhage; there were 31 vesicovaginal fistulas.

Pool (1959) reported his findings in 50 women seen over a 5-year period for radiation cystitis. Of the 31 patients considered to have mild reaction requiring no therapy, two (6 per cent) developed fistulas (one vesicovaginal and one rectovaginal). Of the remaining 19 patients having signs and symptoms severe enough to warrant treatment, three (16 per cent) developed significant complications (two vesicovaginal fistulas and one ureteral obstruction).

Kagan and associates (1979), using their proposed staging system (see earlier discussion), found bladder injuries in 83 of 406 (20 per cent) of patients treated for cervical carcinoma; 16 per cent were reversible (R_1 and R_2) and 4 per cent were severe (S_1 and S_2).

Laboratory Evaluation

Urinalysis

The urine in patients with radiation cystitis may be grossly bloody or merely positive for occult blood when tested with commercially available dipsticks. Proteinuria may accompany heavy hematuria and pyuria. In spite of significant bladder symptoms, the urinalysis may be completely normal. Microscopic examination of the sediment will variably identify leukocytes, erythrocytes, crystals, peculiar epithelial cells, necrotic debris, and bacteria. Each of these elements may occur singly or in combination, depending on the presence or absence of bacterial infection.

Urine Culture

A properly collected urine specimen should be obtained for culture and sensitivity testing. A clean-catch midstream specimen suffices in most patients; if this is negative, there is no need to proceed to a catheterized specimen.

Secondary infection is common with radiation cystitis or fistula, therefore the need for culture to identify the offending pathogen. As with common urinary tract infections, the organisms in radiation cystitis are usually enteric and include *E. coli*, *Pseudomonas aeruginosa*, *Klebsiella-Aerobacter* group, and *Proteus* species. Less commonly identified organisms include *Streptococcus faecalis* and anaerobes. Mixed infection (multiple organisms identified on culture) is common when a radiation-induced urointestinal fistula is present (see later discussion).

Cytologic Examination

Freshly voided urine or a specimen obtained by bladder catheterization should be submitted for cytologic diagnosis, since persistent or recurrent malignancy may be in question. A specimen taken by urethral catheterization or at the time of cystoscopy should be obtained by bladder washings. The urinary bladder is lavaged four or five times with approximately 50 ml. of sterile saline, via the instrument or catheter; the washings produced in this manner are sent for cytologic evaluation. The washings may be submitted to the laboratory fresh or placed in an equal volume of alcohol fixative for examination at a later time. The loose cells and cell clumps exfoliated by this maneuver may lead to a diagnosis of cancer involving the urinary bladder. One pitfall in the cytologic diagnosis of malignancy is the effect of prior radiation therapy on epithelial cells. These altered cells make the diagnosis difficult. Prior or concomitant administration of chemotherapy also produces epithelial changes that may be difficult to distinguish from malignancy and radiation effect.

Complete Blood Count

Hematologic evaluation may be normal unless the patient has complications from persistent malignancy or ureteral obstruction with renal insufficiency. In the latter instance a normocytic, normochhromic anemia may be identified. The presence of severe bacterial infection may result in leukocytosis with a shift to the left. However, the white cell count and platelet count may be on the low side of normal and drop to subnormal range if the patient has had prior radiation therapy, chemotherapy, or a combination of these.

Renal Function Tests

Blood urea nitrogen (BUN) and serum creatinine determinations should be obtained as a baseline measure of renal function. Kidney function can be expected to be normal unless significant bilateral ureteral obstruction with hydronephrosis is present. Any increase in the BUN or serum creatinine levels should be considered a sign of significant renal impairment and should be further evaluated with creatinine clearance and urographic studies to determine anatomic and functional details. Prior studies of renal function and urographic anatomy, if available, are helpful in assessing the degree of change.

Intravenous Pyelogram (IVP)

The intravenous pyelogram will help to identify ureteral injury (stenosis or fistula) rather than details of the bladder mucosa. In the acute phase of radiation cystitis, there may be reduced bladder capacity in the presence of normal emptying ability. The bladder outline may be irregular and contain lucent filling defects, representing either malignancy, inflammatory reaction, bladder calculi, or blood clots.

Cystoscopy

Cystourethroscopy can generally be carried out under topical anesthesia; general or regional anesthesia is used when the patient is extremely uncomfortable or when bladder biopsies are to be taken. The residual urine is usually normal (less than 5 ml.) unless inflammation or urethral obstruction from extensive carcinomatous invasion is present. Total bladder capacity is often reduced and may be under 100 ml. Distention of the bladder can be quite painful to the patient. This poor distensibility and patient discomfort may require general or regional anesthesia.

Changes in the bladder mucosa will be patchy, with normal areas interspersed with areas that are pink to red, containing frank ulceration (Figure 28–8). Severely involved areas will be necrotic and may show calcific debris or encrustations. Cobblestone or polypoid lesions and inflammation are frequent and are variably distributed around the bladder wall. A common site of alterations seen in women treated with intracavitary radium is the posterior midline, superior to the interureteric ridge (see Figure 28–1). A focal collection of such lesions may suggest underlying malignant invasion or fistula, especially a vesicointestinal fistula.

The submucosal vascular pattern may vary from a paucity of vessels to telangiectasia and submucosal hemorrhages. The ulceration and ectatic vessels are often responsible for severe hemorrhage. Fistulous openings may be visible and can be catheterized for injection with contrast material

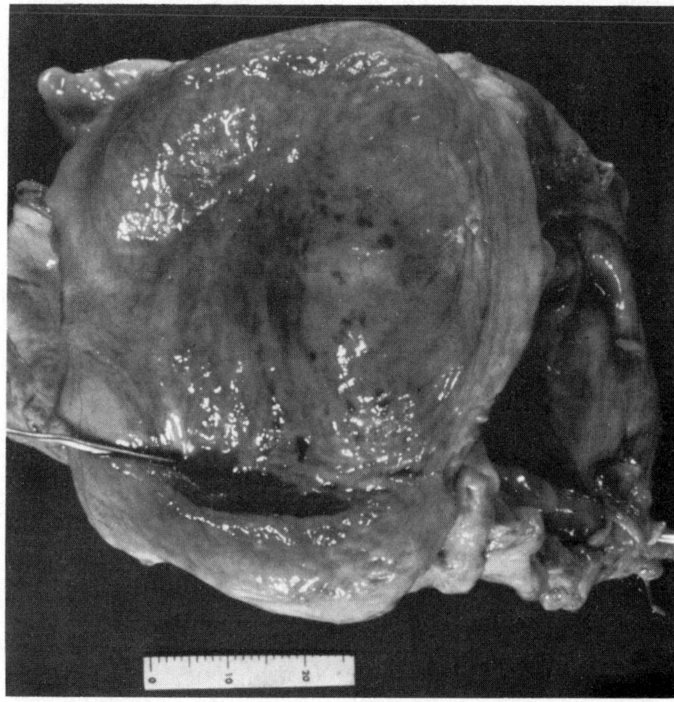

Figure 28–8. Patchy changes of radiation cystitis in an autopsy specimen.

to help identify extent and location. Radiation-induced ulceration may lead to overt fistula formation at a later date. Retrograde pyeloureterography may be indicated to identify the site of ureteral obstruction when the external urogram has demonstrated hydroureteronephrosis with or without a ureteral fistula.

Bladder Biopsy

Transurethral biopsies of the bladder are indicated to rule out the presence of infiltrating pelvic malignancy. There are "cold" and "hot" techniques of bladder biopsy. In the "cold" technique, a rigid or flexible stemmed instrument (especially designed for this purpose) is passed through the cystoscope, and a biopsy is taken, under vision, of the suspicious areas. Some of the biopsy instruments are cup-shaped, whereas others have a more rectangular or alligator jaw. The instrument usually removes mucosa and submucosa, and at most only superficial muscle. The bleeding that follows may require direct coagulation for control but usually stops spontaneously. The "hot" technique utilizes the resectoscope loop used for resection of bladder tumors and prostatic tissue. The high-frequency current usually produces a deeper biopsy of the bladder and may severely distort the specimen because of cautery artifact. In addition, the thermal destructive changes on the adjacent bladder wall may be such that with the existing poor vascularity, delayed healing, persistent bleeding, and infection, perforation or fistula formation may follow (Pool, 1959). In our opinion, biopsies should be taken only with the "cold" instruments, which do less to distort the specimen and cause fewer changes in the adjacent bladder mucosa.

Management

Antimicrobials

Any secondary infection documented by urine culture should be treated with appropriate antimicrobials. Uncomplicated infections can usually be treated by an oral agent such as nitrofurantoin, 50 to 100 mg. four times daily; sulfamethoxazole, 1.0 gm. twice daily; or ampicillin, 500 mg. four times daily. Infecting organisms requiring more toxic or parenteral antibiotics should suggest the possibility of urinary fistula and obstruction.

Antispasmodics

Symptomatic relief of severe irritative bladder symptoms can be achieved with antsipasmodic agents. The majority of these are anticholinergic in their activity and include methantheline bromide (25 to 50 mg., four times daily) and propantheline bromide (15 mg., four times daily). A newer agent, oxybutynin, in doses of 5 mg. three or four times daily, has direct spasmolytic as well as anticholinergic activity. Other bladder sedatives include tincture of belladonna, with or without scopolamine, or small doses of barbiturate. Occasionally, drugs with adrenergic activity, such as ephedrine sulfate, 25 to 50 mg. four times a day, can be added.

Analgesics

The urethral and suprapubic discomfort associated with radiation cystitis can often be severe and debilitating. Phenazopyridine hydrochloride, 1 or 2 tablets four times a day, may give pain relief, but systemic analgesics may be required. Should the discomfort be severe enough to require narcotic drugs, a search for complicating factors is indicated.

Topical Therapy

The removal of necrotic and calcific debris, which act as foreign bodies irritating the bladder, may be helpful in relieving symptoms. Encrusted cystitis can be treated by transurethral resection or scraping of the involved area and light fulguration of the exposed muscle or submucosa. Transurethral fulguration may also be used for related bladder bleeding. Various solutions are available for daily and long-term use in such patients. Instillations of 10 per cent hemiacridin (citric and D-gluconic acids) or urologic solution G are appropriate for patients with considerable calcific debris. Thirty to 100 ml. can be introduced into the urinary bladder one to three times daily and allowed to remain in place for 30 minutes.

These preparations function as chelating agents.

Bacterial infection can also be treated by the intermittent instillation of topical antibiotic solutions containing neomycin, polymyxin, or bacitracin. Silver nitrate solutions of 1:1000 to 1:500 or 5 per cent Argyrol (silver protein) can also be used on a daily basis for chemical cauterization of inflamed bladder mucosa. Another option is the instillation of sodium oxychlorosene (0.1 per cent solution), which acts both as an oxidizing agent on the inflamed mucosa and as an anti-infective.

Hydraulic Dilatation

For patients with contracted bladder secondary to radiation cystitis, with no evidence of persistent or recurrent malignancy, hydraulic dilatation may be tried. Under general or regional anesthesia, the urinary bladder is progressively dilated with the irrigating solution used for cystoscopy. This mechanical expansion of the bladder wall is least effective in severely contracted bladders due to radiation injury. The major disavdvantages are the need for repeated general or regional anesthesia, urosepsis from frequent instrumentation, and the possibility of bladder rupture through a diseased portion of the wall.

Intramural Corticosteroids

Direct injection of anti-inflammatory agents into the diseased bladder wall may occasionally be helpful. Under local, general, or regional anesthesia, a specially designed flexible injection needle is threaded through a cystoscope and a submucosal puncture of the bladder mucosa made under direct vision. Triamcinolone acetonide, in concentrations ranging from 10 to 40 mg. per ml., is the most commonly used preparation. Several areas of the bladder can be injected at one sitting. The total dose can range from 100 to 200 mg. Postinjection bleeding is usually negligible, and systemic corticosteroid effects are rare.

Other Medical Therapies

Oral corticosteroids or antiflammatory agents have not been helpful in the treatment of radiation cystitis. Currently under investigation in the United States, and recently made available for clinical use in Europe, is a new metalloprotein compound (orgotein) manufactured from bovine liver, with a molecular weight of approximately 34,000 (Marberger et al., 1974). This preparation is nontoxic when administered parenterally, intramurally, or topically. Its main mode of action appears to be the high activity of the enzyme superoxide dismutase. This acts as a scavenger for the destructive free radicals produced in tissue injured by irradiation or inflammation (Fridovich, 1975). This agent has been effective in chronic radiation damage but may be more effective in preventing or ameliorating the side effects of acute radiation cystitis. Orgotein is injected directly into the bladder wall through the cystoscope, using the special needle described earlier.

In an Austrian study, 22 women with radiation cystitis following treatment for cervical carcinoma were treated with intramural injections of orgotein (Marberger et al., 1975). The patients were seen 1 to 16 years (average, 4.7 years) after radiation therapy. Evaluation included cystoscopic examination and measurement of voided urine volume. All patients responded to therapy, but many only after 2 or 3 injections of the drug at 2- to 3-month intervals. Seventy-five per cent of the patients were reported free of symptoms and signs up to 2 years following treatment; 25 per cent were considered improved an average of 1 year following the injections.

In Sweden, intramuscular orgotein was administered in a randomized double-blind, placebo-controlled study to 42 patients receiving definitive radiation therapy (6400 to 8400 rads) for bladder carcinoma (Edsmyr et al., 1976). Orgotein or placebo was given after each radiation treatment. There was significant amelioration of undesirable side effects caused by the radiation therapy in the group of patients receiving orgotein. Parameters of response included functional bladder capacity, urinary frequency, urinary incontinence, bladder pain, and dysuria. Additional double-blind and placebo-controlled studies by these investigators (Menander-Huber et al., 1980) suggest that patients who received orgotein had fewer side effects and were able to tolerate higher doses of radiation therapy than those receiving placebo.

MANAGEMENT OF HEMATURIA

Formalin Instillation

Several favorable reports have appeared on the use of intravesical formalin for the control of hematuria in radiation cystitis (Brown, 1969; Servadio and Nissenkorn, 1976; Behnam et al., in press).

The instillation requires a general or regional anesthetic; formalin, applied to the bladder mucosa, causes severe pain. A catheter is passed per urethra, and all clots are evacuated. Depending on bladder capacity, 60 to 150 ml. of a 4 to 10 per cent formalin solution is instilled via gravity and allowed to remain in place 15 to 30 minutes. The formalin is then removed and the bladder irrigated with sterile saline. The catheter may be removed or left indwelling for another 24 hours. The instillation may be repeated in a few days, or months later, depending on the patient's response.

The formalin probably functions by direct coagulation of blood vessels. Potential hazards include further bladder fibrosis and vesicoureteric reflux. For the woman who already has a supravesical urinary diversion, these complications are insignificant. Servadio and Nissenkorn (1976) reported excellent results in seven of eight patients and Behnam and associates (in press) in five of five patients with hematuria secondary to radiation therapy.

Hypogastric Artery Embolization

Embolization of selected arteries for control of bleeding has found increasing application in the last few years (Kadish et al., 1973). Although it is easier to perform than hypogastric artery ligation, it requires special facilities and personnel familiar with the technique. Preliminary contrast injections will demonstrate the abnormal vascular pattern and usually identify the bleeding vessel. Autologous clot and Gelfoam particles are injected as emboli to stop the blood flow bilaterally. Further contrast injections are made to monitor the effect of the embolization.

Hypogastric Artery Ligation

Hypogastric (internal iliac) artery ligation should be considered for the control of *severe* hemorrhage resulting from radiation cystitis after other methods have failed. The procedure can be performed through either an extraperitoneal or a transperitoneal approach; the choice depends on the patient's condition and the effects of any prior surgery and radiation therapy.

AUGMENTATION CYSTOPLASTY

Augmentation cystoplasty — the use of a bowel segment, either ileum or colon, to increase the bladder capacity — can be applied in selected patients with contracted bladder secondary to radiation therapy. A functioning vesical neck mechanism and absence of cancer and vesicovaginal fistula must be documented before such a procedure should be considered. The technique is similar to that for the formation of a conduit: A segment of bowel is utilized; blood supply is maintained by its mesentery.

URINARY DIVERSION

When these measures are ineffective in controlling bladder symptoms or alterations secondary to radiation therapy, urinary diversion should be considered. The most appropriate methods for supravesical diversion are discussed in Chapter 11. In patients with good prognosis who can withstand major surgery, conduit diversion is the procedure of choice. Schmidt and coworkers (1976) have demonstrated the value of the transverse colon conduit in patients with prior radiation therapy (Chapter 11).

VESICOVAGINAL FISTULA

Vesicovaginal fistula represents the highest degree of radiation injury to the bladder and occurs in 0.5 to 2.0 per cent of patients treated for cervical carcinoma (Kottmeier, 1964; Cushing et al., 1968; Boronow and Rutledge, 1971; VillaSanta, 1972). It rarely develops following external beam therapy alone; the radium with its variable dose to the bladder makes the major contribution. Factors that predispose to radiation cystitis probably also play a role in fistula formation: infection and compromise of the blood supply. With tumor invasion, control of the local disease automatically results in a vesicovaginal fistula. The incidence of vesicovaginal fistulas increases fourfold when surgery follows radiation therapy of gynecologic malignancy (Boronow and Rutledge, 1971); re-irradiation markedly increases the likelihood of fistula formation.

Symptoms

The development of a vesicovaginal fistula is generally preceded by a variable period of severe bladder symptoms, including frequency, urgency, dysuria, and hematuria. Bladder capacity is usually reduced, but there is no interference with the voiding mechanism. Kline and co-workers (1972) could find no correlation between the development of major late urinary tract complications and the onset of symptoms, during or immediately following treatment. Most vesicovaginal fistulas develop within 2 years of completion of radiation therapy, though Kottmeier (1964) reported a radiation-induced vesicovaginal fistula developing 28 years after completion of therapy. The average interval from radiation therapy to the development of fistula has been reported as 18 months (range, 4 to 55) and 17 months (range, 7 to 27) (VillaSanta, 1972; Cushing et al., 1968).

Fistulas in patients with prior bladder wall invasion by neoplasm develop earlier than do those resulting from radiation injury. The leakage of urine may be preceded by pelvic pain and temperature elevation. Persistent or recurrent carcinoma must be excluded by examination and biopsy.

Repair

Radiation-induced fistulas never close spontaneously, and their repair is a vexing problem. Only rarely can they be closed by conventional surgical techniques (Chapters 21 and 22). The tissue surrounding the fistula is fibrotic and inelastic, with diminished vascularity as a result of radiation-induced endarteritis obliterans (see Figure 28–5). Inability to mobilize the tissue in an avascular surgical field leads to almost uniform failure with conventional layered closures. Even colpocleisis with its concomitant loss of coital function is generally unsuccessful (Graham, 1965). The lack of success in repair of radiation fistulas results primarily from the diminished blood supply. The successful repair requires increased vascularity at the fistula site by the mobilization of vascular pedicles from adjacent structures. Gluteus maximus, adductor longus, gracilis, sartorius, rectus abdominis, and pubococcygeus muscles, as well as the bulbocavernosus muscle in combination with the labial fat pad (Martius technique, McCall and Bolton, 1956) and the omentum, have all been used.

It is obvious from the variety of procedures that have been used in the repair of these fistulas that no single technique is applicable in all cases. The procedure must be chosen on an individual basis.

Preoperative Considerations

Before repair is attempted, the status of the upper urinary tract must be determined and recurrent malignancy ruled out. This may require biopsy of the fistulous tract from the vagina and the bladder — even at the cost of enlarging the fistula. Repair should be delayed long enough to allow demarcation of necrotic tissue and slough; repair in the presence of edematous friable tissue is likely to fail. In the time required to allow local tissue recovery, the patient should be brought to an optimal nutritional state with the use of oral dietary supplements or hyperalimentation; blood volume and red cell deficits must be corrected and urinary tract infection cleared.

Martius Technique

We have had experience with a number of techniques utilizing a variety of pedicles, including omentum, gracilis muscle, and a combination bulbocavernosus muscle and labial fat pad (Martius technique). We prefer the latter as the procedure of choice. It allows mobilization of vascularized tissue outside the field of irradiation, with minimal displacement of the graft. In addition, the "donor site" is in the prepared operative field, simplifying the procedure and reducing the likelihood of contamination.

A Schuchardt incision is made at the 5 or 7 o'clock position on the perineum, dividing the pubococcygeus, the transverse perineal, and a portion of the levator muscles. The incision can be made on either side of the perineum, but we prefer to make it on the side opposite the bulbocavernosus that will be used for the graft. By doing this, the graft is less likely to be disturbed (Figure 28–9*A*).

Once adequate exposure has been obtained, the fistula is trimmed of scar tissue around its entire circumference. The amount of scar tissue to be removed can be estimated by evaluating the elasticity and blood supply of the tissue. Bleeding is controlled by fine chromic catgut ligatures. A "collar" of tissue is then formed around the fistula by incising the vaginal mucosa above the pubovesical fascia. This incision is made approximately 5 mm. from and parallel to the edges of the fistula. The vaginal mucosa is then widely dissected from the fascia, great care being taken not to buttonhole the mucosa. Such undermining of the vesicovaginal septum is necessary to provide mobilization of the bladder mucosa from the fibrotic and inelastic anterior vaginal wall. The bladder mucosa is also undermined around the fistula tract, thus providing greater surface area for closure of the fistula. After the bladder mucosa has been adequately mobilized to allow closure without tension, interrupted 3–0 chromic catgut sutures are placed horizontally in the bladder wall.

After the bladder defect is closed, attention is turned to the bulbocavernosus muscle and labial fat pad. The labium majus is carefully palpated between thumb and forefinger to identify the muscle and its fat pad. The skin of the labium majus is then incised vertically from the level of the mons pubis to the lower third of the labium. The edge of the labium is chosen for cosmetic reasons. The skin edges are retracted and the muscle and its fat pad are dissected free (see Figure 28–9*A*). Increased vasculature is noted as one dissects the muscle toward its posterior attachments. A length of bulbocavernosus muscle is chosen that will allow the end to easily cover the fistula without undue tension. The fat pad and muscle should be divided high on the mons pubis, thereby providing sufficient length to reach the fistula. Although the length of a similar skin graft should not exceed twice the width, the rich blood supply of this muscle allows greater length and a narrower base.

A tunnel is then formed under the skin between the labium majus and the fistula, through the lateral vaginal wall. The end of the muscle and fat pad is passed through the tunnel and placed over the now closed bladder defect (Figure 28–9*B*). The tunnel must be wide enough to prevent compression of the blood supply of the pedicle. The fat pad is then sutured over the closed fistula site with 3–0 chromic catgut suture (Figure 28–9*C*).

The vaginal mucosa is next closed over the pedicle with chromic catgut sutures. We prefer to close this defect in a vertical fashion, although the vault may be slightly narrowed by this maneuver (Figure 28–9*D*). On occasion there may not be enough vaginal mucosa to close the defect. This presents no problem; the muscle will become completely epithelialized.

A small Penrose drain is then placed at the base of the labial incision, and the skin closed with interrupted sutures of 4–0 nylon (Figure 28–9*E*). The Schuchardt incision can also be drained with a small Penrose drain. (The Penrose drains are removed after 48 hours or when the dressings remain dry.) The nylon sutures on the labium are removed 8 to 10 days postoperatively. The bladder is decompressed with a suprapubic catheter for approximately 3 weeks, and the patient is maintained on antimicrobial therapy. The patient is at bed rest for the first 3 postoperative days and then is allowed physical activities. Sexual intercourse is prohibited for at least 3 months.

Occasionally, a small defect will persist after a large vesicovaginal fistula has been repaired. We prefer to wait a minimum of 3 and generally 6 months before attempting another repair utilizing the other bulbocavernosus muscle and labial fat pad. All signs of inflammation must be cleared prior to reoperation.

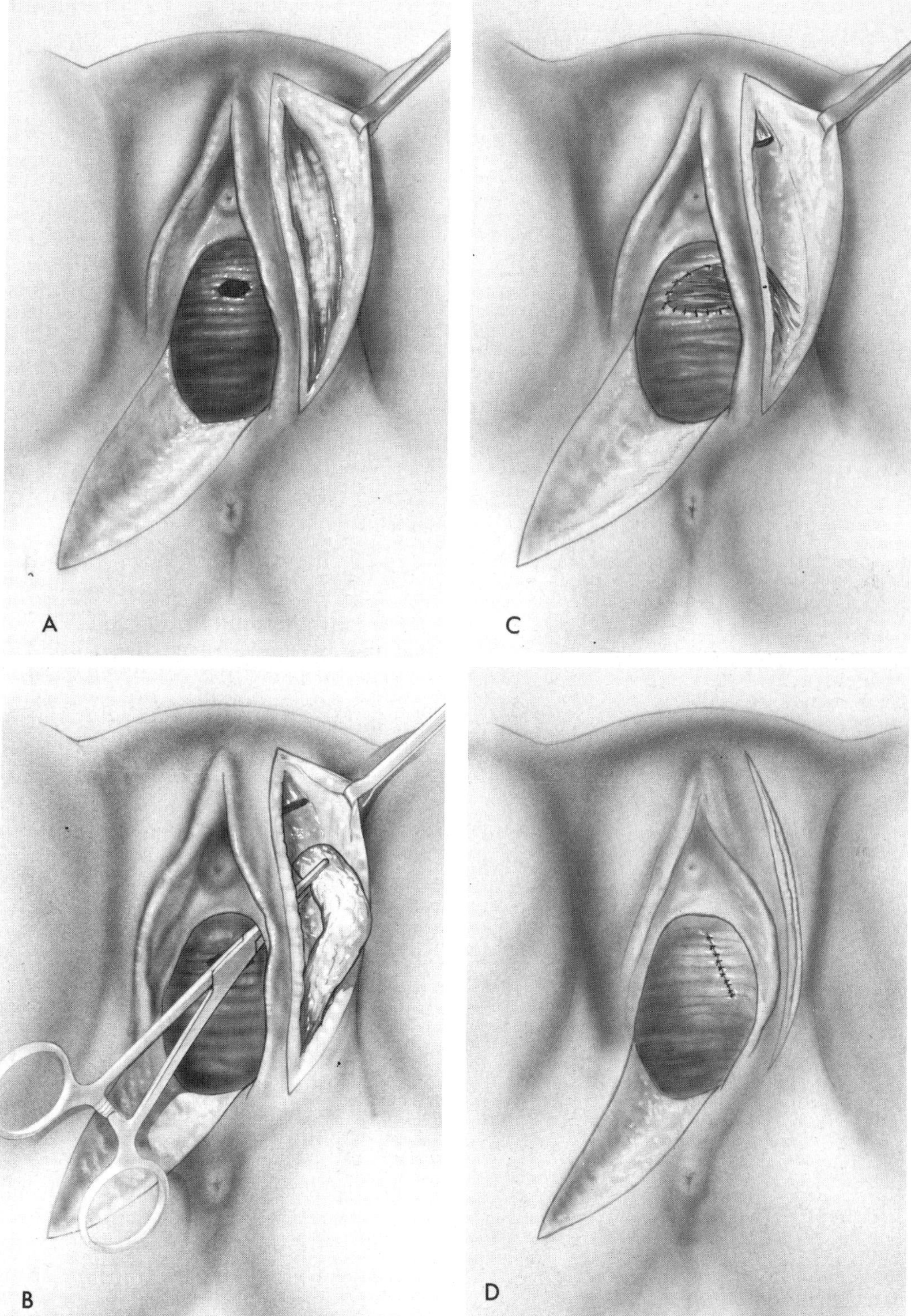

Figure 28–9. Martius technique for repair of vesicovaginal fistula, utilizing bulbocavernosus muscle and labial fat pad.

A, Schuchardt incision in perineum at the 7 o'clock position. Left labium majus has been incised, and bulbocavernosus muscle and labial fat pad have been exposed. Fistula has been excised.

Illustration continued on following page

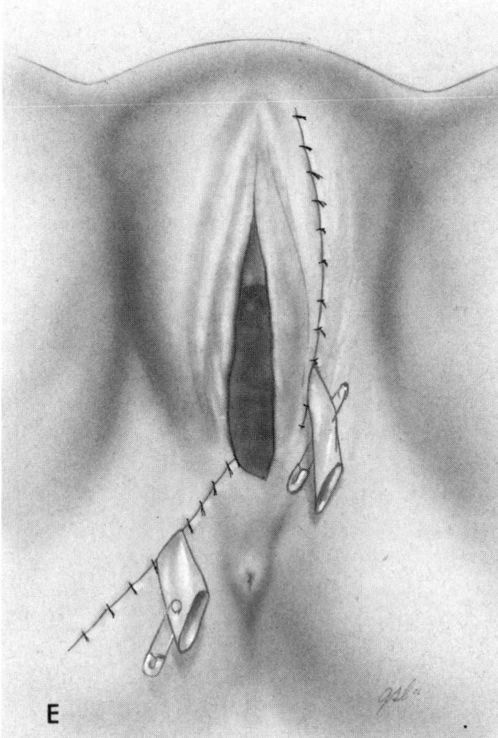

Figure 28–9 *Continued.* *B,* Muscle and labial fat pad have been mobilized, and are shown being passed through tunnel.

C, After closure of bladder wall, bulbocavernosus muscle and labial fat pad are shown sutured over bladder defect.

D, Closure of vaginal mucosa.

E, Labial and Schuchardt incisions closed, with Penrose drains in incisions.

We have used this technique in the repair of eight radiation-induced fistulas, and all have been successfully closed. One patient required a second procedure utilizing the opposite bulbocavernosus muscle and labial fat pad. Satisfactory results utilizing the Martius technique have been reported in the American literature by Betson (1965), Boronow (1971), and Smith and Johnson (1980).

UROINTESTINAL FISTULA

An extreme example of radiation injury is urointestinal fistula, a communication between the urinary and intestinal tracts. This can also communicate with the skin, the vagina, or the perineum (Figure 28–10). These fistulas generally develop when surgery precedes or follows a full course of radiation therapy.

Symptoms

The presence of a urointestinal fistula is suggested by the passage of fecal material or other products of digestion in the urine (fecaluria). The passage of air or gas from the lower urinary tract (pneumaturia) also suggests a urointestinal fistula. In some cases, in the absence of a rectovaginal fistula, the patient may be continent of feces and pass urine from the rectum. In the presence of an intact rectal sphincter there may be intestinal absorption of the pooled urine, which can lead to malaise, nausea and vomiting, diarrhea, general debilitation, and fever.

Diagnostic Aids

The most thorough investigation, including contrast studies of the upper gastrointestinal tract and the colon, intravenous pyelography, cystography, and cystoscopic examination, may not identify the site of communication. The oral administration of medicinal charcoal can be of help in determining transit time from ingestion until the charcoal appears at an orifice. The oral administration of carmine red, with careful examination of fistula drainage, can also be of value in diagnosis. Another method is the intravenous administration of indigo carmine, with careful examination of the stool.

Management

The management of such fistulas must be individualized. The goal of repair should be reconstitution of the intestinal and urinary tracts to restore the patient to full continence. When this is not possible, the procedure that provides the fewest stomas and offers the patient the greater convenience at the lowest nutritional and metabolic price should be chosen. Before any surgical attempt is undertaken, the patient should be brought to optimal nutritional condition compatible with her clinical status.

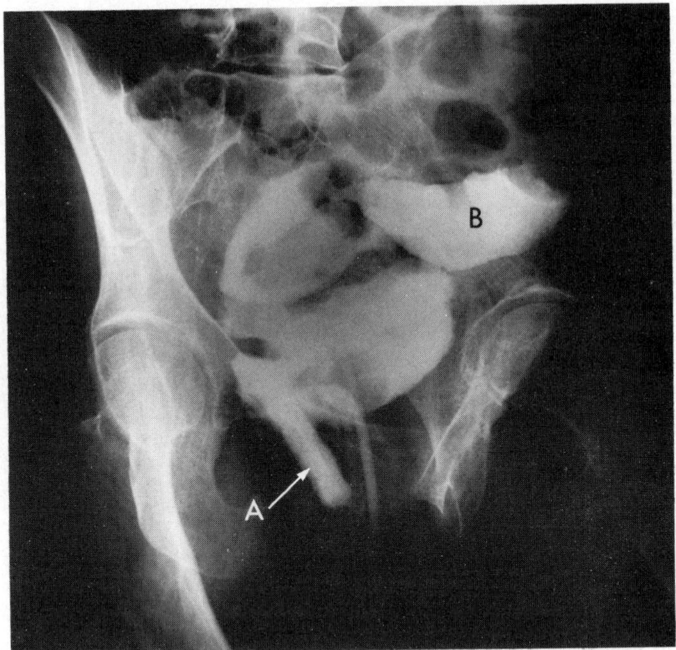

Figure 28–10. Cystogram in patient with vesicosigmoid and vesicovaginal fistulas following radiation therapy for cervical carcinoma. Contrast material can be seen outlining vaginal tampon (A), demonstrating communication between the bladder and vagina, and contrast material is seen in the colon (B).

Cecovesicovaginal Fistula

Figure 28–11*A* demonstrates a cecovesicovaginal fistula in a patient who had had a hysterectomy following a full course of radiation therapy. She noted vaginal leaking of urine and feces approximately one month following surgery. An ileotransverse colon anastomosis and sigmoid colostomy failed to give her any relief. Approximately 2 years following the last surgical procedure, the communication between the cecum, the bladder, and the vagina was still present (Figure 28–11*B*). When we evaluated her, small particles of fecal material were seen in the bladder on cystoscopic examination.

Surgical correction of both fistulas was carried out utilizing an omental graft. After the repair of the vesicovaginal and cecovaginal fistulas, the patient was continent of both urine and feces. The colostomy was eventually closed, and the patient returned to normal continence (Figure 28–11*C*).

Vesicosigmoid Fistula

As with other radiation-induced urointestinal fistulas, vesicosigmoid fistulas generally develop after some form of surgical intervention but may follow severe diverticulitis. If the rectal sphincter is intact and there is no rectovaginal fistula, the patient will note decreased urinary output from the urethra. She may develop electrolyte and acid-base problems related to the presence of pooled urine in the intestinal tract.

We saw a patient who had bilateral tubo-ovarian abscesses removed and a hypogastric artery ligation prior to a full course of radiation therapy for advanced cervical carcinoma. Approximately 2½ years following completion of radiation therapy, the patient noted feces in the vagina. A rectovaginal fistula was found. On cystographic examination, fecal material was noted in the bladder. On intravenous pyelography and cystography, contrast material was noted to pass into the sigmoid colon (Figure 28–12*A*).

The patient's general debilitation was corrected with intravenous hyperalimentation and the anemia corrected with blood transfusions. A bladder biopsy revealed "necrotic tissue and bladder wall with submucosal fibrosis and radiation changes." At celiotomy, a 1.5 × 1.5 cm. communication was found between the dome of the bladder and the sigmoid. The bladder was markedly contracted and fibrotic. Because of the patient's rectovaginal fistula, an end-sigmoid colostomy was performed. The dis-

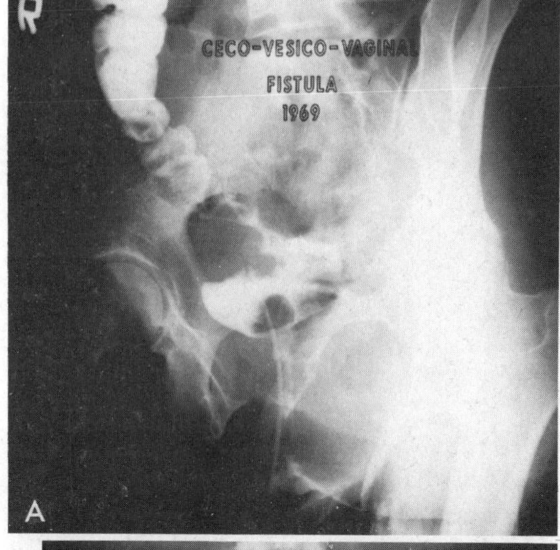

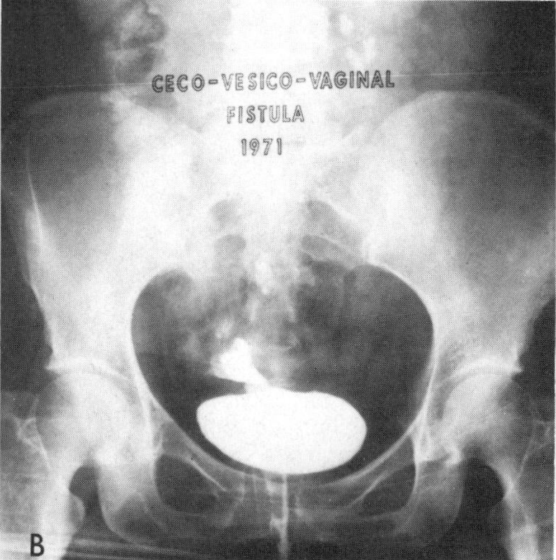

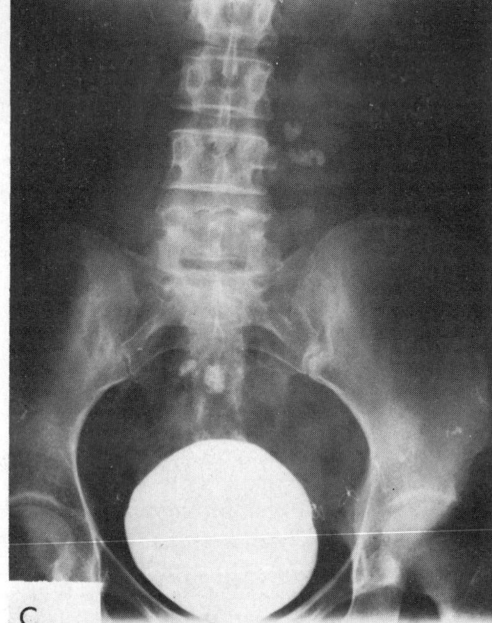

Figure 28–11. Cecovesicovaginal fistula following radiation therapy and hysterectomy in patient with cervical carcinoma.

A, Oblique view of cystogram (1969) demonstrating filling defect in dome of bladder, with contrast material in cecum.

B, Cystogram (1971) following ileotransverse colon anastomosis and colostomy. Contrast material is present in ascending colon and in vagina, demonstrating persistence of fistula.

C, Cystogram after successful repair of cecovesicovaginal fistula. Colostomy was eventually closed, and patient was returned to full continence. From White, A. J., and Buchsbaum, H. J.: Cecovesicovaginal fistula. Urology *2*:559, 1973.)

tal end of the sigmoid was closed and the rectosigmoid distal to the urointestinal communication divided and closed. An augmentation cystoplasty was performed by leaving the segment of rectosigmoid attached to the bladder.

The patient was continent of urine postoperatively and adjusted well to her colostomy. During the postoperative period there has been no deterioration of the upper urinary tracts and she has not developed an electrolyte imbalance (Figure 28–12*B*). However, she has formed bladder stones, managed by transurethral methods.

URETERAL FIBROSIS

Ureteral obstruction by cancer continues to be the most common cause of death in patients with cervical carcinoma (Chapter 27). The risks of ureteral obstruction following radical pelvic surgery have long been recognized; the role of ureteral fibrosis and obstruction following radiation therapy, though first reported by Schmitz in 1920, has only recently been appreciated.

When ureteral obstruction is found following radiation therapy, it behooves the physician to determine whether recurrent

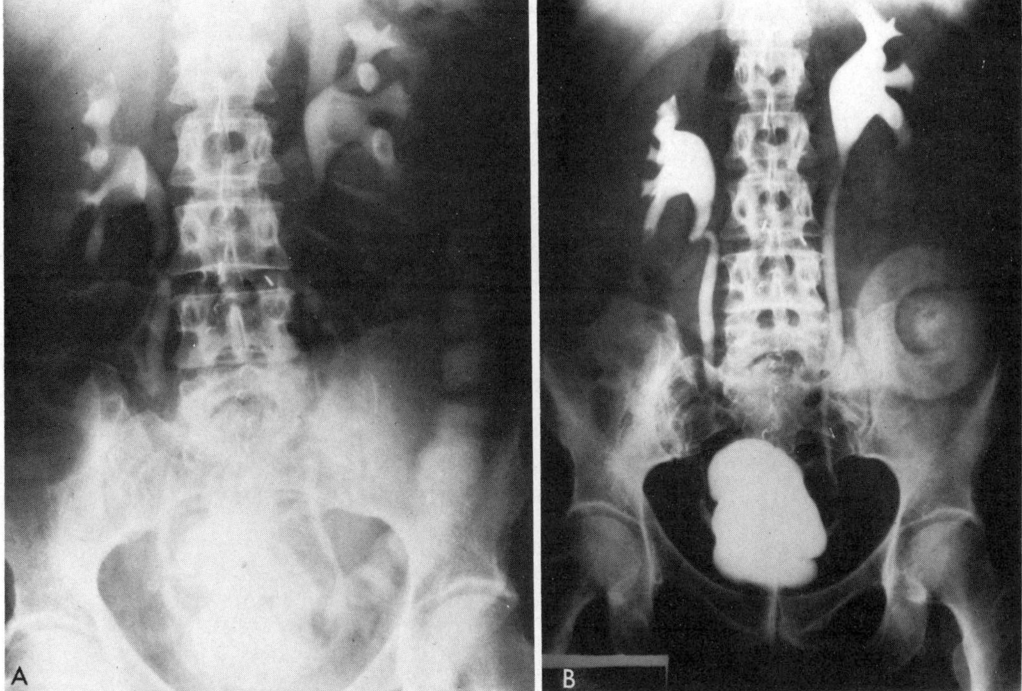

Figure 28–12. Radiation-induced vesicosigmoid fistula.
A, Intravenous pyelogram showing contrast material in sigmoid and ascending colon.
B, Intravenous pyelogram following sigmoid colostomy and augmentation cystoplasty utilizing sigmoid colon.

malignancy or radiation fibrosis is the cause. The radiographic picture (Figure 28–13) is similar to partial or complete obstruction caused by persistent or recurrent carcinoma. The site of obstruction is generally 4 to 6 cm. from the ureterovesical junction.

The frequency with which ureteral fibrosis occurs following radiation therapy has been variously reported, ranging from 0.4 to 2.0 per cent (Rhamy and Stander, 1962; Kottmeier, 1964; Graham and Abad, 1967; Cushing et al., 1968; Shingleton et al., 1969; Kaplan, 1977; Muram et al., 1981). Altvater and Imholz (1960) suggested that ureteral stenosis is a significant factor contributing to the deaths of women treated with radiation therapy. Of 38 women whose deaths were related to genitourinary tract abnormalities following radiation therapy of cervical carcinoma, 24 had ureteral obstruction secondary to cancer, while 12 (31.6 per cent) had no evidence of recurrent disease but died of ureteral fibrosis. Kirchoff (1960), in an autopsy study, found complete or partial obstruction in 17.5 per cent of women previously treated for cervical carcinoma but free of disease.

In a study of 34 patients with ureteral obstruction following radiation therapy for cervical carcinoma, Muram and co-workers (1981) found that the stricture was a result of radiation fibrosis in 12 (35 per cent). The likelihood that the obstruction resulted from paraureteral fibrosis was greatest in patients treated for an early stage of cervical carcinoma: 7 of 9 patients (77 per cent) with Stage Ib and 5 of 16 patients (31 per cent) with Stage II. In all cases of radiation fibrosis, the stricture was in the lower one third of the ureter.

In patients with bilateral ureteral obstruction following radiation therapy, the possibility that one side may be obstructed as a result of recurrent disease, and the other side as a result of radiation fibrosis, should be considered (Sklaroff et al., 1978).

Mechanism of Ureteral Obstruction

The exact mechanism of obstruction following radiation therapy is not known but is

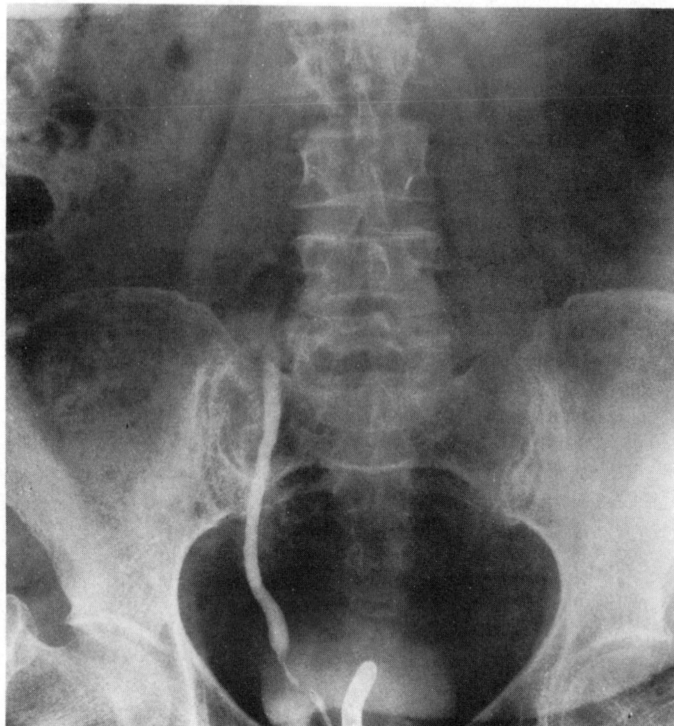

Figure 28–13. Retrograde ureterogram in patient 3 years following radiation therapy for cervical carcinoma. Ureteral obstruction resulting from radiation fibrosis is seen 3 to 4 cm. from ureterovesical junction.

related to fibrosis of the periureteral tissue. The ureter is relatively radioresistant; the susceptibility of the ureteral wall to the effects of radiation therapy is heightened when its blood supply is compromised. The fibrosis is generally periureteral and may represent replacement of tumor by dense scar tissue. Furthermore, tumor may elicit a connective tissue response in the periureteral tissue out of proportion to the space it occupies (Alfert and Gillenwater, 1972). Ureteral fibrosis appears more commonly in patients treated for pelvic inflammatory disease, so that infection and parametritis may predispose the ureter to fibrosis. In Kaplan's series (1977) of 11 cases, three women had pelvic inflammatory disease severe enough to necessitate surgery.

VillaSanta (1972) reported finding ureteral obstruction at an average of 23 months (range, 5 to 63) following therapy; Shingleton and co-workers (1969) at 18 months (range, 13 to 28); and Rhamy and Stander (1962) at 37 months (range, 28 to 52) following radiation therapy. Kirkinen and associates (1980) reported the mean time that elapsed between radiation therapy and the diagnosis of stricture was 53.3 months.

The ureteral fibrosis appears somewhat later than does vesicovaginal fistula. There appears to be no predilection for side, and the obstruction may be bilateral. In one study (Kirkinen et al., 1980) of 19 patients, 9 were found to have unilateral, and 10 bilateral, strictures resulting from radiation fibrosis. Several studies have failed to document any correlation between the bladder mucosal dose and the subsequent development of ureteral fibrosis.

Management

A thorough investigation of the urinary tract should be performed before management of radiation fibrosis of the ureter is undertaken. The status of the opposite ureter, the functional capacity of the bladder and of the ureteral orifices, and the patient's general condition and ability to care for herself must be considered.

When these factors have been assessed, the patient should be explored by a transperitoneal route, and the site of obstruction exposed. Careful dissection should be carried out to expose the ureter and obtain tissue for frozen section examination. The most common cause for ureteral obstruction in patients treated for cervical carcinoma is still recurrent tumor. Depending on the pathology findings, one of several options are open. If the obstruction is secondary to tumor at the ureterovesical junction, pelvic exenteration may be indicated. If the obstruction is secondary to fibrosis, surgical lysis of the fibrotic tissue surrounding the ureter is generally inadequate in managing the problem of ureteral fibrosis. Methods of managing ureteral obstruction secondary to radiation fibrosis include the following:

1. Ureteral Dilatation. This is a conservative technique that is generally unsatisfactory.

2. Ureteral Catheter. Placement of an indwelling catheter through a cystoscope. Appropriate for several months at a time.

3. Ureteroneocystotomy. This technique is fraught with problems of anastomosing a heavily irradiated ureter to an equally heavily irradiated bladder. The irradiated bladder is generally not mobile enough to allow a "psoas hitch" or creation of a bladder tube.

4. Transureteroureterostomy. This technique can be used if the other ureter is patent and there is no great disparity in ureteral size. The orifice of the recipient ureter must be normal and the bladder functional.

5. Conduit. If both ureters are involved or the bladder is markedly compromised secondary to chronic radiation changes or fistula, supravesical diversion by conduit is appropriate (Chapter 11).

6. Ureterostomy, Nephrostomy. These techniques may be used as a temporizing measure but are generally not acceptable for long-term diversion.

7. Ureterosigmoidostomy. This may be satisfactory for a select group of patients, but generally electrolyte and acid-base problems will be encountered. The use of irradiated bowel and ureter increases the incidence of complications.

REFERENCES

Alfert, H. J., and Gillenwater, J. Y.: The consequences of ureteral irradiation with special reference to subsequent ureteral injury. J. Urol. *107*:369, 1972.

Altvater, G., and Imholz, G.: Die Ureterstenosen bein Kollumkarzinom. Geburtsh. Frauenheilkd. *20*:1214, 1960.

Behnam, K., Patil, U. B., and Mariano, E.: Intravesical instillation of formalin for hemorrhagic cystitis secondary to radiation for gynecologic malignancies. Obstet. Gynecol. (in press).

Betson, J. R.: Bulbocavernosus fat-pad transplant. Obstet. Gynecol. *26*:135, 1965.

Bloomer, W. D., and Hellman, S.: Normal tissue responses to radiation therapy. N. Engl. J. Med. *293*:80, 1975.

Boronow, R. C.: Management of radiation-induced vaginal fistulas. Am. J. Obstet. Gynecol. *110*:1, 1971.

Boronow, R. C., and Rutledge, F.: Vesicovaginal fistula, radiation and gynecologic cancer. Am. J. Obstet. Gynecol. *111*:85, 1971.

Bosch, A., Frias, Z.: Complications after radiation therapy for cervical carcinoma. Acta. Radiol. Ther. Phys. Biol. *16*:53, 1977.

Brown, R. B.: A method of management of inoperable carcinoma of the bladder. Med. J. Aust. *1*:23, 1969.

Buchler, D. A., Kline, J. C., Peckham, B. M., et al.: Radiation reactions in cervical cancer therapy. Am. J. Obstet. Gynecol. *111*:745, 1971.

Calame, R. J., and Wallach, R. C.: An analysis of the complications of the radiologic treatment of carcinoma of the cervix. Surg. Gynecol. Obstet. *125*:39, 1967.

Cushing, R. M., Tovell, H. M., and Liegner, L. M.: Major urologic complications following radium and X-ray therapy for carcinoma of the cervix. Am. J. Obstet. Gynecol. *101*:750, 1968.

Dean, A. L.: Injury of the urinary bladder following irradiation of the uterus. Am. J. Obstet. Gynecol. *25*:667, 1933.

Edsmyr, F., Huber, W., and Menander, K. B.: Orgotein efficacy in ameliorating side effects due to radiation therapy. I. Double-blind, placebo-controlled trial in patients with bladder tumors. Cur. Ther. Res. *19*:198, 1976.

Fridovich, I.: Superoxide dismutases. Ann. Rev. Biochem. *44*:147, 1975.

Gowing, N. F. C.: Pathological changes in the bladder following irradiation. Br. J. Radiol. *33*:484, 1960.

Graham, J. B.: Vaginal fistulas following radiotherapy. Surg. Gynecol. Obstet. *120*:1019, 1965.

Graham, J. B., and Abad, R. S.: Ureteral obstruction due to radiation. Am. J. Obstet. Gynecol. *99*:409, 1967.

Hueper, W. C., Fisher, C. V., deCarvajal-Forero, J., et al.: The pathology of experimental roentgen-cystitis in dogs. J. Urol. *47*:156, 1942.

Kadish, L. J., Stein, J. M., Kotler, S., et al.: Angiographic diagnosis and treatment due to pelvic trauma. J. Trauma *13*:1083, 1973.

Kagan, A. R., Nussbaum, H., Gilbert, H., et al.: A new staging system for irradiation injuries following treatment for cancer of the cervix uteri. Gynecol. Oncol. *7*:166, 1979.

Kaplan, A. L.: Postradiation ureteral obstruction. Obstet. Gynecol. Surv. *32*:1, 1977.

Kirchoff, H.: Komplicationsreiche Verädungen am Harnsystem nach Strahlentherapie des Kollumkarzinoms. Geburtsh. Frauenheilkd. *20*:34, 1960.

Kirkinen, P., Kauppila, A., and Kontturi, M.: Treatment of ureteral strictures after therapy for carcinoma of the uterus. Surg. Gynecol. Obstet. *151*:487, 1980.

Kline, J. C., Buchler, D. A., Boone, M. L., et al.: The relationship of reactions to complications in the radiation therapy of cancer of the cervix. Radiology *105*:413, 1972.

Kottmeier, H. L.: Complications following radiation therapy in carcinoma of the cervix and their treatment. Am. J. Obstet. Gynecol. *88*:854, 1964.

Lee, K. H., Kagan, A. R., Nussbaum, H., et al.: Analysis of dose, dose rate, and treatment time in the production of injuries by radium treatment for cancer of the uterine cervix. Br. J. Radiol. *49*:430, 1976.

Marberger, H., Bartsch, G., Huber, W., et al.: Orgotein: A new drug for the treatment of radiation cystitis. Curr. Ther. Res. *18*:466, 1975.

Marberger, H., Huber, W., Bartsch, G., et al.: Orgotein: A new antiinflammatory metalloprotein drug: evaluation of clinical efficacy and safety in inflammatory conditions of the urinary tract. Inter. Urol. Nephrol. *6*:61, 1974.

McCall, M. L., and Bolton, K. A.: Martius' Gynecological Operations. Boston, Little, Brown and Co., 1956, p. 327.

Menander-Huber, K. B., Edsmyr, F., and Huber, W.: Orgotein efficacy in ameliorating side effects due to radiation therapy. Scand. J. Urol. Nephrol. (Suppl.)*55*:219, 1980.

Muram, D., Oxorn, H., Curry, R. H., et al.: Postradiation ureteral obstruction: A reappraisal. Am. J. Obstet. Gynecol. *139*:289, 1981.

Peckham, B. M., Kline, J. C., Schultz, A. E., et al.: Radiation dosage and complications in cervical cancer therapy. Am. J. Obstet. Gynecol. *104*:485, 1969.

Pool, T. L.: Irradiation cystitis: diagnosis and treatment. Surg. Clin. North Am. *39*:947, 1959.

Rhamy, R. K., and Stander, R. W.: Pyelographic analysis of radium therapy in carcinoma of the cervix. Am. J. Roentgenol. *87*:41, 1962.

Rubin, P., and Casarett, G. W.: Urinary tract: The bladder and ureters. *In* Clinical Radiation Pathology. Vol. I. Philadelphia, W. B. Saunders Co., 1968, p. 334.

Schmidt, J. D., Buchsbaum, H. J., and Jacobo, E. C.: Transverse colon conduit for supravesical urinary tract diversion. Urology *8*:542, 1976.

Schmitz, H.: The classification of uterine carcinoma for the study of efficacy of radiation therapy. Am. J. Roentgenol. *7*:383, 1920.

Servadio, C., and Nissenkorn, I.: Massive hematuria successfully treated by bladder irrigations with formalin solution. Cancer *37*:900, 1976.

Shingleton, H. M., Fowler, W. C., Jr., Pepper, F. D., et al.: Ureteral strictures following therapy for carcinoma of the cervix. Cancer *24*:77, 1969.

Sklaroff, D. M., Gnaneswaran, P., and Sklaroff, R. B.: Postirradiation ureteric stricture. Gynecol. Oncol. *6*:538, 1978.

Smith, W. G., and Johnson, G. H.: Vesicovaginal fistula repair — revisited. Gynecol. Oncol. *9*:303, 1980.

Stockbine, M. F., Hancock, J. E., and Fletcher, G. H.: Complications in 831 patients with squamous cell carcinoma of the intact uterine cervix treated with 3000 rads or more whole pelvis irradiation. Am. J. Roentgenol. *108*:293, 1970.

van Nagell, J. R., Parker, J. C., Maruyama, J., et al.: Bladder or rectal surgery following radiation injury for cervical carcinoma. Am. J. Obstet. Gynecol. *119*:727, 1974.

VillaSanta, V.: Complications of radiotherapy for carcinoma of the uterine cervix. Am. J. Obstet. Gynecol. *114*:717, 1972.

Watson, E. M., Herger, C. C., and Sauer, H. R.: Irradiation reactions in the bladder: Their occurrence and clinical course following the use of X-ray and radium in the treatment of female pelvic disease. J. Urol. *57*:1038, 1947.

White, A. J., and Buchsbaum, H. J.: Cecovesicovaginal fistula. Urology *2*:559, 1973.

29

DISEASES OF THE URETHRA

E. JACOBO, M.D.
L. F. GREENE, M.D., Ph.D.

RELATED ANATOMY

An understanding of the anatomy of the female urethra and perineum is essential for correlation of the disease processes affecting this area. (See also Chapters 1 and 2.)

Topographically the perineum may be conveniently divided into two compartments: the anterior or urogenital triangle and the posterior or anal triangle. The urogenital triangle of the female perineum contains the vaginal and urethral openings. The urethral meatus is an irregularly ovoid opening 4 × 5 mm. in diameter located 2 to 3 cm. below the clitoris. Adjacent to this meatus there are several small cryptlike openings that represent the minor vestibular glands, the homologues of the glands of Littré in the male urethra (Figure 29–1).

Urethra

The urethra in the adult female measures from 3.0 to 3.6 cm. in length and in the newborn female about 2.5 cm. Its normal diameter is in the range of 8 mm.

The distal two thirds of the urethra is closely adherent to the anterior vaginal wall, an important fact to remember when performing surgery in this area, whereas the proximal one third of the urethra is clearly separable from the anterior vaginal wall.

Vascular and Nervous Supply

The arterial supply to the upper third of the urethra results from multiple anastomoses of vessels from the bladder, while the middle and lower thirds receive branches directly from the inferior vesical artery as it courses the superior lateral aspect of the vagina. Superiorly, the venous drainage is through the inferior, middle, and superior vesical veins. Inferiorly, the drainage is through the clitoral venous plexus. The nerve supply to the urethra is mainly via the hypogastric plexus.

Lymphatics

Lymphatics in the urethra are numerous. Anteriorly the drainage is into the vestibular plexus with connecting channels to the inguinal nodes. The posterior urethra has three different lymphatic routes: (1) the anterior superior portion towards the bladder wall and external iliac chain; (2) the anterolateral and lateral lymphatic drain into the lateral bladder wall and at this point the channels may turn into the medial group of the external iliac chain or into the hypogastric or obturator group; (3) the posterior portion of the urethra drains into the posterior bladder wall and the uterine channels.

Musculature

The urethra is covered primarily by smooth muscle fibers coursing in two patterns, the circular pattern and the longitudinal pattern, which are interwoven at tangents and merge with the smooth muscle layers of the bladder. Striated muscle appears markedly demarcated from the smooth muscle fibers and is attached to the urethra without forming part of it. The

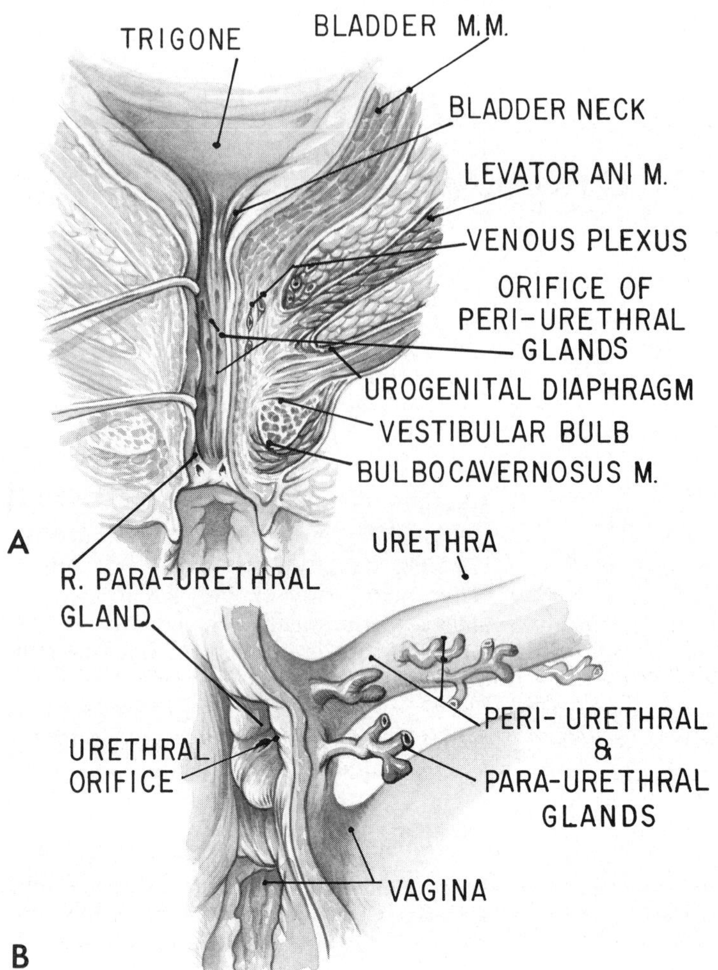

Figure 29–1. *A,* Diagrammatic representation of the anatomy of the female urethra and related structures. *B,* Anatomy of the paraurethral glands and ducts (Skene's glands).

striated muscles are the bulbocavernosus and the ischiocavernosus muscles (Krantz, 1951).

The bulbocavernosus muscle lies lateral to the urethra at the external meatus. It originates from the central tendinous line and mixes with the fibers of the ischiocavernosus muscle. The ischiocavernosus muscle arises along the medial aspect of the ischial ramus and envelops the crus of the clitoris anteriorly and superiorly, whereas inferiorly it courses over the urethra and the midline.

Supporting Structures

The urethra is held in position beneath the pubic symphysis by several structures.

Urogenital Diaphragm

The most superficial of these structures is the urogenital diaphragm, which encloses a slit compartment termed the deep perineal compartment. In this deep perineal compartment, between the superficial and deep layers of fascia attached to the inner aspect of the pubic arc, lie (1) the deep transverse perineal muscle, (2) the sphincter urethrae muscle, and (3) the pudendal vessels and nerves.

The superior fascia of the urogenital diaphragm arises from the pubic bone as two narrow bands that spread out, reaching the urethral wall. These bands are firmly inserted into the urethra and have been called the "pubourethral ligaments." These bands contain a tiny cul-de-sac anterior to the urethra through which the perineal veins communicate with the pelvic venous plexus, constituting a retropubic hiatus of the urogenital diaphragm.

The deep transverse perineal muscle is the separable posterior part of the musculature of the urogenital diaphragm and is located deep to the superficial transverse perineal muscle. This deep transverse perineal muscle passes across the perineum behind the vaginal orifice and sends muscle fibers into the rectum and, posteriorly, behind the rectum into the coccyx. The sphincter of the urethra is contained in the anterior portion and arises from the inner surface of the ischial rami. The main function of the urogenital diaphragm appears to be supportive.

Pelvic Diaphragm

The pelvic diaphragm surrounds the urethra and also provides support. It is composed of the superior and inferior fascial layers with an interposed layer of muscle, made up of two pairs of muscles, the *levator ani* and the *coccygei*. These muscles pass downward toward the midline to meet each other, fusing and surrounding the terminal portions of the rectum, vagina, and urethra. The muscular slings that pass into the urethra do so on the posterior lateral aspect and intermingle with the urethral wall. The muscle is deficient only in an area behind the pubic symphysis, where there exists the retropubic hiatus in which the dorsal clitoral vessels pass.

Cervical Vaginal Fascia

The proximal one third of the urethra remains as a separate structure from the anterior vaginal wall by the continuation of loose connective tissue. This loose connective tissue envelops the vagina and rectum as the cervical vaginal fascia. Recognition of this intimate association of the urethra and vaginal wall allows a better understanding of how vaginal and other gynecologic problems, including hormonal influences on the vaginal epithelium, may affect the urethra and produce symptoms.

Paraurethral Ducts (Skene's Glands)

In 1880 Alexander Skene established the clinical significance of the paraurethral ducts. The importance of these ducts and their exact role in perpetuating gonococcal infection became more apparent when in 1948 Huffman described their anatomy in detail. He concluded then that the Skene's glands do not number only two, as they were described initially, but can be multiple in number. They constitute a complex system of tubuloalveolar structures that branch into the proximal portion of the urethra (Figure 29–2). These glandlike structures are formed by low columnar epithelium, some of them terminating in tubular lacunae without drainage into ducts. Skene's glands represent the homologue of the prostate in the male.

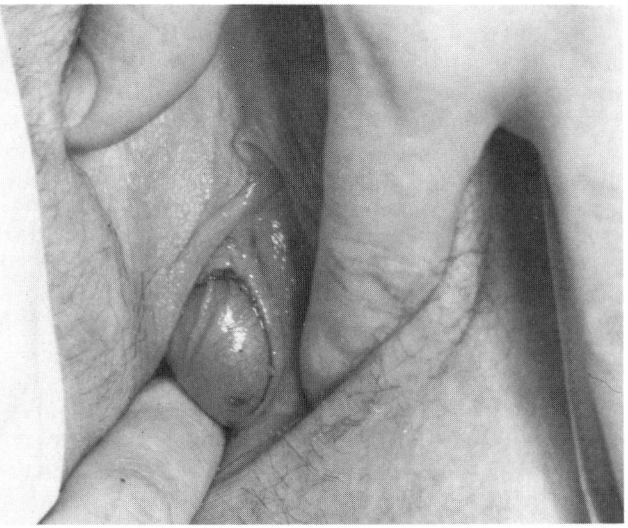

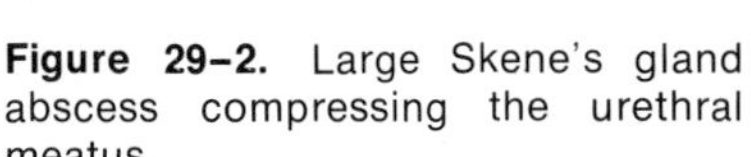

Figure 29–2. Large Skene's gland abscess compressing the urethral meatus.

Obstruction of the narrow outlet of the paraurethral ducts by infection is an important factor in the etiology of abscesses of the anterior vaginal wall as well as the urethral wall itself. Owing to the glandular nature of these ducts, it has been postulated that primary adenocarcinoma of the urethra originates here.

DEVELOPMENTAL ANOMALIES OF THE URETHRA

Epispadias

Epispadias results from a developmental defect involving the cloaca and in its most severe form presents as bladder exstrophy. Female epispadias is classified as follows:

1. Partial or incomplete epispadias, representing involvement of the anterior portion of the distal urethra, occasionally associated with a bifid clitoris. Stress incontinence may occur with this anomaly.

2. Subsymphyseal epispadias, involving the external urinary sphincter and accompanied by deformities of the external genitalia. The labia are widely separated anteriorly; the urethra is absent, presenting as a large defect, allowing the examiner's finger to be passed easily inside the bladder (Figure 29–3) (Muecke and Marshall, 1968).

3. Retrosymphyseal epispadias, the most severe form. Occasionally prolapse of the bladder coexists, and the entire anomaly is considered a variant of exstrophy.

Usually, mild forms of epispadias go undetected. Several successful urethrovesical suspensions have been reported in patients with mild incontinence secondary to the epispadias.

The width of the pubic symphysis correlates fairly well with epispadias. In its most severe form, the symphysis appears wider and the pubes are separated. In the normal adult female, the width of the pubic symphysis should not exceed 10 mm.

When the severe type of epispadias is not corrected at an early age the patients are apt to have, in addition to chronic infection, severe perineal dermatitis from constant contact with urine (Figure 29–3).

The more severe forms of epispadias (types 2 and 3) require repair; the Leadbetter modification of Young-Dee's operation is preferred. It is beyond the scope of this discussion to describe the surgical techniques for the plastic repair of epispadias (Flocks and Culp, 1975).

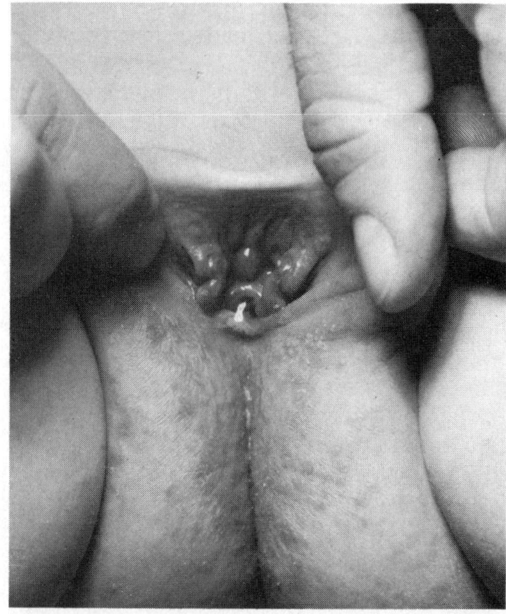

Figure 29–3. Complete epispadias extending to the urinary sphincter, associated with incontinence. Notice the extensive changes on the perineal skin consistent with ammonia dermatitis.

Hypospadias

In this defect, the urethra opens into the anterior vaginal wall. As in epispadias, the defect may range from an opening into the vaginal wall near the usual location of the external meatus to a complete absence of the dorsal portion of the urethra extending close to the bladder neck. Incontinence of urine and repeated urinary tract infections are the most important clinical features of this entity. On voiding, the stream is directed initially towards the vagina. Thus, ascending infections are common. In the vast majority of these patients, urinary tract localization studies reveal bacteriuria of the upper urinary tract with the same organisms as those recovered from the vaginal flora.

URETHRAL OBSTRUCTION AND STENOSIS

A patient frequently encountered by both gynecologists and urologists is the woman with complaints of disturbance in micturition. In some patients the abnormal voiding pattern exists unaccompanied by urinary tract infections. In others it coincides with the onset of bacterial cystitis or urethritis.

Stenosis of the urethra is often a developmental anomaly. Meatal stenosis is thought to be the result of a persistent cloacal membrane. Stenosis may also occur as a sequela of inflammation of the paraurethral ducts and glands.

Symptoms

Symptoms usually point toward recurring episodes of cystitis characterized by a long history of frequency in urination with or without infection. Hesitancy has been reported in over 25 per cent of patients. Surprisingly, many of these patients have a lifelong history of symptoms. Therefore, slow urinary stream goes easily unnoticed by these patients. Dyspareunia is not a very common finding unless there is inflammation of the paraurethral glands.

Urethral Calibration

Residual urine greater than 25 ml. is present in over one third of these patients. Urethral calibration as performed clinically in the nonvoiding state detects areas of stenosis. Indirect but highly useful data regarding the likely areas of resistance to urine flow can be obtained via this technique. The method of calibration involves the passage of graded sizes of bougies à boules (Figure 29–4) via the urethra into the bladder, with subsequent withdrawal. Since the meatus is the seat of the vast majority of strictures, a ring is usually present at this point. The area blanches with the passage of the bougie à boule. Isolated strictures of the middle and distal urethra are not uncommon, but urethral stricture is by far most commonly seen at the level of the meatus.

The caliber of the meatus and urethra has been the subject of extensive studies in regard to age and hormonal influences upon this structure. In 1966 Immergut and coworkers calibrated the urethras of 136 normal girls undergoing tonsillectomy, finding that 92 of these patients had a distal urethral lumen equal to that of the meatus (Table 29–1). The caliber of the urethra ranged from 14 French at age 2 years to an average of 26 French at age 18 to 20 years, increasing in a steep progression until the age of 12 years, at the onset of menarche, at which point a rapid increase in lumen size occurs (Figure 29–5). This rapid change was thought to be a response to physiologic hormonal changes.

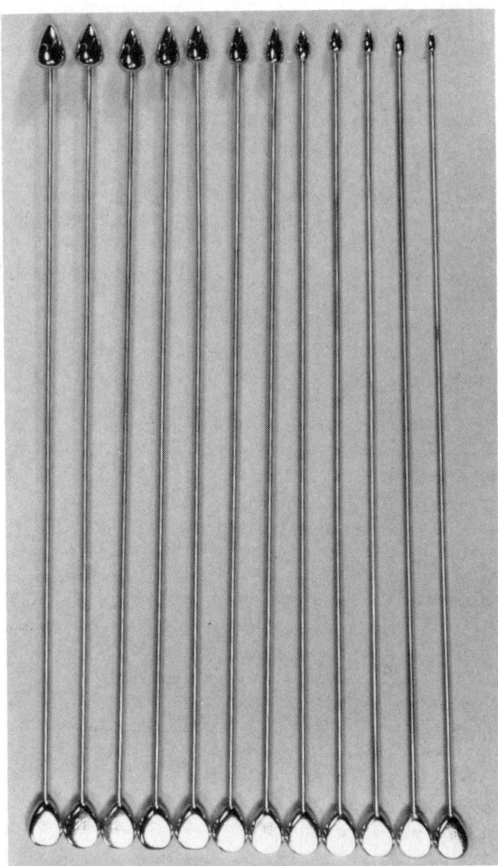

Figure 29–4. Bougies à boules utilized for the calibration of the urethra. Note the acorn shape that allows for easy introduction into the urethral meatus. On withdrawal, the flat, non-coned segment will produce the typical "snap" if a tight ring is present. Bougies à boules range in size from 8 to 40 French.

In another study, the caliber of the urethra in the face of infection was greater in each age group than that of the urethral size of the normal uninfected female child.

TABLE 29–1. CALIBER OF URETHRAL MEATUS AND DISTAL URETHRA IN ASYMPTOMATIC NONINFECTED CHILDREN

	URETHRAL MEATUS		
Age	**Number of Patients**	**Caliber (French)** *Mean*	*Median*
2	14	14	14
4	20	15.6	16
6	27	16.1	16
8	27	16.9	16
10	18	19.6	20
12	6	23.3	22
14	4	24.5	24
16	9	25.8	26
18–20	6	27.3	26
	DISTAL URETHRA		
Age	**Number of Patients**	**Caliber (French)** *Mean*	*Median*
2	15	14	14
4	18	15.3	14
6	23	15.4	16
8	25	16.8	16
10	16	19.5	16
12	6	21.0	20
14	7	23.4	24
16	9	25.6	26
18–20	6	26	24

Note increase in size of the lumen with age.

From Immergut, M., Culp, D., and Flocks, R. H.: The urethral caliber in normal female children. Trans. Am. Assoc. Genitourin. Surg. *58*:25, 1966, with permission.

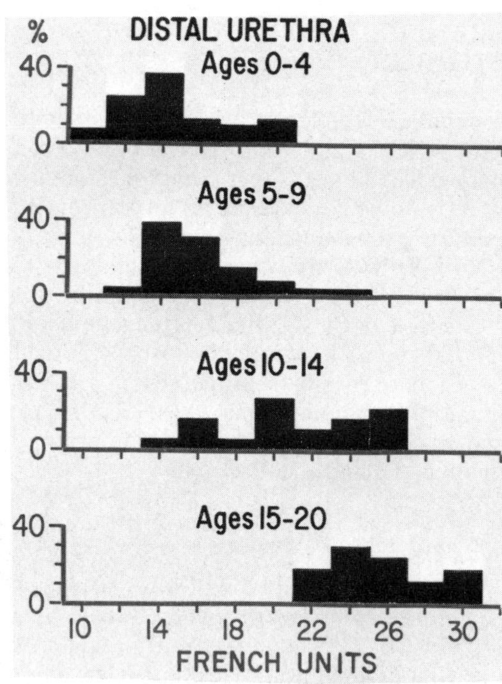

Figure 29–5. The caliber of the distal urethra in normal female children correlates with the caliber of the meatus. A significant shift to the right during menarche is evident. (From Immergut, M., Culp, D., and Flocks, R. H.: The urethral caliber in normal female children. Trans. Amer. Assoc. Genitourin. Surg. *58*:25, 1966, with permission.)

Statistically it appears that a functional abnormality exists, since following a urethral meatotomy and dilatation to approximately 30 French, 84 per cent of the infected children were free of symptoms 4 months later without antibacterial therapy (Walker and Richard, 1973). Hormonal factors influencing urethral widening at the age of menarche could explain why some female patients with a long history of urinary tract infection develop sterile urine and obtain relief of symptoms following puberty. Dilatation of the ureters and hydronephrosis are not uncommon (Figure 29–6).

Lyon and Smith (1963) found a point of consistent urethral narrowing at the most distal third of the urethra in symptomatic children (Lyon's ring). Characteristically the presence of a ring with a snug feel as the bougie is inserted and a tendency to snap as the bougie is forced into its lumen was observed. Whether the reported symptomatic improvement following dilatation of this tight ring is related to this treatment is at the present time the subject of controversy in the understanding of the pathophysiology of lower urinary tract infections in females. As a rule, resistance to the passage of 22 or 24 French bougie in the postpubertal female is suggestive of mechanical obstruction.

Clinically one encounters patients in whom the picture simulates that of mechanical obstruction except that the urethral caliber is wide and normal. These patients are theoretically harboring functional obstruction, and residual urine is commonly present, fostering the subsequent development of infection.

Other Diagnostic Aids

Response to the initial dilatation confirms the working diagnosis, and the favorable response to this initial dilatation in

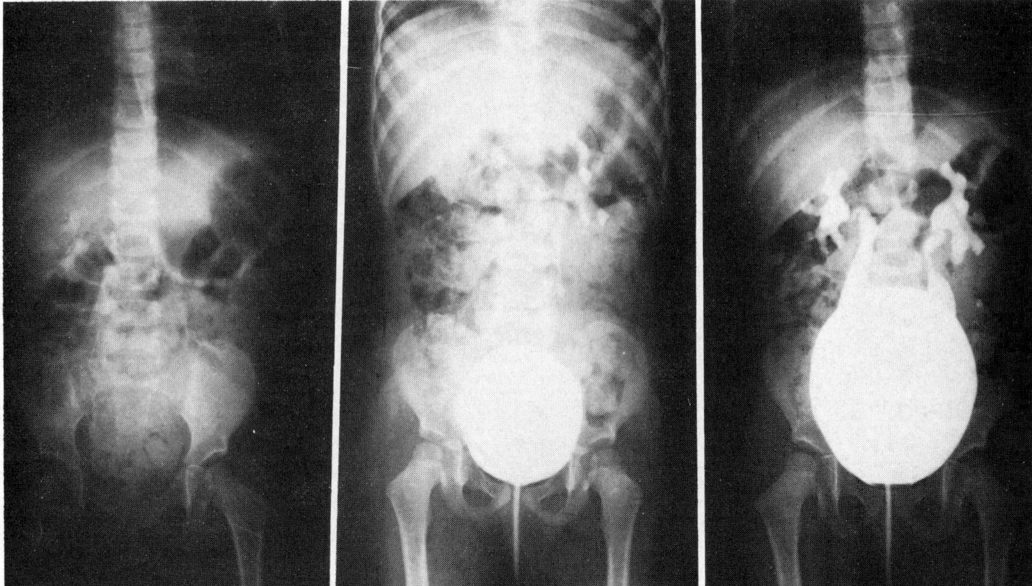

Figure 29–6. Six-year-old white female with meatal stenosis and no other source of obstruction in the urinary tract. *A*, pyelogram shows poor concentration of contrast material with pyelocaliectasis more evident in the right collecting system. Cystogram (*B, C*) reveals massive bilateral vesicoureteral reflux with hydroureteronephrosis. These changes improved following periodic dilatation of the meatal stenosis.

many instances allows the patient to remain free of symptoms for a prolonged period of time. Cystoscopic examination at the time of dilatation should be carried out in order to assess the presence of trabeculation and damage to the detrusor muscle as a result of the distal obstruction. Cystoscopy will rule out polypoid lesions at the level of the bladder neck as well as other sources of symptoms.

Voiding cystourethrography is a helpful diagnostic test to estimate the presence or absence of vesicoureteral reflux not uncommonly present in the face of distal urethral obstruction. In many instances the voiding phase will reveal ballooning and dilatation proximal to the stricture with subsequent narrowing at the level of the stricture (Figure 29–7). Although these findings are suggestive of urethral stricture, they are per se not diagnostic without the calibration using bougies à boules.

"URETHRAL SYNDROME"

The term "urethral syndrome" has been coined because of the gamut of associated complaints that are present with the urologic aspects of this poorly understood entity.

Symptoms

Typically the patient emphasizes that her complaints originate from the urinary tract and expresses very eloquently the symptoms of dysuria, frequency, back pressure, suprapubic discomfort, malaise, and occasionally dyspareunia. Frequently there is a history of hematuria, most commonly seen on the toilet paper after voiding.

Possible Etiologic Factors

In these patients, intravenous pyelography, cystoscopy, urethral calibration, cystourethrography, and perineal electromyography all yield normal findings. Somehow the urethra has been blamed for the syndrome, and the poor correlation of symptoms with physical findings is conspicuous. Allergies, psychic factors, senile atrophy, meatal obstruction, and paraurethral gland infections have all received consideration as the triggering mechanisms. Nowadays "urethral syndrome" is an arena for extensive heated discussions, but few cold facts are available.

In patients with "urethral syndrome," the incidence of hysterectomy and pelvic surgery is at least twice that in the general population. Endometriosis has been con-

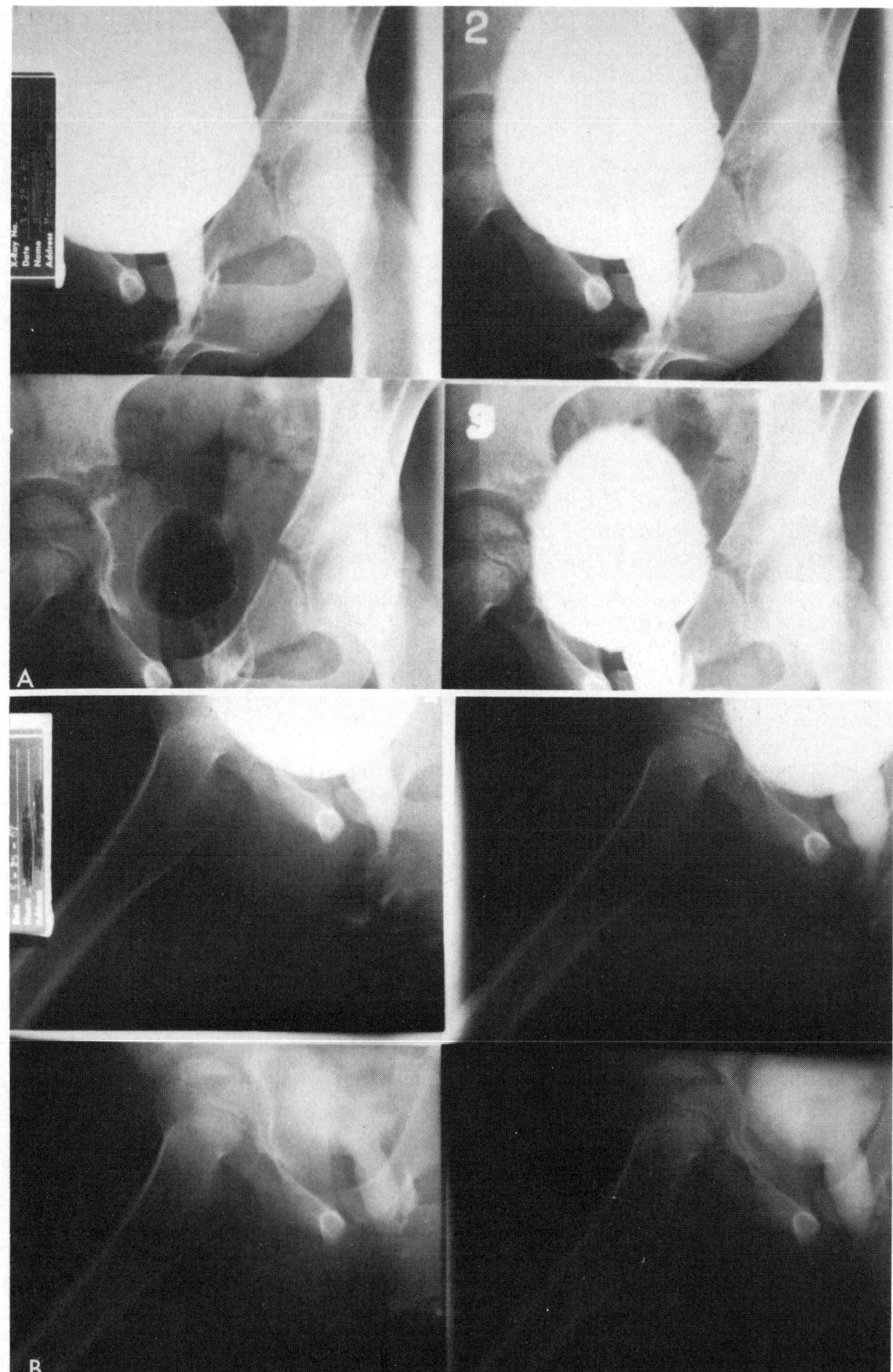

Figure 29–7. Sequential voiding cystourethrograms.

A, Meatal obstruction due to stenosis. Note the progressive ballooning of the urethra and the distal narrowing at the level of the meatus.

B, Three months following dilatation of the urethra, this patient returned with similar symptoms. Illustrated are recurrent progressive dilation of the proximal two thirds of the urethra and narrowing at the level of the meatus.

firmed in about 25 per cent of operated patients.

Of special interest to clinicians has been the correlation of pathogenic organisms present in the vaginal vestibule and urethra in these patients. Bruce and associates (1973), through the use of culture swabs, recovered organisms such as *Streptococcus faecalis* and *Enterobacter* significantly more frequently in patients with "urethral syndrome" than in a control group of asymptomatic patients. Moreover, the organisms recovered from the urethra, vestibule, and vagina were similar in individual patients. Routine urine cultures showed that neither the patients nor the control group had significant bacteriuria. With refinements in urine culture techniques in the female, the first portion of the voided specimen yielded a greater number of organisms, which correlated well with the bacteria of the introitus. Although quantitatively the colony counts were not significant, the same pathogens were present in both urine and vestibule.

In addition, hard data have been accumulated in recent years favoring the concept that "urethral syndrome" is in many instances the result of pathogenic organisms harbored in the vagina, vestibule and urethra (Stamey et al., 1971). It is necessary to reemphasize that these organisms are usually not recovered through routine "clean catch" cultures nor via suprapubic aspiration. Swab cultures of the periurethral areas (introitus) should be obtained for adequate bacteriologic correlation (Elkins and Cox, 1974; Fair et al., 1970).

Stamm and colleagues (1980), in a prospective study of women with urethral syndrome (median age, 25 years), found that 79 of 181 eligible patients had less than 10^5 bacteria per milliliter in midstream urine samples and the remaining 102 patients had greater than 10^5 microorganisms per milliliter. Serial cultures revealed that the two most common organisms associated with the urethral syndrome were *Escherichia coli* and *Chlamydia trachomatis*. The latter was implicated in 10 of the 16 patients with the urethral syndrome who had sterile bladder urine and pyuria. IgG and IgM microimmunofluorescent antibody titers to *C. trachomatis* were elevated, displaying up to fourfold changes. Of interest is the fact that chlamydial urethritis in females was commonly related to recent change in sex partners and use of oral contraceptives. The finding of "low count" urinary tract infection requires reexamination. Eleven of the 59 patients with "negative" cultures (19 per cent) had chlamydial infections, and 10 of these 11 women had pyuria.

Recently, Parsons and co-workers (1981) have shown in experimental studies that bacterial adherence to the bladder urothelium is considerably reduced in the presence of mucin. The use of protamine sulfate produced alterations on the bladder surface enhancing the adherence of bacteria.

The role of immunoglobulin A (IgA) in the vaginal secretions, acting to retard bacterial colonization in the vaginal vestibule, and the Enterobacteriaceae coating action of IgG, are new avenues for studies in the hope of understanding the urethral syndrome.

Tuttle and associates (1978), studying girls from 2 to 10 years of age with recurrent urinary tract infections (UTI), found a correlation between radiologic evidence of pyelonephritis and vaginal IgA deficiency. A cyclic variation of the vaginal levels of these immunoglobulins has been established. They are absent at midcycle, appear shortly after ovulation, reach a peak at the luteal phase and taper off early in the proliferative phase of the next cycle. The primary source of IgG is the secretory endometrium, whereas IgM derives from the endocervix. All three immunoglobulins have been found in the vaginal secretions of patients who have had a hysterectomy, despite the fact that the stratified squamous vaginal epithelium does not produce antibodies. Further studies are in progress to determine the source of the local antibodies in these women.

Treatment

Numerous modalities of treatment have been advocated: cranberry juice, urethral fulguration, periodic urethral dilatations, silver nitrate cauterization, and others. In reality no therapy has been consistently successful.

Zufall and Dover (1963) studied and treated 190 patients and reported that placebos were as effective as any other form of treatment.

The topical application of hexachlorophene (pHisoHex) and povidone-iodine ointment to the introitus and vestibule has been recommended in an attempt to decrease the bacterial count in these areas. Nitrofurazone (Furacin) topical ointment has been useful in reducing aerobic and anaerobic bacteria. Patients are instructed to apply the preparation at bedtime and in the morning.

Unfortunately, in a few cases the eradication of pathogens from the urethra and vestibule does not correlate with the symptomatic improvement, but the average patient reports some benefits for extended periods and remains free of symptoms for an average of 4 to 6 months with this program.

The oral administration of trimethoprim-sulfamethoxazole (TMP/SMX) or trimethoprim (TMP) alone at a dose of 100 mg. at bedtime has a salutory effect by reducing the number of pathogenic organisms in the vaginal flora without affecting the normal fecal anaerobes. The multiple modalities of treatment employed in this syndrome reflect the poor understanding of its pathophysiology and the unpredictable patterns of recurrence.

URETHRITIS

Gonococcal Urethritis

Gonorrheal urethritis is only one aspect of gonorrheal infection in the adult female. As a rule, when gonorrhea affects the urethra, all the organs of the genital tract, e.g., cervix, vagina, tubes, uterus, and Bartholin's and Skene's glands, may become involved. Ascending infection to the upper urinary tract is rare. Dysuria, frequency, urgency, and pruritus are seen, accompanied by a purulent yellowish urethral discharge. The urethral mucosa appears red and swollen and protrudes from the meatus. Likewise, Skene's and Bartholin's glands show inflammation. They are tender, and with minimal pressure an exudate can be elicited. Palpation of the urethra also produces an exudate.

Gram-stain smears will demonstrate intracellular diplococci, but documentation of the organism may require several serial cultures in special media. Serologic tests for syphilis should be done simultaneously, since both conditions coexist occasionally. Penicillin is still the treatment of choice.

Herpes Urethritis (Herpes Progenitalis)

Herpes progenitalis affects more commonly the vulva, but recently several patients have been seen in whom the initial clinical manifestation of the disease is in the urethra. Dysuria, dyspareunia, pain, and itching are the presenting symptoms. Attacks recur in about two thirds of all patients during the year after the first episode. These lesions are restricted to small vesicular, ulcerated areas, usually recurring at the same site. Inguinal lymphadenopathy is present at the first episode and is seen in about 75 per cent of recurring cases.

The disease is self-limiting, and the symptoms disappear approximately 1 week later. Vesicular fluid for inoculation and the use of fluorescent type-specific rabbit antiserum confirm the diagnosis (Chan et al., 1974). Herpesvirus type I has been frequently recovered, presumably due to the orogenital contact practiced by most of these patients. The incidence of type I progenital herpes has increased from 7 to 14 per cent over the past years and involves the cervix less often than those cases reported several years ago. Although the aspects of urethral involvement in this disease await further studies, it seems that type I virus has a predilection for the periurethral and urethral mucosas.

Chemical Urethritis

The rapidly proliferating manufacturing industries have provided the public with new lines of body-cleaning products, mainly cosmetics, soaps, deodorants, and detergents. Also available are soaps and perfume spray deodorants for feminine hygiene. Bubble bath is a well-documented source of chemical irritation and cystourethritis in little girls (Marshall, 1965). Douches have different names, colors, and odors; they also contain chemicals that irritate and dehydrate the skin and mucosa.

Some of the most irritative chemicals are derived from laundry enzymatic detergents and so-called pre-soaks. The necessary phosphates present in the pre-soak may be contaminated with arsenic; the amount of arsenic varies, depending on where the phosphates are mined. The small particles of arsenic remain on clothes and underclothes, and the repeated contact and exposure to the arsenic causes dermatitis and mucositis.

The list of cosmetics and products, including the famous deodorant-impregnated tampon, is extensive, but soaps, enzymes and deodorants are the chief offenders. Only recently has the correlation been recognized between the use of laundry detergents and body soaps and the incidence of recurrent episodes of vulvourethritis, particularly in patients who have had a complete urologic work-up with normal results and repeated urine cultures with negative findings. It is in this group of patients that a change of soaps and detergents and the omission of feminine spray deodorants should be advised. Not surprisingly, in many instances, this change has been the ideal treatment.

SPECIFIC LESIONS

Condylomata Acuminata ("Venereal Warts")

Occasionally condylomata acuminata involve the urethra. These are highly proliferative lesions, and autoinfection is the rule. Condylomata acuminata can grow in an accelerated fashion during pregnancy. Since these lesions are known to bleed easily when they are present in the genital tract and around the urethra, they can produce considerable bleeding during delivery. Therefore, it is of paramount importance to treat these lesions as early as possible. The use of 20 per cent podophyllin in benzoin tincture is recommended in the nonpregnant. To prevent the contact of the solution with the nonaffected areas of the vulva and periurethral areas, a topical solution of mineral oil is applied to the unaffected surrounding areas. For large lesions, local excision and fulguration have been employed with success.

Syphilis

Primary chancre may occur around the urethral meatus, appearing as a flat painless ulcer with sharply demarcated borders and covered by a seropurulent exudate. Painless inguinal lymphadenopathy is commonly present. The primary chancre can cause so much induration and deformity that the meatus of the urethra may be obstructed, causing secondary urinary retention.

Urethral Caruncle

This entity was first described by Sharp in 1750. There has been considerable controversy concerning the etiology, pathology, classification, and treatment of this entity.

Symptoms and Clinical Findings

Caruncle occurs only in the female urethra. Symptoms include intermittent bleeding and enlargement with secondary partial obstruction of the urethral lumen. Infrequently true hematuria is present. Characteristically the bleeding is spotty, present following friction from pads and the use of toilet tissue.

The first finding may be a small tumor mass, well-circumscribed, pedunculated, or sessile, embedded within the mucosa of the distal urethra. It has an irregular surface and a vascular consistency. Size ranges from 1 to 2 cm. (Figure 29–8).

Differential Diagnosis

The term "urethral caruncle" has been applied to a great variety of similar lesions of the distal urethra, such as polyps, papillomas, hemangiomas, and varicose veins, and in particular to the redundant or prolapsed urethral mucosa. The latter conditions are commonly seen in the postmenopausal age group and in multiparas (Palmer et al., 1948).

Marshall and associates (1960) reported 20 primary urethral meatal tumors found in

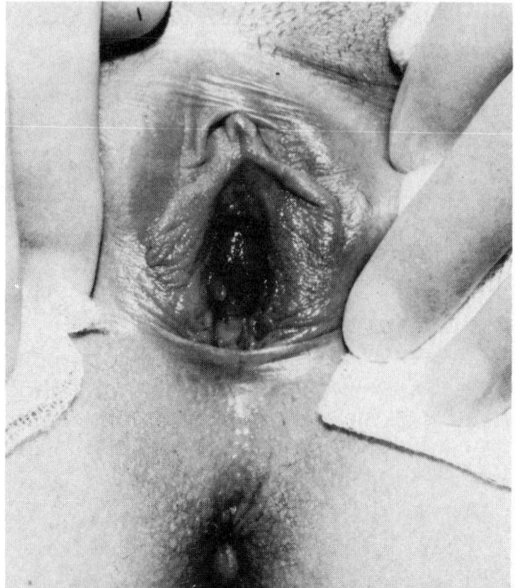

Figure 29–8. Urethral caruncle. Observe the sharply demarcated margins of this lesion as it protrudes from the urethral meatus. The gross appearance of this benign lesion has marked similarities to that of neoplastic processes. In this case, excisional biopsy and microscopic examination confirmed the clinical diagnosis.

394 women operated on for caruncle. In nine patients the lesions were malignant, mainly carcinoma in situ and urothelial neoplasms.

Urethral carcinoma may be grossly indistinguishable from urethral caruncle, particularly in the early stages. The age incidence of carcinoma of the urethra is the same, and the final differential diagnosis requires microscopic confirmation.

Hemangiomas (Figure 29–9), adenomas, and polyps (Figure 29–10) of the urethra are uncommon. For caruncles, excisional biopsy for histologic confirmation of the nature of the lesion is advised.

Treatment

Surgical excision of the caruncle and approximation of the uninvolved urethral mucosa with fine catgut is the treatment of choice. Fulguration of the lesion is not advocated because of the incidence of recurrence, bleeding, and late sloughing of tissue, but most importantly because the only opportunity to identify clearly the nature of this lesion histologically would be hampered by the electrocauterization.

Following excision, a Foley catheter is left indwelling for 24 to 48 hours; subsequently the patient usually voids without further problems. Sitz baths give some symptomatic relief in the weeks following surgery.

After removal of the caruncle, the patient requires no further treatment.

Periurethral Abscess

Periurethral abscess may be present in conjunction with inflammation of the paraurethral glands or Skene's ducts, occluding these glandular orifices by thick inspissated secretions (Figure 29–11). Gonococcal skenitis is not uncommon, but other organisms have been isolated from these glands. Incision and drainage, sitz baths, or electrocoagulation of the involved glands may be necessary as the ultimate treatment to control infection.

URETHRAL TRAUMA

Traumatic injuries to the female urethra are rare because of its privileged protected position underneath the pubic symphysis and on the anterior wall of the vagina. Tears by bone fragments of crushed pelvis resulting from automobile, snowmobile, and motorcycle accidents are the most commonly seen. More rarely, traumatic intercourse and the introduction of foreign bodies for erotic stimulation are responsible for a small number of cases of urethral trauma. In the case of automobile or straddle injury, when extensive hematomas are present and multiple injuries represent a serious threat to the life of the patient, initial management is limited to diverting the urine from the urethra via suprapubic catheter drainage for 12 weeks prior to performing further endoscopic studies and attempting any plastic reconstruction.

URETHRAL PROLAPSE

Over 400 cases of urethral prolapse in females have been reported (Klaus and Stein, 1973; Turner, 1973). Over 50 per cent have been found in girls under 18 years of

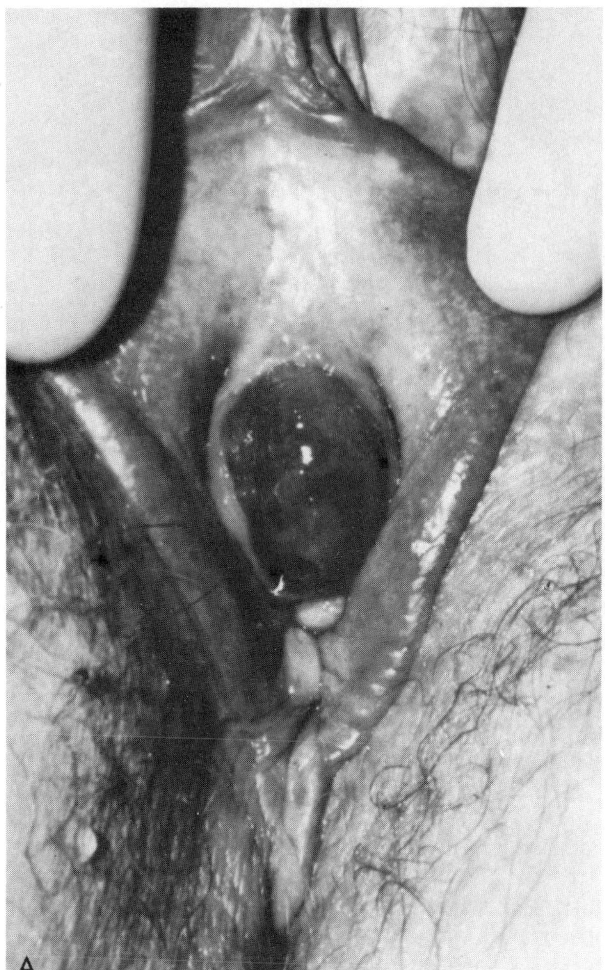

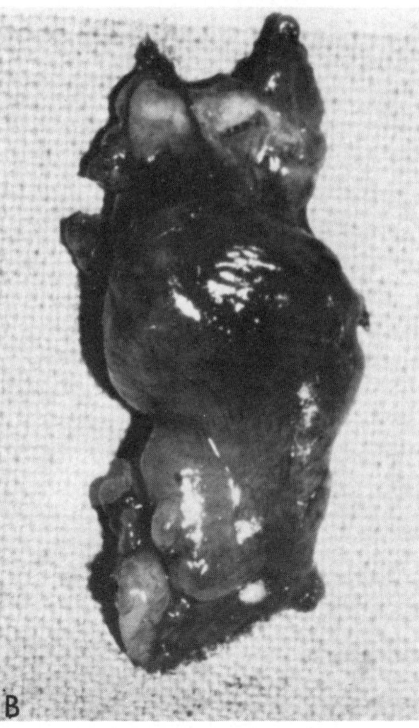

Figure 29–9. *A,* Intermittent bleeding and stranguria were caused by this 4 × 3 cm. hemangioma of the urethra. *B,* The surgical specimen removed "en bloc." A vaginal urethroplasty was performed. Microscopic sections confirmed the nature of this lesion as a benign hemangioma. In this case, no further treatment was required.

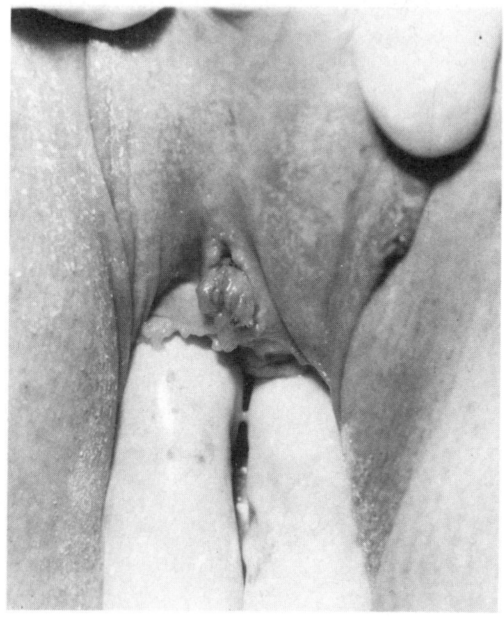

Figure 29–10. Polyp protruding from the urethral meatus. Dysuria and spotty bleeding were this patient's complaints.

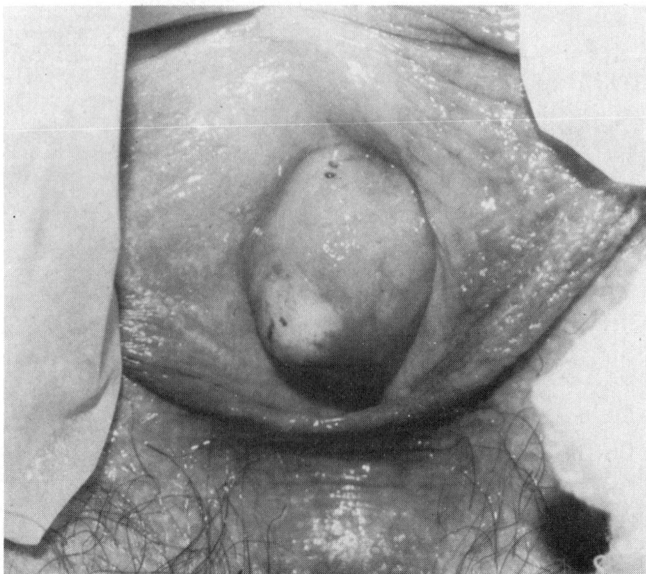

Figure 29–11. Large Skene's gland abscess obstructing the urethral meatus. Bacteriologic studies showed this lesion was due to gonococcal skenitis.

age. This condition is seen more often in the black population. The common presenting symptoms and findings include mild vaginal bleeding, painless vaginal mass (Figure 29–12), hematuria, and dysuria. The etiologic factors are unknown. Stress, coughing, and Valsalva-like maneuvers have been hypothesized. Vaginoscopy is necessary to exclude tumors such as botryoid sarcoma. The differential diagnosis includes polyps, condyloma, cysts, periurethral abscess, and granuloma. Biopsy is required if there is any doubt about the nature of the lesion.

Surgical excision of the redundant prolapsed urethra and suturing of the urethral mucosa to the vaginal vestibule is the treatment of choice (Figure 29–13). Mild and incomplete forms of prolapsed urethra require no surgical treatment (Figure 29–14).

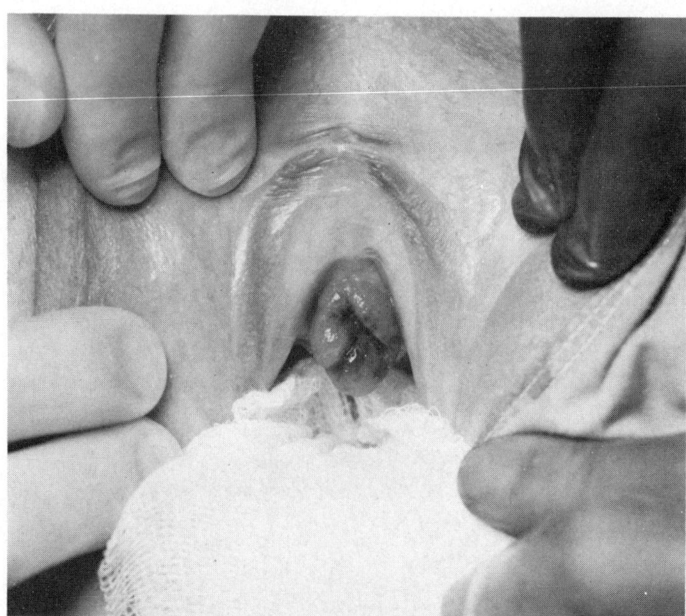

Figure 29–12. Urethral prolapse. Observe the ischemic changes present in this edematous urethral mucosa, particularly on the anterior portion of the prolapsed lesion.

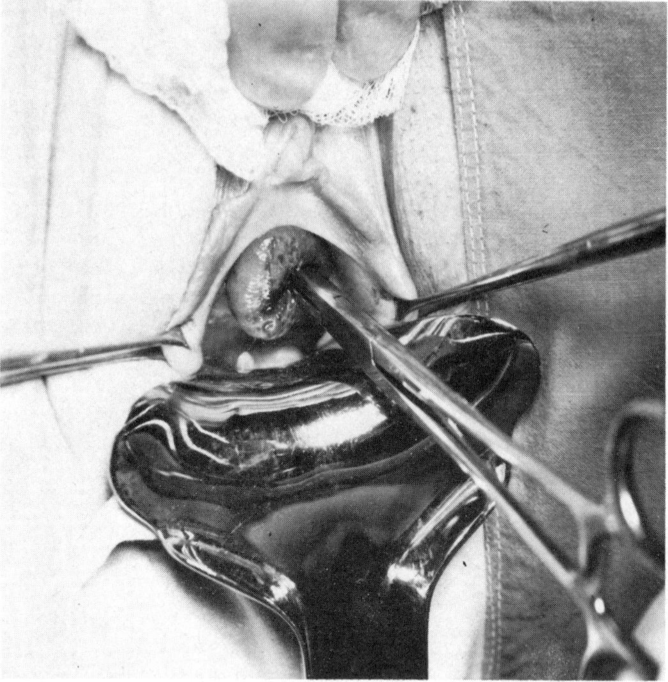

Figure 29–13. Complete prolapse of the urethra. The redundant urethral prolapse was excised, and the fresh edges of the mucosa were sutured to form a new meatus. Illustrated here is the prolapsed urethra prior to its excision.

URETHRAL DIVERTICULUM

Female urethral diverticulum is a rather common entity, having been reported in 3 to 4 per cent of studies by pressure urethrography. The age distribution varies from 20 to 60 years, but it occurs more frequently in the fourth decade and is more common in blacks than in whites, with a ratio of 6:1 (Andersen, 1967).

Etiology

Urethral diverticulum has been reported sporadically in children. Because of this early appearance in life, it has been classified as either congenital or acquired.

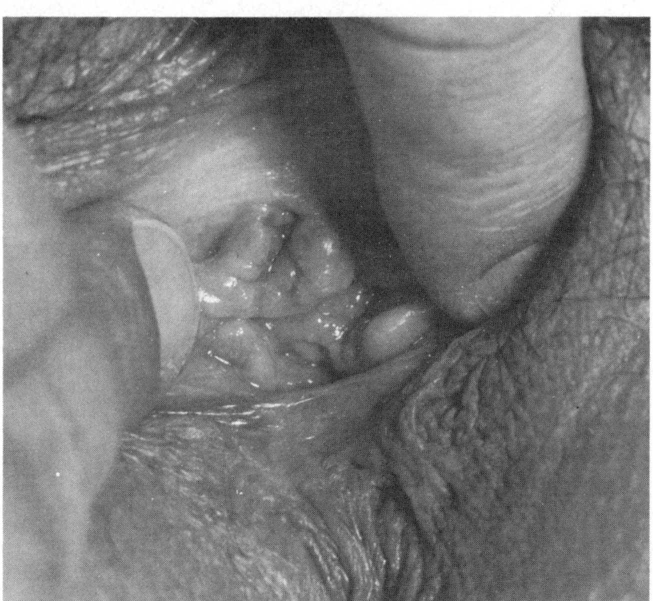

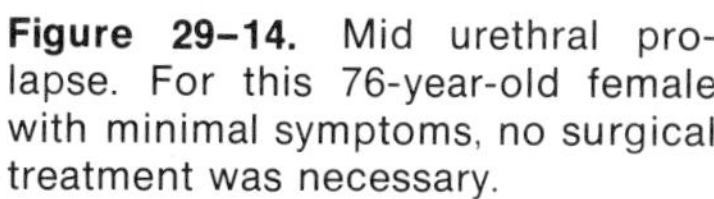

Figure 29–14. Mid urethral prolapse. For this 76-year-old female with minimal symptoms, no surgical treatment was necessary.

Congenital. Documenting the congenital etiology of a urethral diverticulum is a difficult if not impossible task, but the following findings are of interest in this regard. Moore (1952) reported an ectopic right ureter emptying into a urethral diverticulum. Hinman (1963) described a case of Gartner's duct carcinoma (wolffian duct derivative) in a urethral diverticulum. Benjamin and co-workers (1974) reported two patients with diverticula containing cloacogenic rests. Moreover, in our institution one patient with such a histologic aberration embedded in the cystic wall of the urethral diverticulum has been seen and treated surgically.

Acquired. The vast majority of diverticula of the female urethra are acquired. They are the result of repeated infections of the paraurethral glands, leading to subsequent inflammation, irritation, and obstruction, and finally the development of cystic enlargements of the intraepithelial glands and formation of small submucosal lacunae.

In the early part of this century, it was postulated that during parturition, pressure of the fetal head on the dorsal urethral wall ruptured the muscle layers at this level, with consequent weakness and herniation of the urethral mucosa and diverticulum formation. Although this seems possible, there are as many urethral diverticula seen in nulliparas as there are in patients who have one or more deliveries or have had all their deliveries via cesarean section. Moreover, recent evidence obtained through urethral pressure studies suggests that without distal obstruction, outpouching of the urethral mucosa into a diverticulum appears unlikely, even in the light of minor trauma to the outer muscle layers.

Retention Cysts

Routh in 1890 noted that the urethral glands may become retention cysts by obstruction of their orifices as a result of repeated episodes of urethritis or periurethritis. The inflamed cyst ruptures and opens into the urethra, and the "mouth" or opening epithelializes, resulting in continuity between the sac and the urethral lumen. Urine finds access to the diverticular cavity at each voiding. Because of the lack of muscle in the diverticular sac, its contents remain stagnant; with time the cavity increases in size.

Stone Formation

Urethral diverticula are usually located in the middle third of the urethra and directed dorsolaterally. Stone formation within the sac of the diverticulum has been the subject of reports in the literature (Hunner, 1938; Presman et al., 1964). These patients present with a hard palpable mass on the anterior vaginal wall. Stasis of urine, infection, and occasional mucoid desquamation of the epithelial lining in the diverticulum provide ideal conditions for stone formation in these patients.

Symptoms

Symptoms range from minimal local discomfort to the classic "three D's" of diverticula: dribbling, dyspareunia, and dysuria. Dribbling has been seen in a large number of patients.

Diagnosis

The lack of awareness of this entity has resulted in many patients being classified as "neurotics," mentally unstable, and so forth. Because a routine urologic evaluation, which includes urinalysis, culture, and sensitivity, intravenous pyelography and cystoscopy, is not per se diagnostic for urethral diverticulum, normal findings are accumulated through this battery of tests without arriving at the diagnosis. For example, an intravenous pyelogram without a voiding urethrogram and a post-void film is of little help, and, unfortunately, a large number of female patients undergoing intravenous pyelography do not routinely receive the benefits of a post-void film. Moreover, Houser and VonEschenbach (1974) encountered filling of contrast material within the diverticulum in about 70 per cent of the patients with this defect who had a post-void film during the excretory urogram. Cystoscopy alone has no place in the diagnosis of urethral diverticulum, and urethroscopy has relatively little value, since in most instances the neck of the diverticulum is collapsed, and the entire length of the urethra cannot be adequately distended with the irrigant solution in order to visualize the sac.

Other diagnostic methods have been advocated for the localization of the diverticulum:

1. Compression on the anterior vaginal wall to empty the diverticulum; with catheterization of the bladder and instillation of 5 ml. of indigo carmine and 60 to 80 ml. of contrast medium through a Foley catheter. The catheter is removed and the patient is instructed to void, occluding the meatus with one finger. Upon voiding, the diverticulum should fill with the solution. At this point x-rays in the anteroposterior and both oblique projections are obtained. This is followed by urethroscopy; the blue dye should be seen in the mouth of the diverticulum (Borski and Stutzman, 1965).

2. Catheterization with a Davis-TeLinde catheter, which is a double balloon urethral catheter with a hole between the balloons. The balloon closer to the meatus is adjustable in order to tamponade the meatus. Contrast material when injected should distend the entire length of the urethra and thus fill the diverticulum. Appropriate x-ray films are then obtained (Figure 29–15) (Davis and TeLinde, 1958).

3. Voiding cystourethrography, using 25 per cent aqueous barium sulfate suspension (previously autoclaved). This has proved to be an adequate medium, which distends and fills the diverticulum better than the more aqueous contrast medium solutions.

Treatment

The multiplicity of procedures to correct this entity is an indication of the controversies and intense interest in the adequate treatment of this condition. They all attempt to minimize the two most dreaded surgical complications, urinary incontinence and urethrovaginal fistula.

Furniss (1935), through a vaginal approach, incised the diverticulum with electrocoagulation and packed it with gauze. A second stage required the closure of the urethrovaginal fistula created by the first procedure. Hunner in 1938 passed sounds through the urethra into the diverticulum, excising it transvaginally. Later he modified this procedure by using a vaginal flap,

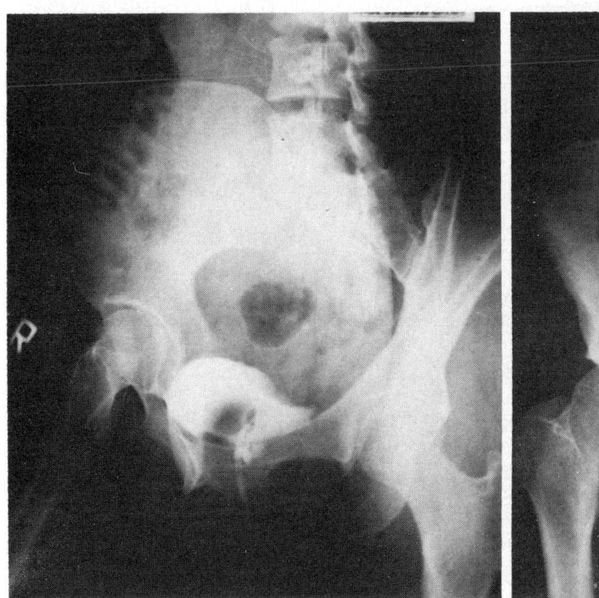

A

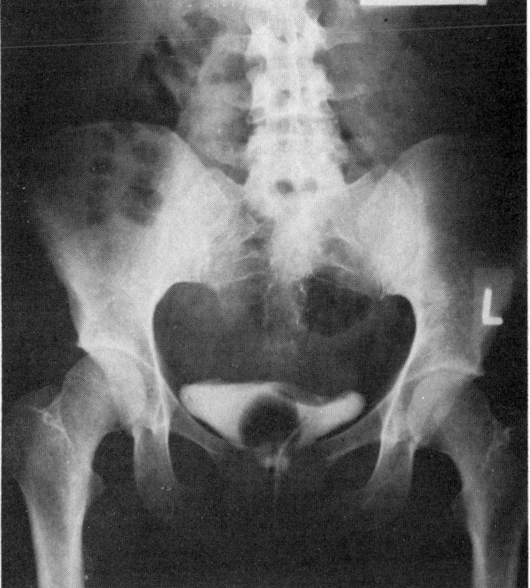

B

Figure 29–15. Cystogram (*A*) and urethrogram (*B*) obtained with a Davis–TeLinde catheter (double balloon), demonstrating a urethral diverticulum. The oblique projection reveals the contrast material distal to the bladder neck and the proximal two thirds of the urethra; the same diverticulum could easily have been missed in an anterior projection.

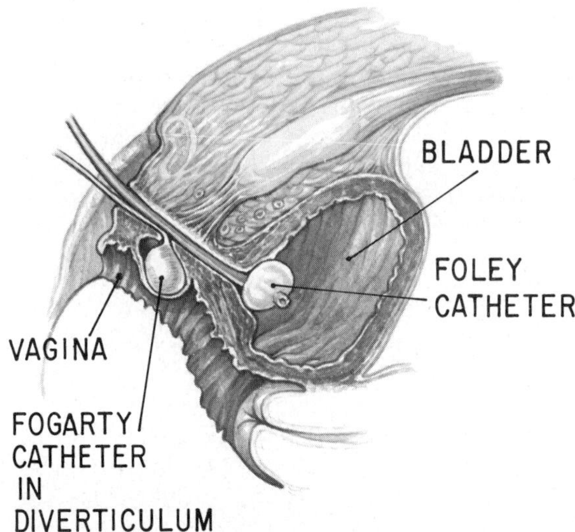

Figure 29-16. Fogarty catheter inserted in the urethral diverticulum and Foley catheter in the bladder. The placement of these catheters facilitates excision of the diverticulum.

taking care that the suture lines were not superimposed.

Hyams and Hyams (1939) packed the diverticulum transurethrally with gauze; with this maneuver they believed that transvaginal excision was facilitated. Cook and Pool (1949) placed a coiling catheter transurethrally to fill the diverticular sac instead of gauze. Moore (1952) exposed the diverticulum transvaginally, creating a small vent in the diverticular sac. A Foley catheter was then placed, and with the aid of an inflated balloon, the sac was better outlined and thus more easily excised.

Ellik (1957) cautioned in regard to the management of diverticula close to the trigone. He recommended a transvaginal excision and packed the cavity with Oxycel, to promote secondary healing by fibrosis. Spence and Duckett (1970) marsupialized the sac of the diverticulum and sutured its wall to the vaginal mucosa but failed to discuss in the description the management of secondary urethral vaginal fistulas that could result from this procedure. Flocks and Culp (1975) emphasized the importance of the identification of the neck of the diverticulum and championed a multilayer

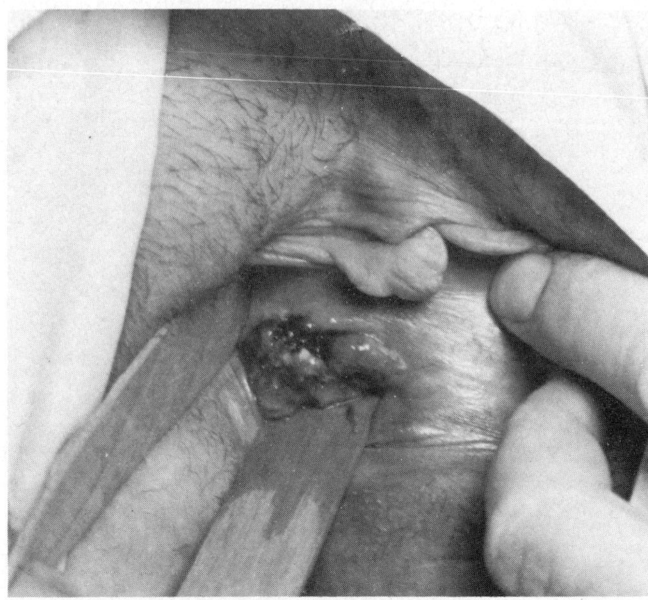

Figure 29-17. Invasive squamous cell carcinoma of the urethra, causing obstruction of the urethral meatus.

closure, avoiding the overlapping of suture lines.

More recently a Fogarty catheter has been placed into the diverticulum prior to surgery, the balloon inflated and a Foley catheter inserted per urethra into the bladder. Surgical excision of the diverticulum is thus facilitated by the easy identification of the sac distended by the Fogarty catheter balloon (Figure 29–16).

NEOPLASMS OF THE URETHRA

Primary Carcinoma

Primary carcinoma of the female urethra constitutes 0.017 per cent of all gynecologic neoplasms (Blath and Boehm, 1973; Desai et al., 1973). Reported cure rates of the diseases have varied, with 5-year survival rates of 20 to 45 per cent.

This entity may be divided into two categories: (1) by cell origin and (2) by clinical stage. Accordingly, epidermoid carcinoma is the most common type seen in the anterior urethra (Figure 29–17). Transitional cell carcinoma is most commonly present in the proximal urethra. Adenocarcinoma (Figure 29–18) represents 12 to 20 per cent of all cases. Lymphoma, sarcoma, melanoma, and the undifferentiated types account for the remainder of the lesions found.

Classification and Staging

The classification of Chau and Green (1965) allows for staging of the disease based on the local extension and metastatic involvement of the neoplasm.

Stage I. Disease limited to the distal one half of the urethra.

Stage II. Disease involving the entire urethra with periurethral extension, but *not* involving vulva or bladder neck.

Stage III. A. Disease involving urethra and vulva.
B. Disease invading vaginal mucosa (Figure 29–19).
C. Disease involving urethra and bladder neck.

Stage IV. A. Disease involving parametrium and/or paracolpium.

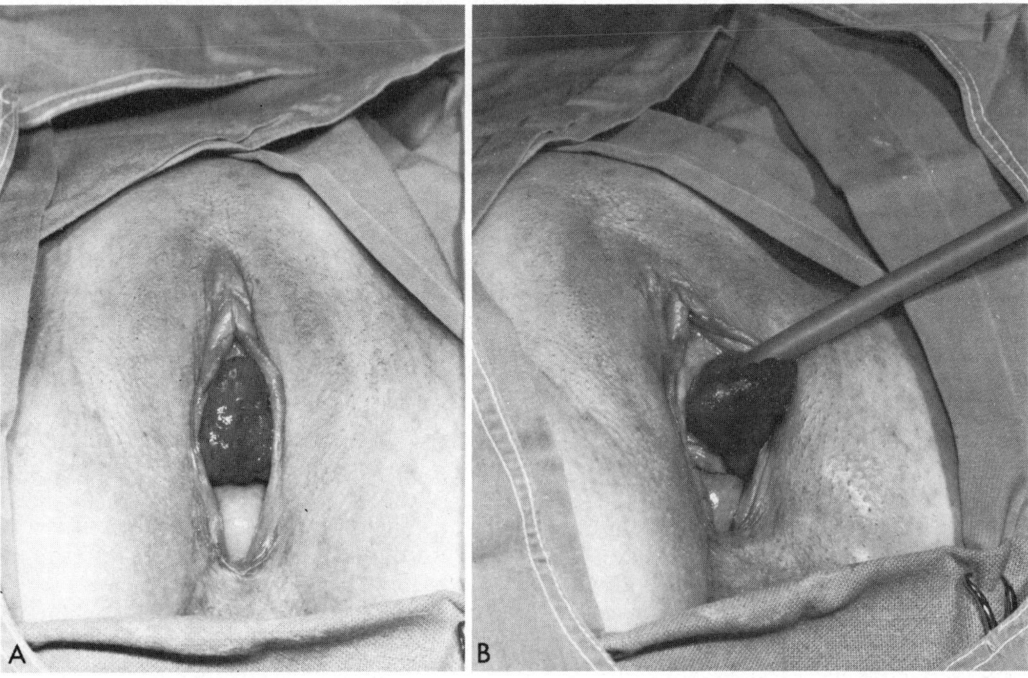

Figure 29–18. *A*, Adenocarcinoma of the urethra with extensive involvement of the vestibule and vagina. *B*, A Foley catheter has been placed into the urethra and bladder prior to the en-bloc removal of this lesion.

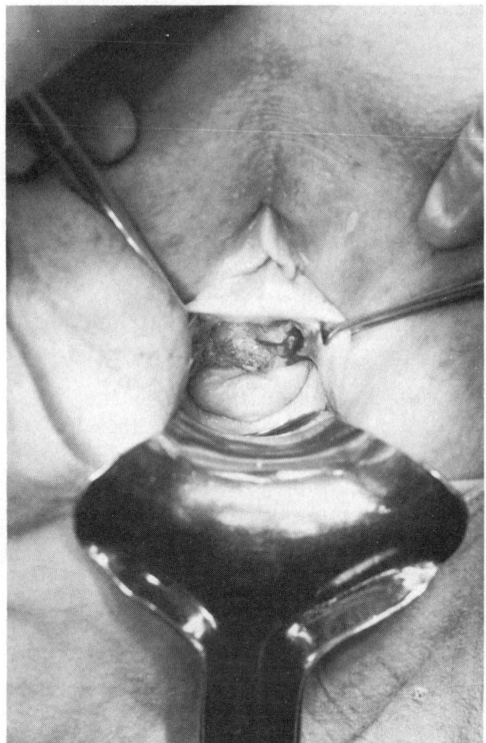

Figure 29–19. Squamous cell carcinoma of the urethra invading the introitus in a 62-year-old patient.

B. Metastatic:
1. Inguinal lymph nodes.
2. Pelvic nodes.
3. Para-aortic nodes.
4. Distant.

Symptoms

Urinary symptoms are the most common initially. Vaginal bleeding is usually present sometime during the course of the disease. Dysuria is conspicuously present in over two thirds of patients. Overflow or stress incontinence has been the presenting symptom in over 25 per cent of patients.

Diagnosis

The initial diagnosis and staging of the disease depend exclusively on a thorough pelvic examination. Once the lesion is identified, histologic diagnosis is of paramount importance. It allows estimation of the depth of invasion, determination of the histology of the disease, and judicious planning of subsequent therapy. Epidermoid carcinoma has less tendency to invade the urethra but commonly metastasizes to inguinal nodes. Transitional cell carcinoma has a tendency to infiltrate the periurethral tissues and metastasize to the iliac chain.

Treatment

Because of the location of the lesion and the fact that carcinoma of the urethra is most commonly seen in the sixth decade and usually involves the vagina, attempts should be made to preserve the anatomy and urinary continence. Therefore, a nonsurgical approach utilizing both radium needle implants and external radiation therapy has gained popularity. Staubitz and co-workers (1955) reported a 28 per cent 5-year cure rate in all stages using interstitial irradiation alone.

Radical anterior exenteration with supravesical urinary diversion and radiation therapy has been championed by Grabstald (1973). Utilizing this combined surgery-radiotherapy approach, a 20 per cent overall 5-year cure rate has been achieved.

Prempree and co-workers (1978) treated 16 patients utilizing radium implants with a dose range of 5500 to 6500 rads in stages I to III; external whole pelvis irradiation (5000 to 8500 rads) followed by radium implants was utilized in the patients with more advanced disease. With these modalities of therapy, excellent local control was reported in stage I disease (anterior urethra), with survival with NED (no evidence of disease) ranging from 2 to 10 years. Three patients with stage IIIA/III B so treated survived 3 to 5 years.

When a combination of external and interstitial radiation was used in more advanced cases, local control was adequate with 50 per cent of the patients exhibiting an objective response of the primary lesion.

At this time it is impossible to determine the superiority of any single method. Regardless of the modality of therapy employed, responses are most favorable when the lesion is confined to the distal part of the urethra, with 5-year survival rates in the range of 50 to 55 per cent, compared with a 9 per cent 5-year survival rate when the lesion involves the entire urethra.

With chemotherapeutic agents such as doxorubicin hydrochloride (Adriamycin), bleomycin, and 5-(3,3-dimethyl-1-triazeno)

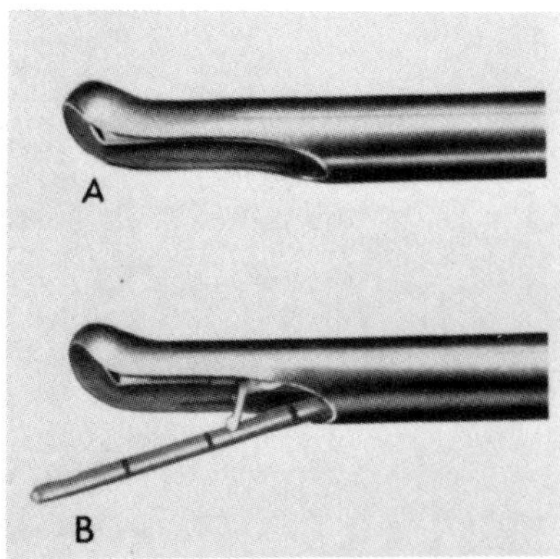

Figure 29–20. *A,* Fenestra at end of cystourethroscopic sheath. *B,* Deflector and catheter within sheath. (From Greene, L. F., and Khan, A. U.: Cystourethroscopy in the female. Urology *10*:461, 1977. Reproduced by permission.)

imidazole-4-carboxamide (DTIC), which have demonstrated activity against some solid tumors and melanomas, the addition of these agents as adjuvants to radiation therapy and surgery in patients with advanced disease should improve the current dismal prognosis for patients with urethral carcinoma.

Secondary Involvement

Secondary malignant involvement of the female urethra is seen infrequently. Sources include adenocarcinoma of the endometrium, transitional cell carcinoma of the urinary bladder, and squamous cell carcinoma at the vulvovaginal areas. Treatment is that of the primary tumor.

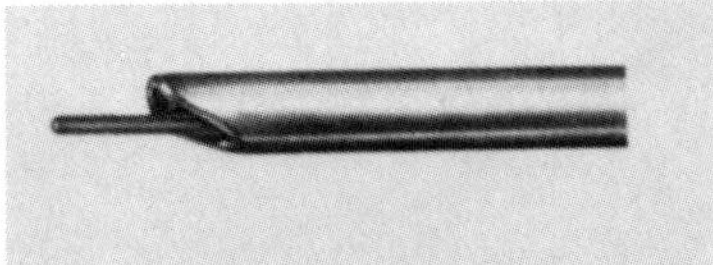

Figure 29–22. Short-beaked urethrocystoscope with ureteral catheter. (From Greene, L. F., and Khan, A. U.: Cystourethroscopy in the female. Urology *10*:461, 1977. Reproduced by permission.)

URETHROSCOPY IN WOMEN

Urethroscopy, an integral part of cystoscopy, is the best method for detecting urethral lesions such as urethritis, fistulas, diverticula, strictures, carcinoma, and ureters that open into the urethra. It is desirable, therefore, that cystoscopes employed for examination of the bladder permit adequate examination of the urethra (Greene and Khan, 1977).

Unfortunately, the urethra of women cannot be examined satisfactorily with the newer cystourethroscopes routinely employed. This derives from the fact that a fenestra is situated on the terminal portion of the sheath to permit use of a deflector (Figure 29–20). The fenestra of the cystoscope of one manufacturer is 27 mm. long and the female urethra is approximately 35 mm. long. Consequently, when urethroscopy is attempted during either introduc-

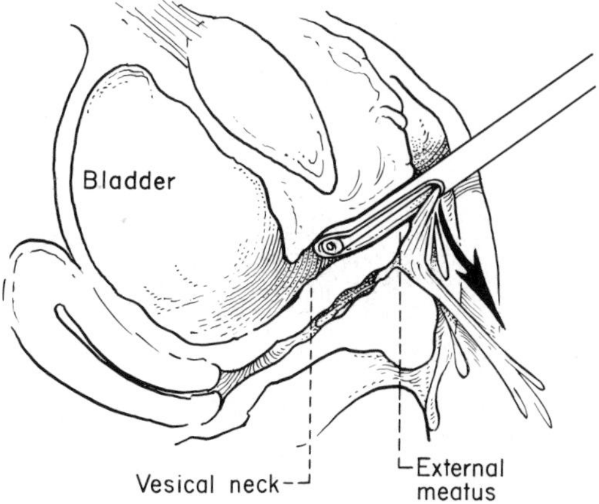

Figure 29–21. Escape of irrigant prevents distension of urethra. (From Greene, L. F., and Khan, A. U.: Cystourethroscopy in the female. Urology *10*:461, 1977. Reproduced by permission.)

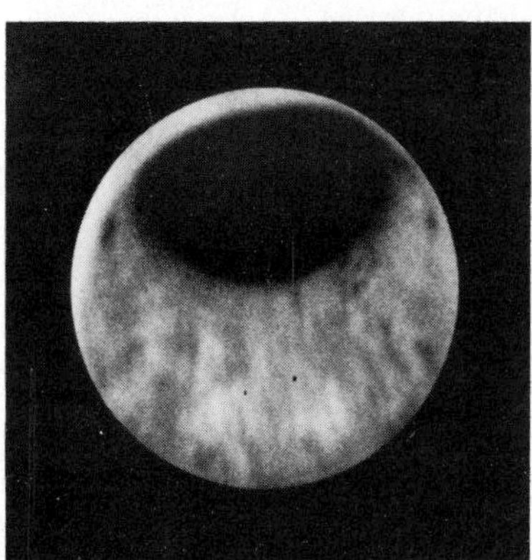

Figure 29–23. Urethrocystoscopic view of distended urethra. (From Greene, L. F., and Khan, A. U.: Cystourethroscopy in the female. Urology *10*:461, 1977. Reproduced by permission.)

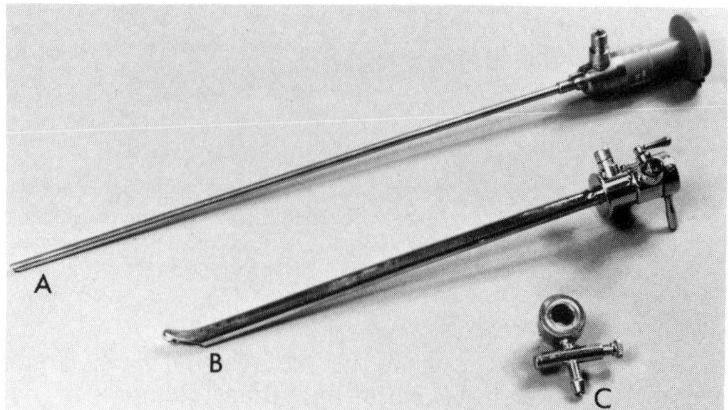

Figure 29–24. Cystourethroscope. *A*, Telescope. *B*, Sheath that carries fiberoptic bundle. *C*, Window. (American Cystoscope Makers, Inc.) (From Greene, L. F., and Khan, A. U.: Cystourethroscopy in the female. Urology *10*:461, 1977. Reproduced by permission.)

tion or withdrawal of the cystoscope, the irrigant escapes around the external meatus and makes distention of the urethra impossible (Figure 29–21). The walls of the urethra then collapse around the objective end of the telescope, and visualization is obscured because the objective image plane is out of the focal plane of the remainder of the optic system.

These instruments permit satisfactory urethroscopic examination of the vesical neck and proximal one fifth of the urethra because the entire fenestra is within the urethra and the urethra can be distended. The terminal four fifths of the female urethra cannot be adequately examined, however, and lesions contained therein may be overlooked. Likewise, lesions in the distal 27 mm. of the male urethra may be missed.

Urethrocystoscopes constructed with short oblique beaks are available (Figure 29–22). Such instruments distend the urethra and permit excellent urethroscopy (Figure 29–23). These sheaths accept right-angle, foroblique, and direct telescopes and thereby permit excellent cystoscopy. Based on discussions with many urologists and with representatives of cystoscope manufacturers, however, it is my impression that such urethrocystoscopes are seldom used. If a urethrocystoscope is not available a short-beaked resectoscope sheath is an acceptable substitute.

A cystoscope designed according to my specifications affords excellent visualization of the bladder and urethra (Figure 29–24). With this instrument the bladder is examined with the customary right-angle and foroblique fiberoptic telescopes. In addition, the sheath carries its own fiberoptic light bundle that permits direct inspection of the bladder and urethra through a window without the use of telescopes. The urethra distends and excellent urethroscopy is possible. Using this cystoscope I have easily detected urethral fistulas, diverticula, and ectopic ureters that could not be visualized with conventional cystourethroscopes despite an awareness of the presence of such lesions.

REFERENCES

Andersen, M. J. F.: The incidence of diverticula in the female urethra. J. Urol. *98*:96, 1967.

Benjamin, J., Elliot, L., Cooper, J. F., et al.: Urethral diverticulum in the adult female. Urology *3*:1, 1974.

Blath, R. A., and Boehm, F. F.: Carcinoma of the female urethra. Surg. Gynecol. Obstet. *136*:574, 1973.

Borski, A. A., and Stutzman, R. E.: Diverticulum of female urethra: a simplified diagnostic aid. J. Urol. *93*:60, 1965.

Bruce, A. W., Chadwick, P., Hassan, A., et al.: Recurrent urethritis in women. Can. Med. Assoc. J. *108*:973, 1973.

Chan, T. W., Fiumara, N. J., and Weinstein, L.: Genital herpes: some clinical and laboratory observations. J.A.M.A. *229*:544, 1974.

Chau, P. M., and Green, A. E.: Radiotherapeutic management of malignant tumors of the vagina. Progr. Clin. Cancer *1*:728, 1965.

Cook, E. N., and Pool, T. L.: Urethral diverticulum in the female. J. Urol. *62*:495, 1949.

Davis, H. J., and TeLinde, R. W.: Urethral diverticulum: an assay of 121 cases. J. Urol. *80*:34, 1958.

Desai, S., Libertino, J. A., and Zinman, L.: Primary carcinoma of the female urethra. J. Urol. *110*:693, 1973.

Elkins, I. B., and Cox, C. E.: Perineal, vaginal and urethral bacteriology of young women: I. Incidence of gram-negative colonization. J. Urol. *111*:88, 1974.

Ellik, M.: Diverticulum of the female urethra: a new method of ablation. J. Urol *77*:243, 1957.

Fair, W. R., Timothy, M. M., Millar, M. A., et al.: Bacteriologic and hormonal observations of the urethra and vaginal vestibule in normal, premenopausal women. J. Urol. *104*:426, 1970.

Flocks, R. H., and Culp, D. A.: Surgical Urology. 4th Ed. Chicago, Year Book Medical Publishers, 1975.

Furniss, H. D.: Diverticulum in the female urethra. Am. J. Surg. *28*:177, 1935.

Grabstald, H.: Tumors of the urethra in men and women. Cancer *32*:123, 1973.

Greene, L. F., and Khan, A. U.: Cystourethroscopy in the female. Urology *10*:461, 1977.

Hinman, F., Jr.: Gartner's duct carcinoma in a urethral diverticulum. J. Urol. *83*:414, 1973.

Houser, L. M., II, and VonEschenbach, A. C.: Diverticula of the female urethra: diagnostic importance of post-voiding film. Urology *3*:453, 1974.

Huffman, John W.: The detailed anatomy of the paraurethral ducts in the adult human female. Am. J. Obstet. Gynecol. *55*:86, 1948.

Hunner, G. L.: A calculus formation in a urethral diverticulum in women. Urol. Cutan. Rev. *42*:336, 1938.

Hyams, J. A., and Hyams, M. N.: A new operative procedure for the treatment of diverticulum of the female urethra. J. Urol. *43*:573, 1939.

Immergut, M., Culp, D. A., and Flocks, R. H.: The urethral caliber in normal female children. Trans. Am. Assoc. Genitourin. Surg. *58*:25, 1966.

Klaus, H., and Stein, R. T.: Urethral prolapse in young girls. Pediatrics *52*:645, 1973.

Krantz, K. E.: The anatomy of the urethra and the anterior vaginal wall. Am. J. Obstet Gynecol. *62*:374, 1951.

Lyon, R. P., and Smith, D. R.: Distal urethral stenosis. J. Urol. *89*:414, 1963.

Marshall, F. C., Uson, A. C., and Melicow, M. M.: Neoplasms and caruncles of the female urethra. Surg. Gynecol. Obstet. *110*:723, 1960.

Marshall, S.: The effect of bubble bath on the urinary tract. J. Urol. *93*:112, 1965.

Moore, T. D.: Diverticula of the female urethra: an improved technique of surgical excision. J. Urol. *68*:611, 1952.

Muecke, E. C., and Marshall, V. F.: Subsymphyseal epispadias in the female patient. J. Urol. *99*:622, 1968.

Palmer, J. K., Emmett, J. L., and MacDonald, J. R.: Urethral caruncle. Surg. Gynecol. Obstet. *87*:611, 1948.

Parsons, C. L., Stauffer, C., and Schmidt, J. D.: Impairment of antibacterial effect of bladder surface mucin by protamine sulfate. J. Infect. Dis. *144*:180, 1981.

Prempree, T., Wizenberg, M. J., and Scott, R. M.: Radiation treatment of primary carcinoma of the female urethra. Cancer *42*:1177, 1978.

Presman, D., Rolnick, D., and Zumerchek, J.: Calculus formation within a diverticulum of the female urethra. J. Urol. *91*:376, 1964.

Spence, H., and Duckett, J. W., Jr.: Diverticulum of the female urethra: clinical aspects and presentation of a simple operative technique for cure. J. Urol. *104*:432, 1970.

Stamey, T. A., Timothy, M., Millar, M., et al.: Recurrent urinary infections in adult women: the role of introital enterobacteria. Calif. Med. *115*:1, 1971.

Stamm, W. E., Wagner, K. F., Amsel, R., et al.: Causes of the acute urethral syndrome in women. N. Engl. J. Med. *303*:409, 1980.

Staubitz, W. J., Garden, L. M., Oberkircher, L. J., et al.: Management of urethral carcinoma in the female. J. Urol. *73*:1045, 1955.

Turner, R. W.: Urethral prolapse in female children. Urology *2*:530, 1973.

Tuttle, J. P., Jr., Sarvas, H., and Koistinen, J.: The role of vaginal immunoglobulin A in girls with recurrent urinary tract infections. J. Urol. *120*:742, 1978.

Walker, D., and Richard, G. A.: Critical evaluation of urethral obstruction in female children. Pediatrics *51*:272, 1973.

Zufall, R., and Dover, N. J.: Treatment of urethral syndrome in women. J.A.M.A. *184*:138, 1963.

SECTION

5

URINARY TRACT IN PREGNANCY

30

MORPHOLOGIC CHANGES IN PREGNANCY

R. M. PITKIN, M.D.

The genital and urinary tracts, on the basis of their common embryologic origin, are intimately related when development is complete. In view of this anatomic proximity, it is hardly surprising that conditions affecting one system usually exert some kind of influence on the other. In particular, pregnancy (the most common genital tract "condition") is associated with substantial morphologic change in the urinary tract.

RENAL PELVIS AND URETER

Dilatation of the renal pelves and ureters represents the most striking morphologic

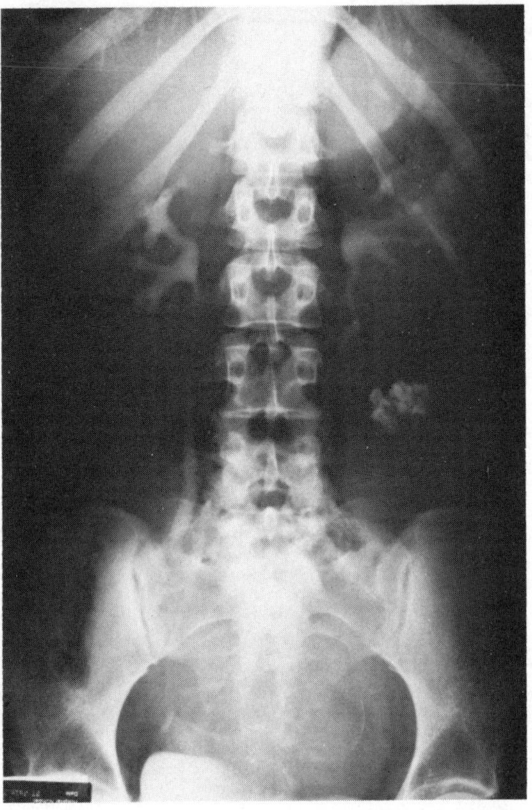

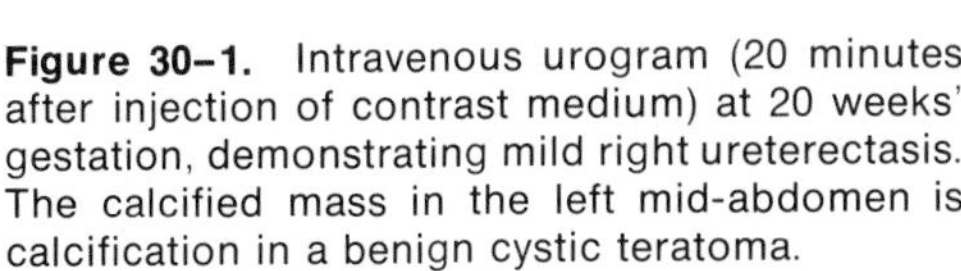

Figure 30–1. Intravenous urogram (20 minutes after injection of contrast medium) at 20 weeks' gestation, demonstrating mild right ureterectasis. The calcified mass in the left mid-abdomen is calcification in a benign cystic teratoma.

change in the urinary tract related to pregnancy. First recognized in autopsy studies well over a century ago, the effect has since been confirmed repeatedly by anatomic and roentgenographic techniques. The term "physiologic hydronephrosis and hydroureter of pregnancy" has been applied widely, emphasizing both the frequency of the changes and their apparent normality.

Characteristics of Pyeloureteral Dilatation

Studies employing intravenous urography have generally indicated that pyeloureteral dilatation appears abruptly at approximately 20 weeks' gestation (Figure 30–1), and both the incidence and severity remain essentially constant from then until term (Schulman and Herlinger, 1975). As illustrated in Figure 30–2, the change typically involves the renal pelvis and upper two thirds of the ureter (i.e., above the brim of the bony pelvis), whereas the pelvic ureter is involved rarely if at all (Dure-Smith, 1970; Harrow et al., 1964; Schulman and Herlinger, 1975). Relatively rapid postpartum resolution is the rule, with most of the changes returning toward normal within 24 to 48 hours after delivery (Figure 30–3), although several weeks may be required for complete resolution (Harrow et al., 1964).

Recent studies utilizing ultrasonic measurement of the kidney and renal pelvis have suggested a somewhat different pattern of onset and progression from that based on earlier radiographic studies. Fried (1979) investigated a large number of asymptomatic gravidas at various stages of gestation and his observations, summarized in Table 30–1, indicate an onset during the first trimester in a substantial proportion and a tendency to increasing severity with progressing gestation.

A major characteristic of pyeloureteral dilatation is the preponderance of right-sided involvement (Figure 30–4). Schulman and Herlinger (1975) examined intravenous urograms of 200 patients in the last half of pregnancy and noted the right side to be fuller than the left in 85.7 per cent, compared with only 10 per cent in which the left

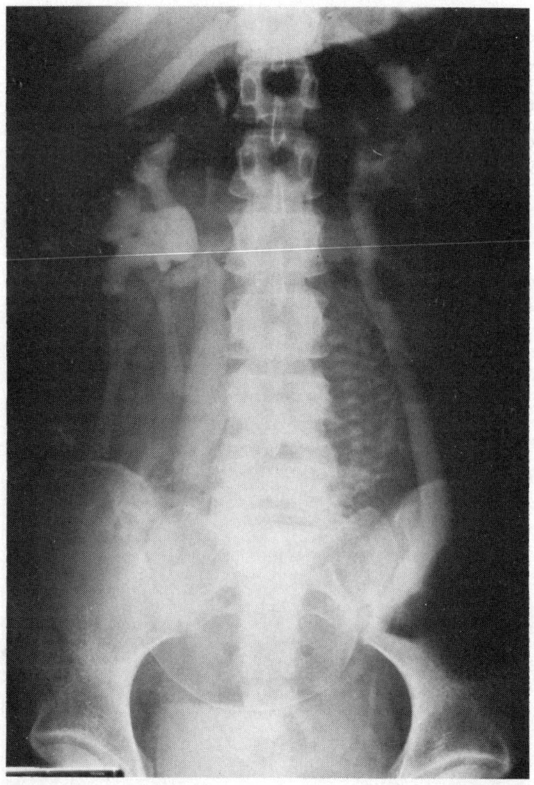

Figure 30–2. Intravenous urogram (20 minutes after injection of contrast medium) at 34 weeks' gestation, with fetal head in the pelvis, demonstrating marked bilateral pyeloureterectasis, "ureteral kinking," and lateral displacement of the left ureter. The radiopaque material in the colon is from a previous cholecystogram.

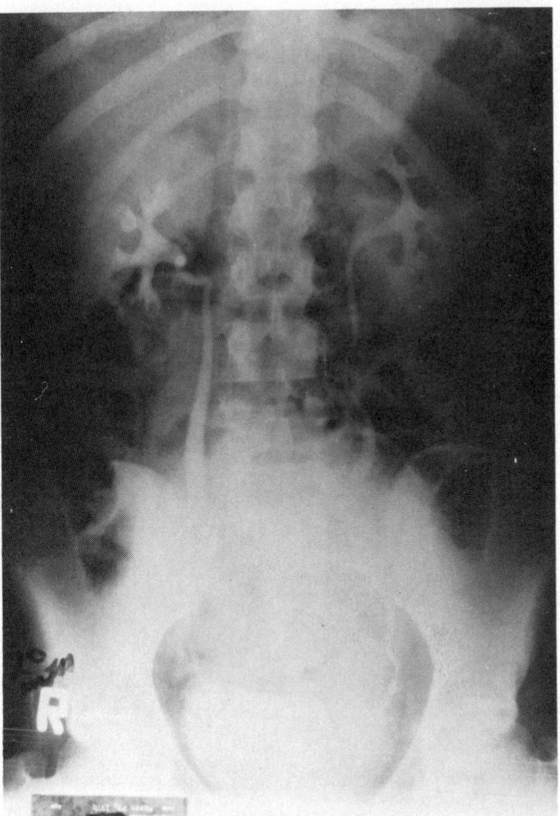

Figure 30–3. Intravenous urogram (20 minutes after injection of contrast medium) on third postpartum day, demonstrating minimal residual right pyeloureterectasis and "kinking" of the right ureter.

side was fuller. Further observations on the side of involvement are summarized in Table 30–2. More than three fourths of patients were judged to have "definite" dilatation on the right, an incidence twice that of the left. The right-sided degree of dilatation estimated on an arbitrary scale averaged more than twice that on the left, and the proportion of subjects with "severe" changes exhibited a fourfold preponderance of right over left. None of the

TABLE 30–1. LATERALITY OF PYELOURETERAL DILATATION

	Right	Left
Incidence of dilatation (per cent)	76	35.1
Extent of dilatation* (mean ± SEM)	2.4 ± 0.1	1.0 ± 0.1
Per cent with severe dilatation (grade 5 or 6)	4.5	1

*Arbitrary scale of 0 to 6, with 6 indicating most marked dilatation.

From data of Schulman and Herlinger (1975).

subjects in this study, strictly speaking, had normal pregnancies, since all had some clinical reason for intravenous urography. However, the most common indication for investigation was antepartum bleeding, a condition not likely to be associated with inherent urinary tract defects, whereas patients known to have previous or subsequent urinary tract disease were excluded. Therefore, the data can be accepted as probably representative of a normal population. Moreover, ultrasound measurements of asymptomatic patients have confirmed the distinct right-sided predominance of pyelocaliceal dilatation (Fried, 1979).

The explanation for the right-sided preponderance of pyeloureteral dilatation is uncertain, though it has been attributed to either a "cushioning" effect of the sigmoid colon on the left that limits impingement of the enlarging uterus on the ureter or to dextrorotation of the uterus, or to both.

Upper urinary tract dilatation has several functional and clinical effects. Bergstrom (1975) studied radioisotopic renography in

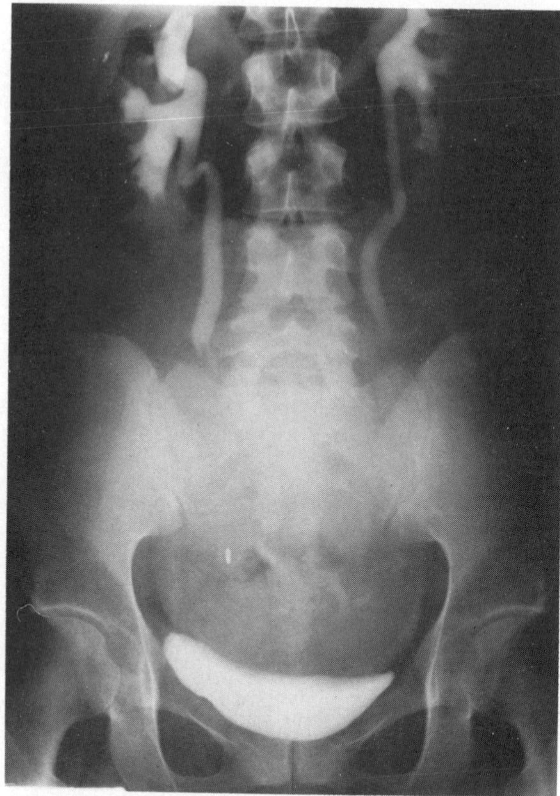

Figure 30–4. Intravenous urogram (20 minutes after injection of contrast medium) at 26 weeks' gestation, demonstrating bilateral pyeloureterectasis, more marked on right, and increased ureteral tortuosity.

patients in late pregnancy with entirely or predominantly right-sided hydronephrosis-hydroureter. There was nearly a five-fold increase in time to peak excretion on the right compared with the left. However, in the majority of cases the ratio of pyelographic dead space on one side to the other was equal to or greater than the ratio of calculated excretion rates, indicating that any renographic delay is due to a "reservoir" effect of the dilated urinary tract rather than to a reduction in urinary flow on the affected side. Thus, urinary stasis does not seem to be a necessary concomitant. From a clinical point of view, the increased incidence of urinary tract infection during pregnancy has been commonly ascribed to pyeloureteral dilatation. However, attempts to relate the incidence and severity of upper urinary tract changes to symptomatic or asymptomatic infection have been unsuccessful (Schulman and Herlinger, 1975).

Etiologic Considerations

The etiology of gestational pyeloureterectasis has been the subject of considerable controversy. Two basic causes — en-

TABLE 30–2. DILATATION OF RENAL PELVIS IN NORMAL PREGNANCY*

		Normal	Mild	Moderate	Severe
First trimester	(N = 18)	39%	61%	0	0
Second trimester	(N = 90)	31%	49%	20%	0
Third trimester	(N = 110)	30%	45%	22%	3%

*Data from ultrasound observations by Fried, A. M.: Hydronephrosis of pregnancy: ultrasonographic study and classification of asymptomatic women. Am. J. Obstet. Gynecol. *135*:1066, 1979.

docrine and mechanical — have been proposed as primary etiologic agents, and each has its advocates.

Fainstat (1963) reviewed the literature and concluded that the primary cause was hormonal in nature, with partial and intermittent ureteral obstruction probably contributing "in an important secondary role." In reaching this conclusion, Fainstat drew heavily on in vitro studies demonstrating diminished ureteral tone and contractility with addition of progesterone and gonadotropins, and on animal experiments indicating ureteral dilatation with various endocrine manipulations. Pointing to the common embryologic origin of the uterus and urinary collecting system from the urogenital ridge and to the well-known ability of progesterone to inhibit uterine motility, he suggested that progesterone and perhaps gonadotropins were primary factors. He also speculated that estrogen might be involved by virtue of its growth-promoting and interstitial fluid-retaining properties, although this hormone tends to stimulate smooth muscle contractility.

Prostaglandins have also been suggested as a mechanism for producing dilatation of the upper urinary tract. Prostaglandin E_1 inhibits ureteral contractility in animals (Boyarsky et al., 1966).

Among factors arguing against a primary endocrine cause (and therefore in favor of mechanical factors) are (1) the generally sharp limitation of dilatation to above the pelvic brim, (2) the tendency to unilaterality, and (3) the customary prompt resolution with delivery. Studies of intraureteral pressure relationships have indicated that advancing pregnancy is accompanied by progressive increases in contractile mean pressure and tonus (but not in contraction frequency) in the upper ureter, while these same parameters all remain low in the pelvic ureter (Sala and Rubi, 1967). Moreover, when a pregnant subject lies on one side, the intraureteral tone of the opposite ureter decreases while that of the same ureter remains high (Rubi and Sala, 1968).

Certain clinical observations tend also to support mechanical obstruction as a primary feature. Hydronephrosis and hydroureter, although common in gravidas with normally situated kidneys, do not occur in pregnant women with pelvic kidneys (Johnson et al., 1967). Moreover, complete ureteral obstruction by a greatly overdistended uterus can occur, albeit rarely (O'Shaughnessy et al., 1980).

On the other hand, the frequent occurrence of some degree of pyelocaliceal dilatation relatively early in gestation (Fried, 1979), when uterine size hardly seems sufficient to cause obstruction, argues against a simple and straightforward mechanical explanation. Similarly, the lack of relationship with fetal presentation, position, or station is difficult to explain on purely mechanical grounds.

Historically, mechanical theories invoking ureteral compression at the pelvic brim by the growing uterus were generally accepted until about 35 years ago, when endocrine factors began to receive greater emphasis. However, during recent years there appears to be a swing back toward obstruction as a basic mechanism, and in addition two new theories involving variations on the mechanical theme have been proposed. Dure-Smith (1970) described a filling defect, termed the "iliac sign," noted on intravenous urography and thought to represent ureteral compression by the iliac vessels. The right-left difference was explained by the observation that the right ureter tends to cross over the common iliac artery, while the left is more likely to lie on the less rigid vein. In addition, the course of the right ureter was said to be more at a right angle to the iliac vessels than is the course of the left ureter. Bellina and associates (1970), on the basis of autopsy dissections, intravenous urography, and pelvic venography, described dilatation of the right ovarian vein complex during pregnancy, and suggested that this anatomic change causes partial ureteral compression with resultant stasis. However, excision of the ovarian vein in other studies in subhuman primates did not affect the course of ureteral dilatation (Roberts, 1971).

In summary, neither mechanical nor endocrine factors alone appear adequate to explain all of the observed characteristics of pyeloureteral dilatation during pregnancy, and it therefore seems likely that both elements are involved. The bulk of the evidence seems to favor partial ureteral compression by some structure (uterus, iliac artery, or ovarian vein) as the primary mechanism, with endocrine effects playing a contributory role.

Other Ureteral Changes

Ureteral alterations less dramatic than dilatation also accompany pregnancy. The ureters tend to elongate and frequently exhibit increased curvature as a consequence. These curves are actually quite gentle when viewed in three dimensions, but in the conventional two-dimensional urogram they may appear acutely angulated (see Figure 30–3), leading to their customary (but inaccurate) designation as "kinks." The ureters may also be located more laterally than usual, probably as a combination of elongation and displacement by the enlarging uterus (see Figure 30–2). Lateral displacement is observed during the last half of pregnancy in 20 to 25 per cent of cases on the left and in 8 to 10 per cent of cases on the right (Schulman and Herlinger, 1975). The right-left difference presumably reflects the position of the sigmoid colon between the uterus and the left ureter.

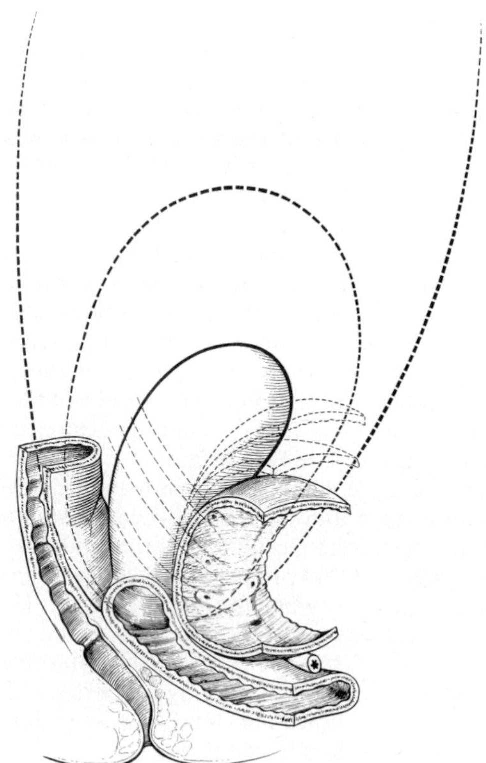

Figure 30–5. Changing relationships of bladder base and ureters with uterine growth in pregnancy. (From Mattingly, R. F., and Borkow, H. I.: Lower urinary tract injuries in pregnancy. *In* Barber, H. R. K., and Graber, E. A. [eds.]: Surgical Disease in Pregnancy. Philadelphia, W. B. Saunders, 1974, p. 442.)

BLADDER AND URETHRA

Bladder

The urinary bladder, because of its intimate anatomic relationship to the cervix and lower uterine segment, is displaced anteriorly and superiorly as the uterus grows. Thus, as pregnancy progresses, the bladder becomes more of an abdominal and less of a pelvic organ. The base of the bladder also broadens (Fig. 30–5), and with descent of the presenting part as term approaches, the cystoscopic appearance of the trigone changes from a concave to a convex surface. The bladder participates in the generalized hyperemia of the pelvic organs, and the mucosal surface often exhibits congestion and increased size and tortuosity of its superficial vessels. Some degree of muscular hypertrophy, presumably as a result of estrogenic stimulation, may be noted in histologic sections, but the effect is not usually evident cystoscopically.

Bladder capacity increases during pregnancy, apparently as a reflection of the well-known atonic effect of progesterone on smooth muscle. However, the extent of the change is unclear. Mattingly and Borkow (1974) described a progressive increase during the second and third trimesters to a capacity of a liter or more. On the other hand, Rubi and Sala (1972) recorded mean bladder volumes of 756 and 838 ml. in nonpregnant and pregnant subjects, respectively, a statistically insignificant difference. These latter investigators also reported significantly less increase in bladder pressure with voiding in pregnant than in nonpregnant patients, although pregnancy did not influence resting pressures.

Urethra

Anatomic changes in the urethra are relatively minor, at least prior to parturition. Upward displacement of the bladder results in a tendency to lengthen the urethra. On urethroscopy, the mucosa appears congested and hyperemic, and cytologically the transitional epithelium becomes more squamous-like under the influence of high estrogen levels.

Recent urodynamic studies by Iosif and colleagues (1980) in nulliparous women in normal late pregnancy and again in the puerperium have documented gestational changes in lower urinary tract function. Urethral length, both absolute and functional, was increased during late pregnancy. Maximal urethral pressure increased by an average of 23 cm. of water compared with a mean increase in bladder pressure of only 11 cm. of water, leading to greater urethral closure pressure during pregnancy. These two effects, increased urethral length and elevated urethral closure pressure, would both tend to promote continence.

SUMMARY

The morphologic changes associated with pregnancy are important to the clinician for two reasons: First, failure to appreciate them as normal concomitants of pregnancy may lead to an erroneous diagnosis of a disease state. Second, some of the changes apparently promote stasis of urine, which accounts for the greatly increased propensity of the pregnant women to develop urinary tract infections. (See Chapter 36.)

REFERENCES

Bellina, J. H., Dougherty, C. M., and Mickal, A.: Pyeloureteral dilation and pregnancy. Am. J. Obstet. Gynecol. *108*:356, 1970.

Bergstrom, H.: Renographic evaluation of renal excretion in hydronephrosis of pregnancy. Acta Obstet. Gynecol. Scand. *54*:203, 1975.

Boyarsky, S., Labay, P., and Gerber, C.: Prostaglandin inhibition of ureteral peristalsis. Invest. Urol. *4*:9, 1966.

Dure-Smith, P.: Pregnancy dilatation of urinary tract: the iliac sign and its significance. Radiology *96*:545, 1970.

Fainstat, T.: Ureteral dilatation in pregnancy: a review. Obstet. Gynecol. Surv. *18*:845, 1963.

Fried, A. M.: Hydronephrosis of pregnancy: ultrasonographic study and classification of asymptomatic women. Am. J. Obstet. Gynecol. *135*:1066, 1979.

Harrow, B. R., Sloane, J. A., and Sulhanick, L.: Etiology of the hydronephrosis of pregnancy. Surg. Gynecol. Obstet. *119*:1042, 1964.

Iosif, S., Ingemarsson, I., and Ulmsten, U.: Urodynamic studies in normal pregnancy and in puerperium. Am. J. Obstet. Gynecol. *137*:696, 1980.

Johnson, D., Immergut, M., and White, C.: Pregnancy, hydronephrosis and renal ectopia. J. Urol. *98*:169, 1967.

Mattingly, R. F., and Borkow, H. I.: Lower urinary tract injuries in pregnancy. *In* Barber, H. R. K., and Graber, E. A. (Eds.): Surgical Disease in Pregnancy, Philadelphia, W. B. Saunders Co., 1974, pp. 440–464.

O'Shaughnessy, R., Wesprin, S. A., and Zuspan, F. P.: Obstructive renal failure by an overdistended uterus. Obstet. Gynecol. *55*:247, 1980.

Roberts, J. A.: The ovarian vein and hydronephrosis of pregnancy. Invest. Urol. *8*:610, 1971.

Rubi, R. A., and Sala, N. L.: Ureteral function in pregnant women. III. Effect of different positions and of fetal delivery upon ureteral tonus. Am. J. Obstet. Gynecol. *101*:230, 1968.

Rubi, R. A., and Sala, N. L.: Ureteral function in pregnant women. VI. Bladder and lower ureteral pressures during voiding. Am. J. Obstet. Gynecol. *113*:335, 1972.

Sala, N. L., and Rubi, R. A.: Ureteral function in pregnant women. II. Ureteral contractility during normal pregnancy. Am. J. Obstet. Gynecol. *99*:228, 1967.

Schulman, A., and Herlinger, H.: Urinary tract dilatation in pregnancy. Br. J. Radiol. *48*:638, 1975.

31

ULTRASOUND IN THE INTRAUTERINE DIAGNOSIS OF FETAL GENITOURINARY TRACT ABNORMALITIES

RIGOBERTO SANTOS-RAMOS, M.D.

The introduction of diagnostic sonography in obstetrics made possible the prenatal detection of soft tissue abnormalities in the fetus. Before the application of ultrasound, only bony abnormalities were detectable by x-rays, after 20 weeks of gestation. Visceral malformations were occasionally suspected — for example, a prominent fetal abdomen visualized on the x-ray films alerted the physicians to the presence of fetal ascites or fetal intra-abdominal tumors. Procedures such as amniography, fetography, and maternal intravenous pyelograms have been used to elucidate some of the fetal problems suspected by clinicians.

Although with classic bistable ultrasound technique the prenatal detection of some fetal malformations was possible, the storage system used with the bistable method was a major shortcoming for the visualization of fetal structures. The sophistication of the modern gray scale system — static and real time — has improved our ability to visualize the pregnant uterus and permits the identification of fetal organs with extreme accuracy. The recent development of real time ultrasound, using linear array of ultrasound transducers or sector scan transducers, has provided us with a constant display of moving images of fetal structures as they are actually occurring. We can observe dynamic physiologic phenomena, such as human fetal breathing movements, motion of fetal heart valves and chambers, filling and emptying of the fetal bladder, fetal body and limb movements, and others. Thus, we now have the potential for the detection of the abnormalities early enough that parents can make the choice between continuation of pregnancy or abortion when the severity of such abnormalities is incompatible with normal extrauterine life. If the pregnancy is permitted to continue, the advantage of establishing the diagnosis prenatally might be life-saving for the neonate requiring surgery immediately after birth.

Sonography is a noninvasive and apparently harmless technique now widely used in obstetrics for assessment of fetal well-being, placental localization, diagnosis of multiple pregnancy, and detection of fetal anomalies. Its success in the diagnosis of open neural tube defects in the early second trimester has encouraged physicians to look for other fetal malformations that can be detected by this method; reports in the literature of diagnosis of gastrointestinal tract abnormalities, skeletal dysplasias, congenital heart anomalies, fetal tumors, abdominal wall defects, and other lesions are becoming more common. While polyhydramnios is almost always associat-

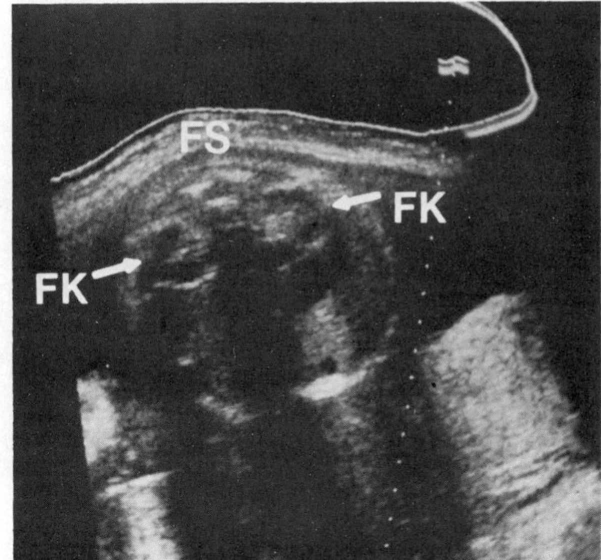

Figure 31–1. Transverse scan of maternal abdomen, showing normal fetal kidneys (*FK*) and fetal spine (*FS*).

ed with open neural tube defects and gastrointestinal atresias, the presence of oligohydramnios requires investigation of the fetal urinary tract.

OBSERVATIONS OF THE NORMAL ANATOMY AND PHYSIOLOGY OF THE FETAL GENITOURINARY TRACT

Kidney. In the normal fetus, the kidneys have a characteristic rounded appearance situated on either side of the lumbar spine (Figures 31–1 to 31–3). The renal pelves containing urine produce a small transonic area lying anteriorly to a more echogenic central structure, which represents fat and connective tissue of the collecting system. Using high-sensitivity gray scale equipment, the kidneys can be identified as early as the end of the first trimester of pregnancy (12 to 14 weeks) (Grannum et al., 1980). It is best to wait until the eighteenth to twentieth weeks of gestation for definitive diagnosis. The kidneys are best visualized in the transverse scans of the fetal abdomen; in the longitudinal cross-sections it is more difficult to demonstrate fetal kidneys routinely even in the last trimester of pregnancy (Figure 31–3).

Assessment of fetal kidney size and preparation of tables of values for normal fetuses at different periods of gestation, using the ratio of kidney circumference to abdominal circumference, has recently been done (Grannum et al., 1980).

Ureters and Bladder. Visualization of the normal fetal ureter, unlike that of the kidneys, is not practical. The fetal bladder, by contrast, when distended, is an easy organ to demonstrate (Figure 31–4). It appears as a sonolucent structure with the

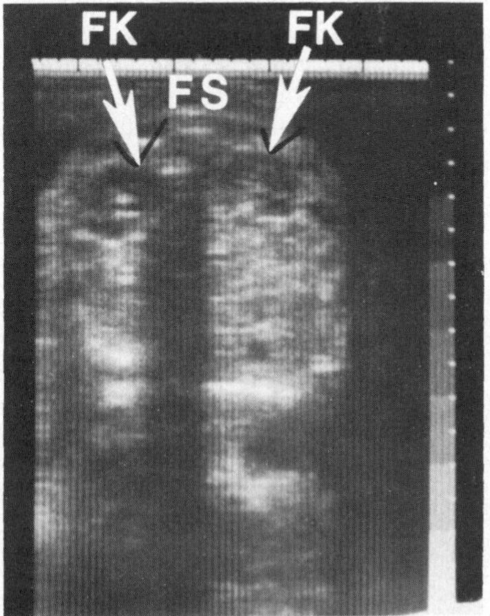

Figure 31–2. Normal fetal kidneys seen on transverse real time scan (linear array). *FS*, Fetal spine; *FK*, fetal kidney.

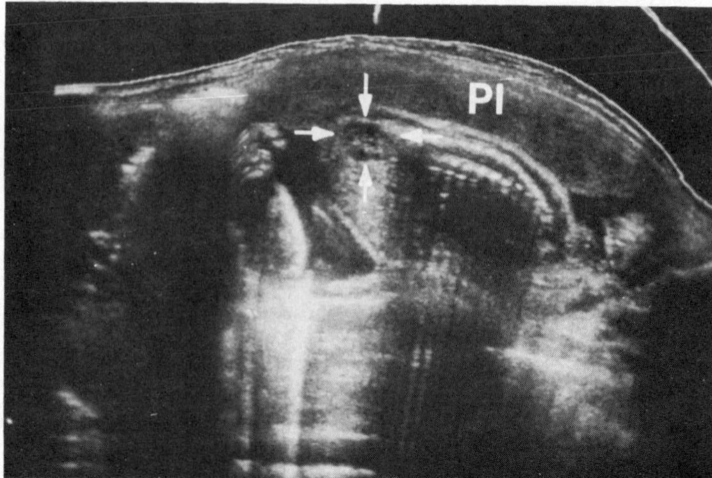

Figure 31–3. Longitudinal scan demonstrating fetal kidney (arrows) and placenta (*Pl*).

shape of an ovoid in the midline of the lower fetal abdomen (Robinson et al., 1968; Garrett and Robinson, 1970).

Several investigations have been performed: the frequency of fetal micturition has been recorded and the fetal urinary output was calculated by Campbell and associates in 1973. The filling and emptying pattern of the fetal bladder was studied by them in 33 patients through a complete cycle. The length of the cycle varied from 50 to 155 minutes. The mean fetal bladder cycle observed was 110 minutes (SD ± 35.8). Filling of the bladder occurred at a constant rate; emptying, however, was more variable. In some fetuses the bladder was emptied in a few seconds, whereas in others it was a slow process that took over 30 minutes. The volume of the fetal bladder at term was estimated to be 39 ml. A gradual increase in the amount of urine produced per hour by the fetus was noted by Campbell and co-workers (1973). At 32 weeks of gestation, the mean volume was 12 ml., whereas at 40 weeks, it was 28 ml. Van Otterlo and colleagues (1977), studying 12 patients with fetal growth retardation, found a reduced fetal urinary output and low amniotic fluid volume.

Visualization of the normal fetal ovaries and uterus is presently beyond our capabilities; however, it is possible to identify the male external genitalia in the third trimester.

DETECTING FETAL GENITOURINARY TRACT ANOMALIES WITH SONOGRAPHY

Fetuses thought to be at risk for urinary tract malformations because of previous family history of affected siblings or be-

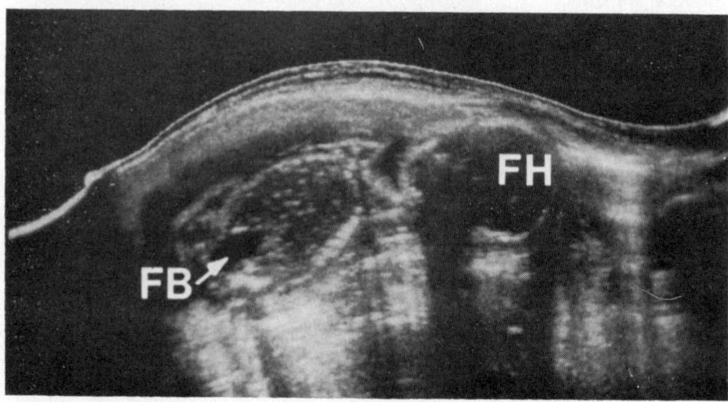

Figure 31–4. Normal fetal bladder (*FB*) shown in a longitudinal cross-sectional view of the fetus at 25/26 weeks of gestation. *FH,* Fetal head.

cause of the presence of oligohydramnios should have a thorough ultrasonic investigation starting in the early second trimester of pregnancy. Sonographic confirmation of oligohydramnios should be followed by careful visualization of fetal kidneys and sequential observations of the changing volume of the fetal bladder. Ordinarily one sonographic study will not be enough; patients with genetic predispositions need serial sonography until fetal abnormalities are either confirmed or ruled out.

RENAL AGENESIS

Fetal renal anomalies should be suspected when there is deviation from the normal ultrasonic pattern in the location or size of renal structures. Bilateral renal agenesis or Potter's syndrome should be suspected when, in the presence of oligohydramnios, sonography fails to demonstrate fetal kidneys and bladder, even after administration of furosemide to the mother (Keirse and Meerman, 1978). According to Warkany (1971), Potter's syndrome is present in 1 in 3000 to 4000 infants and has a 5 to 50 per cent risk of recurrence, depending on which mode of inheritance is operative (autosomal recessive or autosomal dominant with variable expressivity or possible multifactorial inheritance or new mutations of the dominant form).

Bilateral renal agenesis is incompatible with extrauterine life and is usually associated with oligohydramnios. When combined with anencephaly or iniencephaly, amniotic fluid is present. Several reports of bilateral renal agenesis suspected or diagnosed during pregnancy have been published (Kaffe et al., 1977*a,b*; Keirse and Meerman, 1978; Miskin, 1979). All infants presented with oligohydramnios. One patient chose to have therapeutic abortion, two infants died immediately after delivery; the third infant was stillborn. All had hypoplastic underdeveloped lungs and all were growth-retarded. Most recently, Dubbins and co-workers (1981) added three more cases to the literature. They suggest that the examination of the renal tract in severe oligohydramnios should be directed toward the fetal bladder. They believe that the identification of reniform outlines in the sonograms can be misleading.

Unilateral renal agenesis has an incidence of 0.1 to 0.2 per cent in the general population. Sonographic evidence of only one fetal kidney and failure to identify the other does not allow one to make the diagnosis because of the possibility of an ectopic kidney. Since this condition is compatible with normal intra- and extrauterine life, diagnosis would be the result of a very high index of suspicion.

INFANTILE POLYCYSTIC KIDNEY DISEASE (POTTER TYPE I)

This is an autosomal recessive condition attributed to hyperplasia of the interstitial portion of collecting tubules. The cysts are numerous and too small to be seen with present ultrasound equipment. Larger cysts that can be demonstrated by ultrasound are occasionally present. However, as a rule the kidneys, although apparently solid, are disproportionately large for the fetal abdomen, and this finding is quickly noted in the sonograms.

Hobbins and co-workers (1979) studied four pregnancies in two patients at risk and were able to diagnose two affected fetuses at 28 weeks of gestation. Stillborn infants were delivered at term and at 36 weeks; both had the classic Potter's syndrome phenotype, with pulmonary hypoplasia and kidney pathology. Another case of recurrent infantile polycystic disease has been reported by Reilly and colleagues (1979). The disease was diagnosed antenatally by sonography in the second sibling at 31 weeks of gestation. The infant was the product of a doubly consanguineous union in a couple of Palestinian origin. At autopsy, ascites was found to be present, the kidneys were enlarged, with multiple small cysts throughout the parenchyma, a 2 cm. cyst was present in the upper pole of the left kidney, and pulmonary hypoplasia and liver fibrosis were present.

DYSPLASTIC MULTICYSTIC KIDNEY (POTTER TYPE II)

This is the most common cause of unilateral multicystic mass found in the flank of the fetus and newborn. Dysplastic multicystic kidney, unlike infantile polycystic

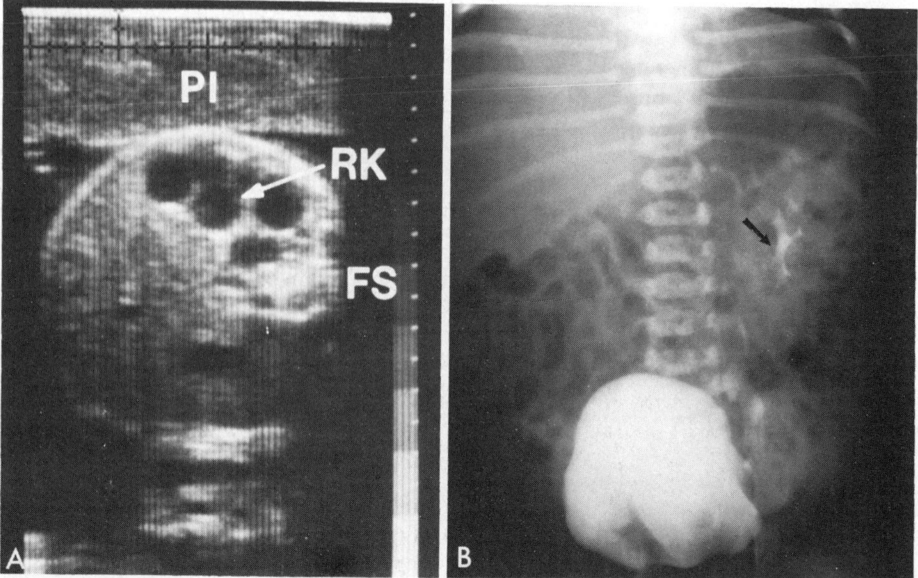

Figure 31–5. *A*, Multicystic right fetal kidney (*RK*), 35 weeks' gestation, transverse real time scan (linear array). Also shown are placenta (*Pl*) and fetal spine (*FS*). *B*, Intravenous pyelogram of the newborn during second day of life. There is no visualization of renal parenchyma or collecting system on the right side.

kidney disease (always bilateral), only rarely affects both kidneys. The abnormality may be associated with Meckel's syndrome, Robert's syndrome, or chromosomal aberrations (Sabbagha, 1980). When only one kidney is involved, the condition is compatible with normal extrauterine life. The affected kidney is enlarged, cystic, and nonfunctional. The ureter is also abnormal, with stricture at the level of the ureteropelvic junction. In sonograms, the multicystic kidney may appear as a unilocular cyst because the fine septa are not always visible. By the same token, sonography is unable to differentiate between fetal hydronephrosis and an apparently unilocular multicystic kidney (Dunne and Johnson, 1979).

Several cases of infants afflicted with this condition, which had been diagnosed or suspected antenatally, have been described since the first case reported in Australia (Garrett et al., 1970; Santos-Ramos and Duenhoelter, 1975; Lee and Blake, 1977; Bartley et al., 1977; Bateman et al., 1980; Henderson et al., 1980). An infant was diagnosed at 24 weeks as having multicystic kidney associated with massive hydramnios by Henderson and co-workers (1980). The infant was delivered at term by cesarean section, had a nephrectomy at 2 days of age, and was discharged from the hospital 5 days later.

Recently we diagnosed another case of multicystic kidney (Figure 31–5*A*,*B*) associated with polyhydramnios at 35 weeks of gestation. The pregnancy had progressed normally until week 39/40, when the patient had spontaneous vaginal delivery; the female infant had an Apgar score of 9/9, with birth weight of 3775 gm. A mass in the right flank was easily palpable in the neonate, and sonography and intravenous pyelogram confirmed the prenatal diagnosis.

INTRAUTERINE DIAGNOSIS OF OBSTRUCTIVE LESIONS OF THE FETAL URINARY TRACT

Obstructive lesions in the fetal urinary tract have been described. The ultrasound findings of a cystic mass may allow one to differentiate between supravesical and infravesical obstructive lesions. Supravesical obstruction is the more common form in the newborn, with obstruction at the ureterovesical rather than at the ureteropelvic

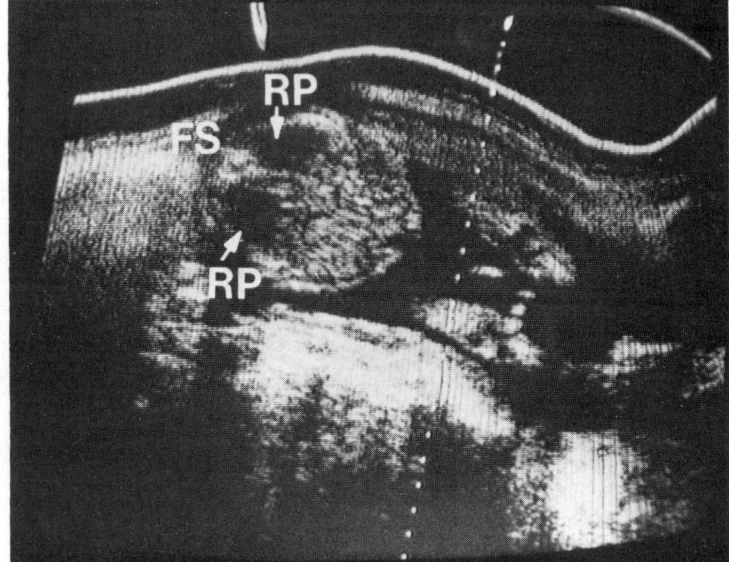

Figure 31–6. Bilateral hydronephrosis, 22/23 weeks' gestation on longitudinal scan 0.5 cm. to the left of midventral line. *FS*, Fetal spine; *RP*, area of dilated renal pelves.

junction (Warkany, 1971). A diagnosis of fetal hydronephrosis and megaureter was made at 34 weeks of gestation by Garrett and colleagues (1975). In this fetus (at 37 weeks), the bladder, although larger than usual, was not grossly dilated. Ultrasound performed 7 days after birth and an intravenous pyelogram obtained 9 weeks later confirmed the antenatal diagnosis. The site of the obstruction and the ultimate fate of the infant were not described. In the same publication, the authors reported a fetus seen at 34 weeks of gestation with a bladder distended by 3500 ml. of urine. A stillborn male infant was delivered the following day, and despite the fact that 2200 ml of fluid had been aspirated from the bladder before delivery, 970 ml. of urine was found in the bladder at autopsy. The fetus had bilateral hydronephrosis and hydroureters. The proximal fetal urethra was patent for 0.5 cm., as was the lower penile urethra. For the remainder there was no lumen demonstrable macroscopically, but sections showed a narrow lumen that was double for a short distance.

We have observed a case of bilateral hydronephrosis (Figure 31–6) at 22/23 weeks' gestation in a fetus with spina bifida. This was apparently a transient phenomenon, since at birth an intravenous pyelogram did not demonstrate dilatation of the renal pelves. In another patient seen in our laboratory, left ureteral obstruction

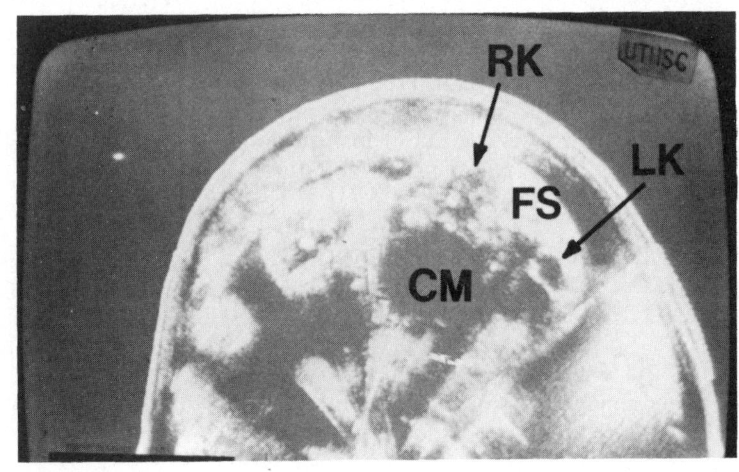

Figure 31–7. Left ureteral obstruction suspected at 34/35 weeks' gestation. Normal right kidney (*RK*), a large cystic mass in region of left kidney (*CM*) and fetal spine (*FS*) are shown. *LK*, Left kidney.

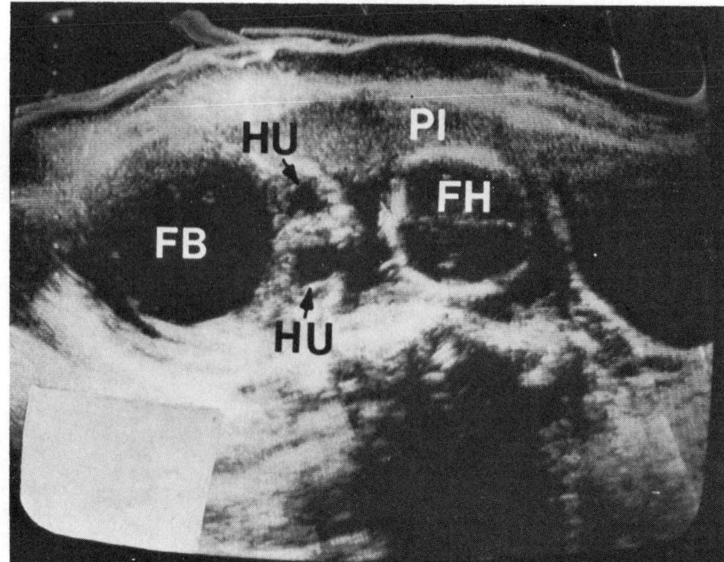

Figure 31–8. "Prune-belly" or Eagle-Barrett syndrome (22/23 weeks' gestation), longitudinal cross-sectional view, 2 cm. to the right of midventral line. *FH,* Fetal head; *FB,* distended fetal bladder; *HU,* hydroureter; *Pl,* placenta.

was suspected (Duenhoelter and Santos-Ramos, 1981). The patient was 34 weeks pregnant, and sonograms showed a large cystic mass in the region of the left kidney (Figure 31–7). On the fourth day of life, the stricture of the ureteropelvic junction was confirmed surgically. Some renal parenchyma was found, and pyeloplasty and nephrostomy were performed.

Another entity that can be detected prenatally by sonography is the absence of abdominal muscles associated with gross dilatation of the urinary tract with or without bladder outlet obstruction. This abnormality is known as the "prune-belly" or Eagle-Barrett syndrome, a condition with no clearly demonstrable mendelian basis, but rather consistently reproduced in many instances (McKusick, 1975). Okulski (1977) published a report of a fetus seen at 20/21 weeks who was followed with serial sonograms and at birth was proved to have the prune-belly syndrome. Another case (Figure 31–8) was observed in our institution in a patient of a comparable gestational age.

INTRAUTERINE DIAGNOSIS OF TUMORS OF THE FETAL GENITOURINARY TRACT

At this time there is little in the literature on the sonographic detection of tumors of the fetal genitourinary tract. Nevertheless, there have been reports of prenatal diagnosis of ovarian cysts (Valenti et al., 1975; Lee and Blake, 1977) and hydrometrocolpos (Coopersberg, 1981). Differential diagnosis of such conditions must include dilatation of the fetal bladder or renal cysts. Absence of oligohydramnios and hydronephrosis might be important clues for better evaluation and diagnosis in these cases.

Recognition of small solid tumors in fetal kidneys with current ultrasound equipment is difficult. The lack of distinctive sonographic texture — unlike cystic masses — accounts for that difficulty. In theory, at least, the presence of larger solid tumors (e.g., Wilms' tumor, congenital neuroblastoma) might be suspected in the presence of enlargement and asymmetry of one kidney. Ascites is expected to coexist with some renal tumors such as congenital renal hamartoma (Coopersberg, 1981).

CONCLUSION

The use of high resolution ultrasound equipment has made possible in utero visualization of several malformations of the fetal urinary tract. Static and real time gray scale sonography *in experienced hands* can detect cystic masses, such as dysplastic kidneys and obstructive lesions of fetal bladder and ureters. Observation of the normal pelvic organs of the female fetus and detection of small solid tumors is still beyond the resolution of present equipment. It is expected, however, that progress in ultrasound technology will allow a more precise evaluation of fetal congenital anomalies and tumors in the future.

REFERENCES

Bartley, J., Golbus, M., Filly, R., et al.: Prenatal diagnosis of dysplastic kidney disease. Clin. Genet. *11*:375, 1977.

Bateman, B., Brenbridge, A., and Buschi, A.: In utero diagnosis of multicystic kidney disease by sonography. J. Reprod. Med. *25*:256–258, 1980.

Campbell, S., Wladimiroff, J. W., and Dewhurst, C. J.: The antenatal measurement of fetal urine production. J. Obstet. Gynaecol. Br. Commonw. *80*:680, 1973.

Coopersberg, P.: Abnormalities of the fetal genitourinary tract. *In* Sanders, R. C., and James, A. E. Jr.: The Principles and Practice of Ultrasonography in Obstetrics and Gynecology. New York, Appleton-Century-Crofts, 1981.

Dubbins, P., Kurtz, A., Wapner, R., et al.: Renal agenesis: spectrum of in utero findings. J. Clin. Ultrasound *9*:189, 1981.

Duenhoelter, J., and Santos-Ramos, R.: Intrauterine diagnosis by ultrasound. *In* Barson, A. J. (Ed.): Laboratory Investigation of Fetal Disease, Bristol, John Wright & Sons, Ltd., 1981, p. 218.

Dunne, M., and Johnson, M.: The ultrasonic demonstration of fetal abnormalities in utero. J. Reprod. Med. *23*:195, 1979.

Garrett, W. J., Grunwald, G., and Robinson, D. E.: Prenatal diagnosis of fetal polycystic kidney by ultrasound. Aust. N.Z. J. Obstet. Gynaecol. *10*:7, 1970.

Garrett, W. J., Kossoff, G., and Osborn, R.: The diagnosis of fetal hydronephrosis, megaureter and urethral obstruction by sonographic echography. Br. J. Obstet. Gynecol. *82*:115, 1975.

Garrett, W. J., and Robinson, D. E.: Ultrasound in Clinical Obstetrics. Springfield, Ill., Charles C Thomas, 1970, p. 66.

Grannum, P., Bracken, M., Silverman, R., et al.: Assessment of fetal kidney size in normal gestation by comparison of ratio of kidney circumference to abdominal circumference. Am., J. Obstet. Gynecol. *136*:249, 1980.

Henderson, S., Van Kolken, R. J., et al.: Multicystic kidney with hydramnios. J. Clin. Ultrasound *8*:249, 1980.

Hobbins, J. C., Grannum, P., Berkowitz, R., et al.: Ultrasound in the diagnosis of congenital anomalies. Am. J. Obstet. Gynecol. *134*:331, 1979.

Kaffe, S., Godmilow, L., Walker, B., et al.: Prenatal diagnosis of bilateral renal agenesis. Obstet. Gynecol. *49*:478, 1977*a*.

Kaffe, S., Ross, J., Godmilow, L., et al.: Prenatal diagnosis of renal anomalies. Am. J. Med. Genet. *1*:241, 1977*b*.

Keirse, M. J., and Meerman, R. H.: Antenatal diagnosis of Potter Syndrome. Obstet. Gynecol. *52*(1 Suppl.):64S, 1978.

Lee, T. G., and Blake, S.: Prenatal fetal abdominal ultrasonography and diagnosis. Radiology *124*:475, 1977.

McKusick, V. A.: Mendelian Inheritance in Man: Catalogs of Autosomal Dominant, Autosomal Recessive, and X-Linked Phenotypes. 5th Ed. Baltimore, The Johns Hopkins University Press, 1975.

Miskin, M.: Prenatal diagnosis of renal agenesis by ultrasonography and maternal pyelography. Am. J. Roentgenol. *132*:1025, 1979.

Okulski, T.: The prenatal diagnosis of lower urinary tract obstruction using B scan ultrasound: a case report. J. Clin. Ultrasound *5*:268, 1977.

Reilly, K., Rubin, S., Blanke, B., et al.: Infantile polycystic kidney disease: a difficult antenatal diagnosis. Am. J. Obstet. Gynecol. *133*:580, 1979.

Robinson, D. E., Garrett, W. J., and Kossoff, G.: Fetal anatomy displayed by ultrasound. Invest. Radiol. *3*:442, 1968.

Sabbagha, R.: Congenital anomalies. *In* Sabbagha, R. (Ed.): Diagnostic Ultrasound Applied to Obstetrics and Gynecology. New York, Harper & Row, 1980, p. 211.

Santos-Ramos, R., and Duenhoelter, J.: Diagnosis of congenital fetal abnormalities by sonography. Obstet. Gynecol. *45*:279, 1975.

Valenti, C., Kassner, E. G., Yermakov, V., et al.: Antenatal diagnosis of a fetal ovarian cyst. Am. J. Obstet. Gynecol. *123*:216, 1975.

Van Otterlo, L. C., Wladimiroff, H. W., and Wallenburg, H.: Relationship between fetal urine production and amniotic fluid volume in normal pregnancy and pregnancy complicated by diabetes. Br. J. Obstet. Gynaecol. *84*:205, 1977.

Warkany, J.: Congenital Malformations. Chicago, Year Book Medical Publishers, Inc., 1971.

32

ALTERATIONS IN RENAL FUNCTION DURING PREGNANCY

E. G. ROBERTSON, M.D.

Pregnancy causes alterations in homeostasis in virtually all systems, particularly the cardiovascular and respiratory systems, and in water and electrolyte control. The kidney has a significant role in these homeostatic changes, not only as a simple excretory organ but also as the organ responsible for coordination of homeostasis in the intact organism. Ideally, the changes in renal function during pregnancy should accommodate the needs of both mother and fetus, through improved control of maternal excretion and recovery in order to provide the proper environment for the fetus, with more accurate regulation than that normally achieved in the nonpregnant woman. Many of the physiologic variations of pregnancy, however, appear to conflict with the needs of the fetus and of the mother and have been ascribed a pathologic role. Before the effects of disease processes can be interpreted, the normal physiology of pregnancy must be understood.

GENERAL HEMODYNAMIC CHANGES IN PREGNANCY

Renal function is affected by changes in other systems and particularly by those that occur in hemodynamic control.

Blood Volume

Blood volume is known to be altered in pregnancy, the increase in total volume being a composite of increments in the plasma volume and red cell volume. Plasma volume increases progressively throughout pregnancy until 34 weeks, when a peak is reached, and a plateau is maintained until term (Lund and Donovan, 1967). In singleton pregnancies, the overall increase in plasma volume in primigravidas is about 1200 ml., representing an increase of nearly 50 per cent above the average level of 2600 ml. in nonpregnant subjects. Following delivery, plasma volume decreases by approximately 1000 ml. within 7 days; available evidence indicates that the volume returns to levels found in nonpregnant subjects by 6 to 8 weeks post partum.

Red cell volume also increases throughout pregnancy but to a lesser extent than plasma volume, leading to hemodilution and a fall in packed cell volume and hemoglobin. The overall average increment is approximately 350 ml., which is less than one third of the increase in plasma volume (Chesley, 1972). Although it is not known for certain how long it takes red cell volume to return to normal pre-pregnancy levels, it is probable that this has occurred, in most subjects, by 8 weeks post partum (Paintin, 1962).

Cardiac Output

The increase in blood volume is accompanied by an increase in cardiac output. Serial studies (Walters et al., 1966; Lees et al., 1967) have established that cardiac out-

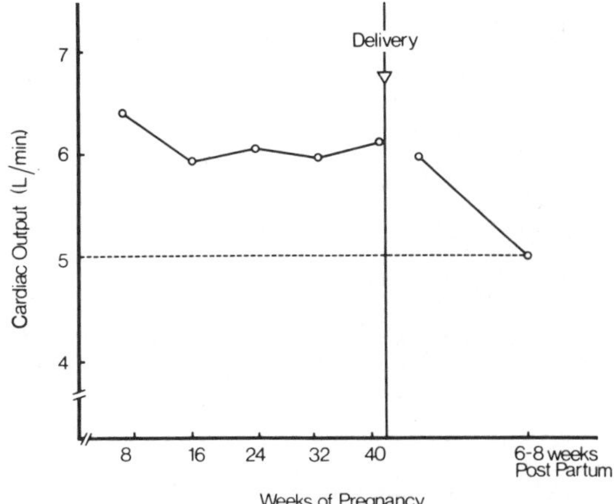

Figure 32–1. Mean cardiac output during pregnancy and the puerperium (derived from the results of Walters, MacGregor, and Hills [1966] and Lees and co-workers [1967].)

put increases early in the first trimester by a mean of 1 to 2 liters per minute from the normal nonpregnant level of 5 to 7 liters per minute (Figure 32–1). This level is maintained throughout pregnancy until delivery has occurred. The frequently observed fall in cardiac output in the last few weeks of the third trimester is a postural effect: The supine position, assumed by the subject when cardiac output is measured, allows the gravid uterus to fall backwards and occlude the inferior vena cava, and thus reduce venous return. During labor, the cardiac output increases with uterine contractions, with a further increase during the first stage of labor of between 15 and 30 per cent. Immediately after delivery, cardiac output and stroke volume remain elevated for at least 30 to 60 minutes, then begin to fall, and usually return to normal levels by 8 to 10 weeks post partum.

Blood Flow

If the peripheral resistance remained unchanged, the increases in blood volume and cardiac output would be accompanied by increases in arterial blood pressure. However, systolic blood pressure, during normal pregnancy, changes little; if anything, it tends to be 3 to 4 mm. Hg below levels found in the nonpregnant subject in the first and second trimesters, with a slight increase to approach normal nonpregnant levels in the third trimester. On the other hand, diastolic blood pressure in early and midpregnancy is significantly lower than in the nonpregnant state. This would suggest that there are marked changes in other organs during pregnancy and that blood flow, in certain systems, must be markedly increased in order to produce this pattern.

Although difficult to measure, uterine blood flow has been estimated to increase from approximately 50 ml. per minute at 10 weeks' gestation to 200 ml. per minute at 28 weeks' gestation (Assali et al., 1960); by term, the total uterine blood flow appears to range between 500 and 700 ml. per minute (Metcalfe et al., 1955). Probably about 80 per cent of the total blood flow to the uterus, at term, is distributed to the chorio-decidual circulation and the remainder to the myoendometrial circulation (Power et al., 1967). This increase does not account for the total change in peripheral blood flow; there must, therefore, be increased circulation to other organs in addition to the uterus. The heightened redness and warmth of the skin of the peripheral parts of the body during pregnancy suggests an increased skin blood flow caused by peripheral vasodilatation. Certainly, general peripheral resistance is lowered, with a resultant fall in central venous pressure. These changes would allow for increased tissue perfusion and for improved water and nutrient exchange at the cellular level.

RENAL HEMODYNAMICS

There are marked changes in renal function during pregnancy, but the effects of pregnancy on renal dynamics are still under investigation. There has been dispute about the size and the timing of changes in renal plasma flow, but all authorities agree that there is indeed an increase during pregnancy. Part of the problem in investigation is that, as with cardiac output, changes in posture are known to influence renal function in nonpregnant subjects, and this effect is exaggerated during pregnancy. For example, when a subject in late pregnancy moves from lying on one side to an upright or supine position, there is an immediate reduction in effective renal plasma flow,

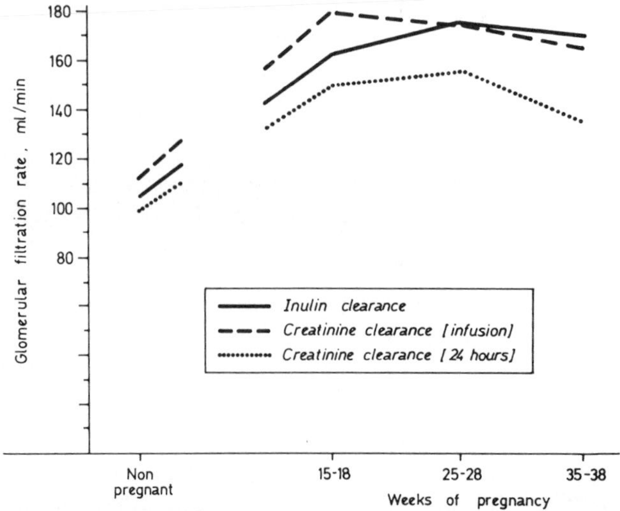

Figure 32–2. Mean glomerular filtration rate in 10 healthy women during pregnancy and 8 to 12 weeks post partum. (Reproduced from Davison, J. M., and Hytten, F. E.: J. Obstet. Gynaecol. Br. Commonw. *81*:588, 1974.)

glomerular filtration rate, and urine flow (Lindheimer and Weston, 1969; Lindheimer, 1970). Thus, renal function tests performed in the third trimester with the subject supine will show decreased values (Figure 32–2). Failure of the subject to maintain a constant position during study results in frequent changes in urine flow rates, leading to incorrect results.

Earlier studies (Sims and Krantz, 1958) demonstrated that glomerular filtration rate (GFR) increased 30 to 50 per cent early in pregnancy and remained elevated until delivery, and that effective renal plasma flow increased 25 per cent during the first half of gestation but declined thereafter. Subsequently, although most authors confirmed the increase in GFR, they could not demonstrate the reduction in renal plasma flow near term.

Chesley and Sloan (1964) suggested that the decline in renal function that occurs during the third trimester is artifactual and attributed it to faulty position. When studies were performed with women positioned in lateral recumbency, both renal plasma flow and GFR remained elevated at term. Conversely, assumption of the supine posture decreased GFR, explaining the previous observations of decreased renal hemodynamics near delivery.

Davison and Hytten (1974*a*) measured renal function serially during and after gestation and confirmed previous studies demonstrating that GFR is already increased during the first trimester and remains elevated until delivery (Figure 32–3). These workers concluded that filtration rate does decline near term, but that the decrease is apparent only when GFR is calculated on a 24 hour basis. They suggest that this decrement may result from the more pronounced effects of upright activity on renal hemodynamics in late pregnancy.

The cause of the increase in renal blood flow during pregnancy is still unknown. Attempts to relate cardiac output, heart size, and blood volume to renal hemodynamics (Gylling, 1961) have not been successful. The endocrine changes accompanying pregnancy may provide a possible explanation. For example, progesterone, when administered over a long period of time to human volunteers, does increase renal plasma flow (Oparil et al., 1974). Administration of the hormone in a single dose, however, fails to increase GFR to the levels noted in pregnant women.

An alternative approach to the mechanism underlying the increased GFR and renal plasma flow of gestation is suggested by Lindheimer and Katz (1975), from studies relating these phenomena to the alterations in extracellular fluid volume that invariably accompany pregnancy. Volume expansion, whether short-lived or existing over a period of time, increases renal hemodynamics in nonpregnant women and in experimental animals. GFR usually increases when vasopressin or exogenous mineralocorticoids are used to produce chronic hypervolemia. In the rat, alter-

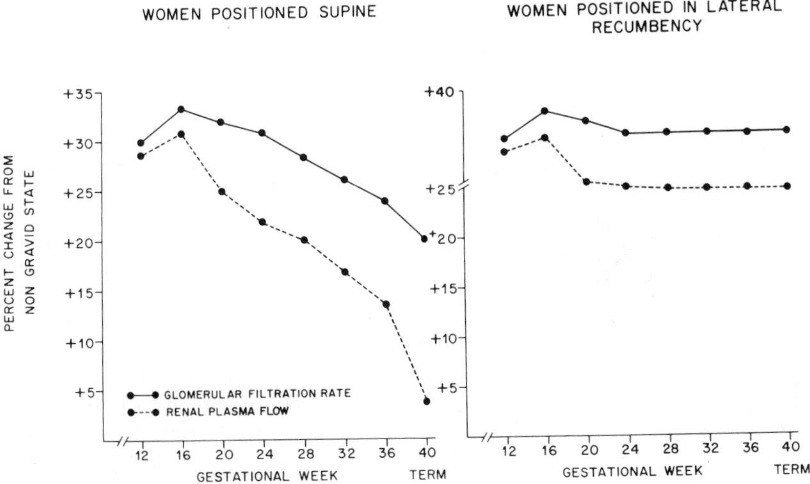

Figure 32–3. Renal hemodynamics in pregnancy. The early increment in glomerular filtration rate and effective renal plasma flow is sustained to term if subjects are tested in lateral recumbency. (Adapted from Pippig, L. C.: Médecine et Hygiène *27*:181, 1969.)

ations in maternal extracellular volume correlate with changes in GFR (Lindheimer and Katz, 1971). Since the physiologic hypervolemia that occurs in women tends to take place at the same time as do the changes in GFR and renal plasma flow, it is reasonable to assume that these phenomena are interlinked.

RENAL HANDLING OF WATER AND ELECTROLYTES

Normal pregnancy is characterized by a gradual cumulative retention of both water and sodium.

Water Retention

Although there are wide individual differences in the amounts of body water stored, most pregnant women will retain water in amounts greater than those required to sustain the product of conception. The most accurate studies, using deuterium oxide as a tracer (Hytten et al., 1966; Seitchik, 1967), have shown that there is an apparent mean increase of 7 to 8.5 liters of water between the beginning and end of pregnancy. The greater part is stored in the product of conception and in added maternal blood and tissue, but, by term, in women with no clinical signs of excessive water storage, there is an excess of some 2.5 to 3 liters that cannot be accounted for in these sites. The work of Hytten and his co-workers showed that this accumulation of excess water is a phenomenon that occurs only in the last 10 weeks of pregnancy, and that up to the thirtieth week of pregnancy there is little or no water stored that cannot be accounted for in known sites.

It is tempting to presume that the excess of water in late pregnancy is entirely extracellular and appears clinically as the commonplace edema of the legs. However, studies of limb volume in pregnancy (Hytten and Taggart, 1967; Robertson, 1971) showed that, even in women with clinically obvious edema, the increase in volume of both legs together was no greater than 500 ml., so that most "excess" water must be stored elsewhere.

The mechanism by which water is stored in the body during pregnancy is not known with any certainty. If judged according to normal nonpregnant homeostatic concepts, the pregnant woman — in terms of electrolyte and water transport and storage — is in a physiologically unstable state. The mechanisms that normally affect water and electrolyte storage are those controlling osmoregulation through the kidney, but in pregnancy, these mechanisms must change considerably. The increase in total body water is accompanied paradoxically by an increase in excretion of water and electrolytes (Parboosingh and Doig, 1973) and by an increased ability to excrete a water load (Hytten and Klopper, 1963). Although these effects tend to reduce towards term, even at that stage the general effect is one of greater than average excretion. Thus, the average fluid and electrolyte intake must be greater throughout pregnancy in order to allow net storage.

Osmolality

The earliest observed changes affecting osmoregulation have been noted shortly after the time of the first missed menstrual period, when there is a fall in total solute concentration of the plasma (Robertson and Cheyne, 1972). Total osmolality falls by about 10 milliosmoles from the normal nonpregnant level and remains at this level throughout pregnancy (Robertson and Cheyne, 1972; MacDonald and Good, 1972). Hytten and Robertson (1971) have suggested that this change occurs by the following mechanism: Because of progesterone-induced overbreathing, the pregnant woman has a reduced P_{CO_2}, and plasma bicarbonate must be lowered to maintain pH. Sodium is excreted with bicarbonate, leading to a fall in plasma osmolality. This does not have much effect on passive diffusion of water because these ions are freely diffusible across the capillary wall, and changes of this nature do not cause an osmotic gradient. However, a fall in solute concentration of this magnitude will be detected by the osmoreceptors in the carotid body and would normally cause complete suppression of antidiuretic hormone (ADH) secretion from the neurohypophysis. Such a change might be expected to lead to a diabetes insipidus–like state, and this may occur transiently in the many women who exhibit polyuria in early pregnancy.

Later, it seems likely that the osmoreceptors are reset to accept and preserve the new low level of osmolality and thus avoid a condition of continuous diuresis. Secretion of ADH should then return to normal and remain within normal nonpregnant limits throughout the rest of pregnancy. However, there is scanty, unpublished evidence that, at least in some patients, ADH secretions may be elevated in late pregnancy (Weir, personal communication, 1974), enhancing the tendency to water retention.

The effect on the kidney of these changes is complex. Even though there are changes in ADH secretion, it is known that glomerular filtration rate, along with solute-load per nephron, increases in pregnancy. This should produce a tendency to lose salt and water that is further promoted by the salt-losing effect of progesterone. On the other hand, this tendency is more or less countered by the marked increases in aldosterone secretion that have been reported (Weir et al., 1971), so that the net effect on water storage of renal changes is probably very limited in the normal woman. The enormously increased activity of the kidney, however, suggests that its margin of safety may be changed and that small disequilibria may have profound effects. There is no doubt that the ability to secrete a water load changes as pregnancy progresses and that there is a marked decrease in the latter part of pregnancy, particularly during the third trimester (Hytten and Klopper, 1963). This reduction in ability to secrete a water load probably accounts for the increase in water retention in later pregnancy in normal women. Exaggeration of this tendency could account for the oliguria that often accompanies preeclampsia.

Sodium Resorption and Excretion

Although the decrease in total osmolality is accompanied by a decrease in plasma sodium concentration (Chesley, 1972; Lindheimer and Katz, 1972; MacDonald and Good, 1972), there is a retention of between 500 and 900 mEq. of sodium distributed between the products of conception and the maternal extracellular fluid (Hytten and Leitch, 1971). This solute storage phenomenon is important since renal sodium handling is a prime determinant of volume homeostasis. We know that glomerular filtration rate increases by up to 50 per cent during pregnancy, resulting in an additional filtered sodium load of 5000 to 10,000 mEq. per 24 hours. This is enormous when compared with a normal nonpregnant excretion of 100 to 200 mEq. per 24 hours. If this increased filtration were not accompanied by a parallel rise in the amount reabsorbed, massive sodium depletion would quickly occur, resulting in circulatory collapse. This increase in tubular sodium resorption represents the largest renal adjustment during pregnancy.

Many factors influence secretion and absorption of sodium by the kidney, and it is not possible to say with any certainty which of these is the most important. Progesterone is known to increase sodium excretion (Landau, 1973), and during pregnancy there is a marked increase in the production of progesterone. Progesterone also relaxes smooth muscle tonus and may produce vasodilatation and decreased renal arterial resistance, which are additional factors favoring natriuresis. The secretion and excretion of aldosterone are also elevated in normal pregnancy (Chesley, 1974). These changes tend to decrease sodium excretion but only to a limited extent. In the nonpregnant state, aldosterone-dependent sodium resorption amounts to less than 2 per cent of the filtered load. Obviously, this rate of resorption if maintained during pregnancy is inadequate to balance the increased sodium load to an appreciable extent. It is highly unlikely that elevated aldosterone levels are a cause of excessive sodium retention during pregnancy, and, in fact, they may represent a compensatory response to changes in sodium content and extracellular volume.

Other factors that have been cited as being responsible for influencing sodium excretion are changes in other salt-retaining hormones — estrogen, cortisol, placental lactogen, and prolactin; changes in maternal posture and in the uteroplacental circulation, which may markedly influence the ability of the kidney to handle sodium; and finally, the influence of the renin–angiotensin system on sodium resorption and excretion, although the mechanism by which this occurs is not known for certain.

THE RENIN–ANGIOTENSIN SYSTEM

Considerable changes occur in the renin–angiotensin system in pregnancy, but these are difficult to interpret with available data. Renin is an enzyme found in the juxtaglomerular cells. There is a considerable increase in plasma activity of renin during pregnancy, from between 5 to 10 times the normal nonpregnant level. This increase in activity is almost certainly due to changes in secretion by the maternal kidney and not due to changes in the fetus or placenta, because the levels remain elevated for at least 24 hours after delivery. Renin substrate is found in the alpha-2-globulin fraction of the plasma and is synthesized in the liver under the influence of the adrenal gland. Renin acts on renin substrate to form angiotensin, and increased amounts of renin substrate have also been demonstrated during normal pregnancy (Helmer and Judson, 1967). An increased substrate concentration does not necessarily mean an increased production of angiotensin; in fact, the available evidence on the levels of angiotensin in pregnancy is confusing. Certainly, there is no indication of an increased pressor effect under normal circumstances, but it is known that the pregnant woman has a greatly reduced sensitivity to angiotensin (Talledo et al., 1968), perhaps due to increased peripheral destruction caused by the raised level of circulating aminopeptidase.

Angiotensin does stimulate aldosterone production; in addition, infusions of angiotensin affect the urinary volume and excretion of sodium. It may be that the major effect of angiotensin is to reduce the excessive secretion of sodium either directly or by increasing aldosterone levels. The significance, however, of the greatly increased activity of the renin-angiotensin system in pregnancy is not understood. Since the pregnant woman is markedly insensitive to angiotensin, it appears that the end product of increased activity is without effect, apart from perhaps a high circulating level of aldosterone.

RENAL NUTRIENT EXCRETION

A rather bizarre feature of the maternal adaptation to pregnancy is the way in which the kidneys appear to waste nutrients, including various sugars, the water-soluble vitamins, and amino acids. Renal excretion involves three discrete processes: glomerular filtration, tubular resorption, and tubular excretion. The glomerular filtrate is essentially plasma that is almost free of protein and lipid and contains various electrolytes and nutrients in solution. It is in the proximal tubule that the nutrients essential to the body economy are reabsorbed. The quantitative contribution of tubular excretion of the total renal nutrient excretion is negligible. A balance normally exists between glomerular and tubular function, leading to conservation of essential nutrients and increased excretion of the useless and sometimes toxic end products of metabolism. These functions are modified during pregnancy; and in certain cases, these modifications are difficult to understand in the physiologic context.

Glucose

Every normal person excretes glucose to some extent, and the proportion of persons designated as glycosuric depends on both the sensitivity of the analytic method and the frequency with which individuals are tested. The development of the hexokinase glucose-6-phosphate dehydrogenase method for urine (Schmidt, 1963) has enabled the true incidence of glucose excretion in the urine to be studied. The first serial study in pregnancy using the hexokinase technique (Lind and Hytten, 1972) showed that the majority of women increased glucose excretion quite markedly during pregnancy; in addition, there was considerable variation in the amount of glucose that was secreted from time to time (Figure 32–4).

In considering the causes of glycosuria in pregnancy, there are two main possibilities. The first is that tubular function is unaltered but is simply overwhelmed by the greatly increased filtered load of glucose consequent to the rise in glomerular filtration rate. The second possible mechanism is a change in the resorptive capacity of the proximal tubule itself. The first view was based on methods and concepts evolved by the classic workers in renal physiology, but a recent study suggests that both their results and their interpretation were in error: Davison (1975) proposes that since the determination of glucose in the urine by the traditional methods grossly underestimated the amount of glucose excreted, the

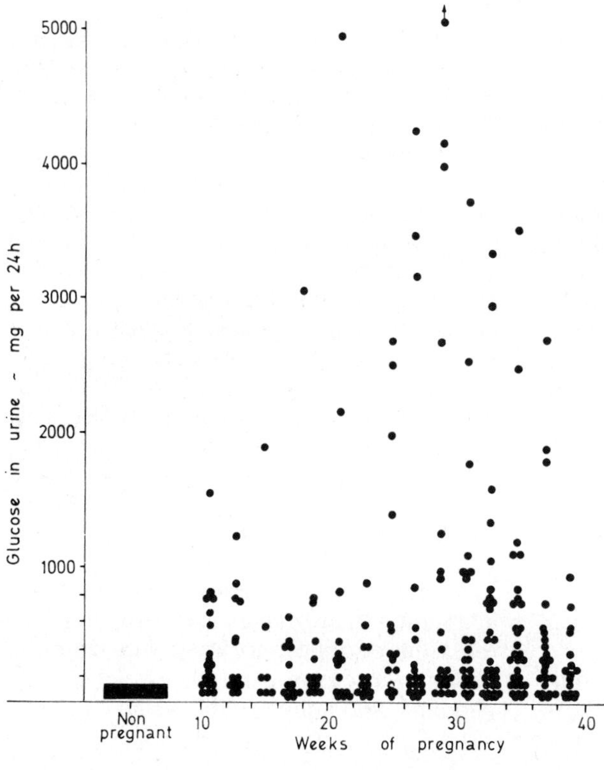

Figure 32–4. Glucose excretion in urine. Overall pattern in 24-hour samples of urine collected serially in pregnancy and at 6 to 8 weeks postpartum in 30 healthy subjects. (From data of Lind and Hytten, 1972.)

kidney was credited with a far greater resorptive capacity than it actually had. Replotting the earlier data on which the concept of a ceiling of glucose resorption (the maximum tubular resorptive capacity) was based shows no evidence of any such ceiling (Davison and Hytten, 1974*b*). It is now obvious that resorption continues to rise, although at a diminished rate, as the filtered load increases.

It has been shown in a group of healthy women that tubular resorption during glucose infusion is less efficient during pregnancy (Davison and Hytten, 1975). This study also revealed that, in general, the greater the amount of glycosuria in pregnancy, the less effective is resorption during the infusion. Plasma and urinary insulin levels were not related to the phenomenon of glycosuria, which is clearly due to an altered renal state specific to pregnancy. Unfortunately, because of this change and because of the intermittent nature of glycosuria, it is difficult to use the measurement of glucose excretion in the urine as an efficient screening procedure for abnormalities of carbohydrate metabolism in pregnancy. However, renal glycosuria may have more significance in the diagnosis of renal disease. It is known that there is diminished tubular function in infants following renal vascular damage (Stark and Geiger, 1973), and congenital anatomic defects have clearly been demonstrated in the proximal tubules of individuals with so-called "renal glycosuria" (Monasterio et al., 1964). Reduced glucose resorption is not found in healthy young men, whereas it is found in young women apparently in good health during pregnancy. The most obvious possibility is inadequate tubular function following damage from renal infection in childhood and adolescence, since minor degrees of damage from even asymptomatic infection may be common in young girls. Patients with recurrent glycosuria and normal glucose tolerance tests should therefore be regarded with suspicion from the point of view of minimal renal damage.

Other Sugars

Lactose, presumably formed by the mammary gland, is excreted in the urine by most pregnant women. Lactosuria of pregnancy is a benign condition of no clinical importance except as a possible source of confusion with glycosuria. Excretion of xylose, ribose, and fructose, but not arabinose, is increased in pregnancy. Some oligosaccharides, presumably of mammary origin, also appear in pregnancy urine. The higher plasma concentration of these compounds plus the elevated GFR during pregnancy may account for their appearance in the urine, but there is also a possibility that less efficient tubular resorption may affect their rates of excretion.

Amino Acids

The pregnant woman excretes much larger quantities of amino acids in the urine than does the nonpregnant woman. A study using column chromatography (Hytten and Cheyne, 1972) has shown that three broad patterns of amino acid excretion exist (Figure 32–5). Glycine, histidine, threonine, serine, and alanine are excreted in greater amounts than are other amino acids in the nonpregnant state. Their excretion rises rapidly in early pregnancy to more than double the nonpregnant level by about 16 weeks' gestation. Thereafter, the urinary loss continues to increase until term, when it reaches four to five times that in the nonpregnant state. The excretion of the second group of amino acids — lysine, cystine, taurine, phenylalanine, valine, leucine, and tyrosine — also rises rapidly in early pregnancy but thereafter tends to fall. Of the remaining six amino acids examined, glutamic acid, methionine, and ornithine were excreted in marginally greater amounts than before pregnancy. The excretion of asparagine and isoleucine was unchanged, and that of arginine tended to fall.

The increased excretion of amino acids together with the generally reduced blood levels and elevated GFR of pregnancy points to a tubular failure to reabsorb. Hytten and Cheyne (1972) calculated that for glycine, the renal tubules may, on occasion, fail to absorb more than half the filtered load. Among those who have investigated the aminoaciduria of pregnancy, the possibility of diminished tubular resorption was first suggested by Page and

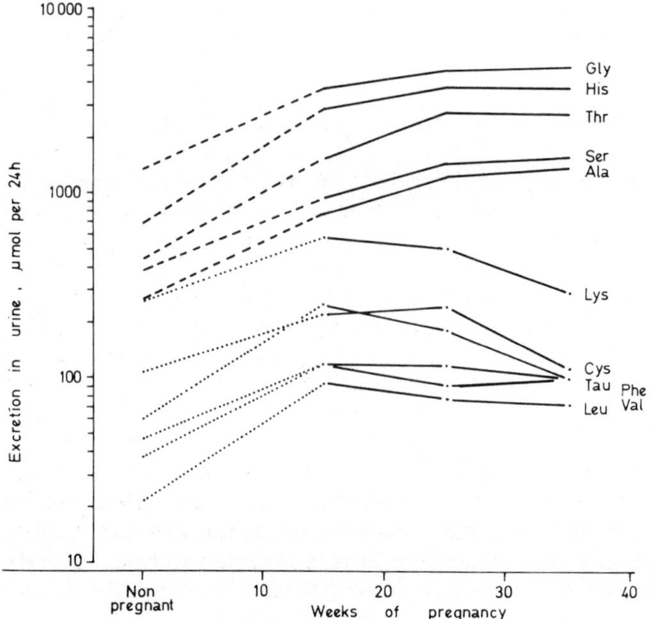

Figure 32–5. The excretion of two groups of amino acids in pregnancy by 10 healthy women. (From data of Hytten and Cheyne, 1972.)

co-workers (1954); they related it to "hormonal changes associated with pregnancy." Zinneman and associates (1963) suggested that it could be related to cortisol-like effects, since ACTH and cortisol can produce changes in amino acid excretion. However, amino acid excretion, like glucose excretion, is significantly increased in early pregnancy, before there is any convincing evidence of increased corticosteroid activity.

Water-Soluble Vitamins

Studies are few, but they all indicate increased excretion of these vitamins during pregnancy. Nicotinic acid and ascorbic acid are excreted at twice the nonpregnant average rate, and an increase in folate excretion is apparent by the end of the first trimester (Landon and Hytten, 1972). Because plasma folate levels are increased during pregnancy, the filtered load of folate is unlikely to be increased. Obviously tubular failure to reabsorb is involved (Fleming, 1972).

Protein

The small protein loss of some 200 to 300 mg. per 24 hours occurring normally in urine is not increased during pregnancy except in the presence of disease processes.

INVESTIGATION OF RENAL FUNCTION IN PREGNANCY

The methods by which renal function can be investigated during pregnancy are limited because of the presence of the fetus. It is also sometimes difficult to determine the significance of changes in those renal function studies that can be used because of the physiologic changes that have been described.

Preliminary Evaluation

In the majority of patients who become pregnant, disorders of renal function are usually asymptomatic; chronic renal disease may be revealed for the first time by the appearance of a hypertensive diathesis in late pregnancy (see Chapter 34). It is therefore very important that all patients who have either hypertension or proteinuria in pregnancy be screened for potential disorders of renal function.

History

The primary investigation is an adequate clinical history, which should include a survey of previous renal complaints, occupations, and drug consumption. Specific inquiry should be made about symptoms suggestive of urinary obstruction and the intake of analgesics, other phenacetin-containing drugs, and methysergide. The history should also include inquiry about renal disease, hypertension and its sequelae, preeclampsia, and other associated problems. Of particular significance in the pregnant patient is a history of recurrent urinary tract infection at or about the time of menarche or the time of first intercourse.

Physical Examination

Although general physical examination does not usually detect any of the long-standing signs of chronic renal disease, it is important to look for signs that might indicate evidence of long-standing cardiovascular involvement. It is particularly important that funduscopy be performed in order to exclude retinal changes which might indicate long-standing hypertension.

Examination of Urine and Blood

As well as a good historical survey and a general physical examination, certain basic investigations should be performed in every pregnant woman. These must include qualitative tests for glycosuria and hematuria and a quantitative test for proteinuria. Urinary microscopy should be performed on a midstream specimen of urine from all patients at the time of the first visit to the prenatal clinic. There are several alternative ways in which urine microscopy can be performed, but the urine should be handled by a constant technique in each case. When many urine samples are being examined, the most acceptable alternative is to allow the urine to settle in a test tube for an hour and withdraw the sediment with a Pasteur pipet. A well-spread, thick drop should be examined under low power for casts and crystals and a thin film under high power for red cells, white cells, and bacteria and for an exact identification of casts. In addition to microscopy, a midstream specimen should also be sent for culture.

If a patient should demonstrate hypertension at the first visit, the following additional investigations should be made of a blood sample: determination of urea, creatinine, sodium, potassium, chloride, bicarbonate, urate, calcium phosphate, alkaline phosphatase, and total protein and electrophoresis.

Contraindicated Procedures

Certain investigations should not be performed during pregnancy; since these investigations are probably some of the most precise methods of assessing renal morphology and function, immediate and accurate determination of the patient's renal status is limited. Infusion pyelography is contraindicated unless there is a suspicion of a life-threatening disease in the renal tract; also contraindicated are renal tomograms and radioisotopic studies of renal function. Although the long-term effects of irradiation to the fetus are as yet unproved, it is obviously not wise to use techniques involving a certain degree of unquantifiable risk. In addition, because of the increased blood flow to the kidney and the general increase in vascularity associated with pregnancy, renal biopsy is also contraindicated as an investigatory procedure.

The 16 hour water deprivation test, either with or without a diuretic, should not be used in pregnancy, and the use of the pitressin-tannate test is absolutely contraindicated.

Even with the restricted testing methods that are available for determining changes in renal function, however, it is possible to assess the likelihood of underlying renal damage in the pregnant woman.

Renal Clearance Studies: GFR and Renal Plasma Flow

Renal clearance studies should be used to assess both glomerular filtration rate and renal plasma flow. If a substance is filtered at the glomerulus in proportion to plasma water and is not reabsorbed or secreted by the tubule, it can be used to estimate glomerular filtration rate because the excretion rate is then determined only by the plasma level and the GFR.

Inulin Clearance

When accurate measures of renal function are required, the one universally accepted marker substance in the nonpregnant state is inulin. This is a mixture of fructose polymers with an average molecular weight of about 5200, but it has the disadvantages of being a variable mixture, of having a low solubility, and of hydrolyzing to fructose during the boiling necessary to dissolve it. The analytic methods for inulin are also difficult, although Robertson and co-workers (1970) showed that a modification of the method described by Heyrovsky (1956) could be used with considerable accuracy in estimation of urinary inulin in the pregnant woman. A further disadvantage of using inulin is that it must be infused at a constant rate for long enough to ensure complete stabilization of the blood level, and then continued until several urine samples can be obtained of sufficient volume to minimize bladder-emptying errors. The need for urine collection can be eliminated if the constant infusion is continued long enough to ensure that plasma levels are completely stable; the infusion rate is then assumed to equal the urinary excretion rate, the very small extra renal loss of inulin being ignored.

Endogenous Creatinine Clearance

The most widely used rough estimate of GFR is the endogenous creatinine clearance using a 24 hour urine collection and a single plasma sample. Estimates by Davison and Hytten (1974*a*) showed that there is a fairly constant relationship in pregnancy between endogenous creatinine clearance and the measurement of GFR by inulin clearance. This technique does, however, have a much greater range of errors than the more accurate exogenous method. It does have the advantage that if renal function is stable, the plasma creatinine varies little during the 24 hours in these circumstances. In the outpatient investigation, it is even permissible to draw the blood sample a few hours after the end of the collection period.

The automated technique used to measure creatinine in most hospitals measures creatinine plus some of the creatinine-like chromogen. Even with the automated method, there is a high interlaboratory variation, particularly when the result is close to normal, which reflects the difficulty in measuring plasma creatinine accurately in the normal range. The analytical error alone is of the order of ±10 per cent, so small changes in creatinine clearance should not be overinterpreted when they are close to normal. Important additional sources of error are loss of urine during defecation, mistiming of collection, incomplete bladder emptying, and washout effects caused by the consumption of diuretics or fluctuations in fluid intake. Careful instruction and good patient cooperation are needed for meaningful results.

Plasma creatinine concentration is determined by its production rate, which is largely a reflection of the muscle mass, and the excretion rate, which is roughly proportional to the GFR. In pregnancy, in which muscle mass is changing rapidly, alterations in plasma creatinine are difficult to interpret, particularly since excretion is greater than in the nonpregnant normal because of the increased renal efficiency. It cannot, therefore, be used with the same degree of confidence as in the nonpregnant state as a guide to the progress of renal function. A raised plasma creatinine level always indicates a depression in GFR, but a normal plasma creatinine level does not exclude renal disease in the pregnant state. Plasma urea values are not a good guide to changes in renal function in pregnancy because they are affected by fluid intake and fluctuate considerably during the 24 hours under the influence of food and drink.

PAH Clearance Rate

During pregnancy, renal blood flow can be estimated only by determination of the clearance rate of para-aminohippurate (PAH). The estimation is based on the assumption that PAH is both filtered at the glomerulus and secreted by the tubules so that it is cleared almost completely from the plasma in a single passage through the kidney. PAH is easy to measure accurately, and it equilibrates in the body more rapidly than inulin, so that the performance of PAH clearance is relatively simple.

From simultaneous measurements of the rates of glomerular filtration and renal plasma flow, one can calculate the proportion of plasma that is filtered off as it passes through the glomeruli, that is, the filtration fraction. The filtration fraction varies in response to several factors. The relative tonus of the afferent and efferent glomerular arterioles regulates the hydrostatic pressure in the glomerular capillaries. Disproportionate constriction on the efferent side raises the filtration pressure while reducing the flow of plasma and thus increases the filtration fraction. This is a characteristic finding in essential hypertension. Conversely, a disproportionate constriction on the afferent side will reduce the filtration pressure and filtration fraction, as may occur in preeclampsia.

Glomerular filtration rate and renal blood flow are both related to body size, and surface area has been found to correlate with them most closely in the nonpregnant adult. Results are often reported by laboratories corrected to a standard surface area of 1.73 square meters for comparison with the normal range. This correction is grossly misleading in pregnancy, for surface area changes continuously; therefore, it is advisable to ensure that the results are reported uncorrected and that the medical staff understands that corrected values are of little use. The correction is, of course, unnecessary in any case when clearances are used serially to follow the progress of disease.

Determination of Urinary Concentration

The ability to concentrate urine is impaired as the population of nephrons declines with disease, and disproportionately so with any disease affecting the loop of Henle or the collecting duct. Traditionally, urine specific gravity has been used as the criterion of urinary concentration. However, as it bears an inconstant relationship to osmolality (which is the best measure of the ability to concentrate urine), particularly in the presence of proteinuria and glycosuria, it should now be abandoned in favor of osmolality, which can be measured more accurately with a much smaller sample, and with modern instruments, almost as quickly. An osmolality of 700 corresponds roughly to a specific gravity of 1.020. The concentration test has often been described as a sensitive index of early renal damage, but the reproducibility is so low and the normal range so wide that it cannot be more than a crude index. To obtain maximal concentration reliably, it is necessary to deprive the patient of fluid for more than 24 hours, which makes the test inapplicable to pregnant women. Of the other simpler tests that can be used, only one is acceptable in pregnancy and that is the testing of early morning urine samples. If one or more of several early morning samples taken without special precautions have an osmolality of 700 milliosmoles per liter, it is unlikely that there is an important defect in urinary concentration.

SUMMARY

Many of the changes in renal physiology appear to contradict the homeostatic needs of the pregnant woman, since pregnancy appears to be characterized by a greater than normal ability to excrete many substances essential for the development of the fetus. In addition, water and electrolytes appear to be able to be removed from the body more efficiently, even though the general tendency in pregnancy is one of fluid retention. In spite of this, the pregnant woman appears to be more capable of withstanding variations in fluid and nutrient intake than she is in the nonpregnant state; thus, as a result, she is capable of providing a more constant environment in which the fetus can develop. Our knowledge of various aspects of renal physiology in pregnancy is limited, but it is becoming obvious that concepts that are accepted for the nonpregnant state cannot be applied to pregnancy without modification.

REFERENCES

Assali, N. S., Rauramo, L., and Peltonen, T.: Measurement of uterine blood flow and uterine metabolism VIII. Uterine and fetal blood flow and oxygen consumption in early human pregnancy. Am. J. Obstet. Gynecol., *79*:86, 1960.

Chesley, L. C.: Plasma and red cell volumes during pregnancy. Am. J. Obstet. Gynecol. *112*:440, 1972.

Chesley, L. C.: Disorders of the kidney, fluids and electrolytes. *In* Assali, N. S. (ed.): Pathophysiology of Gestational Disorders. Vol. 1. New York, Academic Press, 1972, pp. 355–477.
Chesley, L. C.: Renin, angiotensin and aldosterone. Obstet. Gynecol. Annu. *3*:235, 1974.
Chesley, L. C., and Sloan, D. M.: The effect of posture on renal function in late pregnancy. Am. J. Obstet. Gynecol. *89*:754, 1964.
Davison, J. M.: Renal nutrient excretion with emphasis on glucose. Clinics in Obstet. Gynaecol. *2*:365, 1975.
Davison, J. M., and Hytten, F. E.: Glomerular filtration during and after pregnancy. J. Obstet. Gynaecol. Br. Commonw. *81*:588, 1974*a*.
Davison, J. M., and Hytten, F. E.: Renal handling of glucose in pregnancy. *In* Sutherland, H. W., and Stowers, J. M. (Eds.): Proceedings of a Symposium on Carbohydrate Metabolism in Pregnancy and the Newborn. London, Churchill Livingstone, 1974*b*, pp. 2–18.
Davison, J. M., and Hytten, F. E.: The effect of pregnancy on the renal handling of glucose. J. Obstet. Gynaecol. Br. Commonw. *82*:283, 1975.
Fleming, A. F.: Urinary excretion of folate in pregnancy. J. Obstet. Gynaecol. Br. Commonw. *79*:916, 1972.
Gylling, T.: Renal hemodynamics and heart volume in normal pregnancy. Acta Obstet. Gynecol. Scand. *40* (Suppl. 5):1, 1961.
Helmer, O. M., and Judson, W. E.: Influence of high renin substrate levels on renin-angiotensin system in pregnancy. Am. J. Obstet. Gynecol. *99*:9, 1967.
Heyrovsky, A.: A new method for the determination of inulin in plasma and urine. Clin. Chim. Acta *1*:470, 1956.
Hytten, F. E., and Cheyne, G. A.: The aminoaciduria of pregnancy. J. Obstet. Gynaecol. Br. Commonw. *79*:424, 1972.
Hytten, F. E., and Klopper, A.: Response to a water load in pregnancy. J. Obstet. Gynaecol. Br. Commow. *70*:811, 1963.
Hytten, F. E., and Leitch, I.: The Physiology of Human Pregnancy. 2nd Ed. Oxford, Blackwell Scientific Publications, 1971, Chap. 6.
Hytten, F. E., and Robertson, E. G.: Maternal water metabolism in pregnancy. Proc. R. Soc. Med. *64*:1072, 1971.
Hytten, F. E., and Taggart, N.: Limb volumes in pregnancy. J. Obstet. Gynaecol. Br. Commonw. *74*:663, 1967.
Hytten, F. E., Thomson, A. M., and Taggart, N.: Total body water in normal pregnancy. J. Obstet. Gynaecol. Br. Commonw. *73*:553, 1966.
Landau, R. L.: Metabolic influence of progesterone. *In* Handbook of Physiology, Endocrinology Part I. Baltimore, Williams & Wilkins, 1973, pp. 573–589.
Landon, M. J., and Hytten, F. E.: The excretion of glucose during pregnancy. J. Obstet. Gynaecol. Br. Commonw. *78*:769, 1972.
Lees, M. M., Taylor, S. H., Scott, D. B., et al.: A study of cardiac output at rest throughout pregnancy. J. Obstet. Gynaecol. Br. Commonw. *74*:319, 1967.
Lind, T., and Hytten, F. E.: The excretion of glucose during normal pregnancy. J. Obstet. Gynaecol. Br. Commonw. *79*:961, 1972.
Lindheimer, M. D.: Further characterization of the influence of supine posture on renal function in late pregnancy. Effect of rapid saline infusion on renal sodium, water and uric acid metabolism. Gynecol. Invest. *1*:69, 1970.
Lindheimer, M. D., and Katz, A. I.: Kidney function in the pregnant rat. J. Lab. Clin. Med. *78*:633, 1971.
Lindheimer, M. D., and Katz, A. I.: Renal function in pregnancy. Obstet. Gynecol. Annu. *1*:139, 1972.
Lindheimer, M. D., and Katz, A. I.: Renal changes during pregnancy: their relevance to volume homeostasis. Clinics in Obstet. Gynaecol. *2*:345, 1975.
Lindheimer, M. D., and Weston, P. V.: Effect of hypotonic expansion on sodium, water, and urea excretion in late pregnancy: the influence of posture on these results. J. Clin. Invest. *48*:947, 1969.
Lund, C. J., and Donovan, J. C.: Blood volume during pregnancy. Am. J. Obstet. Gynecol. *98*:393, 1967.
MacDonald, H. N., and Good, W.: The effect of parity on plasma, sodium, potassium, chloride, and osmolality levels during pregnancy. J. Obstet. Gynaecol. Br. Commonw. *79*:441, 1972.
Metcalfe, J., Romney, S. L., Ramsey, L. H., et al.: Estimation of uterine blood flow in normal human pregnancies at term. J. Clin. Invest. *34*:1632, 1955.
Monasterio, G., Oliver, J., Muiesau, G., et al.: Renal diabetes as a congenital tubular dysplasia. Am. J. Med. *37*:44, 1964.
Oparil, S., Ehrlich, E. N., and Lindheimer, M. D.: Effects of progesterone on volume homeostasis in man. *In* Fregley, M. J., and Fregley, M. S. (eds.): Oral Contraceptives and High Blood Pressure. Gainesville, Fla., Dolphin Press, 1974, pp. 170–183.
Page, E. W., Glendenning, M. B., Dignam, W., et al.: The causes of histidinuria in pregnancy. Am. J. Obstet. Gynecol. *68*:110, 1954.

Paintin, D. B.: The size of total red cell volume in pregnancy. J. Obstet. Gynaecol. Br. Commonw. *69*:719, 1962.

Parboosingh, J., and Doig, A.: Renal nyctohemeral excretory patterns of water and solutes in normal human pregnancy. Am. J. Obstet. Gynecol. *116*:609, 1973.

Power, C. G., Longo, L. D., Wagner, H. N., Jr., et al.: Uneven distribution of maternal and fetal placental blood flow as demonstrated using macroaggregates and its response to hypoxia. J. Clin. Invest. *46*:2053, 1967.

Robertson, E. G.: Natural history of oedema during pregnancy. J. Obstet. Gynaecol. Br. Commonw. *78*:520, 1971.

Robertson, E. G., and Cheyne, G. A.: Plasma biochemistry in relation to oedema in pregnancy. J. Obstet. Gynaecol. Br. Commonw. *79*:769, 1972.

Robertson, E. G., Hytten, F. E., and Cheyne, G. A.: The measurement of extracellular fluid volume in pregnancy with inulin. J. Obstet. Gynaecol. Br. Commonw. *77*:520, 1970.

Schmidt, F. H.: Enzymatische Methoden zur Bestimmung von Blut-und Hamzucker nuter Berucksichtigung von Vergleichsuntersuchungen mit klassichen Methoden. Internist *4*:554, 1963.

Seitchik, J.: Total body water and total body density of pregnant women. Obstet. Gynecol. *29*:155, 1967.

Sims, E. A. H., and Krantz, K. E.: Serial studies of renal function during normal pregnancy and the puerperium in normal women. J. Clin. Invest. *37*:1764, 1958.

Stark, H., and Geiger, R.: Renal tubular dysfunction following vascular accidents of the kidneys in the newborn period. J. Pediatr. *83*:933, 1973.

Talledo, O. E., Chesley, L. C., and Zuspan, F. P.: Renin-angiotensin system in normal and toxemic pregnancies. 3. Differential sensitivity to angiotensin II and norepinephrine in toxemia of pregnancy. Am. J. Obstet. Gynecol. *100*:218, 1968.

Walters, W. A. W., MacGregor, W. G., and Hills, M.: Cardiac output at rest during pregnancy and the puerperium. Clin. Sci. *30*:1, 1966.

Weir, R. J., Paintin, D. B., Brown, J. J., et al.: A serial study in pregnancy of the plasma concentrations of renin, corticosteroids, electrolytes, and proteins and of the haematocrit and plasma volume. J. Obstet. Gynaecol. Br. Commonw. *78*:590, 1971.

Zinneman, H. H., Johnson, J. J., and Seal, U. S.: Effect of short-term therapy with cortisol on the urinary excretion of the free amino acids. J. Clin. Endocrinol. *23*:996, 1963.

33

CLINICAL AND OPERATIVE OBSTETRICS

H. J. BUCHSBAUM, M.D.

OBSTETRICS

The genitourinary structures undergo rather extensive anatomic changes in accommodating to pregnancy (see Chapter 30). In spite of these changes the proximity of the ureters, bladder, and urethra to the pregnant uterus and the birth canal exposes them to pathologic processes in the genital tract and makes them susceptible to injury during labor and delivery.

Height of the uterine fundus, although not valid for estimation of gestational age, is used to identify intrauterine growth retardation, multiple gestation, or oligo- and polyhydramnios. Worthen and Bustillo (1980), utilizing ultrasound techniques, found significant differences in fundal height when measured with a full or empty bladder. The differences varied with gestation, but averaged 2 to 3 cm.

Incarcerated Uterus

Under rare circumstances the enlarged and gravid uterus can cause urethral obstruction. A retroflexed and retroverted uterus can become incarcerated in the true pelvis and in the third month of gestation markedly displace the bladder anteriorly. The cervix presses against the trigone, obstructing the urethra and causing frequency and overflow incontinence. If untreated, the bladder becomes overdistended and can rupture. The bladder should be emptied by suprapubic aspiration before any attempt is made to displace the incarcerated uterus (Moir and Myerscough, 1971).

Placenta Percreta

Placenta percreta is a rare defect of placentation in which chorionic villi penetrate the entire thickness of the uterine wall and can even penetrate the serosa. When such a placenta is implanted low on the anterior wall it can invade the bladder. Patients with this condition present with painful hematuria. This rare entity should be suspected when a bleeding granular lesion is seen on the posterior wall on cystoscopic examination in a pregnant patient (Grabert et al., 1970; Taefi et al., 1970). Total hysterectomy and partial cystectomy are often necessary to control the bleeding.

Labor and Delivery

Although a full bladder may cause mechanical dystocia, Read and co-workers (1980) concluded that moderate amounts of urine (less than 300 ml.) have no effect on uterine contractions, cervical dilatation, or the course of labor.

The bladder is traumatized in normal labor and delivery, and the risks of injury are greatly increased in operative obstetrics and by obstructed prolonged labor. Normal labor and delivery result in some edema of the bladder wall but rarely cause hematuria and detrusor injury severe enough to produce postpartum bladder dysfunction. Postpartum bladder dysfunction sufficient to require catheterization occurs in slightly less than 10 per cent of deliveries (Sherline and Danforth, 1962). Urinary retention is generally of short duration, averaging 2.2 days.

Prolonged Labor and Vesicovaginal Fistula

Obstetric fistulas have been identified in Egyptian mummies dating from the 11th Dynasty, 250 B.C.E. (Mahfouz, 1957).

Incidence. Obstetric vesicovaginal fistula is now extremely rare in the United States and developed nations, but it continues to be a serious problem in emerging countries, where labor and delivery may be conducted by untrained personnel. The experience at the Margaret Hague and Los Angeles County Hospitals with obstetric vesicovaginal fistulas reflects the changing incidence of this complication (McCausland et al., 1960). There were six vesicovaginal fistulas in over 30,000 deliveries (0.00018 per cent) during the period 1931–1935, and two in approximately 95,000 deliveries (0.00002 per cent) in 1951–1955. During the earlier period the average length of labor was 40.6 hours. This was reduced to 12 hours in the later period, with a ninefold reduction in the incidence of vesicovaginal fistulas. This reduction was accompanied by a decreased incidence of hematuria and postparum urinary retention necessitating indwelling catheters. In keeping with the national experience, only 5.6 per cent of the vesicovaginal fistulas seen at these two institutions were pregnancy-related.

In contrast to the experience with women in industrialized countries, pregnancy-related urinary fistulas continue to be a major problem in developing nations, accounting for approximately 90 per cent of all vesicovaginal fistulas (Foda, 1959; Coetzee and Lithgow, 1966; Massoudnia, 1972). This great disparity between industrial and developing countries is related to the incidence of prolonged obstructed labor.

Mechanism of Injury. Bladder injuries usually develop in the first stage of labor when the bladder, distended or empty, is pressed against the bony pelvis by the fetal head. In cases in which vesicovaginal fistulas develop, the fetus need not be excessively large, but one can anticipate that the bladder has not been elevated out of the pelvis. The common denominator in these cases is prolonged obstructed labor, often secondary to cephalopelvic disproportion. Although bladder injury is the most common type of injury following prolonged labor, the ureters and urethra can also be injured. Pure ureteral injury rarely follows prolonged labor; ureterovaginal fistulas generally follow extensive pelvic necrosis. Complete evaluation must be carried out to avoid overlooking a second and perhaps more serious fistula.

In Linke and co-workers' (1971) series of 10 cases of extensive bladder and urethral injury, the duration of labor averaged nearly 80 hours. The mechanism of bladder injury is: pressure, ischemia, necrosis. The loss of urine may not be evident immediately following delivery and may be delayed until the necrotic tissue sloughs. The damage can be quite extensive, destroying the trigone, the ureters, or urethra. For the management of uncomplicated vesicovaginal fistulas see Chapter 21. Extensive necrosis of the bladder base with urethral destruction is rarely seen in the Western world. For discussion of surgical management the reader is referred to the excellent reports of Ingelman-Sundberg (1954), McCall and Bolton (1956), Moir (1967), and Hamlin and Nicholson (1969).

Uterine Rupture

Like other complications of pregnancy, uterine rupture is becoming a rarity in the United States but continues to be a major obstetric problem in developing nations. In Asia and Africa, uterine rupture is reported to occur as frequently as 1 in 93 deliveries (Rendle-Short, 1960). Rupture occurs most commonly in the unscarred uterus as the result of prolonged labor with cephalopelvic disproportion. In the United States, inappropriate administration of oxytocin is the leading cause of uterine rupture.

When rupture occurs through the lower uterine segment (below the peritoneal reflection) in the presence of a distended bladder, bladder and ureteral injury can occur. The degree of bladder injury ranges from contusion, with edema and ecchymosis, to perforation. Serious bladder injury occurs in approximately 10 per cent of patients with uterine rupture (Hassim, 1968). A major bladder injury involving all layers of the vesical wall was present in 8 per cent, and less extensive tears in 14 per cent of 100 cases of uterine rupture reported by Raghavaiah and Devi (1975). The injury is usually a transverse laceration, and the patient presents with hematuria.

An extreme example of uterine rupture with bladder perforation involves escape of the fetus into the bladder. The bladder must be distended at the time of rupture of the lower uterine segment to facilitate entry of the fetus into the bladder. Approximately 10 such cases have been reported. These patients present in shock, generally following long labor. Approximately half had significant hematuria; some had meconium-stained urine, and the presence of vernix in the urine has been reported. The peritoneal cavity can be unsoiled, with the whole fetus or a part (body, head or extremities) present in the bladder.

While primary ureteral injury can occur with uterine rupture, hysterectomy following rupture presents the greater risk to the ureters (see later discussion). It is interesting to note that none of the survivors in Raghavaiah and Devi's (1975) series of 100 patients with uterine rupture developed vesicovaginal fistulas after repair of the bladder; but four developed what were probably iatrogenic ureterovaginal fistulas.

The bladder tear should be closed in two layers utilizing interrupted or continuous 2–0 chromic catgut sutures. Unlike surgical entries into the bladder, uterine rupture presents a significant degree of blunt trauma with hematoma and detrusor muscle injury. This compromises postoperative bladder function, requiring prolonged bladder drainage.

Forceps Delivery

Most forceps deliveries traumatize the bladder; the degree of trauma varies, ranging from mild contusion to severe injury with hematuria and postpartum dysfunction. Bladder and ureteral lacerations are fortunately rare. McCausland and coworkers (1960) reported 15 of 23 (65 per cent) pregnancy-related fistulas resulted from forceps deliveries.

The use of high forceps applied to the floating head, which requires considerable intrauterine manipulation, has been totally abandoned. Mid-forceps delivery presents the greatest risk to the bladder, with the Kielland forceps being the major offender. The commonly used outlet forceps rarely cause bladder or urethral problems.

The bladder must be emptied prior to any forceps application and delivery. When the Kielland forceps are used in mid-pelvic arrest, with the head in the occiput transverse, two methods of applying the anterior blade can be used: the classic and the wandering method. In the classic application the anterior blade is inserted with the cephalic concavity pointing up. The toe of the blade is directed behind the symphysis into the cervix. The blade is then advanced into the fundus, at which point the tip can be palpated through the mother's abdominal wall. Since the cephalic concavity of the forceps is directed upward, the blade must be rotated 180 degrees so that the cephalic curve becomes applied to the convexity of the fetal head.

In this method of application, bladder injury can occur at two points: (1) If the toe of the anterior blade is not in the cervical canal when the blade is advanced, it can be introduced directly into the bladder through the anterior fornix; and (2) when the anterior blade is rotated 180 degrees in a tight uterus, the blade can shear through the thin uterine wall and injure the bladder. To minimize the risk of bladder injury, most authorities recommend applying the anterior blade over the face or brow of the fetus and then gliding or wandering it to its anterior position.

The Kielland forceps are contraindicated in the flat pelvis, where the Barton forceps are more appropriate. Traction applied to the Kielland forceps in the flat pelvis, prior to rotation, brings the cephalic bulge of the anterior blade against the bladder, compressing it against the symphysis. A similar mechanism of bladder injury is present if traction is applied to the Barton forceps in the axis of the handles.

Parry-Jones (1952) reported the occurrence of five urinary fistulas (four vesicovaginal and one urethrovaginal) in 233 cases of occiput posterior or transverse arrest delivered with Kielland forceps. In his personal series, nearly 20 per cent (11 of 60) of patients delivered with Kielland forceps developed postpartum hematuria. In the series of McCausland and co-workers (1960) 60 per cent of the forceps-induced fistulas followed delivery with Kielland forceps.

Lest one think that the Kielland forceps are the only offenders, Klein and Malinconico (1955) reported five vesicovaginal fistulas and one bladder laceration in a review of 3198 mid-forceps operations in which a variety of instruments were used. In their own series of 351 mid-forceps deliveries, there were three urinary tract injuries among 41 women delivered with Kielland forceps, and two injuries in 112 cases (1.7 per cent) when delivery was accomplished by a Scanzoni maneuver.

In contrast, Dunlop (1969) reported 292 mid-forceps deliveries utilizing a variety of forceps (including 42 Kielland applications) without a urinary tract injury. Postoperative urinary retention and urinary tract infection commonly follow mid-forceps delivery. Cooke (1967) reported urinary tract complications in 6.3 per cent (27 of 427) of patients. Eighteen women had bladder atony requiring drainage for a period of from 34 hours to 14 days; transient hematuria was present in three, and six developed urinary tract infections.

The incidence of bladder injury in mid-forceps delivery is related to several factors: (1) indications; (2) experience of the operator; (3) shape of the pelvis; and (4) type of forceps utilized. An important factor is the predisposing condition. Tissue exposed to prolonged pressure is more likely to be injured during forceps delivery. In Coetzee and Lithgow's series (1966), nearly 20 per cent of the pregnancy-related fistulas followed forceps delivery. However, all patients had prolonged and neglected labors, which undoubtedly traumatized the tissue and made it more susceptible to injury. Furthermore, Dudley and coworkers (1971) showed a marked difference in the incidence of postpartum urinary retention and urinary tract infection in indicated and elective forceps deliveries. The former carried a higher rate of urinary tract complications.

Cesarean Section

Cesarean section is one of the oldest surgical procedures. In antiquity it was performed on the dead mother in an attempt to save the infant. Since the end of the nineteenth century, the procedure has been modified and made safer, so that it is now performed in approximately 15 to 20 per cent of all deliveries. On some obstetric services the incidence of cesarean section may be even higher (Pritchard and McDonald, 1980). There are 300,000 such procedures performed annually for a variety of indications, often under emergent conditions. They are performed by individuals with greatly varied surgical training and skill, and as a result, the incidence of urinary tract injuries following cesarean section varies greatly.

EXTRAPERITONEAL CESAREAN SECTION

This procedure was popular before the introduction of antibiotics. By displacing the bladder, the advocates of this form of cesarean section hoped to avoid soiling the peritoneal cavity. In practice the peritoneal cavity was often entered and the incidence of bladder and ureteral injuries unacceptably high, so that the procedure is now obsolete.

CLASSIC AND LOW SEGMENT CESAREAN SECTIONS

The two main types of cesarean section, classic and low segment transverse, present different risks to the urinary tract. Several precautions can reduce the overall incidence of urinary complications. The bladder should be emptied and an indwelling catheter placed prior to surgery, for continuous drainage.

Surgical Precautions

The most appropriate abdominal incision is a midline vertical incision below the umbilicus. The peritoneum is opened vertically and entered at the cephalad end of the incision near the umbilicus. If a transverse or Pfannenstiel incision is used, the peritoneum should also be incised in a vertical fashion. The urinary bladder becomes an abdominal organ in later pregnancy (von Schubert, 1929) and injury can be avoided by starting the peritoneal incision at the cephalic end.

In classic cesarean section, a longitudinal incision is made into the anterior wall of the fundus. The classic incision in the fundus is unlikely to cause injury to urinary tract structures. The more common lower segment transverse incision and the low vertical incision require development of the bladder flap with caudal displacement of the bladder. In order to do this, the vesicouterine fold of the visceral peritoneum is elevated with a tissue forceps and opened laterally. The bladder flap is incised in a V-shaped incision between the round ligaments. It is safest to undermine the tissues by inserting a Metzenbaum scissors and opening the blades prior to cutting the peritoneum. After the peritoneum is incised, the bladder can safely be mobilized by blunt dissection with one or two layers of gauze over a finger. A sweeping motion supinating the hand effectively dissects the areolar tissue and displaces the bladder.

Considering the close proximity of the bladder and the haste to deliver the infant, bladder injury is rare in cesarean section, occurring in less than 1 per cent of elective and emergency procedures (Jones, 1976; Evrard et al., 1980).

In patients with previous cesarean section, the bladder flap may be considerably higher on the fundus of the uterus, and the peritoneum must be incised at an appropriate point. In such cases mobilization of the bladder off the lower uterine segment requires sharp dissection, since tissue planes have been obliterated by scarring.

Bladder Injury

If the bladder is lacerated in the course of dissection, the site of injury is marked by a suture, which is left long and tagged. The cesarean section should be completed and the baby delivered, the placenta and membranes removed, and the uterine incision repaired, before bladder repair is undertaken.

If any doubt exists about the integrity of the bladder, several hundred milliliters of methylene blue-colored saline should be instilled into the urinary bladder via the indwelling catheter. The escape of any blue-colored saline identifies the site of injury.

If the bladder has been entered, the edges of the incision are identified and stay sutures placed. The bladder is closed in two layers utilizing 2–0 chromic catgut on atraumatic needles. An indwelling catheter should be left in place for 7 to 10 days, and administration of urinary antimicrobials started.

Bladder Fistula. Unrecognized bladder injury is likely to result in vesicovaginal fistula. If the patient becomes incontinent following cesarean section, evaluation should be undertaken to rule out fistula. If the loss of urine is evident within 2 to 3 days following surgery, immediate repair of the defect can be attempted. If the fistula becomes evident after a longer period of time, repair should be delayed 2 to 3 months to allow tissue reaction to subside. With continuous bladder drainage, spontaneous closure of uncomplicated vesicovaginal fistulas can be anticipated in 20 to 30 per cent of cases.

VESICOCORPOREAL FISTULA. A rare form of bladder fistula is vesicocorporeal fistula, in which the communication is between the bladder and the uterine corpus (Figure 33–1 *A*, *B*). The patients are continent of urine and have cyclic hematuria (Frankel and Buchsbaum, 1971). Youssef (1957) believes that these patients have a "functional" uterine sphincter. All the menstrual blood flows into the bladder and exits via the urethra during menses (menouria). If the communication is between the bladder and the cervix, patients are incontinent with urine discharged through the cervical os (Warren, 1979). The menstrual flow is normal.

Ureteral Injury

More serious than bladder laceration is injury of the ureter. As a result of dextrorotation of the pregnant uterus, the left ureter is at particular risk. The left lateral aspect of the uterus is moved anteriorly, bringing the ureter closer to the dilated cervix. In one case in which cesarean section was performed on a patient with a markedly

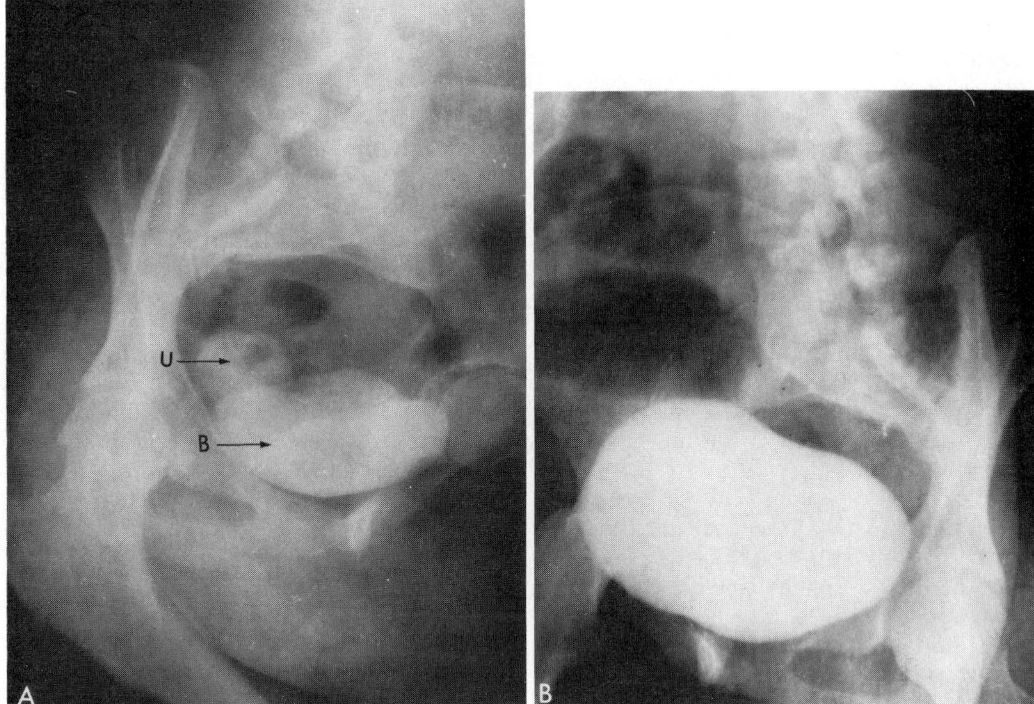

Figure 33–1. Vesicocorporeal fistula.

A, Retrograde cystogram in patient with menouria following cesarean section. Oblique view demonstrates contrast material in the bladder (B) and uterus (U).

B, Cystogram following spontaneous closure of vesicocorporeal fistula.

(From Frankel, T., and Buchsbaum, H. J.: Vesicocorporeal fistula with menouria. J. Urol. *106*:860, 1971. Copyright © 1971 The Williams & Wilkins Co., Baltimore. Reproduced by permission.)

deformed pelvis, the ureter was located anterior to the uterus. The ureter was injured in performing a transverse incision, and the defect was not recognized. The ureter communicated with the uterine corpus, creating a ureterocorporeal fistula with urine passing from the cervical os (El Mahgoub and El Zeniny, 1971). In these unusual cases of urinary fistulas, a hysterogram, intravenous pyelogram, cystogram, and cystoscopic examination can establish the proper diagnosis.

The ureters can be protected in cesarean section by dissecting the bladder flap further than the operator would anticipate, and by the placement of a broad retractor.

Control of Bleeding. Perhaps the greatest risk to the ureters is lateral extension of a lower segment transverse uterine incision, when increased bleeding occurs. Attempts to control bleeding with clamps placed lateral to the cervix can result in ureteral injury. The proximity of the ureter to the uterine artery is shown in Figure 8–4. Active bleeding and clots obscure the anatomy. Direct pressure with a sponge stick will often control bleeding enough to allow the ureter to be identified. The lateral peritoneum between the round and infundibulopelvic ligaments can be opened and the ureter identified at the pelvic brim just medial to the bifurcation of the common iliac artery. Hypogastric or uterine artery ligation can then be performed to establish hemostasis. The course of the ureter can be identified and traced to the area of bleeding. If multiple sutures were used to control bleeding, the surgeon should dissect out the ureter to ensure that it has not been crushed or ligated. Bulky pedicles ligated close to the ureter present special problems. They can kink and displace the ureter, causing partial obstruction.

Bilateral Obstruction. An extreme example of ureteral injury is bilateral obstruction. Lloyd-Davies (1969) reported a patient with this complication. The critical feature of the report, describing the low segment transverse cesarean section, was the considerable bleeding requiring multiple ligatures.

CESAREAN HYSTERECTOMY

Cesarean hysterectomy presents special problems related to the urinary tract. The procedure can be performed for "indicated" (e.g., ruptured uterus, placenta accreta) or "elective" (sterilization) reasons. The frequency of complications generally relates to the indication for the hysterectomy. If the hysterectomy is done for bleeding from a ruptured uterus, the emergent nature of the procedure dictates the speed with which it is performed. Bleeding into the broad ligament with hematoma formation often obscures vital structures.

Mickal and coworkers (1969) reported urinary complications in 3.3 per cent of patients (bladder lacerations and ureteral trauma) and a 0.4 per cent fistula rate in a literature review of 3166 cases of cesarean section hysterectomy. Their own 384 cases reflected the broader experience: 20 instances of bladder entry (5.2 per cent). All injuries were repaired with resultant fistula in only one case. There were two additional vesicovaginal fistulas in unrecognized bladder injuries, and one case of ureteral injury (0.2 per cent). Barclay (1970) reported 41 cases in which the bladder was entered in 1000 consecutive cesarean section hysterectomies at the Charity Hospital. Thirty-seven were recognized and repaired — all but one healed. There were five vesicovaginal fistulas that resulted from unrecognized bladder injury for a total of six vesicovaginal fistulas (0.6 per cent). There were four unilateral ureteral injuries, two in the 200 emergency and two in the 800 cases done for elective indications.

In recent series, bladder injury during cesarean hysterectomy has been reported, varying from 1.7 per cent (Britton, 1980) to 6 per cent (Haynes and Martin, 1979), with most recognized and repaired at surgery. Vesicovaginal fistulas are extremely rare.

Cesarean hysterectomy therefore presents heightened risks to the urinary tract. Following completion of the operation, the bladder should routinely be distended with 300 to 400 ml. of methylene blue-colored saline, to ensure its integrity. In cesarean section hysterectomy, as in other gynecologic surgery, the recognized and repaired bladder injury is unlikely to result in the formation of a fistula; it is the unrecognized injury that results in a fistula.

Version and Extraction

Internal version and extraction of an infant is an extremely difficult procedure. Few obstetricians have been taught the technique, and even fewer have applied it clinically. It carries significant risks to maternal genital structures and the urinary bladder. Version and extraction (except for a second twin) has been replaced in clinical practice by cesarean section.

Destructive Operations

With the exception of craniotomy in a hydrocephalic infant, destructive operations are rarely performed today. Embryotomy and decapitation require the use of a variety of instruments including hooks, scissors, and cranioclasts, and present obvious risks to the urinary tract.

REFERENCES

Barclay, D. L.: Cesarean hysterectomy. A thirty years' experience. Obstet. Gynecol. *35*:120, 1970.

Britton, J. J.: Sterilization by cesarean hysterectomy. Am. J. Obstet. Gynecol. *137*:887, 1980.

Coetzee, T., and Lithgow, D. M.: Obstetric fistulae of the urinary tract. J. Obstet. Gynaecol. Br. Commonw. *73*:837, 1966.

Cooke, W. A. R.: Evaluation of midforceps operation. Am. J. Obstet. Gynecol. *99*:327, 1967.

Dudley, A. G., Markham, S. M., and McNie, T. M.: Elective versus indicated midforceps delivery. Obstet. Gynecol. *37*:19, 1971.

Dunlop, D. L.: Midforceps operations at the University of Alberta Hospital (1965–1967). Am. J. Obstet. Gynecol. *103*:471, 1969.

El Mahgoub, S., and El Zeniny, A.: Uretero-uterine fistula after cesarean section. Am. J. Obstet. Gynecol. *110*:881, 1971.
Evrard, J. R., Gold, E. M., Cahill, T. F.: Cesarean section: a contemporary assessment. J. Reprod. Med. *24*:147, 1980.
Foda, M. S.: Evaluation of methods of treatment of urinary fistulas in women: report of 220 cases. J. Obstet. Gynacecol. Br. Emp. *66*:372, 1959.
Frankel, T., and Buchsbaum, H. J.: Vesicocorporeal fistula with menouria. J. Urol. *106*:860, 1971.
Grabert, H., Mossa, A., Oliveira, S. F., et al.: Placenta percreta with penetration of the bladder. J. Obstet. Gynaecol. Br. Commonw. *77*:1142, 1970.
Hamlin, R. H. J., and Nicholson, E. C.: Reconstruction of the urethra totally destroyed in labour. Br. Med. J. *2*:147, 1969.
Hassim, A. M.: Uterine rupture with extrusion of the fetus into the bladder. Int. Surg. *49*:130, 1968.
Haynes, D. M., and Martin, B. J., Jr.: Cesarean hysterectomy: a twenty-five year review. Am. J. Obstet. Gynecol. *134*:393, 1979.
Ingelman-Sundberg, A.: Repair of vesicovaginal and rectovaginal fistula following fulguration of recurrent cancer of the cervix after radiation. *In* Meigs, J.: Surgical Treatment of Cancer of the Cervix. New York, Grune & Stratton, 1954.
Jones, O. H.: Cesarean section in present-day obstetrics. Am. J. Obstet. Gynecol. *126*:521, 1976.
Klein, J., and Malinconico, L. L.: The midforceps operation. Am. J. Obstet. Gynecol. *70*:952, 1955.
Linke, C. A., Linke, C. L., and Worden, A. C.: Bladder and urethral injuries following prolonged labor. J. Urol. *105*:679, 1971.
Lloyd-Davies, R. W.: A case of bilateral ureteric obstruction following obstetrical trauma. Br. J. Urol. *41*:689, 1969.
Mahfouz, N.: Urinary fistulae in women. J. Obstet. Gynaecol. Br. Emp. *64*:23, 1957.
Massoudnia, N.: Female genital fistulas in Iran. Etiology, incidence, and treatment. Geburtsh. Frauenheilkd. *32*:903, 1972.
McCall, M. L., and Bolton, K. A.: Martius's Gynecological Operations. Boston, Little, Brown & Co., 1956, Chap. 3.
McCausland, A. M., Cailloutte, J. C., Beunallack, D. A., et al.: A comparative study of vesicovaginal fistulas following delivery. Am. J. Obstet. Gynecol. *79*:1110, 1960.
Mickal, A., Begneaud, W. P., and Hawes, T. P., Jr.: Pitfalls and complications of cesarean section hysterectomy. Clin. Obstet. Gynecol. *12*:660, 1969.
Moir, C.: The Vesico-Vaginal Fistula. 2nd Ed. London, Baillière Tindall and Cassell, 1967, Chap. 10.
Moir, J. C., and Myerscough, P. R.: Munro Kerr's Operative Obstetrics. 5th Ed. London, Baillière Tindall and Cassell, 1971, p. 455.
Parry-Jones, E.: Kielland Forceps. London, Butterworth and Co., 1952.
Pritchard, J., and McDonald, P.: Williams Obstetrics. 16th Ed. New York, Appleton-Century-Crofts, 1980.
Raghavaiah, N. V., and Devi, A. I.: Bladder injury associated with rupture of the uterus. Obstet. Gynecol. *46*:573, 1975.
Read, J. A., Miller, F. C., Yeh, S. Y., et al.: Urinary bladder distention: effect on labor and uterine activity. Obstet. Gynecol. *56*:565, 1980.
Rendle-Short, C. W.: Rupture of the gravid uterus in Uganda. Am. J. Obstet. Gynecol. *79*:1114, 1960.
Sherline, D. M., and Danforth, D. N.: Effects of labor, delivery and anesthesia on postpartum bladder function. Obstet. Gynecol. *19*:808, 1962.
Taefi, P., Kaiser, T. F., Scheffer, J. B., et al.: Placenta percreta with bladder invasion and massive hemorrhage. Obstet. Gynecol. *36*:686, 1970.
von Schubert, E.: Topographie der Harnblase in Schwangerschaft, Geburt und Wochenbett. Zeut. Gynaecol. *53*:2541, 1929.
Warren, J. M.,Jr.: Conservative management of vesicouterine fistulas. South. Med. J. *72*:938, 1979.
Worthen, M., and Bustillo, M.: Effect of urinary bladder fullness on fundal height measurements. Am. J. Obstet. Gynecol. *138*:759, 1980.
Youssef, A. F.: Menouria following lower segment cesarean section: A syndrome. Am. J. Obstet. Gynecol. *73*:759, 1957.

34

RENAL CHANGES IN TOXEMIA

E. G. ROBERTSON, M.D.

The term "toxemia of pregnancy" has been used to describe gestational hypertension associated with proteinuria and edema. However, the term is misleading because it suggests a single disease entity associated with a specific pathogenicity, whereas in fact the hypertensive disorders associated with gestation have many causes, including one specific to pregnancy. This specific hypertensive disorder consists of two phases, preeclampsia and eclampsia. A major aim of prenatal care is the prevention of eclampsia, which is easy to recognize by the characteristic development of seizures and coma. Preeclampsia, on the other hand, is a diagnosis of exclusion unless it is followed by eclampsia. In this regard, pregnancy hypertension of unknown etiology is often treated as preeclampsia.

Whatever its cause, hypertension occurring during pregnancy is a major factor in maternal and fetal mortality and may also be associated with considerable morbidity in both mother and fetus. Both mortality and morbidity rates vary, depending on the underlying cause for the hypertension; therefore, it is important that an effort be made to determine whether a specific lesion exists when the patient presents with an elevated blood pressure.

DEFINITION AND CLASSIFICATION OF PREGNANCY HYPERTENSION

A major difficulty in assessing hypertension in pregnant women lies in determining whether it is in fact present. As yet there are no universally accepted criteria defining the hypertensive disorders. Since blood pressure is a continuous variable, the diagnosis of hypertension can be made only if an arbitrary level is defined above which hypertension is said to exist. In pregnancy, the situation is further complicated because the diastolic blood pressure normally falls in mid pregnancy and then rises again toward the end of the third trimester, whereas the systolic blood pressure essentially remains unchanged throughout pregnancy. One widely accepted definition of hypertension takes this phenomenon into account and suggests that any patient with an elevation from her midpregnancy blood pressure of more than 20 mm. Hg systolic and 30 mm. Hg diastolic, whatever the final level, should be regarded as having hypertensive disease. Page (1972) prefers to utilize the mean arterial blood pressure derived from the following equation:

$$\frac{(\text{systolic pressure}) + (\text{diastolic pressure} \times 2)}{3}$$

as suggested by Burton (1965). He designates an elevation of 20 mm. Hg in the mean arterial pressure from the midpregnancy value as significant; if previous blood pressures are not available, hypertension is defined as a mean arterial pressure of 105 mm. Hg or greater. An alternative in the absence of previous blood pressures is to consider "raw" blood pressure levels of 140/90 mm. Hg or greater on two occasions separted by at least 48 hours as indicative of hypertensive disease.

Once hypertension has been diagnosed, further classification is essential. The classification recommended by the American College of Obstetricians and Gynecologists consists of four groups: (1) preeclampsia-eclampsia; (2) chronic hypertension of whatever cause; (3) chronic hypertension with superimposed preeclampsia; and (4) late or transient hypertension. In the evaluation of individual patients, the physician must expand group 2 in order to complete a differential diagnosis. This group is composed of those patients with essential hypertension and those who have hypertension secondary to other diseases. The diagnosis of essential hypertension can be made only if the patient is known to be hypertensive in the absence of any other disease state outside of pregnancy or, alternatively, if she has been found to be hypertensive in early pregnancy and all investigations at that time disclosed no abnormality. Secondary hypertension may be due to pathologic processes affecting the kidney, e.g., chronic pyelonephritis or glomerulonephritis, or the adrenal, e.g., pheochromocytoma, or may be associated with other abnormalities such as diabetic nephropathy, coarctation of the aorta, lupus nephritis, and other, rarer conditions.

Although the physician must be aware of the possible underlying disease states, because of the restrictions placed on investigation of the patient during pregnancy, the final diagnosis sometimes cannot be made until after delivery. The commonest causes of hypertensive disease, however, are preeclampsia in the primigravida and essential hypertension and chronic renal disease in the multigravida. For a rigid definition of preeclampsia, the patient should be a primigravida, should have hypertension, proteinuria and a reduction in renal plasma flow and glomerular filtration rate, and, in addition, should have evidence of a specific glomerular lesion demonstrated on renal biopsy (Page, 1972). Since, however, renal biopsy is not a procedure that should be employed in routine clinical practice, use of the criteria is not always practical.

PATHOPHYSIOLOGIC CHANGES IN PREGNANCY HYPERTENSION

Renal Histologic Changes in Preeclampsia–Eclampsia

A number of histologic changes in the kidney have been described in patients with preeclampsia–eclampsia, and it is now agreed by most workers that there is an associated renal lesion not duplicated in its entirety by any other disease.

"Glomerular Capillary Endotheliosis"

As early as 1918, Löhlein suggested that the major lesion of preeclampsia occurred in the glomerulus; subsequent to that, light microscopists described thickening of the glomerular basement membrane, which was believed to be the specific lesion. In 1959, Farquhar reported the first electron microscopy study of the renal lesion in preeclampsia, and her findings were subsequently confirmed by Spargo and coworkers (1959). They described a marked swelling of the endothelial cells of the glomerular capillaries with deposition of an electron-dense fibrinoid material within and under the endothelial cells. The capillary basement membrane epithelium and epithelial foot processes were normal. This lesion was described as ''glomerular capillary endotheliosis.''

Altchek (1961) suggested that three changes are pathognomonic of preeclampsia–eclampsia: swelling of the endothelial cells, deposits of electron-dense material, and an increase in the intercapillary cells that reduce the capillary lumens (Figure 34–1). Faith and Trump (1966) compared the renal lesions of acute glomerular nephritis, systemic lupus erythematosus, and preeclampsia. Aside from the specific differences, they found the elements of the glomerulus to show certain general changes in all three diseases, with more or less characteristic exaggerations of one change or the other in each disorder. They theorized that the major differences were not in the endothelial cells but in the site and appearance of the deposits.

It has been proposed that intravascular coagulation plays a role in the etiology of preeclampsia, and Faith and Trump (1966) suggested that the endothelial cells of the glomerular capillaries act as phagocytes and ingest fibrin. Renal lesions resembling those in preeclampsia have been produced in rabbits by thromboplastin infusion, presumably resulting in the formation of fibrin that is subsequently taken up by the endothelial cells of the glomerular capillaries

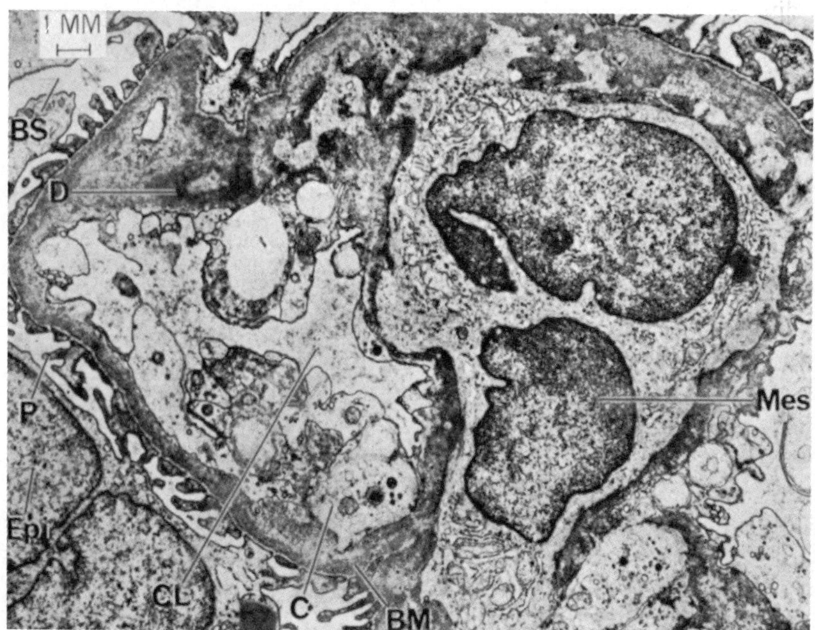

Figure 34–1. The glomerular capillary lesion of preeclampsia. BS = Bowman's space; D = electron-dense deposit, probably a derivative of fibrinogen; P = podocytes or foot processes of epithelial cell; Epi = nucleus of epithelial cell; CL = lumen of capillary; C = markedly swollen endothelial cytoplasm; BM = basement membrane; Mes = nucleus of mesothelial cell. (Courtesy of Charles P. McCartney and Benjamin Spargo.)

and by other cells in the reticuloendothelial system. A major difference between preeclampsia and other renal lesions is that immunofluorescent methods have been unable to demonstrate deposits of immunoglobulins or complement within the glomerular endothelial cells, as are seen in lupus erythematosus and glomerular nephritis, suggesting that immunologic injury does not play a role in the etiology of preeclampsia.

Diagnostic Significance

This specific glomerular lesion does not occur in all patients labeled clinically as having preeclampsia. McCartney and colleagues (1964) performed renal biopsies on 214 women who had acute hypertension in late pregnancy. Of 152 multiparas, only 14 per cent had glomerular endotheliosis. Of 62 primigravidas, the preeclamptic lesion was found in 71 per cent; 26 per cent were found to have chronic renal disease, the majority having chronic glomerulonephritis. Pollack and Nettles (1960) had also found that the clinical diagnosis accorded with the renal biopsy in about 70 per cent of their cases. Other studies have shown similar results. Thus, although it is far from proved that every patient with preeclampsia has the characteristic lesion, it seems obvious that the clinical diagnosis of preeclampsia in the multiparous patient is usually wrong and that unrecognized renal disease is often mistaken for preeclampsia. This is especially true in the young primigravida. There is, however, a difference between the renal lesion of preeclampsia and that of chronic renal disease in that the lesion of preeclampsia has been shown to be completely reversible following delivery.

Changes in Renal Hemodynamics

In normal pregnancy, there is an increase in body water composed mainly of an increase in the extracellular compartment. The expansion of the extracellular fluid volume is accompanied by an increase in plasma and red cell volume, and by an increase in cardiac output. Paradoxical

TABLE 34–1. CHANGES IN RENAL HEMODYNAMICS (COMPARED WITH NONPREGNANT STATE)

	Normal Pregnancy	Preeclampsia
Renal blood flow	increased	decreased
Renal plasma flow	increased	decreased
Glomerular filtration rate	increased	decreased
Filtration fraction	increased	decreased

changes occur in patients with gestational hypertension. Hytten and Thompson (1966) have shown that total body water is increased in patients with preeclampsia in late pregnancy, but this increase is within the normal range for patients who had edema but did not have hypertension. Dieckmann and Pottinger (1955) described how, in a patient with mild hypertension, there is an initial expansion of the plasma volume which may be even greater than normal for the period of pregnancy, but when the hypertension becomes severe, the patient develops a relative or absolute concentration of the blood. Thus, fluid appears to have diffused from the vascular space into an already enlarged interstitial space. In addition, there has been little difference determined in cardiac output in late pregnancy between patients who are normal and those who have hypertension. Therefore, it is almost certain that, in preeclampsia, the distribution of blood flow changes markedly and that some organs will be at greater risk than others.

The effect of this redistribution of blood flow on renal hemodynamics has been difficult to interpret because of the practical problems involved in investigating renal function in pregnancy.

Renal Blood Flow

Early work in this field suggested that renal blood flow was within normal limits, but at that time it was not appreciated that even normal pregnancy affected renal function. More recent studies indicate that, in pregnant women with hypertension, the circulation to the kidney is reduced, but whether this is a primary or secondary effect is as yet unknown.

Renal Plasma Flow

Following the observation by Sims and Krantz (1958) that glomerular filtration rate was increased in normal pregnancy, it was recognized that renal plasma flow was also increased; because of this, the information on renal hemodynamics in preeclampsia needed to be reevaluated. There is now evidence that women with preeclampsia, when compared with normal pregnant women at the same stage of gestation, have a reduction in effective renal plasma flow.

GFR and Filtration Fraction

McCartney and his co-workers (1964) showed, in a study of 22 patients who developed hypertension during pregnancy, that glomerular filtration rate (GFR) and the filtration fraction are reduced in patients with preeclampsia. In this study, each patient underwent renal biopsy and renal function studies; from these values, the quantity of free water extracted per unit of glomerular filtration could be calculated. This value was reduced in patients with nephrosclerosis or glomerulonephritis but strikingly increased in patients with preeclampsia. The degree of reduction of renal plasma flow and glomerular filtration rate in uncomplicated preeclampsia is equivalent to the severity of the disease. In severe disease, the reduction in circulating blood volume is sufficient to produce marked changes in renal plasma flow and quite profound depression of the glomerular filtration rate.

Considerations in Chronic Renal Disease

In patients with underlying renal disease responsible for the hypertension, the situation is, of course, more complicated. In the first place, if the renal disease is severe enough, these patients may already have depressed renal plasma flow and glomerular filtration before pregnancy. In the second place, the effect of pregnancy on the expansion of renal function may be entirely different. Bucht and Werko (1953) studied renal function in patients with chronic renal disease, and found that the clearances of inulin and para-aminohippuric acid (PAH) were, in early pregnancy, usually greater than in late pregnancy, in the puerperium, or at a later date. In two patients whose clearances were measured before conception, increases were found during pregnancy, although these were much less than would be expected in normal pregnant women.

Changes in Water and Electrolyte Excretion

Changes in sodium and water balance are characteristic of pregnancies complicated by hypertension. Larger quantities of sodium are retained in preeclampsia than in normal pregnancy, and water is retained in excess of sodium (Little, 1965).

Sodium Retention

In women with preeclampsia, some of the factors favoring the excretion of sodium during pregnancy are reversed: (1) the filtration rate is depressed, sometimes severely; (2) the renal vascular resistance is increased; (3) the plasma flow in the peritubular capillaries is reduced; and (4) the plasma volume is less than normal. Presumably, these changes play a part in the retention of sodium in preeclampsia. It has been shown that the urine of preeclamptic women is nearly free of chloride and that these women do not concentrate sodium normally. In addition, they appear to excrete a sodium load much more slowly than do normal pregnant women. Nonpregnant patients with essential hypertension normally respond to a sodium load with exaggerated natriuresis. Studies in which the state of sodium balance was carefully defined have demonstrated the same phenomenon in pregnant patients with essential hypertension, but patients with preeclampsia have a lower peak rate of sodium excretion after saline infusion than do subjects with essential hypertension (Sarles et al., 1968). Since the load of sodium presented to the tubules is much greater during pregnancy, the effect of even minor reductions in the ability of the tubules to handle this load is to produce a marked retention of sodium; this occurs in preeclampsia.

Water Retention

The retention of sodium is also associated with retention of water. In addition to being unable to excrete a load of sodium in the normal way, the pregnant woman with hypertension also has a reduced ability to handle a water load. Thus, the hypertensive patient presents with oliguria and the secretion of concentrated urine. Although several factors affect the concentration of urine, normally the major one is vasopressin (antidiuretic hormone, ADH). The exact mechanism of the action of ADH is uncertain, but it appears to act at the level of the distal tubules. The simplest hypothesis is that ADH increases the permeability of the distal tubules and collecting ducts to water. In consequence, the osmotic removal of water from the fluid within the ducts brings the urine into equilibrium with the highly concentrated papillary interstitial fluid. However, in early pregnancy, what little evidence there is suggests that the ADH secretion is normally suppressed and the normal nonpregnant levels are higher than those in the latter part of pregnancy.

Several workers have reported that the blood of preeclamptic women contains pressor substances and that this may be indicative of antidiuretic activity. If that is so, a simple explanation exists for the retention of water in patients who have preeclampsia, but edema is not characteristic of syndromes or diseases in which excessive vasopressin is excreted. When there is an effect, it is usually profound hyponatremia, which seldom occurs in preeclampsia.

There is no doubt that the hypertensive pregnant woman will store water and salt in excess of the amounts required to maintain the pregnancy. The reasons for this retention are not known with certainty at present.

Proteinuria

The development of edema in patients with hypertension does not appear to be associated with any decrease in reproductive efficiency (Robertson, 1975), but the appearance of proteinuria in a hypertensive patient is regarded as an indicator of increased risk to both mother and fetus. Although proteinuria is a grave sign in preeclampsia, this may not be true in pregnancies complicated by chronic renal disease in which proteinuria may be present in the first trimester of pregnancy. There are difficulties in distinguishing the self-limiting condition of preeclampsia from chronic renal disease, since both processes are characterized by renal lesions that lead to the excretion of protein.

Definition

Proteinuria should be defined quantitatively rather than qualitatively. It has been advocated by the American College of Obstetricians and Gynecologists (Hughes, 1972) that proteinuria should be regarded as significant if it is present in amounts of 0.3 gm. per 100 ml. of urine or more. In addition, the possibility of contamination from either urinary tract or genital tract infection should be excluded.

Mechanisms of Protein Excretion

Proteinuria can be produced by the following mechanisms: (1) the escape of normal plasma proteins through a defective glomerular basement membrane; (2) failure of renal tubular function in which low molecular weight proteins, normally present in the glomerular filtrate, are not reabsorbed by the damaged tubule; (3) a loss of tissue protein from the renal parenchyma, ureter, and bladder; and (4) the loss of abnormal plasma proteins, such as Bence Jones proteinuria in multiple myeloma. Immunoelectrophoretic techniques of analysis have enabled the description of the protein fractions in various "toxemic" states.

Studd (1973), using the Laurell immunoelectrophoretic technique, showed that the proteinuria in preeclampsia seems to be the result of a glomerular leak of normal plasma proteins of intermediate molecular weight and is not a failure of tubular resorption of low molecular weight proteins. No tissue proteins or "pregnancy proteins" have been demonstrated in the urine of patients with preeclampsia. This finding is similar to the type of leakage found in patients with chronic renal disease, particularly chronic glomerulonephritis.

Studd also performed differential protein clearance studies in patients with a histologic diagnosis of nephrotic syndrome and compared them with patients with a clinical diagnosis of preeclampsia. The measurement of differential protein clearances enables the determination of the selectivity of the defect in the filtering mechanism of the glomerulus. Large protein molecules being passed through the damaged basement membrane suggest a large leak with severe irreversible pathology, whereas the passage of small protein molecules suggests that the lesion is potentially reversible. The cases of primary renal disease demonstrated the range of protein clearances that would be expected with mixed renal pathology. Some were selective, but the majority with proliferative or membranous glomerulonephritis were poorly selective. With the preeclamptic group, protein clearances were without exception poorly selective to a degree usually associated with advanced chronic renal disease. This is despite the fact that the renal changes in preeclampsia are morphologically different and regress some weeks after delivery.

Although this work suggests that the proteinuria in preeclampsia is due to a glomerular leak, no such break in the continuity of the basement membrane has been found on electron microscopy. The available evidence suggests that the nephropathy of preeclampsia can be regarded as a diffuse intrarenal fibrination that produces a functional defect in the glomerular basement membrane through which the protein may escape.

Proteinuria and Fetal Outcome

Further studies have shown that the renal leakage of proteins in hypertensive disease has effects in terms of fetal outcome (Studd et al., 1972). Maternal serum protein concentrations are normally lower in pregnancy, but in preeclampsia there is a further fall in albumin and IgG, and an elevation of α_2-M globulin and β-lipoprotein. These protein changes are identical to those found in the protein-losing nephropathies of the nephrotic syndrome and appear to be the result of molecular sieving of serum proteins of intermediate molecular weight with retention of the macromolecules of α_2-M globulin and β-lipoprotein.

A study of the nephrotic syndrome in pregnancy (Studd and Blainey, 1969) showed the unexpected association of fetal growth retardation with the severity of proteinuria and maternal hypoalbuminemia. This association might be due to hypoalbuminemia leading to hypovolemia and diminished placental circulation, but alternatively, it could be the result of chronic protein malnutrition of the fetus. However, there is little, if any, transplacental passage of albumin, as this is mainly produced by the fetal liver; the maintenance of fetal serum albumin seems to be a biochemical priority that is not modified by maternal hypoalbuminemia. The fetus is affected by depression of maternal serum IgG since, unlike the other proteins studied, the fetus obtains all of its IgG from the mother. There is some evidence for chronic protein malnutrition in fetal growth retardation; it can be postulated that chronic maternal protein loss, as well as diminished transfer of amino acids across the damaged placenta of preeclampsia, is a factor in the causation of fetal dysproteinemia and dysmaturity.

The excretion of protein by the kidney in patients with preeclampsia is similar to that in patients who have the more common chronic renal diseases. The effect of protein excretion appears to be a serious one in terms of fetal outcome; thus, proteinuria should always be considered an important manifestation in pregnancy complicated by hypertension.

Changes in Renal Humoral Mechanisms

Although it has been shown that preeclampsia is accompanied by retention of water and electrolyte and by a specific renal lesion that gives rise to proteinuria, these are probably not causes but effects of the disease. The basic pathologic lesion is probably an increased responsiveness of the arterial system to pressor substances, which causes the generalized vasoconstriction common to all forms of pregnancy hypertension.

Although the renin–angiotensin–aldosterone system is clearly involved in pressure-volume homeostasis, the importance of this system in initiating and sustaining various forms of hypertension in pregnancy is not clear. Animal studies (Miller et al., 1972) have shown that renin plays a major role in the genesis of renovascular hypertension, but similar experimental models have not been examined for other forms of hypertension. There is general agreement that renin substrate concentration, renin activity, and aldosterone levels all rise during normal pregnancy. During the first trimester, renin concentration is also elevated (Boonshaft et al., 1968). Although chorionic tissue produces large amounts of renin which is released into the amniotic fluid, the relation of this source to plasma renin activity during pregnancy is unknown (Skinner et al., 1968).

Studies of the renin-angiotensin system in subjects with preeclampsia have yielded conflicting results. In one study, renin activity was found to be increased while renin concentration apparently decreased (Bonnar et al., 1966). Renin concentration, however, was found by one group of workers to be elevated in "toxemic" pregnancy (Maebashi et al., 1965). Renin substrate and angiotensin II levels were found to be increased by Massani and colleagues (1967). Another study has found decreased concentrations of renin, renin substrate, angiotensin II and aldosterone in hypertensive pregnancies (Weir et al., 1973). Most studies have failed to show any increase in pressor substances during pregnancy; it has therefore been postulated that the primary etiology of the generalized vasoconstriction is an increased responsiveness of the arterial wall. In normal human pregnancy, there is a decreased blood pressure response to pressor agents, but in preeclampsia there is a marked increase in response to angiotensin and to norepinephrine (Talledo et al., 1968), and the increased pressor response to angiotensin in pregnant women precedes the development of hypertension (Gant et al., 1973).

Unfortunately, it is not known what causes this increased sensitivity. Page (1972) proposed that it may be due to the presence of increasing concentrations of sodium within the arterial wall. Studies of isolated blood vessels have indicated that an increased sodium content could be brought about by a combination of general sodium retention and the influence of steroid hormones. There has, however, been little evidence of abnormal mineralocorticoid activity in patients with hypertensive disease: Patients with preeclampsia have been found to excrete less aldosterone than do subjects with normal pregnancies (Watanabe et al., 1965).

Thus, available evidence suggests that the changes in renal humoral mechanisms do not directly contribute to the primary lesion of pregnancy hypertension, but there are many unanswered questions regarding the role of pressor substances in the production of the generalized vasoconstriction.

MANAGEMENT OF HYPERTENSIVE DISEASE

Since the diagnosis of preeclampsia in a patient presenting with acute hypertension in pregnancy must be one of exclusion, the investigation of that patient must be directed to determining whether an underlying chronic renal lesion exists. Since, in the majority of instances, the basic etiologic mechanism will be unknown at the time of diagnosis, the treatment can be only symptomatic, directed toward maintaining renal function and uteroplacental function.

Prevention

Considerable attention has been directed toward those factors that might prevent the development of preeclampsia. There is no doubt that a well-constructed program of prenatal care will reduce the incidence of hypertensive disease in pregnancy, particularly if the patient is advised about limitation of physical activity, given good dietary advice, and watched carefully for the development of excessive weight gain, water retention, or an upward trend in diastolic blood pressure. Early hospitalization also plays a major role in preventing the more severe aspects of hypertensive disease.

Diagnostic Considerations

Once a patient has developed hypertension, the stage of pregnancy should indicate the likelihood of underlying chronic renal disease. For example, if a patient presents in the first trimester or is multiparous, there is a high likelihood that a chronic lesion exists and causes the elevation of blood pressure. In this group, the investigation should be directed toward determining whether there is renal involvement and the degree of limitation of renal function. If, on the other hand, the patient presents in the latter part of pregnancy as a primigravida with hypertensive disease, she probably does not have a chronic lesion and the diagnosis is most likely preeclampsia. In this instance, the investigation should be directed toward determining whether the hypertensive disease has affected renal function on an acute basis. If a specific disease process is diagnosed, the management is that of the disease with the addition of symptomatic therapy directed toward management of the hypertension. If no underlying disease is determined, the treatment is directed solely towards preserving the integrity of the patient and her baby.

Treatment

Preeclampsia is insidious in onset and once established may increase in severity at a rapid rate. Severe preeclampsia and eclampsia are diseases that threaten the life of mother and fetus but should be preventable by early diagnosis and treatment. Once the diagnosis has been made, the only successful approach to therapy involves early admission to hospital; delay in admission usually leads to progression of the disease. Although the major therapy is usually directed toward control of hypertension, the renal system is particularly at risk, and management plans should take this into account. Initial treatment for mild preeclampsia is bed rest and sedation to depress increased neuromuscular excitability. If this controls the disease, delivery should not be delayed beyond 38 weeks. If there is an increase in severity of hypertension and proteinuria develops, therapy should be directed toward the prevention of eclampsia and toward the avoidance of permanent organ damage to the kidneys, liver, and central nervous system. In addition to management of hypertensive disease, the condition of the fetus must be monitored by placental function studies and by more dynamic methods of assessment, such as non-stress testing. Evidence of deteriorating fetal status will indicate premature induction, irrespective of maternal condition.

Severe preeclampsia is an acute obstetric emergency and is characterized by changes in cardiovascular dynamics that are, as yet, only poorly understood. Therapy to date has been symptomatic and empiric. Early delivery remains the only treatment that will cure the disease, but without intensive supportive therapy during the acute phase, even this may not be enough to protect the patient from long-term sequelae and possible death. Recent studies have led to an improved understanding of the cardiovascular changes in the severe form of the disease and may lead to more successful treatment.

Soffronoff and associates (1977) have confirmed that blood volumes in patients with severe preeclampsia are only 75 per cent of those found in normotensive nulliparas. Until recently the effect on hemodynamics of this relative hypovolemia was unknown because of the practical difficulties involved in monitoring severely ill patients. In 1970, Swan and co-workers developed a multiple-lumen, flow-directed pulmonary artery catheter that could be inserted percutaneously and reliably passed from the venous system into the pulmonary artery without fluoroscopy. The device permits reliable monitoring of cardiopulmonary hemodynamic characteristics in severely ill patients and has been used for this purpose in both medical and surgical intensive care units. This can now be used to monitor the condition of women with severe preeclampsia and there are reports of its usage for this purpose. Benedetti and associates (1980) described their findings in 10 patients. They found that pregnancy with severe preeclampsia does not appear to affect pulmonary artery pressures. However, cardiac output was higher than had previously been shown in normal patients but there was no significant increase in output when early labor was compared with the early puerperium. They suggested that the failure of preeclamptic patients to demonstrate an increase in cardiac output with delivery may be related to the blood volume deficit combined with excess blood loss at delivery. They found that the systemic vascular resistance was increased when compared with normal pregnancy. The correlation between Swan-Ganz catheter measurements and central venous pressure (CVP) monitoring was poor, and this has also been confirmed by Strauss and co-workers (1980) in patients with preeclampsia and pulmonary edema. In the absence of severe cardiopulmonary dysfunction, CVP monitoring will reflect right ventricular function, but in cases with hemorrhage, pulmonary edema, or prolonged oliguria, a Swan-Ganz catheter will give more reliable information regarding the ability of the heart to tolerate fluid loads.

Therapy should take these findings into account. Initial treatment of the patient with severe preeclampsia must include monitoring of cardiac function and renal output. The patient should have continuous electrocardiographic monitoring and a central venous pressure line should be used where Swan-Ganz catheterization is not available. An indwelling urinary catheter will measure urinary output accurately. Magnesium sulphate is given intravenously to control neuromuscular excitability and to reduce peripheral vascular resistance; magnesium acts to block acetylcholine release in peripheral nerves and ganglia. The rate of infusion should be controlled by assay of magnesium levels and by changes in clinical status. Hydralazine may also be used, since this is a weak arteriolar vasodilator and will reduce the cardiac afterload, with subsequent improvement in cardiac output; although hydralazine increases cardiac output, it does not increase placental perfusion in experimental animals and should be used only for short-term therapy. Inotropic stimulation with digoxin is unnecessary, since there is no evidence to suggest marked impairment of intrinsic contractibility. Since patients with toxemia are already relatively hypovolemic, the use of diuretics will reduce intravascular volume still further and jeopardize cardiac output and tissue perfusion. Decreased urinary output should be treated by increased volume infusion controlled by central cardiac monitoring, rather than by diuretic therapy.

Once the patient has a stable blood pressure, delivery should be accomplished as soon as possible by the most appropriate route. For at least 12 to 24 hours following delivery, the kidney is at most risk because of reduced tissue perfusion. Intensive treatment and monitoring must be continued until diuresis occurs. Sodium nitroprusside has been suggested as an effective agent for use in the severely ill patient in the puerperium, but this is a potent arteriolar vasodilator and continuous arterial blood pressure monitoring is required, implying the placement of a Swan-Ganz catheter. If afterload reduction using vasodilator therapy accompanied by adequate fluid replacement is used as the primary mode of treatment, the risk of permanent organ damage is considerably reduced.

If Swan-Ganz catheters are not available, magnesium sulfate and hydralazine will remain the standard therapeutic regime. Therapy with other hypotensive agents, such as methyldopa, in the prenatal period is only appropriate to patients with chronic hypertension; their usage is contraindicated in preeclampsia, since acute changes in renal function may occur, leading to chronic renal damage.

Underlying Renal Disease

Previous work has suggested that about 30 per cent of primigravidas and the majority of multigravidas with acute hypertensive disease in the latter part of pregnancy will have underlying chronic renal changes. If the patient presents with hypertension and proteinuria, the plan of management must include evaluation of the patient's renal tract 8 to 12 weeks after delivery in order to exclude the possibility of permanent renal damage. The renal changes associated with preeclampsia return to normal within 6 weeks of delivery, and there are usually no long-term effects from an acute episode of this nature. If, on the other hand, renal function studies are abnormal 3 months after delivery, any residual changes that are present are unlikely to be due to pregnancy-specific hypertension. If either a stillbirth or a neonatal death occurred as a result of hypertensive disease, adequate counseling cannot be given to the patient unless she has had a thorough evaluation to exclude underlying renal disease.

Prognostic Implications

In a patient with chronic renal disease, although the disease adversely affects pregnancy, there is little evidence that pregnancy affects the long-term prognosis for the disease. If the patient develops symptoms only during pregnancy, it is unlikely that she will have symptomatic renal failure during her reproductive years. However, she should be advised that obstetric problems will increase as she becomes older, and it would therefore be advisable for her to complete her family as soon as possible. In a patient with established chronic renal disease whose renal function deteriorates during pregnancy, the question of sterilization should be raised, particularly if she already has an established family unit. When the diagnosis of renal disease is made for the first time either during pregnancy or following delivery, future management of this patient, both between and during pregnancies, should be undertaken in association with a nephrologist.

REFERENCES

Altchek, A.: Electron microscopy of renal biopsies in toxemia of pregnancy. J. Clin. Invest. *32*:44, 1961.

Benedetti, T. J., Cotton, D. B., Read, J. C., and Miller, F. C.: Hemodynamic observations in severe pre-eclampsia with flow-directed pulmonary artery catheter. Am. J. Obstet. Gynecol. *136*:465, 1980.

Bonnar, J., Brown, J. J., and Davies, D. L.: Plasma renin concentration in American Negro women with hypertensive disease of pregnancy. J. Obstet. Gynaecol. Br. Commonw. *73*:418, 1966.

Boonshaft, B., O'Connell, J. M. B., and Hayes, J. M.: Serum renin activity during normal pregnancy. J. Clin. Endocrinol. *28*:1641, 1968.

Bucht, H., and Werko, L.: Glomerular filtration rate and renal blood flow in hypertensive toxemia of pregnancy. J. Obstet. Gynaecol. Brit. Emp. *60*:157, 1953.

Burton, A. C.: Physiology and Biophysics of the Circulation. Chicago, Year Book Publishers, 1965.

Dieckmann, W. J., and Pottinger, R.: Etiology of preeclampsia-eclampsia V. Extra- and intracellular fluid changes and electrolyte balances. Am. J. Obstet. Gynecol. *70*:822, 1955.

Faith, G. C., and Trump, B. F.: The glomerular capillary wall in human kidney disease: Acute glomerulonephritis, systemic lupus erythematosus, and preeclampsia–eclampsia. Lab. Invest. *15*:1682, 1966.

Farquhar, M.: Ultrastructure of the nephron disclosed by electron microscopy. Section A — Review of normal and pathologic glomerular ultra structure. *In* Metcoff, J. (Ed.): Proceedings of the Tenth Annual Conference on the Nephrotic Syndrome. New York, National Kidney Disease Foundation, 1959, pp. 2–7.

Gant, N. F., Paley, G. L., and Chand, S.: A study of angiotensin II pressor response throughout primigravid pregnancy. J. Clin. Invest. *52*:2682, 1973.

Hughes, E. C. (Ed.): Obstetric-Gynecologic Terminology. Philadelphia, F. A. Davis Company, 1972.

Hytten, F. E., and Thomson, A. M.: Body water in preeclampsia. J. Obstet. Gynaecol. Br. Commonw. *73*:714, 1966.

Little, B.: Water and electrolyte balance during pregnancy. Anesthesiology *26*:400, 1965.

Löhlein, M.: Zur Pathogenese der Nierenkrankheiten II. Nephritis and Nephrose, mir besonderer Berucksichtigung der Nephropathia Gravidarum. Dtsch. Med. Wschr. *44*:1187, 1918.

McCartney, C. P.: Renal structure in pregnancy patients with acute hypertension. Circulation *29*(Suppl. 2): 32, 1962.

McCartney, C. P., Spargo, B., Lorincz, A. B., et al.: Renal structure and function in pregnant women with acute hypertension. Osmolar concentration. Am. J. Obstet. Gynecol. *90*:579, 1964.

Maebashi, M., Aida, M., and Yoshinaga, K.: Estimation of circulatory renin in normal and toxemic pregnancies. Tohuku J. Exp. Med., *84*:55, 1965.

Massani, Z. M., Sanguinetti, R., and Gallegos, R.: Angiotensin blood levels in normal and toxemic pregnancies. Am. J. Obstet. Gynecol. *99*:315, 1967.

Miller, E. D., Samuels, A. I., and Haber, E.: Inhibition of angiotensin conversion in experimental reno-vascular hypertension. Science *177*:1108, 1972.

Page, E. W.: On the pathogenesis of preeclampsia and eclampsia. J. Obstet. Gynaecol. Br. Commonw. *79*:883, 1972.

Pollack, V. E., and Nettles, J. B.: The kidney in toxemia of pregnancy: A clinical and pathological study based on renal biopsies. Medicine *39*:469, 1960.

Robertson, E. G.: Water metabolism. Clinics in Obstet. Gynaecol. *2*:431, 1975.

Sarles, H. E., Hill, S. S., LeBlanc, A. L., et al.: Sodium excretion patterns during and following intravenous sodium chloride loads in normal and hypertensive pregnancy. Am. J. Obstet. Gynecol. *102*:1, 1968.

Sims, E. A. H., and Krantz, K. E.: Serial studies of renal function during normal pregnancy and the puerperium in normal women. J. Clin. Invest. *37*:1764, 1958.

Skinner, S. L., Lumbers, E. R., and Symonds, E. H.: Renin concentration in human fetal and maternal tissues. Am. J. Obstet. Gynecol. *101*:529, 1968.

Soffronoff, E. C., Kaufmann, B. M., and Connaughton, J. F.: Intravascular volume determination and fetal outcome in hypertensive disease of pregnancy. Am. J. Obstet. Gynecol. *127*:4, 1977.

Spargo, B., McCartney, C. P., and Winemiller, R.: Glomerular capillary endotheliosis in toxemia of pregnancy. Arch. Pathol., *68*:593, 1959.

Strauss, R. G., Keefer, J. R., Burke, T., and Civetta, J. M.: Hemodynamic monitoring of cardiogenic pulmonary edema complicating toxemia of pregnancy. Obstet. Gynecol. *55*:170, 1980.

Studd, J.: The origin and effects of proteinuria in pregnancy. J. Obstet. Gynaecol. Br. Commonw. *80*:872, 1973.

Studd, J. W. W., and Blainey, J. D.: Pregnancy and the nephrotic syndrome. Br. Med. J., *1*:276, 1969.

Studd, J. W. W., Shaw, R. W., and Bailey, D. E.: Maternal and fetal serum protein. Circulation in normal pregnancy and pregnancy complicated by proteinuric preeclampsia. Am. J. Obstet. Gynecol. *114*:582, 1972.

Swan, H. J. C., Ganz, W., Forrester, J., et al.: Catheterization of the heart in man with use of a flow-directed balloon tipped catheter. N. Engl. J. Med., *283*:447, 1970.

Talledo, O. E., Chesley, L. C., and Zuspan, F. P.: Renin-angiotensin system in normal and toxemic pregnancies. Am. J. Obstet. Gynecol. *100*:218, 1968.

Watanabe, M., Murker, C. L., and Gray, M. J.: Aldosterone secretion rates in abnormal pregnancy. J. Clin. Endocrinol. *25*:1665, 1965.

Weir, R. J., Fraser, R., and Lever, A. F.: Plasma renin, renin substrate angiotensin II, and aldosterone in hypertensive disease of pregnancy. Lancet *1*:291, 1973.

35

ASYMPTOMATIC BACTERIURIA DURING PREGNANCY

F. GARY CUNNINGHAM, M.D.
PEGGY J. WHALLEY, M.D.

Pregnant women are particularly susceptible to acute urinary tract infections, and physicians caring for these women have long demonstrated concern for gravidas who develop acute pyelonephritis or cystitis (Chapter 36). Conversely, there are pregnant women who demonstrate significant bacteriuria without symptoms, and until the past few decades, these patients received relatively little attention. There were no recognized risks associated with *asymptomatic bacteriuria*. This was due in part to imprecise urine culture techniques that did not allow for differentiation between bacterial contamination inherent in urine collection and the presence of actively multiplying organisms as a consequence of urinary tract colonization.

In 1956 Kass devised a technique for distinguishing true bacteriuria from bacterial contamination using the clean voided method of urine collection and quantitative culture techniques. These innovations made possible the detection of asymptomatic bacteriuria in large population groups without having to resort to urethral catheterization. This technique prompted a revival of interest in the investigation of bacteriuria and its relationship to urinary tract infections.

Bacteriuria usually remains silent unless an element of urinary tract obstruction is superimposed. In normal pregnancy, physiologic relaxation of the ureters and renal pelves occurs, presumably as the result of progesterone of placental origin (Chapter 30). The enlarging uterus soon contributes an element of mechanical obstruction, and the net effect of these two processes, i.e., loss of ureteral tone and mechanical obstruction, is *urinary stasis*. This stasis is in itself harmless; however, asymptomatic bacteriuria in combination with pregnancy-induced urinary obstruction produces a milieu that allows bacterial replication. The production of significant numbers of uropathogens may then cause symptomatic urinary tract infection. Infection may occur either in the lower urinary tract, where it manifests itself as cystourethritis, or in the upper tract, producing the more serious complication of acute pyelonephritis. Frequently lower tract infection appears to occur first and may then be followed by ascending bacteriuria with resultant parenchymal infection.

Since Kass' original work, much time and effort have been expended to determine not only the frequency of maternal bacteriuria but also its relationship to a variety of pregnancy complications. In spite of several extensive investigations, there still exists much general disagreement as to the significance of asymptomatic bacteriuria and some of its alleged adverse effects on pregnancy — in particular, prematurity, anemia, and hypertension. Furthermore, although there is general agreement that a relationship exists between recurrent urinary tract infections, chronic pyelonephritis, and chronic renal disease, the long-term sequelae of bacteriuria have been only partially defined.

The purpose of this chapter is to analyze the known and suspected effects of asymptomatic bacteriuria on pregnancy and the immediate puerperium. Treatment of maternal bacteriuria and its effect on acute urinary infections, as well as its possible effects on other pregnancy complications, will be considered. Finally, the long-term prognosis for gravidas with asymptomatic bacteriuria will be briefly discussed.

DEFINITION OF ASYMPTOMATIC BACTERIURIA

By definition, the term *asymptomatic bacteriuria* implies that the patient in whom significant bacteriuria is demonstrated has no symptoms referable to the urinary tract. Close questioning will reveal that approximately one fifth of all women, with or without bacteriuria, have experienced one or more symptoms related to the urinary tract within the past year. For example, Waters (1969) reported that 22 per cent of 2933 nonpregnant women questioned during a routine examination complained of dysuria during the previous year. McFadyen and co-workers (1973) reported that 30 per cent of pregnant women with significant bacteriuria had urinary frequency, nocturia, dysuria or stress incontinence; however, these symptoms were also found in 26 per cent of women with sterile urine.

Methods of Urine Collection

The definition of bacteriuria itself is more complex. The word merely indicates the presence of bacteria in urine. Since bacteria normally reside in the terminal portion of the female urethra as well as in the contiguous genital structures, all urine specimens obtained by voiding or by catheterization will contain some bacteria from contamination incident to urine collection itself. For these reasons, quantification of bacteria is necessary to determine significance. If bacteriuria is defined as the presence of a *significant* number of microorganisms in urine, the number considered "significant" will depend on the method of collection.

Suprapubic Aspiration and Urethral Catheterization

Urine obtained by suprapubic bladder aspiration is completely sterile, and any bacterial growth indicates urinary infection. In a specimen obtained by urethral catheterization, the count must be between 10,000 and 100,000 organisms per ml. of urine to be considered "significant."

Suprapubic aspiration has not been widely employed because of patient discomfort as well as technical difficulties associated with specimen collection. *Urethral catheterization is not recommended for routine screening because bacteria may be introduced into an otherwise sterile bladder.*

Clean Voided Technique

The most commonly accepted method for detection of asymptomatic bacteriuria is by the *clean voided technique.* When performed correctly, the technique is harmless and the results obtained are extremely reproducible. Care must be taken to cleanse the external urethral meatus with an antiseptic solution. The labia should be spread apart before the woman is instructed to void. For a midstream culture the first portion of the urine is discarded and the midportion of the voided specimen is collected in a sterile container. However, we have found it unnecessary to collect a midstream specimen. Most urine specimens that are contaminated during collection contain less than 10,000 bacteria per ml. of urine. Moreover, women with significant infection frequently have bacterial counts in excess of 1 million organisms per ml.

By current accepted definition, significant bacteriuria is present when 100,000 or more colony-forming organisms are demonstrated per milliliter of urine obtained by the clean voided technique. As with any other laboratory test, the accuracy is dependent on the methods employed to collect and process the specimen. The use of the value of 100,000 or more organisms per milliliter of urine to differentiate significant bacteriuria from contamination during collection is based on statistical probabilities.

Kass (1956) demonstrated that when 100,000 or more bacteria are found per milliliter in urine obtained by catheterization, the next specimen obtained from the same patient by catheterization will show the same concentration of bacteria 96 per cent of the time. When the initial urine specimen is obtained by the clean voided technique, the likelihood that a second specimen will also contain 100,000 or more organisms per milliliter decreases to 80 per cent. However, if each of two consecutive clean voided urine specimens contains these numbers of organisms, so will the third specimen 96 per cent of the time. These data indicate the reliability of clean voided specimens in demonstrating significant bacteriuria. Furthermore, the reproducibility of this procedure has been proved in pregnancy.

Since the use of routine urethral catheterization for the detection of bacteriuria is neither practical nor safe, a specimen should be obtained by the clean voided technique. From a practical point of view, obtaining three consecutive specimens is both time-consuming and expensive. It can be recommended that only two specimens be obtained; if both demonstrate significant bacteriuria, treatment should then be given. Furthermore, in large clinics in which care is given for indigent women in whom there is an increased incidence of bacteriuria, it seems even more practical to obtain only one specimen. Indeed, this is our policy for detection of bacteriuria in women attending the Prenatal Clinics at Parkland Memorial Hospital, Dallas. From a purist point of view, 20 per cent of women receive unnecessary therapy, but from a practical point of view, the remaining 80 per cent with significant bacteriuria are treated earlier and with less expense.

Bacterial colony counts between 10,000 and 100,000 per ml. of clean voided urine are of questionable significance and may or may not indicate infection. Colony counts in this range fortunately are infrequent, and when they occur, a second specimen should be collected to determine if significant bacteriuria is present. In our experience the finding of a single species of bacteria within this "intermediate" numerical range indicates significant bacteriuria approximately one half of the time. Therefore, if it is inconvenient to repeat the urine culture or if expense is of concern, treatment should be given. If any doubt exists, it is far wiser to treat the woman rather than risk pyelonephritis developing during the pregnancy. Likewise, if a second specimen is collected and contains the *same* organism, again with an "intermediate" colony count, treatment is recommended.

Processing of Urine Specimen

The processing of the urine specimen requires special consideration. Urine is usually an excellent culture medium, and most bacterial contaminants will double in number every 20 to 30 minutes unless the specimen is refrigerated. *Escherichia coli*, for example, divides every 18 minutes under ideal circumstances. Theoretically this rate of replication could produce 60,000 to 80,000 colony-forming bacteria from only one bacterium at room temperature in 8 hours. To prevent these false high colony counts, the urine specimen ideally should be plated immediately, or at least within a short time following collection. If a delay between collection and plating is anticipated, the urine should be stored at 4° C.

Summary

In summary, the term *asymptomatic bacteriuria* implies that a woman without urinary tract symptoms is demonstrated to have 100,000 or more colony-forming organisms per milliliter of urine on two and preferably three consecutive clean voided urine specimens. Routine urethral catheterization should be discouraged; however, if such a sample is tested, a count of 10,000 to 100,000 colonies per ml. of urine is considered significant. In each instance the organism isolated must be the same in all samples. Lower colony counts by either method may imply significant bacteriuria or may merely represent contamination from the distal urethra. When a specimen contains these smaller numbers of organisms the culture should be repeated to positively identify the woman at risk. If any doubt exists as to the significance of a positive urine culture, it is recommended that the woman be treated.

PREVALENCE OF MATERNAL BACTERIURIA

Predisposing Factors

The prevalence of significant bacteriuria during pregnancy ranges from 2 to 10 per cent. Factors that have been implicated as having a positive influence on maternal bacteriuria include socioeconomic status, race, age, parity, and the sickle cell trait. Of these factors, only the first and the last are universally agreed upon as having a definite correlation with an increased prevalence of bacteriuria.

Socioeconomic Status

Prevalence of maternal bacteriuria is directly related to socioeconomic status, with the highest rates found in women attending public clinics for the indigent and the lowest rates found in private obstetric patients. Several investigators have studied the influence of socioeconomic status on prevalence of bacteriuria. Bacteriuria was found in 2 to 3 per cent of nonindigent patients and in 6 to 10 per cent of indigent women. Why these factors influence bacteriuria is not exactly known; however, Monto and Rantz (1963) suggested that economically affluent women are more likely to seek medical aid when they develop relatively minor genitourinary symptoms. These women therefore would receive earlier treatment, which may prevent persistent bacteriuria that would otherwise be discovered later during pregnancy. Since there is little evidence that earlier treatment reduces chronic recurrent bacteriuria, this supposition seems unlikely. Most importantly, it must be emphasized that regardless of the social status of the pregnant woman with bacteriuria, the per cent incidence of antepartum pyelonephritis that occurs is identical if bacteriuria is not treated (Brumfitt, 1975).

Racial Factors

Although some investigators have found that the prevalence of asymptomatic urinary tract infection is increased in pregnant black women compared with white women, the effects of social factors were not clearly defined. On the basis of controlled studies it seems likely that differences in the prevalence of bacteriuria between ethnic groups are related to socioeconomic status. For example, Turck and co-workers (1962) demonstrated that the prevalence of bacteriuria did not differ significantly among black and white women within the same socioeconomic groups. Studies of large numbers of women at Parkland Memorial Hospital of essentially the same socioeconomic status indicate that race has no influence on prevalence of bacteriuria (Whalley, 1965). McFadyen and colleagues (1973) likewise demonstrated no difference in ethnic groups studied in England when patients were matched by the social classification of the Registrar General.

Age and Parity

A wide diversity of opinion exists over whether age and parity can be considered related to the prevalence of maternal bacteriuria. Opinion is equally divided between those who claim that neither age nor parity influences bacteriuria and those who claim that increasing age or greater parity is associated with higher rates of bacteriuria. Although difficult to prove, it seems logical that bacteriuria would increase as a function of both increased age and parity; however, these factors are not mutually exclusive.

Sickle Cell Trait

One host factor that has been shown unequivocally to have a significant influence on the frequency of maternal bacteriuria in black women is sickle hemoglobin. The experiences from Parkland Memorial Hospital (Whalley et al., 1965; Pritchard et al., 1973) have demonstrated this. Asymptomatic bacteriuria is twice as common in black pregnant women with the sickle cell trait as in black pregnant women of the same socioeconomic status whose red cells contain no sickle hemoglobin. The reasons for this difference have not been clarified.

Pregnancy and Bacteriuria

Aside from those factors already mentioned, the role that pregnancy itself plays in the acquisition of bacteriuria must be considered. It has been shown that some women acquire bacteriuria prior to beginning sexual activity. Beginning with sexual intercourse, the prevalence of bacteriuria increases presumably owing to attendant urethra and bladder trauma. These studies offer convincing evidence that in the majority of instances, the acquisition of bacteriuria antedates conception, and indeed, if bacteriuria is sought early in pregnancy the majority of cases will be detected. Approximately 1 per cent of those women demonstrated to be abacteriuric when initially screened will acquire significant bacteriuria later in the same pregnancy.

Critical analysis of data regarding the effect of pregnancy on the prevalence of bacteriuria suggests that pregnancy per se does not cause an increase in bacteriuria, although it may create a situation in which instrumentation of the urethra and bladder is more likely to be performed. Routine urethral catherization at the time of delivery is still widely practiced, as is the placement of an indwelling catheter prior to cesarean section. These procedures may result in bacteriuria, which may persist and go undetected until a later pregnancy. The observations of several investigators that the prevalence of bacteriuria increases with parity may well be the consequence of such instrumentation. Another factor that may lead to urinary bacterial colonization is bladder distention incited by urethral trauma associated with normal delivery.

DIAGNOSTIC TECHNIQUES

Detection of Bacteriuria

There are several reliable and simple methods for detection of significant bacteriuria as a routine screening procedure. In most cases the physician will use the services of the hospital bacteriology laboratory. Again, it must be emphasized that the handling of the urine specimen after collection is of utmost importance if reliable results are to be obtained. Preferably the specimen should be taken immediately to the laboratory for culture. However, in most cases this is not feasible. The urine should then be refrigerated at 4° C and processed on the day of collection. Overnight storage of specimens decreases the accuracy of bacterial recovery and is not recommended.

Calibrated Bacteriologic Loop Technique

Many laboratories, including ours, use the calibrated bacteriologic loop technique, which delivers 0.01 ml. of urine. Several types of agar are suitable; we prefer eosin–methylene blue (EMB) or MacConkey's media. After appropriate sterilization the loop is dipped into the urine and is then brought down the center of the plate from one side to the other. A zig-zag motion is then used from side to side at right angles to the center line. Enumeration of bacterial colonies is done 18 to 24 hours following inoculation. Actual colony counting may be performed; however, after experience with the technique the number of colonies present can be accurately estimated. Figure 35–1 demonstrates this technique.

If a pure culture is obtained, the microorganism is identified using standard biochemical tests. Antimicrobial sensitivities can also be performed using any one of several standard methods.

This technique of enumerating urinary bacterial counts may seem cumbersome, but in reality it is simple. The clinician with access to an incubator can easily perform screening cultures in all prenatal patients by following the procedures outlined previously. Identification of species as well as antimicrobial sensitivities is more difficult and is not recommended for the office laboratory. The loop method can be used in the office for screening, and if the results indicate significant bacteriuria, a second specimen may be obtained and sent to the microbiology laboratory for identification of the organism and its antimicrobial sensitivities. The loop technique may also be employed for "test of cure" cultures following treatment for bacteriuria as well as symptomatic urinary tract infection.

Commercial Testing Systems

Several commercial testing systems for bacteriuria screening are available to the physician. The Greiss test, for example, is a dipstick method for quantification of bacteria by indirect chemical reactions. The re-

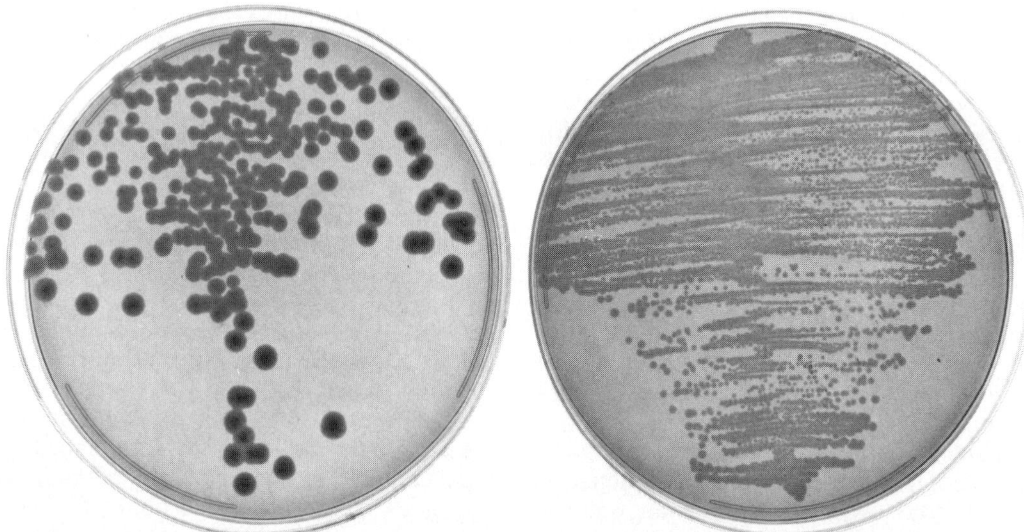

Figure 35–1. Bacterial colony enumeration. The plate on the left has approximately 300 colonies. Because the calibrated loop delivers 0.01 ml of urine this number is multiplied by 100, and in this specimen there are therefore 30,000 bacteria per ml. of urine. On the right is a plate with greater than 1,000 colonies, which indicates a urine bacterial count of greater than 100,000 per ml.

sults of this test have been compared with the plate method described previously. Unless an early morning urine specimen is collected, the probability of false-negative reactions is rather high, ranging from 10 to 40 per cent. For routine screening of large populations, the Greiss test, as well as other chemical tests, is not recommended (Andriole, 1975).

For women at high risk for bacteriuria, e.g., those previously treated during pregnancy, self-testing at home may prove beneficial. Kunin and Degroot (1975) showed that testing of three successive daily first-voided specimens using Microstix-Nitrite (Ames Company) detected 88 per cent of cases of bacteriuria. Furthermore, there were no false-positive tests and only 11 per cent were false-negative.

The Testuria Kit (Ames Company) uses the same principles as the calibrated loop technique. A dipstick is saturated with urine and lightly touched to a small agar plate. This is placed in a "mini-incubator," and the colonies are counted to determine if significant bacteriuria is present. Our experience with this system has been that it is accurate enough for routine screening. Another system with which we have had experience is the Bacturcult (Wampole Laboratories). In addition to providing an estimation of the colony count, this test kit differentiates groups of species of commonly encountered uropathogens by means of a color reaction. Our limited experience with Bacturcult shows it to be accurate both in enumeration of bacteria and in grouping species. It is suitable for office screening and "test of cure" cultures.

These kits as well as many others not named here are convenient for bacteriuria *screening* in a prenatal population. If significant bacteriuria is demonstrated by these methods, or if an "intermediate" number of organisms is detected, it is recommended that a clean voided specimen be sent to the microbiology laboratory. If this is not feasible, treatment should be given on the basis of these test results.

Direct Examination of Urine

A frequently neglected but simple rapid screening procedure is to examine a drop of *uncentrifuged* urine with the 43× microscope objective. If any bacteria are seen, one can anticipate a colony count of greater than 100,000 organisms per ml. of urine.

TABLE 35–1. METHODS FOR LOCALIZATION OF BACTERIA IN THE URINARY TRACT*

Direct	Indirect
1. Ureteral catheterization	1. Serum antibodies
2. Renal biopsy	2. Urine concentration
3. Bladder washout technique	3. Creatinine clearance
	4. Antibody-coated bacteria

*From Sanford, 1973.

We, as well as Andriole (1975), recommend this simple screening test, although it should be kept in mind that a 20 per cent *false-negative* error is associated with the technique (Norden and Kass, 1968).

Localization of Bacteriuria

Although there is general agreement that acute and chronic pyelonephritis may ultimately lead to the development of chronic renal disease, the relationship between these entities has not been precisely defined. It is assumed that infection expressly confined to the lower urinary tract does not directly cause chronic renal disease. This is not to say, however, that lower tract infection cannot lead to renal infection either by ascension or by resultant obstructive uropathy. The major question therefore has been: How frequently do patients with urinary tract infections have evidence of renal parenchymal involvement?

Reeves and Brumfitt (1968) state: "We consider that a major advance in the understanding of urinary tract infection will occur when a simple and reliable method is available for the localization of infection within the urinary tract of the individual."

Several methods are currently used for localization of urinary infection; these are summarized in Table 35–1.

DIRECT METHODS

Ureteral Catheterization

Of the direct methods, the most reliable is recovery of bacteria by ureteral catheterization. This technique has been used since the resurgence of interest in quantitative bacteriology of urine (Sanford et al., 1956). Stamey and co-workers (1965) have utilized this technique extensively to differentiate between renal and lower tract infection. The invasiveness of this method obviously limits its utility.

Renal Biopsy

Renal biopsy not only is a relatively dangerous method of determining parenchymal involvement but also may be unreliable because of the patchy distributions of lesions found in chronic pyelonephritis (Freedman, 1960).

Bladder Washout Technique

Fairley and associates (1967) developed the bladder washout technique, which allows for collection of ureteric urine without ureteral catheterization. This method involves bladder catheterization with a triple-lumen Foley catheter. After collection of a specimen of bladder urine the bladder is emptied and irrigated. After 45 minutes the bladder is again emptied and washed, and urine is collected thereafter every 10 minutes for quantitative bacterial counts. Serial specimens that contain increasing bacterial counts indicate renal bacteriuria. This procedure has been used quite extensively and correlates well with ureteric catheterization. However, it is not only invasive but also too cumbersome for routine use.

INDIRECT METHODS

Measurement of Serum Antibodies

Of the indirect methods, one that has been used widely is the measurement of serum antibodies against the O antigen of the infecting microorganism. When infection involves the renal parenchyma, antibodies may be demonstrable, but these antibodies are absent when infection is confined to the lower tract. Although antibody determination may be useful in studying groups of patients, there is much individual variation, and overall the method is rather imprecise.

Renal Function Tests

The results of renal function tests to measure urine concentrating ability and to estimate glomerular filtration rate may correlate with the site of infection. Neither of these determinations, however, is sufficiently predictive of subtle differences in a given individual to be of clinical utility.

Antibody-Coated Bacteria Immunofluorescence Test

In 1974, Thomas and coworkers described a relatively simple technique for the detection of antibody-coated bacteria by using an immunofluorescence test. Fresh urine sediment is mixed with fluorescein-conjugated antihuman globulin; the presence of fluorescent bacteria indicates that they are renal in origin. Evidence of the reliability of this method was established by Jones and co-workers (1974), who compared results using the bladder washout technique with antibody-coated bacteria. Some imprecision has been reported by Harding and colleagues (1978), who showed that antibody-coated bacteria correlated in all cases with renal infection determined by bladder washout. However, if bacteria did not fluoresce, 20 per cent of patients were still found to have renal infection. Because of the simplicity and apparent reliability of this test, it is the best method now available for localization of bacteriuria. Bacteria that exhibit fluorescence are presumably renal in origin, whereas those that do not fluoresce indicate "bladder bacteriuria."

The direct immunofluorescence test has been evaluated by Thomas and Harris and their co-workers in pregnant women with asymptomatic bacteriuria as well as in those with cystitis and pyelonephritis. Thomas and associates (1975) demonstrated antibody-coated bacteria in the urine of 12 of 15 pregnant women with acute pyelonephritis but in none of 13 women in whom cystitis was diagnosed. Data from Harris (1976) as well as those from Parkland Memorial Hospital (Leveno et al., 1981; Gilstrap et al., 1981*b*) indicate that approximately one half of pregnant women with asymptomatic bacteriuria have antibody-coated bacteria, implying renal parenchymal infection. These results correlate well with the findings of Boutros and co-workers (1972) and of Fairley and associates (1973), who employed the bladder washout technique in pregnant women with significant bacteriuria and reported that 40 to 50 per cent of bacteriuria was renal in origin.

CLINICAL SIGNIFICANCE OF MATERNAL BACTERIURIA

Although asymptomatic bacteriuria in pregnancy has been recognized for many years, it stimulated little investigation until Kass (1960) presented his initial observations at the First International Symposium on Pyelonephritis in 1959. Since then a voluminous literature has accumulated, and there is evidence both to corroborate and to refute Kass' original contention on the deleterious effect of asymptomatic bacteriuria in pregnancy. Some of the proved as well as some of the alleged effects of bacteriuria on pregnancy will now be considered.

Asymptomatic Bacteriuria and Symptomatic Urinary Tract Infection

ANTEPARTUM URINARY INFECTIONS

Kass (1960) found that 40 per cent of pregnant bacteriuric women treated with a placebo developed pyelonephritis. He further demonstrated that treatment with antimicrobial agents throughout gestation prevented acute pyelonephritis during pregnancy. This relationship of maternal bacteriuria to symptomatic clinical urinary tract infection, either cystitis or pyelonephritis, remains undisputed.

In 1967, Whalley reviewed the literature and reported that 14 to 63 per cent of

TABLE 35–2. ASYMPTOMATIC BACTERIURIA AND ANTEPARTUM SYMPTOMATIC URINARY TRACT INFECTION (UTI)

	Bacteriuric Patients			**Non-Bacteriuric Patients**		
	Total	*Symptomatic UTI*		*Total*	*Symptomatic UTI*	
Author	*Patients*	*Number*	*Per Cent*	*Patients*	*Number*	*Per Cent*
Kass (1962)	95	18	19	1,000	0	0
Sleigh et al. (1964)	100	43	43	100	14	14
Kincaid-Smith & Bullen (1965)	55	20	37	4,000	48	1.2
Norden & Kilpatrick (1965)	110	25	23	105	1	1.0
Whalley (1965)	179	46	26	179	0	0
Little (1966)	141	35	25	4,735	19	0.4
Brumfitt (1975)	179	55	31	–	–	–
Total	858	242	28	10,119	82	0.8

patients with bacteriuria during pregnancy developed acute antepartum urinary tract infections, compared with 0 to 14 per cent of pregnant women who were abacteriuric at the first prenatal visit. This wide variation in reported incidence can be accounted for by the various criteria used to diagnose acute pyelonephritis. For example, renal infection was diagnosed on the basis of fever and flank pain by some, whereas others required only dysuria and frequency to make this diagnosis. It has been emphasized previously that both of these latter symptoms are common complaints during normal pregnancy and do not necessarily indicate urinary tract infection.

When several clinical studies are compared (Table 35–2), it can be seen that symptomatic clinical urinary tract infections develop in approximately 30 per cent of patients with *untreated* maternal bacteriuria. Conversely, less than 1 per cent of women without bacteriuria developed urinary tract infection.

Overall, 25 to 30 per cent of cases of pyelonephritis in pregnancy occur in women who had sterile urine cultures on their first prenatal visit. It can logically be concluded from these data that antepartum pyelonephritis cannot be completely eradicated even by screening and treating all cases of bacteriuria identified in pregnancy. These observations have led some to question or even condemn routine screening for maternal bacteriuria (Dixon and Brant, 1967; Lawson and Miller, 1971, 1973). In our opinion, such arguments are untenable, since 60 to 70 per cent of cases of severe maternal renal infection can be prevented. An argument for detection and eradication of maternal bacteriuria is emphasized by the report from Parkland Memorial Hospital by Gilstrap and associates (1981*a*). More than 2 per cent of 24,000 pregnant women during a 4½ year period developed severe antepartum pyelonephritis. Theoretically, with proper screening and treatment for bacteriuria, over 350 of these 534 cases would have been prevented. Similar experiences from Charity Hospital of New Orleans, in which 3 per cent of pregnant women with severe pyelonephritis developed endotoxin shock, attest to the seriousness of this disease (Cunningham et al., 1973).

Postpartum Urinary Infections

Symptomatic urinary tract infections in the puerperium are more frequent in women who have had antepartum bacteriuria or symptomatic infections. Recurrent pyelonephritis developing post partum may be seen in as many as 10 per cent of women who suffered antepartum pyelonephritis (Cunningham et al., 1973; Gilstrap et al., 1981*a*). Many of these infections, however, arise de novo and may be iatrogenic, i.e., related to bladder catheterization performed at delivery. The significance of catheterization is well illustrated in a report by Brumfitt and co-workers (1961), who studied a group of women who were abacteriuric just prior to delivery and who had no history of urinary tract infection. Significant bacteriuria appeared during the puerperium in 4.7 per cent of women with uncomplicated labor who were not subjected to catheterization; however 9.1 per cent of a similar group who were catheterized simply to obtain a urine specimen developed postpartum bacteriuria. In still another group of patients who received an indwelling catheter for valid indications (e.g., cesarean section), the prevalence of subsequent bacteriuria was 22.8 per cent. Clinical urinary tract infections occurred in one half of all of these women who developed puerperal bacteriuria. These important data emphasize the significant immediate problems that may develop from routine catheterization, and also illustrate how bacteriuria may be acquired as a result of delivery.

Asymptomatic Bacteriuria and Prematurity and Perinatal Mortality

Whether or not bacteriuria is causally associated with premature labor and increased perinatal mortality is controversial, and as pointed out by Zinner (1979), there are multiple reasons for this. Kass (1960) reported an increased prematurity rate as well as increased perinatal mortality in women with bacteriuria. In addition he observed that prematurity and perinatal mortality could be reduced significantly with antimicrobials given throughout gestation. Other workers have failed to confirm these observations, however.

Most investigators have defined prematurity as a birth weight of less than 2500 gm. Modern obstetric concepts dictate that low birth weight per se does not indicate prematurity. The gestational or chronologic age of the fetus determines prematurity, and many infants weighing less than 2500 gm are not premature but rather *growth retarded.* These infants are variously classified as *light for dates, small for gestational age,* or *dysmature.* In some cases it is impossible to differentiate between prematurity and fetal growth retardation because of lack of reliable obstetric criteria for assessing gestational age. The confusion about these two conditions and its relatively recent clarification make it impossible to determine from earlier reports whether infants born to mothers with bacteriuria were premature, dysmature, or both.

If the hypothesis is correct that bacteriuria causes prematurity, this effect should be apparent in bacteriuric women when compared to abacteriuric women, provided that in all other respects the two groups are comparable. This means that any group of women studied should be matched for variables known to influence prematurity as well as to produce growth-retarded infants, e.g., age, race, parity, socioeconomic status, smoking habits, pregnancy hypertension, and previous delivery of low birth weight infants.

Two large studies using data from the Collaborative Perinatal Project suggest a positive correlation between urinary tract infection and adverse perinatal outcome. Naeye (1979) showed a relationship with urinary tract infection and increased infant mortality from *noninfectious* complications — e.g., gestational hypertension. Urine cultures, however, were not done in many of these women. Sever and colleagues (1979) analyzed *symptomatic* urinary tract infections in the same women from the Collaborative Perinatal Project and partially confirmed these findings; however, as pointed out by Zinner (1979), neither study was prospectively designed to analyze these effects.

Some who report a positive relationship between bacteriuria and prematurity disagree on the efficacy of antimicrobial drugs in reducing the incidence of prematurity. As mentioned previously, Kass (1960) showed a reduction in prematurity in bacteriuric women treated throughout gestation. Although the work of LeBlanc and McGanity (1964) confirmed these observations, Kincaid-Smith and Bullen (1965) as well as Brumfitt (1975) were unable to significantly reduce the prematurity rate with antimicrobial therapy.

From the foregoing it is apparent that confusion and disagreement exist about the relationship of maternal bacteriuria and prematurity. Earlier data from Parkland Memorial Hospital (Whalley, 1967; Whalley and Cunningham, 1977) did not demonstrate an increased incidence of preterm delivery or dysmaturity in bacteriuric women. With introduction of the antibody-coated bacteria test for noninvasive localization of the site of bacteriuria, it was possible to analyze pregnancy outcome in

TABLE 35–3. GESTATIONAL AGE, PRETERM DELIVERY, BIRTH WEIGHT, AND FETAL GROWTH RETARDATION IN WOMEN WITH PREGNANCY BACTERIURIA VERSUS CONTROLS*

	Renal Infection		**Bladder Infection**	
	Bacteriuria	*Control*	*Bacteriuria*	*Control*
Gestational age (weeks ± S.E.M.)	39.9 ± .18	39.1 ± .2	39.9 ± .22	39.5 ± .14
Preterm delivery (< 37 weeks)	5	7	11	5
Mean birth weight (grams ± S.E.M.)	3254 ± 581	3077 ± 558	3073 ± 604	3121 ± 489
Growth retardation	9	7	10	13

*From Gilstrap, L. C., Leveno, K. J., Cunningham, F. G., et al.: Renal infection and pregnancy outcome. Am. J. Obstet. Gynecol., *141*:709, 1981*b*.

these women with regard to whether they had renal or bladder infection. We recently completed a prospective matched-control study in which 256 pregnant women with confirmed bacteriuria were matched with abacteriuric controls and carefully followed throughout their pregnancies (Gilstrap et al., 1981*b*). The results of this study are presented in Table 35–3 and show no differences in adverse perinatal outcome in either group. Moreover, there were no differences when these groups of women were analyzed for adverse pregnancy outcome according to the site of infection.

Asymptomatic Bacteriuria and Pregnancy Hypertension

The alleged relationship between maternal bacteriuria and pregnancy hypertension is also controversial. Investigators who have addressed this subject have not used a standard definition of pregnancy hypertension, making comparisons between studies difficult. For example, in some reports patients with edema and proteinuria but *without hypertension* were included in the "hypertensive" group. In another report, pregnancy hypertension was diagnosed only if hypertension and excessive weight gain persisted after diuretic therapy.

Brumfitt (1975) found no significant increase in the incidence of pregnancy hypertension or "toxemia," or both, in women with maternal bacteriuria. However, McFadyen (1973) did demonstrate a twofold increase in the incidence of pregnancy hypertension in bacteriuric women compared with those without bacteriuria. Kincaid-Smith and Bullen (1965) found that the incidence of pregnancy hypertension was identical in bacteriuric women whether or not treatment was given. Although all of the patients in McFadyen and co-workers' study were treated, these authors hypothesized that treatment may have reduced the incidence of hypertension.

Here again, studies utilizing localization of bacteriuria may prove to be of value when investigating the possible relationship of bacteriuria and pregnancy hypertension. It seems reasonable to assume that if there is an increased incidence of pregnancy hypertension associated with bacteriuria, it would occur in women with renal bacteriuria. However, data from the prospective study from Parkland Memorial Hospital failed to show any association between pregnancy hypertension and maternal bacteriuria. As shown in Table 35–4, the incidence of hypertension in women with renal bacteriuria was almost identical to that of women with bladder bacteriuria. Similarly, when hypertension in nulliparous women was compared with that in multiparous women, there were no significant differences when the site of infection was compared nor when either group was compared with abacteriuric controls.

Asymptomatic Bacteriuria and Maternal Anemia

The relationship between maternal bacteriuria and anemia also remains controversial. As with prematurity, several factors

TABLE 35–4. PREGNANCY HYPERTENSION IN 256 BACTERIURIC WOMEN AND NONINFECTED CONTROLS*

	Renal Infection (%)		**Bladder Infection (%)**	
	Bacteriuria	*Control*	*Bacteriuria*	*Control*
Nulliparous	14/49 (29)	10/49 (20)	10/52 (19)	12/52 (23)
Multiparous	0/66	7/66 (11)	10/86 (12)	7/86 (8)
Totals	14/115 (12)	17/115 (15)	20/138 (15)	19/138 (14)

*From Gilstrap, L. C., Leveno, K. J., Cunningham, F. G., et al.: Renal infection and pregnancy outcome. Am. J. Obstet. Gynecol., *141*:709, 1981*b*.

must be analyzed when this association is investigated. In the etiology of maternal anemia, one important factor is the woman's socioeconomic status and related nutritional state, especially with regard to iron and whether or not iron supplements were taken during pregnancy. One factor definitely associated with the development of anemia in pregnancy is an episode of acute pyelonephritis. Brumfitt (1975) reported that the frequency of anemia was the same in abacteriuric control patients as in those with treated bacteriuria; however, he pointed out that *untreated* asymptomatic bacteriuria increases the likelihood of anemia. This latter observation is related in great part to the superimposition of pyelonephritis occurring in the untreated women. Brumfitt showed that 45 per cent of patients with untreated bacteriuria who developed pyelonephritis had anemia. The data from Parkland Hospital are similar (Gilstrap, Cunningham, and Whalley, unpublished observations). Of 435 women with acute antepartum pyelonephritis, 30 per cent had a hematocrit of less than 30 per cent when admitted for acute infection. Our preliminary studies indicate that anemia is due to increased red cell destruction as well as decreased production (Cunningham and Pritchard, 1977).

In the prospective study from Parkland Memorial Hospital, we demonstrated that women with asymptomatic bacteriuria have slightly—albeit significantly—lower mean hematocrit values than women without bacteriuria. Although one might predict that this would hold true for women with *renal bacteriuria,* this was not the case. As shown in Table 35–5, this slight difference was observed in all women with bacteriuria. More importantly, however, anemia (hematocrit less than 30 per cent) was not observed more frequently in those women treated for bacteriuria. The significance of these observations is not known.

Long-Term Prognosis

The long-term prognosis of women with asymptomatic bacteriuria first detected during pregnancy deserves attention. Should bacteriuria persisting beyond pregnancy be considered a benign process or a manifestation of continuing active renal infection? Several investigators have shown that women who demonstrate bacteriuria during pregnancy will frequently continue to have bacteriuria following delivery. For example, Whalley and co-workers (1965) detected significant bacteriuria two or more

TABLE 35–5. ANEMIA AND MEAN HEMATOCRIT VALUES IN 253 BACTERIURIC WOMEN COMPARED WITH NON-INFECTED CONTROLS*

	Renal Infection			**Bladder Infection**		
	Bacteriuria (N=115)	*Control (N=115)*	*P*	*Bacteriuria (N=138)*	*Control (N=138)*	*P*
Anemia	3	3	N.S.	5	2	N.S.
Mean hematocrit	34.9	35.8	<0.05	35.4	36.1	<0.05

*From Gilstrap, L. C., Leveno, K. J., Cunningham, F. C., et al.: Renal infection and pregnancy outcome. Am. J. Obstet. Gynecol., *141*:709, 1981*b*.

months post partum in 81 per cent of 111 women with *untreated* pregnancy bacteriuria. Other investigators have reported similar results.

There is evidence to strongly suggest that many women with maternal bacteriuria do indeed have renal involvement. Most of these investigations unfortunately were done without the benefit of bacteriuria localization. Whalley (1967) summarized the results of several reports in which women with maternal bacteriuria were studied with intravenous pyelography remote from pregnancy. Many of these women continued to have persistent bacteriuria post partum. Only subjects with major urinary tract abnormalities were included, and 30 to 40 per cent of the women had changes in the urinary tract suggestive of renal parenchymal disease. Stanley and Muldowney (1974) have also recently demonstrated that recurrent bacteriuria in pregnancy is associated with underlying structural disease of the kidneys or lower urinary tract in 40 per cent of women.

Further support for the thesis that bacteriuria is associated with renal parenchymal disease is provided by the observations that serum antibody titers to uropathogens are elevated in pregnant women with asymptomatic bacteriuria. In addition, the inability to concentrate urine can be demonstrated in approximately one half of pregnant women with bacteriuria, suggesting renal parenchymal involvement.

In long-term follow-up studies, Zinner and Kass (1971) found that 38 per cent of women with bacteriuria during pregnancy had significant bacteriuria when examined 10 to 14 years later, regardless of intervening therapy. Furthermore, they showed that radiographically demonstrable renal abnormalities were more frequent in the persistently bacteriuric women than in women who subsequently had sterile urine. Although Zinner and Kass concluded that their data were inadequate to state the magnitude of risk of renal involvement related to a single episode of pregnancy bacteriuria, they demonstrated evidence of chronic pyelonephritis in 10 per cent of patients who had *recurrent* or *persistent* bacteriuria.

Similar data have accrued from long-term follow-up studies done in women cared for at Parkland Memorial Hospital (Gilstrap et al., 1981*a*). In this study, 208 women cared for during 1964 through 1969 were reviewed for adverse sequelae through 1977. Of these 208 women, 42 per cent were given treatment while they were not pregnant for one or more episodes of symptomatic urinary tract infection. Of 140 women who had at least one subsequent pregnancy cared for at Parkland Hospital, 38 per cent had one or more urinary tract infections in at least one of these pregnancies. These results are summarized in Table 35–6 and show that 29 per cent had acute pyelonephritis whereas another 9 per cent had either asymptomatic bacteriuria or cystitis.

Neither chronic pyelonephritis nor renal insufficiency will develop in many women with bacteriuria during pregnancy. Current evidence suggests that end-stage renal disease from chronic pyelonephritis is rare, and in two large series this was the presumed cause of death in only 13 patients in more than 8000 consecutive autopsies (Freedman, 1967; Farmer and Heptinstall, 1970). Furthermore, the data are insufficient to draw conclusions regarding the role

TABLE 35–6. LONG-TERM (8 TO 13 YEAR) FOLLOW-UP OF 208 WOMEN WITH ACUTE ANTEPARTUM PYELONEPHRITIS*

Recurrent Infection		Number	Per Cent
Infection in subsequent pregnancy		53/140	38
Acute pyelonephritis	40/53		
Bacteriuria or cystitis	13/53		
Urinary infection, nonpregnant state		91/208	42

*From Gilstrap, L. C., Cunningham, F. G., and Whalley, P. J.: Acute pyelonephritis in pregnancy: an anterospective study of 656 women. Reprinted with permission from the American College of Obstetricians and Gynecologists (Obstet. Gynecol. *57*:409, 1981).

TABLE 35–7. EFFECT OF CONTINUOUS ANTIMICROBIAL THERAPY ON ANTEPARTUM PYELONEPHRITIS IN WOMEN WITH ASYMPTOMATIC BACTERIURIA

	Untreated Bacteriuric Patients			Patients Treated for Bacteriuria		
		With Pyelonephritis			*With Pyelonephritis*	
Author	*Total*	*Number*	*Per Cent*	*Total*	*Number*	*Per Cent*
Kass (1962)	95	18	19	84	0	0
Kincaid-Smith & Bullen (1965)	55	20	37	61	2	3.3
Little (1966)	141	35	25	124	4	3.2
Condie et al. (1968)	86	20	23	87	9	10.0
Total	377	93	25	356	15	4.2

of long-term drug therapy in preventing chronic renal lesions. With the advent of a simple test for localization of bacteriuria, well-designed long-term follow-up studies should be conducted to determine the prognostic significance, if any, of renal versus bladder bacteriuria.

ANTIMICROBIAL THERAPY

As previously discussed, it is undisputed that detection and eradication of maternal bacteriuria will appreciably decrease the incidence of antepartum symptomatic urinary tract infections. The effect of treatment of bacteriuria on the incidence of other pregnancy complications remains controversial.

In Table 35–7, data from four representative studies are compared for the effect of no treatment and effective therapy on the subsequent development of urinary tract infections. The incidence of antepartum symptomatic urinary tract infection is drastically altered by treatment of bacteriuria. In these studies, antimicrobial agents were given continuously throughout pregnancy. Approximately 25 per cent of untreated patients with bacteriuria developed clinical disease compared with 4.2 per cent of treated patients.

Therapeutic Considerations

Continuous versus Short-Term Therapy

Kass (1960) and Kincaid-Smith and Bullen (1965) were unable to eradicate maternal bacteriuria with short-term antimicrobial agents. Conversely, Williams and co-workers (1965) reported an initial cure rate of bacteriuria in 77 per cent of pregnant women treated with an 8 day course of sulfonamide chemotherapy. Amplifying their earlier work, Williams and associates (1968) later demonstrated a cure rate of 85 per cent in 240 pregnant women 1 week after completing 8 days of sulfonamide therapy. Six weeks after therapy 77 per cent of these women remained abacteriuric. Short-term ampicillin administration effected a similar cure rate when evaluated by these same investigators. Furthermore, McFadyen and associates (1973) demonstrated that a 10 day course of antimicrobial therapy with either sulfamethizole or ampicillin eliminated bacteriuria initially in 62 per cent of pregnant women; another 21 per cent responded to a second 10 day course.

Data from Parkland Memorial Hospital (Whalley and Cunningham, 1977) indicate that therapy for 2 weeks with either a short-acting sulfonamide (sulfamethizole) or nitrofurantoin is effective in eradicating bacteriuria for the duration of pregnancy in 65 per cent of patients. Initial comparative results of long- versus short-term therapy are shown in Table 35–8. Another 19 per cent of women in the short-term group were cured by a second 14 day course of therapy. The combined 84 per cent cure rate of short-term therapy compares favorably with the 92 per cent cure rate effected by continuous administration of these same two drugs.* Antepartum pyelonephritis oc-

*In the continuous treatment group, bacteriuria in an additional 5 per cent of patients (shown as relapse and reinfection in Table 35–8) cleared when the agent was changed.

TABLE 35–8. INITIAL COMPARATIVE RESULTS OF SHORT-TERM VERSUS CONTINUOUS ANTIMICROBIAL THERAPY IN ERADICATION OF MATERNAL BACTERIURIA

Therapy	Number of Patients	Results (Per Cent)			
		Cured†	*Relapse*	*Reinfection*	*No Response*
Short-term*	199	65	24	2	9
Continuous	95	87	3	2	8

†For remainder of gestation.
*14-day therapy.
Both groups of patients received either sulfamethizole, 1 gm. four times daily, or nitrofurantoin, 100 mg. twice daily.

curred in the short-term and continuous therapy groups with the same incidence (2 and 3 per cent, respectively), and at a rate that compares favorably with that in previous investigations in which continuous antimicrobial therapy was given.

More recently, we completed studies (Leveno et al., 1981) in which nitrofurantoin, 100 mg. given at bedtime for 10 days, was compared to empiric treatment with one of four antimicrobials given four times daily for 21 days. Following one course of treatment, these women were carefully monitored and the results showed that bacteriuria was eradicated for the remainder of gestation in 60 per cent of those women given 10 day therapy and in 68 per cent of those given 21 day therapy.

It is our opinion that sufficient data have been accumulated to recommend a short course (10 to 14 days) of antimicrobial therapy with continued surveillance to assure sterility after therapy. Short-term therapy would be most acceptable to asymptomatic patients. Costs, drug toxicity, and potential teratogenic effects could also be reduced by short-term therapy.

Selection of Antimicrobial Agent

Initial selection of an antimicrobial agent for treatment of asymptomatic bacteriuria in pregnancy is empiric. Regimens that have been shown to be effective include (1) a short-acting sulfonamide, 1 gm. four times daily; (2) nitrofurantoin, 100 mg. given either twice daily or once at bedtime; or (3) ampicillin or cephalexin, 250 mg. four times daily. A combination of sulfamethoxazole and trimethoprim has been shown to be superior to the sulfonamide alone in eradication of bacteriuria in nonpregnant as well as pregnant women (Williams et al., 1969); however, trimethoprim has not been approved by the Food and Drug Administration for use during pregnancy.

Recurrent or Persistent Bacteriuria

If bacteriuria recurs after one course of short-term therapy (and it can be expected to in one third of cases), a second course should be given using an antimicrobial selected after reveiwing the in vitro sensitivities of the organism. In the majority of cases one of the drugs cited earlier will prove appropriate. In some women, bacteriuria will again recur, and a third course of therapy will be required.

In the 5 to 10 per cent of pregnant women who demonstrate *persistent* or *recurrent* bacteriuria after adequate therapy, continuous "suppressive" therapy should be given for the remainder of pregnancy. In these cases, repeat culture surveillance during drug administration is mandatory to ensure that the urine remains sterile. One drug regimen that we have found effective in achieving these results with a minimum of side effects is 100 mg. of nitrofurantoin given at bedtime. Alternative regimens of continuous suppression, often dictated by antimicrobial sensitivities, include either 500 mg. of ampicillin or an oral cephalosporin derivative given at bedtime.

If acute antepartum pyelonephritis develops in a woman receiving treatment or who has been treated for bacteriuria, immediate hospitalization is mandatory, and parenteral antibiotic therapy is required. Once again, the choice of antimicrobial therapy is dictated by previously obtained in vitro sensitivities. Usually intravenous ampicillin or cephalothin will be sufficient, but occasionally bacterial resistance will require the addition of an aminoglycoside.

Precautions

In the majority of instances, bacteriuria is not identified until after the first trimester of pregnancy, when embryonic organogenesis is completed. For this reason, administration of antibacterial drugs is considerably safer. In the unusual case when asymptomatic bacteriuria is detected prior to the twelfth week of gestation, it would seem prudent to delay therapy until the first trimester is completed. Obviously if acute pyelonephritis develops prior to this time, treatment is mandatory; however, symptomatic urinary tract infections very rarely occur before the second trimester.

Results of Therapy in Bladder versus Renal Bacteriuria

It seems logical to assume that bladder bacteriuria is more amenable to cure than is renal bacteriuria. During studies to localize the site of maternal bacteriuria, Boutros and co-workers (1972) demonstrated that more than half of women with bladder bacteriuria were cured simply by the topical antimicrobial used in the bladder washout procedure. Conversely, all patients with renal bacteriuria who were treated only with topical antibiotics eventually demonstrated recurrent bacteriuria. These same investigators (Ronald et al., 1976) later demonstrated that a single 500 mg. dose of intramuscular kanamycin effected a cure rate of 77 per cent in women with bladder bacteriuria tested 4 weeks later. However, only 30 per cent of women with renal bacteriuria were cured using this regimen. At 6 weeks, 43 per cent of all the women remained cured, but 94 per cent of the relapses were in the group with renal bacteriuria.

We have recently investigated the utility of localization of bacteriuria by the antibody-coated bacteria test in selection of treatment (Leveno et al., 1981). The incidence of renal bacteriuria in these 233 women was 42 per cent. Regardless of the site of infection, following one course of short-term (10 day) or long-term (21 day) antimicrobial therapy, almost two thirds of these women were abacteriuric for the remainder of gestation. Women given short-term treatment were more likely to have a recurrence within 2 weeks of completing therapy (relapse) compared with women given long-term therapy. Moreover, these early recurrences were more frequent in women given short-term treatment for renal bacteriuria. Conversely, recurrences 6 weeks or more after completing therapy (reinfection), regardless of the site of infection, were more common in women given long-term treatment. Although the timing of recurrence varied significantly in relation to duration of treatment and site of infection, the ultimate recurrence risk was not related

TABLE 35–9. RECURRENCE OF BACTERIURIA: RELAPSES AND REINFECTIONS IN RELATION TO DURATION OF THERAPY AND SITE OF BACTERIURIA*

	Relapses (%)			Reinfections (%)		
	Renal	*Bladder*	*Total*	*Renal*	*Bladder*	*Total*
10 day therapy (N=129)	16/55 (29)	10/74 (14)	26/129 (20)	2/39 (5)	10/64 (16)	12/103 (12)
	$P < 0.05$ (renal vs. bladder)		$P < 0.001$ (10 day vs. 21 day)			$P < 0.01$ (10 day vs. 21 day)
21 day therapy (N=81)	2/34 (6)	1/47 (2)	3/81 (4)	10/32 (31)	13/46 (28)	23/78 (29)

*From Leveno, K. J., Harris, R. E., Gilstrap, L. C., et al.: Bladder versus renal bacteriuria during pregnancy: recurrence after treatment. Am. J. Obstet. Gynecol. *139*:403, 1981.

to either. From these data, summarized in Table 35–9, we have concluded that localization of bacteriuria does not contribute to its management during pregnancy.

SUMMARY

The pregnant woman is particularly susceptible to the development of acute pyelonephritis from asymptomatic bacteriuria, which in most cases antedates pregnancy. Hormonal and mechanical changes of pregnancy result in urinary stasis that favors bacterial replication and development of symptomatic urinary tract infection.

The prevalence of significant maternal bacteriuria ranges from 2 to 10 per cent. Increased prevalence is particularly associated with lower socioeconomic status and the presence of sickle hemoglobin. Other factors that have been implicated in having a positive influence on the prevalence of bacteriuria are race, age, and parity, although their effects are less clear. Pregnancy itself may contribute to the acquisition of bacteriura by trauma to the lower urinary tract or, more importantly, by catheterization performed either with normal delivery or during cesarean section.

The one irrefutable complication of untreated bacteriuria during pregnancy is the development of symptomatic urinary infection. It has been unequivocally demonstrated that treatment of maternal bacteriuria dramatically reduces the incidence of these infections. Alleged associations between maternal bacteriuria and increased prematurity and perinatal mortality, as well as increased pregnancy hypertension and anemia, remain controversial at this time.

The possible link between bacteriuria and these latter conditions may now be clarified with the simple method of direct immunofluorescence for bacteriuria localization. Recent studies using this method have indicated no link between maternal bacteriuria and adverse pregnancy outcome, regardless of the site of infection. It is anticipated that further investigations will be confirmatory.

The long-term prognosis for women having bacteriuria during pregnancy appears to be that of recurrent infection, both while pregnant and while not pregnant. Although those women with persistent or recurrent bacteriuria over several years have a higher incidence of associated radiographic renal abnormalities, the majority of data suggest that end-stage renal insufficiency from chronic pyelonephritis is rare unless infection is due to structural abnormalities and is manifest early in childhood.

Initial treatment recommended for asymptomatic bacteriuria in the pregnant woman is a 10 to 14 day course with one of several antimicrobials. One of several drugs may be selected; these include short-acting sulfonamides, nitrofurantoin, cephalexin, and ampicillin. After initial treatment there must be continued urine culture surveillance, since in at least one third of cases, bacteriuria recurs, and acute pyelonephritis may follow this recurrence. A second short-term therapeutic course will eradicate bacteriuria in another 20 per cent of women. Occasionally bacteriuria will persist or recur in spite of three short courses of antimicrobial therapy. In these cases, the woman should be treated with suppressive therapy for the remainder of the pregnancy; urine culture studies should be performed while the patient is receiving medication.

REFERENCES

Andriole, V. T.: Urinary tract infections in pregnancy. Urol. Clin. North Am. *11*:485, 1975.

Boutros, P., Mourtada, H., and Ronald, A. R.: Urinary infection localization. Am. J. Obstet. Gynecol. *112*:379, 1972.

Brumfitt, W., Davies, B. I., and Rosser, E. I.: Urethral catheter as a cause of urinary tract infection in pregnancy and puerperium. Lancet *2*:1059, 1961.

Brumfitt, W.: The effects of bacteriuria in pregnancy on maternal and fetal health. Kidney Int. *8* (Suppl.):113, 1975.

Condie, A. P., Williams, J. D., Reeves, D. S., et al.: Complications of bacteriuria in pregnancy. *In* O'Grady, F., and Brumfitt, W. (eds.): Urinary Tract Infection. London, Oxford University Press. 1968, pp. 148–159.

Cunningham, F. G., and Pritchard, J. A.: Hematologic disorders in pregnancy. *In* Bolognese, R. J., and Schwarz, R. H. (Eds.): Perinatal Medicine. Baltimore, Williams & Wilkins Co., 1977, 246–264.

Cunningham, F. G., Morris, G. B., and Mickal, A.: Pyelonephritis in pregnancy — A clinical review. Obstet. Gynecol. *42*:112, 1973.

Dixon, H. G., and Brant, H. A.: The significance of bacteriuria in pregnancy. Lancet *1*:19, 1967.

Fairley, K. F., Bond, A. G., Brown, R. B., et al.: Simple tests to determine the site of urinary tract infections. Lancet *2*:7513, 1967.

Fairley, K. F., Whitworth, J. A., Radford, N. J., et al.: Pregnancy bacteriuria: The significance of site of infection. Med. J. Aust. *2*:424, 1973.

Farmer, K. F., and Heptinstall, R. H.: Chronic non-obstructive pyelonephritis: a reappraisal. *In* Kincaid-Smith, P., and Fairley, K. F. (Eds.): Renal Infection and Renal Scarring. Melbourne, Mercedes, 1970, p. 233.

Freedman, L. R.: Prolonged observations on a group of patients with acute urinary tract infections. *In* Quinn, E. L., and Kass, E. H. (eds.): Biology of Pyelonephritis. Boston, Little, Brown and Co., 1960, pp. 345–353.

Freedman, L. R.: Chronic pyelonephritis at autopsy. Ann. Intern. Med., *66*:697, 1967.

Gilstrap, L. C., Cunningham, F. G., and Whalley, P. J.: Acute pyelonephritis in pregnancy: an anterospective study of 656 women. Obstet. Gynecol. *57*:409, 1981*a*.

Gilstrap, L. C., Leveno, K. J., Cunningham, F. G., Whalley, P. J., and Roark, M. L.: Renal infection and pregnancy outcome. Am. J. Obstet. Gynecol., *141*:709, 1981*b*.

Harding, G. K. M., Marrie, T. J., Ronald, A. R., et al.: Urinary tract infection localization in women. J.A.M.A. *240*:1147, 1978.

Harris, R. E.: Infections of the urinary tract during pregnancy: Use of fluorescent antibody as an aid in patient evaluation. South. Med. J. *69*:1429, 1976.

Jones, F. R., Smith, J. W., and Sanford, J. P.: Localization of urinary tract infections by detection of antibody-coated bacteria in urine sediment. N. Engl. J. Med. *290*:591, 1974.

Kass, E. H.: Asymptomatic infections of the urinary tract. Trans. Assoc. Am. Physicians, *69*:56, 1956.

Kass, E. H.: *In* Quinn, E. L., and Kass, E. H. (Eds.): Biology of Pyelonephritis. Boston, Little, Brown and Co., 1960, p. 399.

Kass, E. H.: Pyelonephritis in bacteriuria. A major problem in preventive medicine. Ann. Intern. Med. *56*:46, 1962.

Kincaid-Smith, P., and Bullen, M.: Bacteriuria in pregnancy. Lancet *1*:395, 1965.

Kunin, C. M., and Degroot, J. E.: Self screening for significant bacteriuria. J.A.M.A. *231*:1349, 1975.

Lawson, D. H., and Miller, A. W. F.: Screening for bacteriuria in pregnancy. Lancet *1*:9, 1971.

Lawson, D. H., and Miller, A. W. F.: Screening for bacteriuria in pregnancy: A critical reappraisal. Arch. Intern. Med. *132*:904, 1973.

LeBlanc, A. L., and McGanity, W. J.: The impact of bacteriuria in pregnancy — a survey of 1300 pregnant patients. Tex. Rep. Biol. Med. *22*:336, 1964.

Leveno, K. J., Harris, R. E., Gilstrap, L. C., et al.: Bladder versus renal bacteriuria during pregnancy: recurrence after treatment. Am. J. Obstet. Gynecol. *139*:403, 1981.

Little, T. J.: The incidence of urinary infection in 5,000 pregnant women. Lancet *2*:925, 1966.

McFadyen, I. R., Eykyn, S. J., Gardner, N. H. N., et al.: Bacteriuria in pregnancy. J. Obstet. Gynaecol. Br. Commonw. *80*:385, 1973.

Monto, A. S., and Rantz, L. A.: The development and character of bacteriuria in pregnancy. Experience with non-indigent population. Ann. Intern. Med. *59*:186, 1963.

Naeye, R. L.: Causes of the excessive rates of perinatal mortality and prematurity in pregnancies complicated by maternal urinary-tract infections. N. Engl. J. Med. *300*:819, 1979.

Norden, C. W., and Kilpatrick, W. H.: *In* Kass, E. H. (Ed.): Progress in Pyelonephritis. Philadelphia, F. A. Davis Co., 1965, p. 64.

Norden, C. W., and Kass, E. H.: Bacteriuria of pregnancy: A critical appraisal. Ann. Rev. Med. *19*:431, 1968.

Pritchard, J. A., Scott, D. E., Whalley, P. J., et al.: The effects of maternal sickle hemoglobinopathies and sickle cell trait on reproductive performance. Am. J. Obstet. Gynecol. *117*:662, 1973.

Reeves, D. S., and Brumfitt, W.: Localization of urinary tract infection. A comparative study of methods. *In* O'Grady, F., and Brumfitt, W. (Eds.): Urinary Tract Infection. London, Oxford University Press, 1968, pp. 53–67.

Ronald, A. R., Boutros, P., and Mourtada, H.: Bacteriuria localization and response to single-dose therapy in women. J.A.M.A. *235*:1854, 1976.

Sanford, J. P., Favour, C. B., Mao, F. H., et al.: Evaluation of the "positive" urine culture. An approach to the differentiation of significant bacteria from contaminants. Am. J. Med. *20*:88, 1956.

Sanford, J. P.: Urinary tract symptoms and infections in the adult. Medical Grand Rounds. Parkland Memorial Hospital, Dec. 20, 1973.

Sever, J. L., Ellenberg, J. H., and Edmonds, D.: Urinary tract infections during pregnancy: maternal and pediatric findings. *In* Kass, E. H., and Brumfitt, W. (Eds.): Infections of the Urinary Tract. Chicago, University of Chicago Press, 1979, 12–21.

Sleigh, J. D., Robertson, J. G., and Isdale, M. H.: Asymptomatic bacteriuria in pregnancy. J. Obstet. Gynaecol. Br. Commonw. *71*:74, 1964.

Stamey, T. A., Govan, D. E., and Palmer, J. M.: The localization and treatment of urinary tract infections: The role of bactericidal urine levels as opposed to serum levels. Medicine *44*:1, 1965.

Stanley, J. C., and Muldowney, F. P.: A follow-up study of recurrent urinary tract infection in pregnancy. J. Ir. Med. Assoc. *67*:74, 1974.

Thomas, V., Shelokov, A., and Forland, M.: Antibody-coated bacteria in the urine and the site of urinary tract infection. N. Eng. J. Med. *290*:588, 1974.

Thomas, V. L., Harris, R. E., Gilstrap, L. C., et al.: Antibody-coated bacteria in the urine of obstetrical patients with acute pyelonephritis. J. Infect. Dis. *131* (Suppl.):57, 1975.

Turck, M., Goffe, B. S., and Petersdorf, R. G.: Bacteriuria of pregnancy. Relation to socioeconomic factors. N. Engl. J. Med. *266*:857, 1962.

Waters, W. E.: Prevalence of symptoms of urinary tract infection in women. Br. J. Prev. Soc. Med. *23*:263, 1969.

Whalley, P. J., *in* Kass, E. H. (Ed.): Progress in Pyelonephritis. Philadelphia, F. A. Davis Co., 1965, p. 50.

Whalley, P. J., Martin, F. G., and Peters, P. C.: Significance of asymptomatic bacteriuria detected during pregnancy. J.A.M.A. *193*:879, 1965.

Whalley, P. J.: Bacteriuria of pregnancy. Am. J. Obstet. Gynecol. *97*:723, 1967.

Whalley, P. J., and Cunningham, F. G.: Short-term versus continuous antimicrobial therapy for asymptomatic bacteriuria in pregnancy. Obstet. Gynecol. *49*:262, 1977.

Williams, J. D., Brumfitt, W., Leigh, D., et al.: Eradication of bacteriuria in pregnancy by a short course of chemotherapy. Lancet *1*:831, 1965.

Williams, J. D., Reeves, D. S., Condie, A. P., et al.: The treatment of bacteriuria in pregnancy. *In* O'Grady, F., and Brumfitt, W. (Eds.): Urinary Tract Infections. London, Oxford University Press, 1968, pp. 160–169.

Williams, J. D., Brumfitt, W., Condie, A. P., et al.: The treatment of bacteriuria in pregnant women with sulphamethoxazole and trimethoprim. Postgrad. Med. J. *45* (Suppl.):71, 1969.

Zinner, S. H., and Kass, E. H.: Long-term (10 to 14 years) follow-up of bacteriuria of pregnancy. N. Engl. J. Med. *285*:820, 1971.

Zinner, S. H.: Bacteriuria and babies revisited. N. Engl. J. Med. *300*:853, 1979.

36

SYMPTOMATIC URINARY TRACT INFECTION DURING PREGNANCY

LARRY C. GILSTRAP, III, M.D.

INTRODUCTION

Symptomatic urinary tract infections occur commonly during pregnancy. There are several features of pregnancy that predispose to the development of acute symptomatic urinary tract infection, paramount among which is the presence of asymptomatic bacteriuria, occurring in 2 to 10 per cent of pregnancies (Whalley, 1967) (see Chapter 35). Moreover, Whalley (1967) has reported that when bacteriuria is present, it is invariably present at the first prenatal visit. It has been well documented that if untreated, 25 per cent of women with bacteriuria will develop symptomatic urinary tract infection (Pritchard and MacDonald, 1980). However, as Cunningham and Whalley have pointed out in Chapter 35, not all patients who develop symptomatic urinary tract infections have preexisting bacteriuria at their first prenatal visit, and thus symptomatic infection cannot be completely prevented by an initial screening culture. In this latter circumstance, the medical history may be useful in deciding who is at significant risk for developing symptomatic urinary tract infection. For example, Gilstrap and co-workers (1981*a*) reported that approximately one third of women with acute pyelonephritis during pregnancy had a history of prior documented pyelonephritis. Thus, patients with a past history of frequent urinary tract infections or known urinary tract anomalies should be screened more often during gestation for the presence of infection.

Other factors associated with the development of acute urinary tract infection during pregnancy include obstruction and stasis. Obstruction may be secondary to hormonal and mechanical changes. Obstruction, in turn, causes stasis, which, in the presence of significant bacteriuria, may lead to acute, symptomatic urinary tract infection.

Symptomatic urinary tract infection may either involve the upper urinary tract — i.e., acute pyelonephritis — and produce systemic symptoms, or be restricted to the lower urinary tract as acute cystitis. Although much has been written concerning the association of asymptomatic bacteriuria and acute pyelonephritis and pregnancy, little has been written concerning acute cystitis during pregnancy. Acute cystitis is frequently mentioned only briefly or is not included at all in discussions of symptomatic urinary tract infections during pregnancy. However, these two entities are distinct clinical syndromes, and although cystitis may lead to pyelonephritis if untreated, maternal morbidity and risk are much less when infection is confined to the lower tract without systemic symptoms. Cunningham and associates (1973) reported that upper urinary tract involvement (acute pyelonephritis) may cause significant maternal morbidity: 3 per cent of their patients developed septic shock. In contrast, Harris and Gilstrap (1981) found no significant maternal morbidity in 126 pregnant patients with acute cystitis.

Although Kass (1973) pointed out that

there is no standardized definition of symptomatic urinary tract infection and that the diagnosis is often subjective, in this chapter an attempt is made to define and describe the two clinical and bacteriologic entities of cystitis and pyelonephritis and their association with pregnancy.

ACUTE CYSTITIS

Although the literature is replete with articles concerning asymptomatic bacteriuria and acute pyelonephritis during pregnancy, there is a paucity of information concerning the association of acute cystitis and pregnancy.

Incidence

Over a 6-year period at our institution, we found 126 women with acute cystitis following 9734 deliveries, for an incidence of 1.3 per cent (Harris and Gilstrap, 1981). This is similar to the incidence of acute pyelonephritis we found during pregnancy (Table 36–1). This incidence of cystitis has remained relatively constant over the 6-year study period.

Two thirds of patients with acute cystitis had negative initial screening cultures. In comparison, it has been reported that one third of patients with acute pyelonephritis do not have bacteriuria early in pregnancy (Whalley, 1967). Again, it must be emphasized that a negative screening urine culture does not preclude the subsequent development of symptomatic urinary tract infection, either cystitis or pyelonephritis.

TABLE 36–1. INCIDENCE OF URINARY TRACT INFECTIONS OVER A SIX-YEAR PERIOD

	Per Cent
Acute cystitis	1.3
Acute pyelonephritis	1.0
Asymptomatic bacteriuria	5.1

Reprinted with permission from the American College of Obstetricians and Gynecologists (Obstet. Gynecol. *57*:579, 1981).

Signs and Symptoms

Patients with acute cystitis during pregnancy present with essentially the same signs and symptoms as nonpregnant patients with cystitis. However, the diagnosis of cystitis is more difficult during pregnancy. Most pregnant women have urinary urgency and frequency, and many experience suprapubic discomfort and pressure, especially in late gestation, from compression of the bladder by the fetal head. Moreover, pregnant patients may complain of difficulty in urinating during the first trimester if the uterus is retroverted and incarcerated in the pelvis. Patients may also complain of "painful urination" if significant vulvovaginitis is present, especially if the urine comes in contact with irritated, cracked skin. For these reasons, the diagnosis of cystitis during pregnancy is based on the presence of significant dysuria or gross hematuria, a positive urine culture, and the absence of systemic symptoms, such as fever or chills. Signs of upper urinary tract involvement, such as costovertebral angle (CVA) tenderness and pain, are absent. Nausea and vomiting are common symptoms of early gestation and are of little help in distinguishing upper from lower tract involvement.

Laboratory

In women with cystitis, the urinalysis generally shows both leukocytes and erythrocytes. These findings may also be present in women with acute pyelonephritis; more importantly, leukocyturia is present in up to 30 per cent of normal pregnant women.

The urine culture is the confirmatory laboratory test and is invariably positive. *Escherichia coli* is the most common microorganism isolated and is recovered in 71 per cent of patients with acute cystitis, followed by Proteus (8 per cent), Klebsiella (8 per cent), Streptococcus (8 per cent) and Staphylococcus (5 per cent).

Harris and Gilstrap (1981), utilizing the antibody-coated bacteria test, found that 94 per cent of the patients with acute cystitis had infection limited to the bladder, compared to almost half of the patients with asymptomatic bacteriuria and almost two thirds of the patients with acute pyelonephritis. Although of academic interest, localization techniques provide little clinically useful information.

Treatment and Follow-up

Pregnant patients with acute cystitis can usually be treated with oral medication as outpatients. Any one of several antibiotics can be used, including nitrofurantoin macrocrystals (50 to 100 mg. q.i.d.), ampicillin (250 to 500 mg. q.i.d.), sulfamethoxazole (500 mg. b.i.d.), or one of the cephalosporins (250 mg. q.i.d.). The usual duration of therapy is 10 to 14 days. Clinical response to treatment is dramatic, and the patients are usually asymptomatic within 48 hours. Tetracyclines are not used during the last half of pregnancy because of the potential for discoloration of fetal deciduous teeth. Other potential side effects of treatment include hyperbilirubinemia in the newborn secondary to sulfamethoxazole and hemolytic anemia in women with glucose-6-phosphate dehydrogenase deficiency given nitrofurantoin macrocrystals.

Harris and Gilstrap (1981) reported that 17 per cent of their patients with acute cystitis had a subsequent positive urine culture during the pregnancy and half had a history of urinary tract infection. The majority of these recurrences were asymptomatic infections.

There are no long-term follow-up studies of women with acute cystitis during pregnancy, although one would predict that future infection would probably be common.

Adverse Effects

There were no cases of subsequent acute pyelonephritis in the cystitis series reported by Harris and Gilstrap (1981). However, the absence of acute pyelonephritis was probably related to prompt treatment after symptoms and frequent follow-up. In that population, consisting of military dependents, patients present soon after symptoms appear, and the majority return for scheduled follow-up visits.

In summary, symptomatic lower urinary tract infection, or acute cystitis, occurs in approximately 1 per cent of pregnancies and is characterized by urgency, frequency, and dysuria in the absence of signs of systemic involvement. The most common bacterial isolate is *Escherichia coli*. Patients can usually be treated as outpatients, and clinical response is rapid. Subsequent upper urinary tract involvement is rare if treatment is initiated early. Moreover, there is no evidence of an increased risk of adverse effects on pregnancy in these patients.

ACUTE PYELONEPHRITIS

Acute pyelonephritis is the most common of the serious medical complications of pregnancy and may result in serious maternal morbidity. In the preantibiotic era acute pyelonephritis was a cause of maternal death (Dodds, 1932). However, with early antibiotic treatment, it has become a rare cause of maternal mortality.

Incidence

With the widespread acceptance of screening for asymptomatic bacteriuria, the reported incidence of acute pyelonephritis has decreased over the last 20 years. Harris (1979) reported a decrease from 4 per cent to a low of only 0.8 per cent over a 20-year period, which he attributed to the identification and eradication of bacteriuria and frequent antepartum follow-up.

The majority of cases of acute pyelonephritis occur in the last two trimesters of pregnancy (Cunningham et al., 1973; Harris and Gilstrap, 1974). Gilstrap and coworkers (1981*a*) in a review of 656 obstetric patients with acute pyelonephritis, found that 75 per cent of cases occurred during the antepartum period, 19 per cent during the postpartum period, and 8 per cent during the intrapartum period. Moreover, of the 482 cases of antepartum pyelonephritis, 9 per cent occurred during the first trimester, with the remainder almost evenly divided between second and third trimesters (Table 36–2). The higher incidence of acute pyelonephritis in the last two trimesters is no doubt related to increasing obstruction of the urinary tract, with resulting stasis as pregnancy progresses. Moreover, acute pyelonephritis in early pregnancy may be un-

TABLE 36–2. INCIDENCE OF ACUTE PYELONEPHRITIS BY TRIMESTER

Author	Number of Patients	Trimester		
		First	*Second*	*Third*
Cunningham et al. (1973)	99	4%	46%	50%
Harris and Gilstrap (1974)	97	11%	56%	33%
Gilstrap et al. (1981*a*)	482	9%	46%	45%
Total	678	8%	48%	44%

derreported in studies of pyelonephritis due to early pregnancy losses (i.e., early spontaneous abortion).

Signs and Symptoms

In general, the history and physical findings of the pregnant patient with acute pyelonephritis are similar to those found in the nonpregnant patient. However, occasionally acute pyelonephritis may be confused with other acute complications of pregnancy, such as appendicitis, placental abruption, renal calculi, and premature labor. Moreover, renal calculi may present with acute pyelonephritis (Chapter 38).

The most common symptoms include fever, chills, nausea and vomiting, and flank pain. Patients may also complain of lower tract symptoms, such as urgency, frequency, and dysuria. In the series of Gilstrap and co-workers (1981*a*), 82 per cent of the patients had flank pain and chills at presentation, 40 per cent had lower tract symptoms, and about 25 per cent had nausea and vomiting. These findings are similar to those reported by Harris and Gilstrap (1974).

The two most common physical findings are fever and costovertebral angle (CVA) tenderness. The temperature is commonly 101° F. or greater, and the CVA pain occurs predominantly on the right side, although it may occur on either or both sides. In the series by Cunningham and associates (1973), two thirds of the patients had a temperature of 102° F. or greater. Gilstrap and coworkers (1981*a*) found a temperature of 101° F. or greater in 84 per cent of their patients and 104° F. or greater in 12 per cent (one patient had a temperature of 107° F.).

Laboratory Findings

The urine culture is invariably positive for bacterial growth and confirms the clinical diagnosis. However, the culture may be negative if the patient has started taking antibiotics prior to the collection of the culture specimen. It is not uncommon for patients who have had urinary tract infections in the past to take left-over medications when they think they have a recurrent infection. As with asymptomatic bacteriuria and cystitis, *Escherichia coli* is the most common microorganism isolated by urine culture, accounting for approximately 70 per cent of all isolates in several series. Organisms of the Klebsiella-Enterobacter group are the second most common isolates (Table 36–3).

Examination of the urinary sediment almost always reveals many leukocytes and

TABLE 36–3. BACTERIOLOGY OF ACUTE PYELONEPHRITIS

Author	Microorganism		
	Escherichia coli	*Klebsiella-Enterobacter*	*Other*
Hibbard et al. (1967)	69%	12%	19%
Cunningham et al. (1972)	70%	20%	10%
Harris and Gilstrap (1974)	73%	15%	12%
Gilstrap et al. (1981*a*)	72%	23%	5%
Total	72%	22%	6%

bacteria. The identification of bacteria on a slide of a drop of unspun urine correlates with a positive culture. Clumps of leukocytes and characteristic white cell casts may also be seen.

Another important laboratory test is measurement of the serum creatinine or creatinine clearance, as a significant number of pregnant women with acute pyelonephritis will have an elevated serum creatinine or a marked decrease in creatinine clearance. Whalley and colleagues (1974) reported that 25 per cent of their group of pregnant patients with acute pyelonephritis developed a transient decrease in glomerular filtration rate as measured by the endogenous creatinine clearance test. Although the exact pathogenesis of this renal dysfunction remains unclear, the authors postulated that nephrotoxicity secondary to an endotoxin from gram-negative organisms might be responsible. This decrease in glomerular filtration rate is only transient and the rate returns to near normal levels 3 to 8 weeks post therapy. Regardless of the pathogenesis of the transient renal dysfunction, it is important to recognize the possibility of decreased glomerular filtration when choosing antimicrobial therapy. Whalley and co-workers (1964, 1970) have reported that tetracycline may cause pancreatitis, azotemia, and acute liver damage in women with acute pyelonephritis and impaired renal function and suggested this drug not be used.

Frequently there is a leukocytosis with a shift to the left. However, evaluation of the hematocrit may be of more interest. Brumfitt (1975) as well as Gilstrap and associates (1981*b*) has reported an increase in frequency of anemia in pregnant patients with acute pyelonephritis.

Adverse Pregnancy Effects

Cunningham and co-workers (1973) have pointed out that acute pyelonephritis may result in dehydration and maternal septic shock. Other adverse effects reported to be associated with symptomatic urinary tract infection include anemia, hypertension, and low birth weight in infants. For example, Sever and colleagues (1975) found a significantly higher incidence of both anemia and hypertension in 1906 pregnant women with symptomatic urinary tract infection than in noninfected controls. As mentioned previously, Brumfitt (1975) also found a high incidence of anemia in pregnant patients with pyelonephritis. In addition, Gilstrap and associates (1981*b*) found a significantly lower mean predelivery hematocrit in 435 pregnant women with acute pyelonephritis when compared with controls.

The association of symptomatic urinary tract infection with maternal hypertension is less clear. Although Sever and colleagues (1975) did report such an association, Gilstrap and co-workers (1981*b*) were unable to demonstrate an association of acute pyelonephritis and the development of hypertension in either the primigravida or multigravida. Hypertension was actually higher in controls than patients. This was similar to the findings reported by Hibbard and others (1967).

A higher incidence of low birth weight in infants has been reported to be associated with urinary tract infections; however, most of these reports dealt with asymptomatic bacteriuria. Exceptions to this are the studies of Hibbard and co-workers (1967) and Sever and colleagues (1975), who reported a higher incidence of low birth weight in infants born to mothers with symptomatic urinary tract infections. In contrast, Gilstrap and associates (1981*b*) found no increase in the incidence of low birth weight in infants in 435 patients with acute pyelonephritis compared with noninfected controls. Likewise, Wilson and collaborators (1966) were unable to demonstrate a significant increase in the incidence of low birth weight in infants born to 85 women with symptomatic urinary tract infection.

Treatment

Pregnant women with acute pyelonephritis should be hospitalized for close observation. These women frequently have severe nausea, vomiting, and anorexia combined with pyrexia, which leads to significant dehydration. As many as 10 per cent of these patients have septicemia and some develop septic shock. Therapy includes vigorous rehydration with intravenous crystalloids and appropriate antimicrobials.

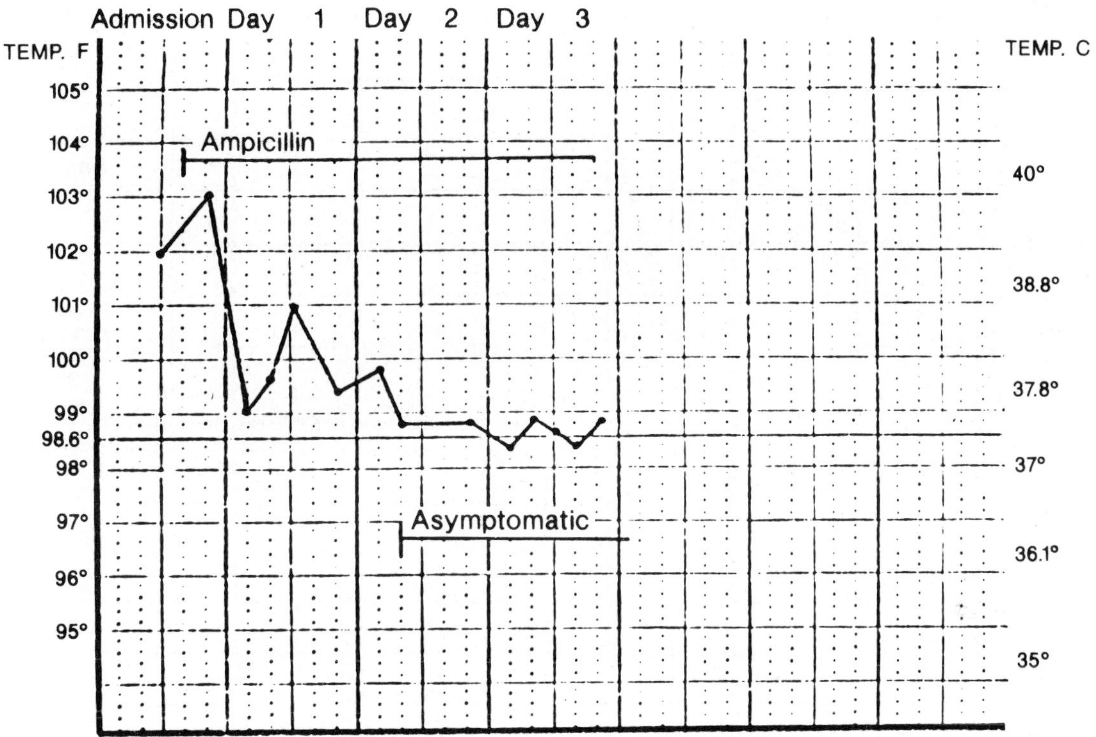

Figure 36–1. Patient with acute pyelonephritis and positive culture for *Escherichia coli.* She was afebrile and asymptomatic within 48 hours.

Patients should be given from 1 to 3 liters of intravenous fluids in order to establish a diuresis of 30 to 60 ml. of urine per hour.

There are a number of suitable antimicrobials available for treatment, and although a urine specimen should be taken for isolation and bacterial sensitivity studies prior to initiation of treatment, the initial selection of antibiotics is usually empiric. Since more than 90 per cent of women with acute pyelonephritis have infection due to the Enterobacteriaceae, especially *Escherichia coli*, initial therapy should consist of either ampicillin or a cephalosporin in doses of 2 to 4 gm. per day. In patients with a documented allergy to penicillin, an aminoglycoside can be used; in these patients it is important to evaluate the status of renal function because of the potential nephrotoxicity of these drugs. The majority of patients with acute pyelonephritis demonstrate a rapid clinical response. The clinical response of a patient with acute pyelonephritis secondary to infection with penicillin-sensitive *Escherichia coli* is summarized in Figure 36–1. Cunningham and associates (1973) reported that 85 per cent of patients with acute pyelonephritis were afebrile and essentially asymptomatic by 48 hours after initiation of therapy. Ninety-five per cent of the patients were afebrile by 72 hours, and only 5 per cent were febrile for longer than 72 hours.

It may be necessary to add one of the aminoglycosides to either ampicillin or the cephalosporin. Guidelines for either the addition of or the primary therapy with an aminoglycoside include the following: (1) a positive urine culture 24 hours following initiation of antibiotics, (2) poor clinical response after 48 hours of therapy, (3) evidence of sepsis, (4) previous screening culture showing resistance to penicillin or cephalosporins, and (5) recurrent disease. An example of a situation in which the patient requires the addition of an aminoglycoside is shown in Figure 36–2. When drugs that are potentially nephrotoxic are used — e.g., aminoglycosides — impaired renal function should be ruled out. A single film intravenous pyelogram (IVP) should be considered for patients who remain febrile

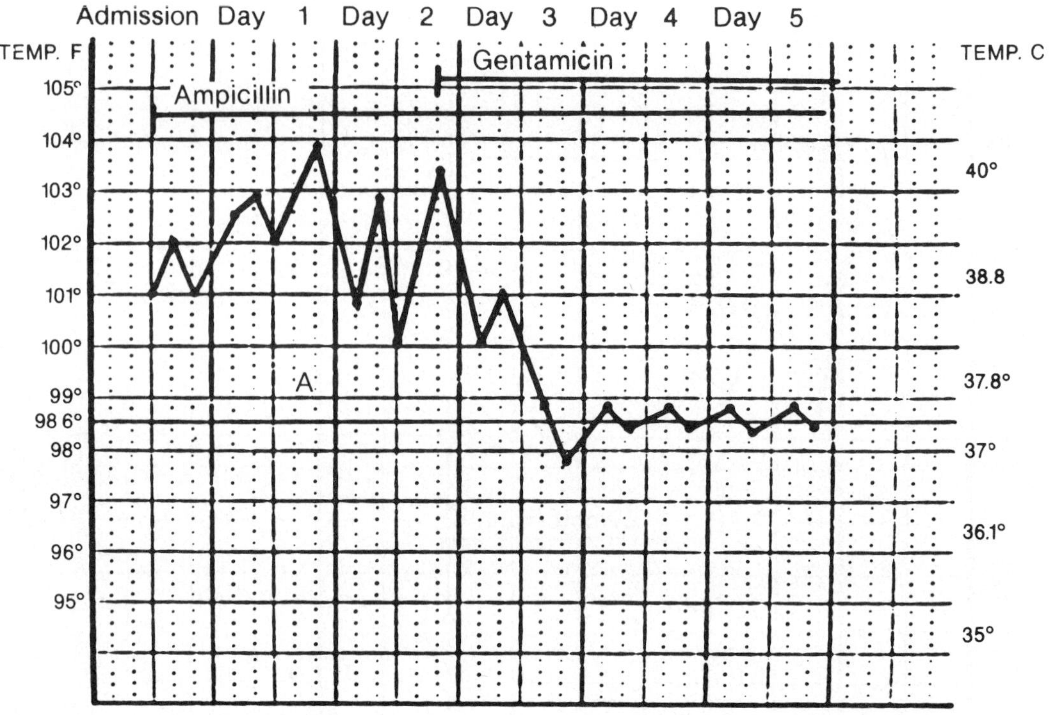

Figure 36–2. Patient with acute pyelonephritis and a positive urine and blood culture for *Escherichia coli* subsequently shown to be resistant to ampicillin. Culture taken at point A was positive for growth at 12 hours.

for 96 hours or longer, especially if the infecting organism is sensitive to the antibiotic(s) being used. An IVP might also be helpful in the patient who has multiple relapses of acute pyelonephritis in a short period of time.

Administration of antibiotics is usually changed to the oral route when the patient has been afebrile for 24 hours and is tolerating a diet. Antibiotics are continued to complete a 10 to 14 day course of therapy.

Recurrent acute renal infection is common. Gilstrap and co-workers (1981*a*) reported a recurrence rate of 23 per cent, half occurring during the antepartum period and half during the postpartum period. In an earlier report, Harris and Gilstrap (1974) reported an overall incidence of recurrence of 18.5 per cent. In general, the same organisms that caused the initial episode of pyelonephritis are involved in subsequent infections. Thus, it is often helpful to review the culture and sensitivity report of the initial infection when deciding on antimicrobial therapy.

In addition, Harris and Gilstrap found that if patients with acute pyelonephritis were treated with suppressive antibiotic therapy for the remainder of pregnancy, the recurrence rate was only 2.7 per cent, compared with 60 per cent in the nonsuppressed patients. Although Cunningham and associates (1973) did not find such a high incidence of recurrent pyelonephritis, they did find that 30 per cent of the patients had a subsequent positive urine culture. From these data, it becomes apparent that if the pregnant patient is not maintained on antibiotic suppression, she is at significant risk of developing recurrent infection, either asymptomatic bacteriuria or acute pyelonephritis. She needs to be seen frequently and monitored with urine cultures. If bacterial surveillance is not feasible, patients with acute pyelonephritis should be given suppressive therapy for the remainder of pregnancy. Several different antibiotics can be used for chronic urinary suppression, such as ampicillin, sulfamethoxazole, nitrofurantoin macrocrystals, or a cephalosporin. An effective, relatively inexpensive regimen for chronic suppression is nitrofurantoin macrocrystals (Macrodantin), 50 to 100 mg.

once a day at bedtime. This regimen also has good patient acceptance and compliance.

Long-Term Prognosis

Much has been written about urinary tract infections and the high incidence of both radiographic urinary tract abnormalities and subsequent urinary tract infections when patients are studied at a remote time from the initial infection. Whalley (1967) reported that 30 to 40 per cent of women with infection during pregnancy had radiologic evidence of renal disease. Likewise, Zinner and Kass (1971) found renal anomalies in a significant number of patients who had bacteriuria in pregnancy when followed 10 to 14 years later, and many had persistent bacteriuria. Parker and Kunin (1973) reported similar findings in women with acute pyelonephritis when followed for 10 to 20 years.

Gilstrap and associates (1981*a*) reported that 38 per cent of the women with subsequent pregnancies had at least one other episode of urinary tract infection in pregnancy. Moreover, during an 8- to 13-year follow up, 42 per cent of the patients who had been seen at least once (nonpregnant) were treated for symptomatic urinary tract infection.

Several authors have alluded to the possibility of long-term morbidity, such as chronic renal disease following acute renal infection. However, although patients who have acute pyelonephritis during pregnancy do have a high incidence of radiographic renal abnormalities and a high rate of recurrent urinary tract infection (Gilstrap et al., 1981*a*), there are few data to suggest that either acute pyelonephritis or bacteriuria alone leads to end-stage renal disease. Zinner and Kass (1971) found little, if any, progression of bacteriuria during pregnancy to end-stage renal disease in a 10- to 14-year follow-up study. Moreover, data presented by Freedman (1967) as well as Farmer and Heptinstall (1970) indicate that acute pyelonephritis very rarely is associated with end-stage renal disease.

In summary, acute pyelonephritis in pregnancy is a common medical problem that may result in significant maternal morbidity. Patients should be hospitalized and treated with intravenous fluids and antibiotics. Clinical response is usually rapid; recurrent urinary tract infection is common. With the exception of lower mean hematocrits and possibly overt anemia, the association of acute pyelonephritis and other complications of pregnancy, such as low birth weight in infants and maternal hypertension, remains controversial.

REFERENCES

Brumfitt, W.: The effects of bacteriuria in pregnancy on maternal and fetal health. Kidney Int. *8* (Suppl.):113–119, 1975.

Cunningham, F. G., Morris, G. B., and Mickal, A.: Acute pyelonephritis of pregnancy: A clinical review. Obstet. Gynecol. *42*:112–117, 1973.

Dodds, G. B.: The immediate and remote prognosis of pyelonephritis. J. Obstet. Gynaecol. Br. Emp. *39*:46–59, 1932.

Farmer, K. K., and Heptinstall, R. H.: Chronic non-obstructive pyelonephritis, a reappraisal. *In* Kincaid-Smith, P., and Fairley, K. F. (Eds.): Renal Infection and Renal Scarring. Melbourne, Australia, Mercedes, 1970, p. 233.

Freedman, L. R.: Chronic pyelonephritis at autopsy. Ann. Intern. Med. *66*:697–710, 1967.

Gilstrap, L. C., Cunningham, F. G., and Whalley, P. J.: Acute pyelonephritis in pregnancy. I. An anterospective study of 656 women. Obstet. Gynecol. *57*:409, 1981*a*.

Gilstrap, L. C., Leveno, K. J., Cunningham, F. G., Whalley, P. J., and Roark, M. L.: Renal infection and pregnancy outcome. Am. J. Obstet. Gynecol., *141*:709, 1981*b*.

Harris, R. E.: The significance of eradication of bacteriuria during pregnancy. Obstet. Gynecol. *53*:71–73, 1979.

Harris, R. E., and Gilstrap, L. C.: Prevention of recurrent pyelonephritis during pregnancy. Obstet. Gynecol. *44*:637–641, 1974.

Harris, R. E., and Gilstrap, L. C.: Cystitis during pregnancy: A distinct clinical entity. Obstet. Gynecol. *57*:579, 1981.

Hibbard, L., Thrupp, L., Summeril, S., et al.: Treatment of pyelonephritis in pregnancy. Am. J. Obstet. Gynecol. *98*:609–615, 1967.

Kass, E. H.: The role of unsuspected infection in the etiology of prematurity. Clin. Obstet. Gynecol., *16*:134–152, 1973.

Parker, J., and Kunin, C.: Pyelonephritis in young women (a 10 to 20 year follow-up). J.A.M.A. *224*:585–590, 1973.

Pritchard, J. A., and MacDonald, P. C.: Medical and surgical illnesses during pregnancy and the puerperium. *In* Williams Obstetric. 16th Ed. New York, Appleton-Century-Crofts, 1980, pp. 701–707.

Sever, J. L., Ellenberg, J. H., and Edmonds, D.: Urinary tract infections during pregnancy: Maternal and pediatric findings. *In* Kass E. H., and Brumfitt, W. (Eds.): Infections of the Urinary Tract. Chicago, University of Chicago Press, 1975, pp. 19–21.

Whalley, P. J.: Bacteriuria of pregnancy. Am. J. Obstet. Gynecol. *97*:723–738, 1967.

Whalley, P. J., Adams, R. H., and Combes, B.: Tetracycline toxicity in pregnancy. J.A.M.A. *189*:357–360, 1964.

Whalley, P. J., Cunningham, F. G., and Martin, F. G.: Transient renal dysfunction associated with acute pyelonephritis of pregnancy. Obstet. Gynecol. *46*:174–177, 1974.

Whalley, P. J., Pritchard, J. A., Martin, F. B., et al.: Disposition of tetracycline by pregnant women with acute pyelonephritis. Obstet. Gynecol. *36*:821, 1970.

Wilson, M. G., Hewitt, W. D., and Monzon, O. T.: Effect of bacteriuria on the fetus. N. Engl. J. Med. *274*:1115–1118, 1966.

Zinner, S. H., and Kass, E. H.: Long-term (10 to 14 years) follow-up of bacteriuria of pregnancy. N. Engl. J. Med. *285*:820–824, 1971.

37

GYNECOLOGIC AND OBSTETRIC PROBLEMS IN RENAL ALLOGRAFT RECIPIENTS

J. R. SCOTT, M.D.

The first successful blood transfusion, a tissue graft in every sense of the term, was administered by an obstetrician to his postpartum patient who was bleeding. The first clinical attempt at human renal transplantation was in a young woman who, while pregnant, had developed an intrauterine infection followed by shock and anuria (Scott and Beer, 1974). Obstetricians and gynecologists were minimally involved with organ transplantation until the past decade, when a tremendous upsurge of interest in maternal-fetal immunology developed. More physicians are now being confronted with disorders encountered in allograft recipients, since over 50,000 kidney transplants have been performed and the number is rapidly increasing. By 1984, more than 55,000 patients in the United States alone will be on dialysis treatment for chronic renal failure or end-stage renal disease (ESRD), with over 5200 likely to receive transplants. This chapter is aimed at establishing practical guidelines for the clinician. It is based on a review of the literature as well as experience in the management of over 200 women at the University of Iowa and the University of Utah Medical Center who have received renal allografts during the past 10 years.

GYNECOLOGIC PROBLEMS

Disorders involving the reproductive tract in nonpregnant transplant patients, although more frequent, have not attracted the same publicity nor received the same emphasis in the literature as have the pregnancies in these women. With the standard technique for renal transplantation (Figure 37–1), the kidney is placed in the iliac fossa just outside the true pelvis and the renal artery is anastomosed to the hypogastric, common, or external iliac artery. The graft is easily palpable abdominally and on bimanual pelvic examination. Because of its location it can sometimes interfere with an optimum pelvic examination, and symptoms secondary to pelvic disease can be mistakenly attributed to the kidney. Female renal allograft recipients may have any gynecologic disease that afflicts the general population, but a number of problems are specifically related to the immunosuppressive drugs they are receiving (Table 37–1). The physician caring for these patients is therefore wise to review the side effects of the drugs to determine whether they can account for the symptoms the patient is experiencing or whether they will affect the management plan.

Psychosexual Problems

Sexual dysfunction is among the many problems created by chronic renal disease. Young women often find that male companions and fiancés are apprehensive about the seriousness of their disorder and question the potential for a successful and happy

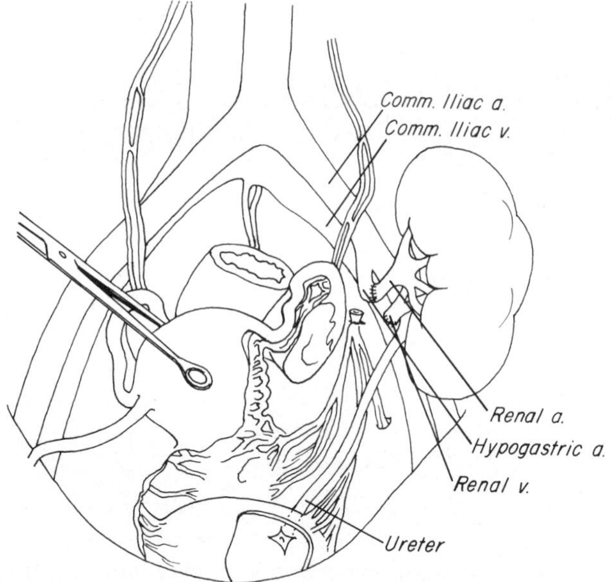

Figure 37–1. The usual technique of renal transplantation. The renal artery is anastomosed to the hypogastric artery, and all branches of the iliac vein are ligated and tied. The periurethral tissue is left intact, and the ureter is placed into the bladder through a tunnel.

marriage. It cannot be denied that a chronic disease such as this places increased demands on the husband, and these couples deserve support and sympathetic counseling. The psychologic aspects of the home environment and individual response to illness are important in evaluating and treating marital problems that sometimes arise.

TABLE 37–1. PROPERTIES OF IMMUNOSUPPRESSIVE AGENTS COMMONLY USED IN RENAL TRANSPLANTATION

Agent/Class	Principal Action	Maintenance Dose/Day	Hazards* I. Immunosuppression	II. Other Activities	III. Idiosyncrasy Hypersensitivity
Prednisone Corticosteroid	Anti-inflammatory	5–25 mg.	Infection Neoplasia(?)	Fluid and electrolyte disturbances, myopathy, osteoporosis, peptic ulcer, impaired wound healing, carbohydrate intolerance, cataracts, glaucoma, negative nitrogen balance	Pancreatitis
Azathioprine (Imuran) Purine antimetabolite	↓ Primary immune response	75–150 mg.	Infection Neoplasia	Bone marrow depression, mutagenesis, anorexia	Drug fever, rash, myopathy, arthralgia, pancreatitis, hepatic cholestasis or fibrosis
Cyclophosphamide (Cytoxan) Alkylating agent	↓ Ongoing immune responses	50–150 mg.	Infection Neoplasia	Bone marrow depression, mutagenesis, teratogenesis, hemorrhagic cystitis, gonadal suppression, alopecia, anorexia	Inappropriate ADH secretion
Antilymphocyte globulin Immune serum	↓ Lymphocytes	2.5 mg./kg.	Infection Neoplasia	Reversed anaphylaxis, thrombocytopenia	Serum sickness, fever, anaphylaxis

*Three major categories of unwanted side-effects are: I, those resulting from immunosuppression per se; II, those arising from unexpected biologic activities related to immunosuppression; and III, those unrelated to the agent's prime biologic effect and due either to its contamination with other materials, to biologic activities other than the prime one, or to an idiosyncratic or hypersensitivity response on the part of the drug's recipient.
(Modified from Weinberg, 1974.)

Diminished libido is most often associated with the general malaise and debilitation before and during hemodialysis. This usually improves following transplantation provided that general health and renal function are satisfactory. In fact, persistent decreased libido is sometimes a symptom of depression that may be caused or aggravated by corticosteroids, or it may be a side effect of antihypertensive medications such as methyldopa (Aldomet). The pelvic location of the kidney does not ordinarily cause pain or any particular difficulty with intercourse. Excluding psychologic reasons, the occasional case of dyspareunia is usually due to candidal or atrophic vaginitis, which disappears with appropriate treatment.

Menstrual Disorders

During Hemodialysis

Menstrual abnormalities are a frequent concomitant of chronic renal disease, and amenorrhea is usual when the serum creatinine level rises to between 5 and 10 mg./deciliter (dl.). Anovulation and amenorrhea persist during hemodialysis treatment, and the most common serum gonadotropin pattern is a normal concentration of follicle-stimulating hormone (FSH) and a moderately elevated level of luteinizing hormone (LH) similar to the tonic LH profile characteristic of females with polycystic ovary syndrome (Strickler et al., 1974). However, mean basal FSH and FSH response to LRH is normal. In hemodialysis patients serum 17-β-estradiol, progesterone, and testosterone levels are low, but following transplantation only testosterone levels remain reduced (Morley et al., 1979). Of those women on long-term hemodialysis not receiving prolactin-enhancing drugs, 73 per cent have consistently elevated basal prolactin (PRL) levels and all patients receiving α-methyldopa have marked prolactinemia (Gomez et al., 1980). Hyperprolactinemia is one of the major factors in hypogonadism of these patients. Therefore, treatment with dopamine agonists could potentially normalize PRL levels, resulting in relief of such symptoms as decreased libido and amenorrhea with subsequent psychologic benefits.

More of a clinical problem are those women who develop dysfunctional uterine bleeding, particularly hypermenorrhea (Rice, 1973). In addition to the anovulatory cycles, these patients receive heparin with each dialysis treatment and are often taking oral anticoagulants, which may contribute to the menometrorrhagia. Active therapy is necessary because dialysis patients are invariably anemic, with hematocrit levels in the range of 15 to 30 per cent. Since maintenance of reproductive function is not of primary concern, one of the regimens outlined in Table 37–2 can be used either to decrease the frequency and quantity of menstrual bleeding or to produce therapeutic amenorrhea.

Despite some apprehension about the use of oral contraceptives in this situation, there is no convincing evidence to date that these patients have increased cannula clotting or other thromboembolic episodes. Moreover, by suppressing pituitary gonadotropins, the oral contraceptive agents tend to prevent hemorrhagic functional ovarian cysts, a frequent and troublesome syndrome in women with irregular menstrual periods who take anticoagulants while undergoing intermittent dialysis (Thaysen et al., 1975). Rupture of a cyst can cause severe abdominal pain and intra-

TABLE 37–2. HORMONAL CONTROL OF DYSFUNCTIONAL UTERINE BLEEDING IN DIALYSIS OR RENAL TRANSPLANT PATIENTS

A. *To produce cyclic, lighter menses:*

Norethynodrel-mestranol (Enovid E, Enovid, Enovid-10) or norethindrone-mestranol (Ortho-Novum 1/35, 1/50, 1/80, 2 mg., 10 mg.). Combination pills are given for 21 days and stopped for 5 to 7 days in the lowest dose that controls the abnormal bleeding.

B. *To produce amenorrhea:*

Depo-medroxyprogesterone acetate (Depo-Provera), administered intramuscularly 150 mg. weekly for 4 weeks; 150 mg. every 2 weeks, for a total of 4 injections; then 150 mg. once every 3 to 4 weeks. Breakthrough bleeding is treated by increasing the frequency of injections and adding oral conjugated estrogen tablets (Premarin) 1.25 mg. daily for 1 week as necessary.

peritoneal bleeding, necessitating exploratory laparotomy and suture, or removal of the ovary.

Post Transplant

Following renal transplantation, menstruation appears between 1 and 14 months, with a mean of 4.2 months (Board et al., 1967, Abramovici et al., 1971). Recovery of ovulatory cycles and regular menses correlates very closely with the level of renal function and the frequency and severity of rejection episodes (Merkatz et al., 1971). With less successful grafts, more women continue to have absent or irregular menstrual periods.

Most renal allograft recipients receive corticosteroids, azathioprine, and, less often, antilymphocyte serum, none of which appreciably affects ovarian function. However, a few patients are immunosuppressed with cyclophosphamide, a drug known to produce gonadal suppression. This effect appears to be proportional to the dosage and duration of therapy. Persistent amenorrhea occurs in at least 50 per cent of women within 1 to 33 months after beginning the drug, and this is not always a reversible process (Warne et al., 1973). The majority of these amenorrheic women have hormonal patterns consistent with ovarian failure; ovarian biopsies often reveal a complete disappearance of ova. When this is the case, conventional oral estrogen replacement therapy is indicated to alleviate menopausal symptoms such as hot flashes and atrophic vaginitis.

Fertility Regulation

Contraception

Since the realization that libido improves and ovulatory cycles return soon after renal transplantation, adequate contraceptive advice is now reducing the number of unplanned pregnancies in these women. Although pregnancies have occasionally occurred in women receiving hemodialysis, the amenorrheic patient has little risk of pregnancy and can often be managed with contraceptive techniques least likely to be associated with health hazards, such as spermicidal vaginal foam or cream, condom, diaphragm, or a combination of these methods. However, oral contraceptives are more reliable in any patient who may be ovulating. It is advisable to start with a combination pill containing 50 micrograms or less of estrogen. The patient should be monitored closely for the development of thromboembolic problems, hypertension, or other serious side effects. The prevalence of menstrual disorders, as well as the susceptibility to serious infections associated with the immunosuppressive drugs, has in our opinion been a relative contraindication to the use of intrauterine devices (IUD). Nevertheless, when this is the only reasonable option, we have successfully used the IUD in many transplant patients with no apparent increase in infections or other complications.

Sterilization

In addition to contraception, sexually active female transplant recipients should be counseled regarding pregnancy and its hazards and offered permanent sterilization as an option, either at the time of transplantation or electively thereafter. Individualization based on the wishes of the patient and her husband is desirable, and in some cases the sterilization procedure may be better delayed, since decisions regarding future childbearing are often dependent on the success of the kidney graft. Although the grafted kidney is located extraperitoneally, it is easily palpable from the peritoneal cavity, projecting from the lateral pelvic wall, often surprisingly close to the adnexal structures on that side. Because of the danger of inadvertently puncturing the kidney by the laparoscopic method and the increased risk of infection by the vaginal route, tubal sterilization using a small midline lower abdominal incision is the recommended technique.

Pelvic Infections

Concern about potential genital tract infections is based on the knowledge that the normal flora of the vagina includes a number of organisms that have caused severe systemic infections in immunosuppressed patients. Generally these organisms are nonpathogenic and, when encountered by hosts with a normal immune surveillance system, are disposed of quite rapidly and cause no difficulties. However, opportunistic viral, bacterial, and fungal infections are quite frequent following renal transplantation and account for most of the deaths in these patients. Symptoms and signs may be obscured by the steroid therapy.

Treatment

Urinary infections are relatively common in renal allograft recipients and require meticulous management. Adequate therapy should include appropriate antibiotics and follow-up urine cultures. Fortunately, pelvic inflammatory disease seems to be very rare in these patients; no cases are reported in the literature. We have encountered one woman with unilateral salpingitis that responded to removal of her intrauterine device and treatment with antibiotics. The incidence of trichomonal and candidal vaginitis does not appear to be increased, and both can be managed satisfactorily with conventional therapy. However, viral infections such as herpes progenitalis and condylomata acuminata are more resistant to the usual methods of treatment and are troublesome to both patient and physician.

Gynecologic Neoplasms

Incidence

The incidence of cancer in renal transplant patients is approximately 100 times greater than that observed in the general population of the same age (Penn, 1975). The association with malignancies has been noted with all of the immunosuppressive agents, and at the present time it is not possible to offer any concrete explanation for the development of these neoplasms. The immunologic surveillance function of the lymphoreticular system may be impaired, allowing potentially malignant cellular mutations to become established as overt cancers. If this theory is correct, one would expect the distribution of tumors to be similar to that in the general population. However, it does not account for the prevalence of lymphomas and squamous cell carcinomas in these patients. Another possibility is that immunosuppressive therapy may activate oncogenic viruses. Herpesvirus infections are very common in organ transplant recipients and may be of particular relevance in view of current speculation concerning the role of Herpesvirus hominis 2 in the etiology of carcinoma of the cervix (Vestergaard et al., 1972).

It is not possible to determine accurately the incidence of gynecologic neoplasms in renal allograft recipients, but those reported are shown in Table 37–3. Nearly a 14-fold increase in the incidence of intraepithelial carcinoma of the cervix has been noted in renal transplant patients compared with an age-matched group in the general population (Porreco et al., 1975). The mean age of patients described in this report at the time of diagnosis was 36 years (range, 22 to 50 years), and the mean time interval from renal transplantation to diagnosis was 38 months (range, 6 to 97 months). In our experience the most common cervical lesion is dysplasia; therefore, it is mandatory that any woman requiring immunosuppressive agents be followed closely with pelvic examinations and cervical cytology studies at least at yearly intervals. Periodic colposcopic examinations have also been recommended (Donohue, 1974). Although this is an excellent method of evaluating cervical abnormalities, it should not be

TABLE 37–3. GYNECOLOGIC NEOPLASMS REPORTED IN RENAL ALLOGRAFT RECIPIENTS

Location	Type	Number
Vulva	Carcinoma in situ	1
Vagina	Carcinoma in situ	2
	Reticulum cell carcinoma	1
Cervix	Carcinoma in situ	32
	Invasive epidermoid	3
Fallopian tube	Adenomatoid	1
Uterus	Adenocarcinoma	3
Ovary	Dysgerminoma	1
Total		44

performed to the exclusion of cervical cytology.

Management

When abnormal cytology is present, biopsies should be obtained and the lesion handled promptly with conventional therapy without stopping the immunosuppressive drugs. Rigid asepsis and meticulous surgical technique are necessary to avoid infectious complications and delayed wound healing following surgery on these immunosuppressed women. Catheterization of the bladder should be done only after a 10 minute preparation of the perineum, and the catheter should be removed within 24 hours after the operation. Because of the risk of infection, total abdominal hysterectomy is preferred over vaginal hysterectomy, and a lower abdominal midline incision will avoid injury to the kidney. Gentle retraction and appropriate packing are used to avoid injury to the allograft ureter and the patients' own ureters. Although many of the patients have diseased kidneys removed, the ureters are often preserved in case they are needed for anastomosis to the allograft ureter or renal pelvis. Care must be taken to obtain absolute hemostasis. Fine, nonabsorbable suture materials are preferable, except for the apex of the vaginal vault, where catgut is employed. Careful wound closure is necessary, with attention to obliteration of dead space and avoidance of stay sutures.

OBSTETRIC PROBLEMS

Since the first successful pregnancy in 1963 in a patient who received a kidney transplant from her monozygotic twin (Murray et al., 1963), over 500 women with renal allografts from living donors or cadavers have become pregnant (Rudolph et al., 1979; Waltzer et al., 1980). In contrast, only 12 patients have been reported who conceived and delivered while receiving regular dialysis treatment for kidney failure (Trebbin, 1979). The most common underlying disease in these women has been glomerulonephritis or chronic pyelonephritis. A review of the records of our female transplant patients shows that a significant number have had toxemia or evidence of underlying hypertensive or renal disease and a high perinatal mortality rate during previous pregnancies. Obstetricians should feel an obligation to refer such patients for an adequate work-up for hypertension, since the proper therapeutic regimen can prevent further renal damage.

The use of living donors is widespread in the United States, accounting for 40 per cent of renal transplants. Although the donation procedure is assumed to be relatively safe, there was a complication rate of 28 per cent among 287 screened kidney donors from one institution (Spanos et al., 1974). Although pregnancy following nephrectomy may be safely undertaken (Schaefer and Markham, 1968), the ultimate risks of kidney donation and living with a solitary kidney after donation are clearly not known. It is very important for large centers to obtain accurate long-term follow-up data to answer this question.

The general tone of reports in the literature regarding pregnancy in renal transplant patients is one of optimisim. However, careful analysis of maternal and fetal complications makes it apparent that the pregnant allograft recipient presents a high risk and requires expert obstetric care as well as superior perinatal facilities.

Pre-Pregnancy Assessment and Advice

The decision concerning pregnancy is extremely difficult for the woman with renal disease and for her family. The ultimate prognosis in chronic renal disease is quite changed as a result of hemodialysis and transplantation. In general, we have discouraged pregnancy in our patients just as we do in any situation involving a serious medical disorder. The 50 to 60 per cent long-term graft survival rate makes the prognosis for these women somewhat guarded. It is likely that some transplant recipients may not live long enough to raise their children to adulthood and may leave the surviving spouse the problem of raising the child or children unaided. Interestingly, previous blood transfusions and pregnancies both seem to decrease the risk of renal allograft rejection (Fauchet et al., 1979).

There is unanimous agreement that a good graft is essential before pregnancy should be considered. Adequate assessment of renal function requires that the patient be followed for at least 1 to 2 years after transplant. Pregnancy should probably not be attempted in any patient with a serum creatinine level above 2.0 mg./dl. Other medical problems, such as diabetes mellitus, recurrent infections, or serious side effects from the immunosuppressive drugs, also weigh against pregnancy. It is becoming increasingly apparent that long-term complications in these patients include hypertension, duodenal ulcer, pancreatitis, viral hepatitis, secondary hyperparathyroidism with avascular bone necrosis, serum lipid abnormalities, and unusual and exotic infections.

Ideally, histocompatibility testing should be performed by comparing white blood cell antigens from the recipient, the potential father, and the kidney donor. Theoretically, if both the donor and fetus share leukocyte antigens that are not present in the mother, fetal to maternal transplacental transfer of cells could result in a maternal immune response directed against the kidney graft. There are at present insufficient data to determine whether this is a practical clinical problem.

Thus, in counseling women the physician must keep in mind that the decision to attempt pregnancy should be made by the patient and her husband after a tactful but honest presentation of the facts. The physician should be willing to accept the patient's decision to bear some risk in an attempt to have a successful pregnancy, just as her wish is accepted if she desires termination of pregnancy.

Abortion

The rates of spontaneous abortion (8.7 per cent) and stillbirth (1.9 per cent) are the same as those seen in the normal pregnant population (Rudolph et al., 1979). However, in at least some cases, abortion has occurred in patients whose renal function was abnormal as measured by very low creatinine clearance values. We have had one patient with an ectopic pregnancy who was managed satisfactorily by conventional unilateral salpingectomy.

Precautions

Many patients have pregnancies terminated at their or their physician's request. No particular technical problems have been encountered with suction curettage during the first trimester. However, because of the danger of infection and potential effects on hypertension and fluid and electrolyte balance, midtrimester instillation of saline or prostaglandin $F_2\alpha$ should be avoided if possible.

Prenatal Care

Maternal Considerations

False immunologic pregnancy tests (which can occur in the presence of proteinuria and menstrual irregularities) may make accurate dating of conception difficult. Nevertheless, early diagnosis of pregnancy should be attempted in these patients so that an accurate estimated date of delivery can be calculated. This is important because there may be a need to intervene should complications arise. The patient should be observed closely (Table 37–4) at three-week intervals until the twenty-eighth week and at weekly intervals thereafter. Immediate hospitalization should be considered if any complications arise.

Renal Graft Rejection. Much has been written recently about the immunologic relationship between mother and fetus, and there is some evidence to indicate that pregnancy results in a mildly diminished capacity for rejection of tissue by the mother (Billingham and Silvers, 1971). Renal graft rejection has become a severe problem in 25 reported cases (Rudolph et al., 1979), but at times immunosuppressive therapy has been decreased and even stopped during pregnancy (Walsh and O'Dwyer, 1970) with no apparent adverse effects. Nevertheless, azathioprine and corticosteroids should usually be continued in the same doses used prior to pregnancy to assure maximal renal function and avoid any chance of rejection. In view of its

TABLE 37–4. SUGGESTED ROUTINE PRENATAL CARE REGIMEN FOR RENAL TRANSPLANT PATIENTS

A. First Antepartum Visit

1. Routine prenatal history
2. Physical and pelvic examination: establish estimated date of confinement (EDC) and that uterine size is compatible with last menstrual period (LMP).
3. Record weight
4. Baseline laboratory values
   a. urinalysis
   b. urine culture
   c. total protein (24-hour urine specimen)
   d. creatinine clearance
   e. complete blood count
   f. blood type and Rh
   g. VDRL
   h. serum sodium, potassium, chloride, carbon dioxide, blood urea nitrogen, creatinine, glucose, SGOT, alkaline phosphatase, bilirubin
   i. cervical cytology

B. Subsequent Visits (at Least Every Three Weeks Until 28 Weeks' Gestation, Then Weekly)

1. Note general health and evaluate any infections
2. Record weight and blood pressure
3. Record fundal height and fetal heart tones
4. Creatinine clearance, urinary protein, glucose
5. Ultrasound for placental localization and biparietal diameter of fetal head at 28 weeks' gestation. Repeat for biparietal diameter at 32 and 36 weeks.
6. Cervical culture for viruses at 28 weeks
7. "Rollover test" (Gant, 1974) at 28 to 32 weeks
8. Repeat complete blood count, cervical cytology at 32 weeks
9. Non-stress test weekly beginning at 32 weeks
10. Fetal maturity studies and hospitalization as necessary

marked teratogenicity in the human, cyclophosphamide should be discontinued prior to any pregnancy.

Reduction in GFR. Normal pregnancy is associated with an elevated glomerular filtration rate (GFR) from about 8 to 10 weeks, which persists until term. In transplant patients, very few have shown even a moderate enhancement of the GFR, and in most it decreased during the third trimester (Merkatz et al., 1971; Sciarra et al., 1975). Fortunately, this deficit is completely reversible after delivery in most cases (Kopsa et al., 1976; Sciarra et al., 1975) and is not usually reflected in a deterioration of creatinine clearance rates. The course of one of our patients is illustrated in Figure 37–2. The patient and her baby are shown in Figure 37–3.

Preeclampsia. Proteinuria, usually less than 1 gm./day, has been commonly observed during the last trimester, often independent of any change in renal function or arterial blood pressure (Rifle and Traeger, 1975). Nevertheless, a clinical picture compatible with preeclampsia has been noted in primigravidas with renal allografts (Merrill et al., 1973; Tagatz et al., 1975; Penn et al., 1971), and the incidence might even be higher if more of these patients did not deliver prematurely. Eclampsia has now also been reported in a transplant patient (Williams and Jelen, 1979).

The management of preeclampsia should not differ appreciably from that in nontransplant patients, and iatrogenic problems introduced by the use of unnecessary drugs should be avoided. If the preeclampsia is severe, the only therapeutic regimen proved to be of value is delivery of the infant.

Renal Failure. Although decreased renal function during the third trimester may be reversible and recovery may occur in the postpartum period, the clinician must be concerned that this renal deterioration may ultimately lead to more extensive renal compromise and renal failure. Renal failure leading to death has been noted (Caplan et al., 1970; Moore and Hume, 1969) and renal failure may have been contributory in the death of at least three other patients (Caplan et al., 1970; Gevers et al., 1971; Merrill et al., 1973). Therefore, an appropriate conservative approach would be to consider any renal compromise appearing during pregnancy as potentially deleterious to the continued survival of the transplant and an indication for termination of the pregnancy or for premature delivery.

Maternal Infections. Bacterial, viral, and fungal infections, primarily urinary tract and pulmonary, are common. Cases of pneumonia and sepsis with such organisms

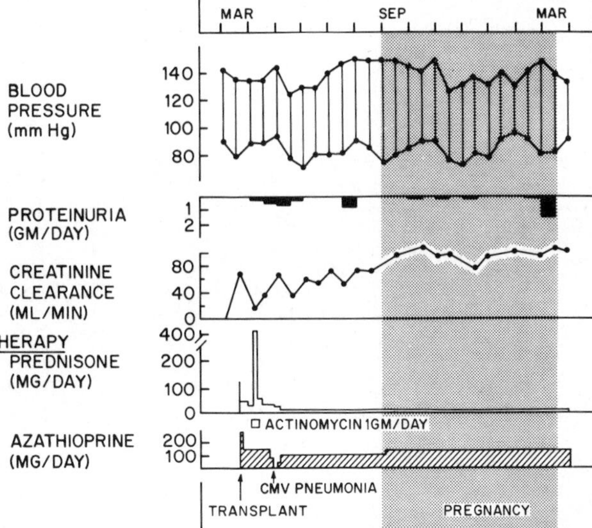

Figure 37–2. Blood pressure, renal status, and immunosuppressive therapy prior to and during pregnancy.

as pneumocystis, aspergillus, *Mycobacterium tuberculosis,* and *Listeria monocytogenes* (also a potential cause of recurrent abortion, amnionitis, and premature labor) have been reported (Rudolph et al., 1979). Fungal complications related to intensive immunosuppression are now reported less frequently as transplant teams have learned more about the limits of immunosuppressive medication. One woman developed gastroenteritis at 6 months of gestation, and she and the infant died.

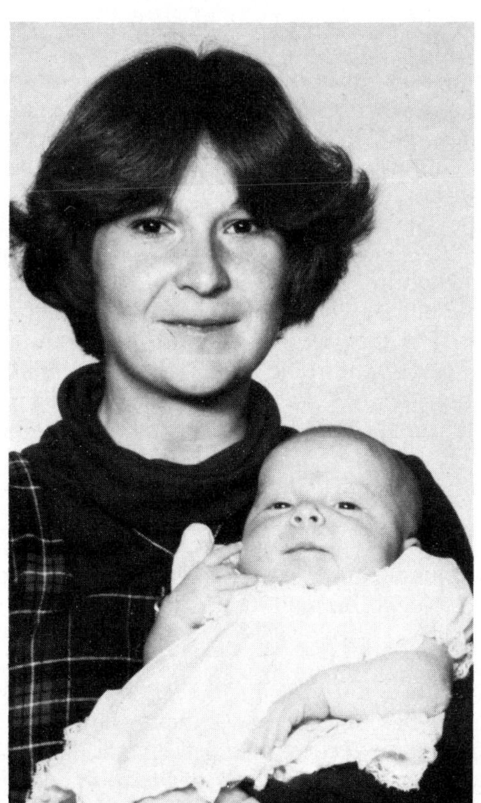

Figure 37–3. Healthy mother and infant at 6 weeks post partum.

Prematurity and Fetal Growth Retardation

Although data regarding last menstrual period, birth weight, and duration of pregnancy are missing from many reports, premature rupture of membranes, prematurity, and intrauterine growth retardation or small for gestational age (SGA) infants are frequent (Nolan et al., 1974). Figure 37–4 illustrates the week of delivery and the birth weight of the infants of our patients and of mothers with renal allografts reported in sufficient detail in the literature. Of those pregnancies that progressed to the third trimester, the percentage of premature births (occurring before the thirty-seventh week) was 33 per cent in 42 pregnancies. Excluding the two sets of twins, 35 (88 per cent) of the infants were below the 50th percentile for weight, and 18 (45 per cent) below the 10th percentile were definitely SGA. Although animal experiments (Scott, 1976) suggest that immunosuppressive drugs decrease both placental and fetal weight, it is not clear in the human

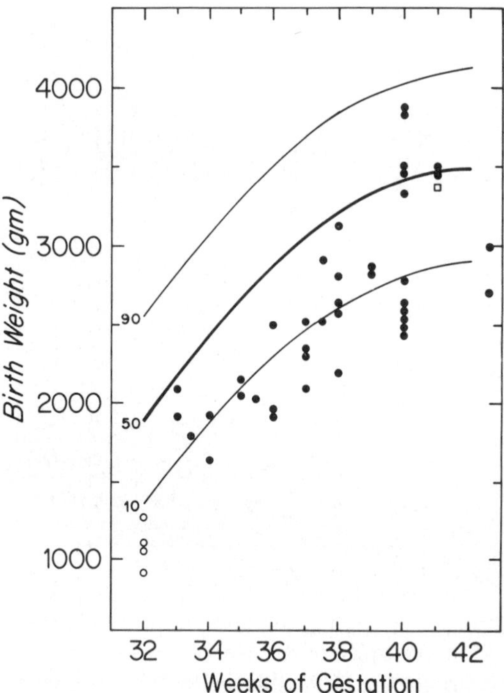

Figure 37–4. Birth weight and week of gestation of infants born to renal allograft recipients. The fetal growth curve is modified from Thomson et al., 1968. ●, Mothers receiving azathioprine and prednisone; ○, twins; □, infants born to a mother who received her renal allograft from an identical twin and required no immunosuppressive drugs.

whether the drugs or the underlying maternal disease is the mechanism responsible for this phenomenon. Excluding cesarean sections performed before term, prematurity and fetal growth retardation seem independent of the source of the transplant and have been observed in normotensive as well as hypertensive patients (Rifle and Traeger, 1975). Prematurity is, however, more frequent in the latter group, as well as in those women whose creatinine clearance is less than 70 ml./min. It is also postulated from studies of the effects of corticosteroids upon connective tissue that chronic corticosteroid therapy may weaken tissues and contribute to the increased incidence of premature rupture of membranes in these patients. Thus, it seems likely that a combination of factors is responsible for the increased incidence of premature delivery.

Maternal Urinary Estriol Assays. Monitoring of fetal well-being in utero has been stressed by many authors, but serial assays of maternal urinary excretion of estrogens have not been particularly helpful. Whether or not the baby is of low birth weight, urinary estriol (E_3) excretion is invariably below the normal range and is usually less than 12 mg./day at the time of delivery (Robertson et al., 1974; Horbach et al., 1973; Rifle and Traeger, 1975; Thiery et al., 1970). Suppression of precursor products of the fetal adrenal by glucocorticoids administered to the mother, and/or inadequate E_3 excretion by the transplant kidney, probably accounts for this finding.

Ultrasound Measurements. Serial ultrasound measurements of the biparietal diameter of the fetal head correlate well with fetal weight and are a useful method for monitoring intrauterine growth, placental localization, and the diagnosis of polyhydramnios, abnormal fetal presentations, or twins (Figure 37–5).

Amniocentesis. In certain situations (Tagatz et al., 1975), assessment of fetal maturity by analysis of amniotic fluid can be of critical importance. The concentration of creatinine in amniotic fluid probably parallels the development of fetal renal function and correlates well with fetal maturity when maternal renal function is normal. However, elevated maternal serum creatinine results in an increased concentration in the amniotic fluid and may negate the usefulness of this measurement in some of these patients. The ratio of lecithin to sphingomyelin (L/S ratio) in amniotic fluid is a uniquely valuable index of fetal maturity. The L/S ratio reflects the concentration of surfactant in the fetal lung and correlates with the risk of the fetus developing respiratory distress syndrome. Pulmonary function is often the critical determinant in fetal survival (Gluck et al., 1971).

Nevertheless, aseptic technique and a healthy respect for the possibility of introducing infection at the time of amniocentesis must be maintained.

Termination of Pregnancy

Amniocentesis and other studies have not been needed in most instances, since the decision to deliver the baby has been based largely on maternal considerations. If severe maternal complications arise, such as fulminating preeclampsia or deteriorat-

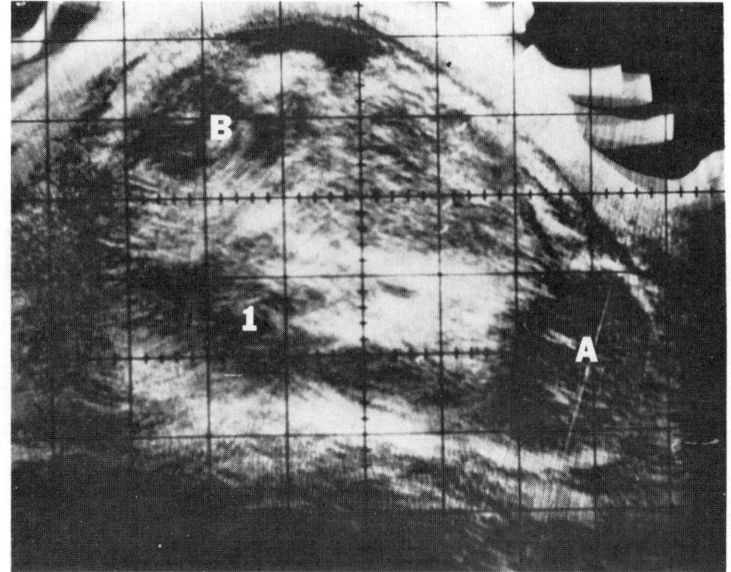

Figure 37-5. Ultrasonogram showing posterior placenta (*1*), presenting vertex of twin A in pelvis (*A*), and cross section of torso of twin B, which was in transverse lie in upper fundus (*B*).

ing renal function, termination of the pregnancy is indicated regardless of fetal maturity. Intrauterine fetal death during the third trimester has been reported, and elective intervention is sometimes necessary because of poor fetal growth or evidence of fetal distress.

Premature Labor. Premature labor occurs spontaneously in a high percentage of cases. Because of this tendency toward premature labor, oxytocin challenge tests should be avoided unless there is a definite indication that the fetus is in distress and would survive delivery at that point in gestation. However, resting tracings of fetal heart rate patterns are not contraindicated.

Labor and Delivery

The position of the kidney in the pelvis does not usually offer a major obstacle to normal vaginal delivery and the kidney is not likely to be damaged. If the fetal head is not engaged when labor begins, the possibility of soft tissue dystocia (Kaufman et al., 1967; Eslami et al., 1976) can be evaluated by simultaneous x-ray pelvimetry and intravenous pyelography (Figure 37–6). However, we now consider ultrasonography to be a very reliable method of assessing the status of the pelvic kidney and fetal position and presentation (Figure 37–7) without exposing the mother and fetus to the hazards of irradiation (Bhakthavathsalan et al., 1979). In order to decrease the chance of infection, prolonged ruptured membranes, multiple vaginal examinations,

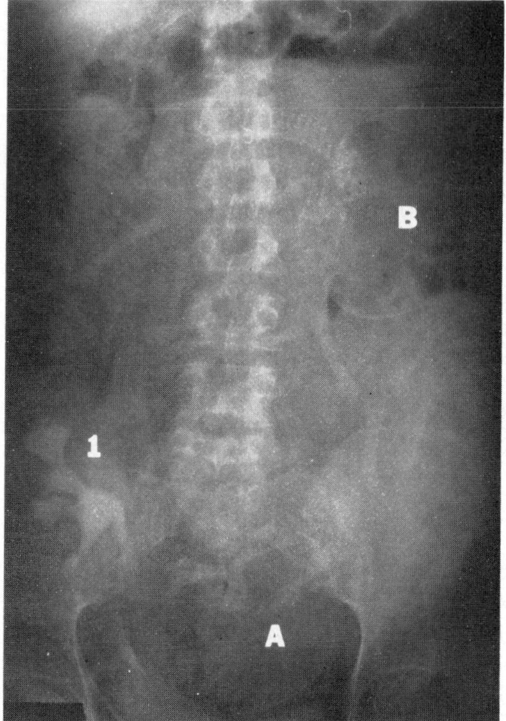

Figure 37-6. Simultaneous x-ray pelvimetry and intravenous pyelogram of same patient as in Figure 37–5. Kidney in right iliac fossa (*1*) is in good position with no obstructive dilatation of the drainage tract, and the fetal head of twin A is engaged (*A*).

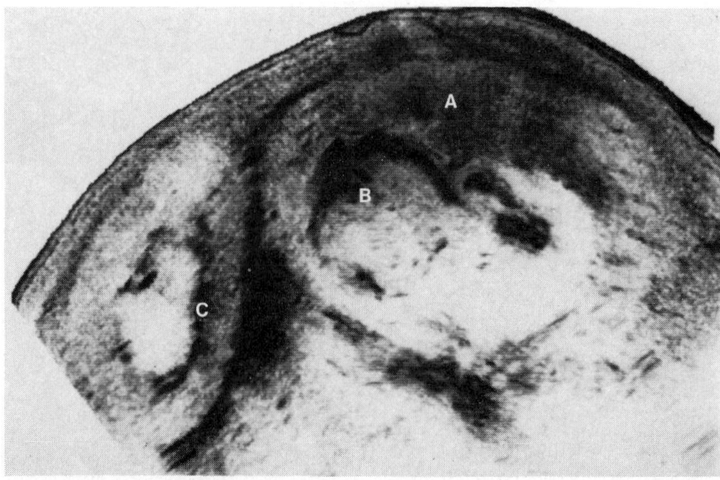

Figure 37–7. Transverse sonogram at 22 weeks' gestation, below the level of the iliac crest, showing anterior placenta (*A*), fetal trunk (*B*), and mild hydronephrosis of the transplanted kidney (*C*).

and possibly internal fetal monitoring should be avoided in these patients.

Uterine Rupture

Uterine rupture has been reported in a 40-year-old grand multipara who had had a tumultuous labor (Merrill et al., 1973). The authors postulated that prednisone may have contributed to the uterine rupture, and therefore stimulation of labor with oxytocin in these women should be done cautiously.

Cesarean Section

Indications for cesarean section must be studied for each individual and a decision made primarily on obstetric factors. A low transverse cervical cesarean section through a lower abdominal midline incision is the procedure of choice. During and after surgery, supplementation with intravenous hydrocortisone has been usual, but we have not found this to be necessary with normal vaginal deliveries.

Neonatal Problems

Congenital Anomalies

Aside from the problems related to prematurity and fetal growth retardation, the clinical condition of the newborns at birth has been for the most part satisfactory. Nevertheless, pregnancy continues to be a relative contraindication to the use of cytotoxic and immunosuppressive drugs because of their potential ability to induce birth defects as well as chromosomal damage. Three of four infants born to mothers who had taken cyclophosphamide during the first trimester of pregnancy for hematologic disorders or glomerulonephritis had multiple congenital anomalies. These included ectrodactylia, umbilical hernia, cutaneous hemangioma, a single coronary artery, grooved palate, flattened nasal ridge, abdominal skin tag, and bilateral hernia sacs (Greenberg and Tanaka, 1964; Lacher and Gelles, 1966; Coates, 1970). Despite studies on lower animals that support the concern for anomalies in the offspring secondary to maternal ingestion of corticosteroids and azathioprine (Rosenkrantz et al., 1967), there has been no statistical increase in congenital abnormalities attributed to these agents in the human. However, one mother who had been on therapy with these two immunosuppressants delivered an infant with pulmonary artery stenosis (Penn et al., 1971). Transient hypoparathyroidism and tetany have been reported in an infant delivered from a transplant mother who was subsequently shown to have hyperparathyroidism herself (Schoenike et al., 1978).

Chromosomal Changes

There have also been reports of infants with chromosomal changes born to mothers receiving azathioprine and prednisone during pregnancy (Leb et al., 1971; Gevers et al., 1971). These changes included bridging, deletions, translocations, and breaks.

Chromosome study 3 months later was within normal limits for one infant, but the other two demonstrated abnormal karyotypes for one and one-half years.

Twins

It is also interesting that two sets of twins have been reported (Lower et al., 1971; Sciarra et al., 1975). We have delivered two more mothers with twins, suggesting that the incidence of twinning in transplant patients receiving prednisone and azathioprine may be higher than the usual ratio of 1:90 pregnancies. Moreover, one renal transplant mother has now delivered triplets (Davidson, 1979)!

Infection

Viral infections in patients treated with immunosuppressive agents may pose an added risk for pregnancy. There is a higher incidence of viral hepatitis, and infants of affected mothers have been born with clinical disease, even when the mother is an asymptomatic carrier (Horstmann, 1969). Cytomegalovirus infection in renal transplant recipients is also common, and one infected infant has been reported (Evans et al., 1975). Although the child developed normally and experienced no untoward infections, impaired T-lymphocyte function and subnormal serum IgA were noted. Both herpes simplex and varicella-zoster have been observed frequently in transplant recipients, and these infections, when present in a pregnant woman, can result in significant neonatal disease.

Immunologic Deficiency

Although most reports have emphasized that the infants from transplant mothers receiving immunosuppressive agents are grossly normal at birth, there is very little in the literature regarding follow-up on these children. Serial lymphocyte counts, T and B cells, antibody titers, serum IgG, IgA, and IgM levels, and other in vitro tests performed through 2 years of age in the infant of one transplant patient revealed no abnormalities of either the cellular or humoral immune systems (Berant et al., 1976), and 10 other offspring who have been followed carefully for as long as 6 years are reportedly physically and psychologically normal (Korsch et al., 1980). Of theoretical concern are possible delayed effects that could result from the transplacental passage of these drugs (Saarikoski and Seppala, 1973) during the crucial development of the fetal immune systems. Most cytotoxic drugs can be found in maternal milk, so that breast feeding should probably be avoided (Stirrat, 1976). The development of vaginal adenosis and vaginal carcinoma in daughters of women treated with diethylstilbestrol adequately demonstrates that adverse effects from in utero exposure to drugs may not surface until years later (Herbst et al., 1971). Since the increased incidence of infections and neoplasms associated with primary immunologic deficiencies and administration of immunosuppressive drugs is well known, it is imperative that any child that has been exposed to these agents in utero have a careful evaluation of the immune system (Table 37–5) and long-term follow-up (Cote et al., 1974). Moreover, if any chromosome damage has occurred in the primordial ova that have undergone haploid division by birth, the occurrence of abnormalities in the next generation is a possibility. Therefore, the long-term prognosis for offspring of renal transplant recipients is unknown, and this should be shared with the patient.

TABLE 37–5. MINIMAL WORKUP FOR INFANTS BORN TO FEMALE RENAL ALLOGRAFT RECIPIENTS

A. At Birth
1. Physical examination
2. Complete blood count
3. Serum immunoglobulin concentration
4. Viral antibody titers (CMV)
5. Bacterial cultures
6. Chest film for thymic shadow
7. Chromosome examination
8. Serum calcium, phosphorus

B. Follow-up Examinations
1. History and physical examination
   a. Recurrent infections
   b. Somatic development
   c. Mental development
2. Complete blood count
3. Serum immunoglobulin concentration
4. Immunizations and antibody titers

REFERENCES

Abramovici, H., Brandes, J. M., Better, O. S., et al.: Menstrual cycle and reproductive potential after kidney transplantation. Obstet. Gynecol. *37*:121, 1971.

Berant, M., Wagner, Y., Jacob, E. T., et al.: Immunologic status of the offspring of a cadaver kidney recipient. Clin. Pediatr. *15*:815, 1976.

Bhakthavathsalan, A., Bree, R., Shapiro, R., et al.: The pregnant renal transplant patient: ultrasound to aid in the choice of delivery. Dialysis Transplant. *8*:910, 1979.

Billingham, R., and Silvers, W.: The Immunobiology of Transplantation. Englewood Cliffs, N.J., Prentice-Hall, Inc., 1971, pp. 168–186.

Board, J. A., Lee, H. M., Draper, D. A., et al.: Pregnancy following kidney homotransplantation from a non-twin. Report of a case with concurrent administration of azathioprine and prednisone. Obstet. Gynecol. *29*:318, 1967.

Caplan, R. M., Dosseter, J. B., and Maughan, G. B.: Pregnancy following cadaver kidney homotransplantation. Am. J. Obstet. Gynecol. *106*:644, 1970.

Coates, A.: Cyclophosphamide in pregnancy. Aust. N.Z. J. Obstet. Gynaecol. *10*:33, 1970.

Cote, C. J., Meuivissen, H. J., and Pickering, R. J.: Effects on the neonate of prednisone and azathioprine administered to the mother during pregnancy. J. Pediatr. *85*:324, 1974.

Davidson, H.: Kidney mum's triplets making good progress. Nurs. Mirror *148*:3, 1979.

Donohue, L. R.: Colposcopic and cytologic evaluation of women undergoing immunosuppressive therapy. J. Reprod. Med. *12*:194, 1974.

Eslami, H., Ribot, S., and Pedowitz, P.: Parenthood in recipients of kidney transplants. J. Med. Soc. N. J. *73*:211, 1976.

Evans, T. J., McCollum, J. P. K., and Valdimarsson, H.: Congenital cytomegalovirus infection after maternal renal transplantation. Lancet *1*:1359, 1975.

Fauchet, R., Wattelet, J., Genetet, B., et al.: Role of blood transfusions and pregnancies in kidney transplantation. Vox Sang. *37*:222, 1979.

Gant, N. F., Chand, S., Worley, R. J., et al.: A clinical test useful for predicting the development of acute hypertension of pregnancy. Am. J. Obstet. Gynecol. *12*:1, 1974.

Gevers, R. H., Hintzen, A. H. J., Kalff, M. W., et al.: Pregnancy following kidney transplantation. Europ. J. Obstet. Gynecol. *4*:147, 1971.

Gluck, L., Kulovich, M. V., Borer, R. C., Jr., et al.: Diagnosis of the respiratory distress syndrome by amniocentesis. Am. J. Obstet. Gynecol. *109*:440, 1971.

Gomez, F., de la Cueva, R., Wauters, J. P., et al.: Endocrine abnormalities in patients undergoing long-term hemodialysis. The role of prolactin. Am. J. Med. *68*:522, 1980.

Greenberg, L. H., and Tanaka, K. R.: Congenital anomalies probably induced by cyclophosphamide. J.A.M.A. *188*:423, 1964.

Herbst, A. L., Ulfelder, H., and Poskanzer, D. C.: Adenocarcinoma of the vagina: Association of maternal stilbestrol therapy with tumor appearance in young women. N. Engl. J. Med. *284*:878, 1971.

Horbach, J., van Liebergen, F., Mastboom, J., et al.: Pregnancy in a patient after cadaveric renal transplantation. Acta Med. Scand. *194*:237, 1973.

Horstmann, D. M.: Viral infections in pregnancy. Yale J. Biol. Med. *42*:99, 1969.

Kaufman, J. J., Digman, W., Goodwin, W. E., et al.: Successful normal childbirth after kidney homotransplantation. J.A.M.A. *200*:338, 1967.

Kopsa, H., Schmidt, P., Mayr, W. R., et al.: Abtossung des Nierentransplantats nach Schwangerschaft und Geburt. Schweiz, med. Wschr. *106*:58, 1976.

Korsch, B. M., Klein, J. D., Negrete, V. F., et al.: Physical and psychological follow-up on offspring of renal allograft recipients. Pediatrics *65*:275, 1980.

Lacher, M., and Gelles, W.: Cyclophosphamide and vinblastine sulfate in Hodgkin's disease during pregnancy. J.A.M.A. *195*:192, 1966.

Leb, D. E., Weisskopf, B., and Kanovitz, B. S.: Chromosome aberrations in the child of a kidney transplant recipient. Arch. Intern. Med. *128*:441, 1971.

Lower, G. D., Stevens, L. E., Najarian, J. S., et al.: Problems from immunosuppressives during pregnancy. Am. J. Obstet. Gynecol. *111*:1120, 1971.

Merkatz, I. R., Schwartz, G. H., David, D. S., et al.: Resumption of female reproductive function following renal transplantation. J.A.M.A. *216*:1749, 1971.

Merrill, L. K., Board, J. A., and Lee, H. M.: Complications of pregnancy after renal transplantation including a report of spontaneous uterine rupture. Obstet. Gynecol. *41*:270, 1973.

Moore, T. C., and Hume, D. M.: The period and nature of hazard in clinical renal transplantation: II. The hazard to transplant kidney function. Ann. Surg. *170*:12, 1969.

Morley, J. E., Distiller, L. A., Epstein, S., et al.: Menstrual disturbances in chronic renal failure. Horm. Metab. Res. *11*:68, 1979.

Murray, J. E., Reid, D. E., and Harrison, J. H.: Successful pregnancies after human renal transplantation. N. Engl. J. Med. *269*:341, 1963.

Nolan, G. H., Sweet, R. L., Laros, R. K., et al.: Renal cadaver transplantation followed by successful pregnancies. Obstet. Gynecol. *43*:732, 1974.
Penn, I.: The incidence of malignancies in transplant recipients. Transplant. Proc, *7*:323, 1975.
Penn, I., Makowski, E., Droegemueller, W., et al.: Parenthood in renal homograft recipients. J.A.M.A. *216*:1755, 1971.
Porreco, R., Penn, I., Droegemueller, W., et al.: Gynecologic malignancies in immunosuppressed organ homograft recipients. Obstet. Gynecol. *45*:359, 1975.
Rice, G. C.: Hypermenorrhea in the young hemodialysis patient. Am. J. Obstet. Gynecol. *116*:539, 1973.
Rifle, G., and Traeger, J.: Pregnancy after renal transplantation: An international survey. Transplant. Proc. *7*:723, 1975.
Robertson, J. G., Cockburn, F., and Woodruff, M.: Successful pregnancy after cadaveric renal transplantation. J. Obstet. Gynaecol. Br. Commonw. *81*:777, 1974.
Rosenkrantz, J. G., Githens, J. H., Cox, S. M., et al.: Azathioprine (Imuran) and pregnancy. Am. J. Obstet. Gynecol. *97*:387, 1967.
Rudolph, J. E., Schweizer, R. T., and Bartus, S. A.: Pregnancy in renal transplant patients. A review. Transplantation *27*:26, 1979.
Saarikoski, S., and Seppala, M.: Immunosuppression during pregnancy: Transmission of azathioprine and its metabolites from the mother to the fetus. Am. J. Obstet. Gynecol. *115*:1100, 1973.
Schaefer, G., and Markham, S.: Full-term delivery following nephrectomy. Am. J. Obstet. Gynecol. *100*:1078, 1968.
Schoenike, S. L., Kaldenbaugh, H. H., Kaplan, A. M., et al.: Transient hypoparathyroidism in an infant of a mother with a renal transplant. Am. J. Dis. Child. *132*:530, 1978.
Sciarra, J. J., Toledo-Pereyra, L. H., Bendel, R. P., et al.: Pregnancy following renal transplantation. Am. J. Obstet. Gynecol. *123*:411, 1975.
Scott, J.: Immunologically induced fetoplacental growth retardation. Gynecol. Invest. *7*:8, 1976.
Scott, J. R., and Beer, A. E.: Reproductive Immunology. *In* Wynn, R. M. (Ed.): Obstetrics and Gynecology Annual. New York, Appleton-Century-Crofts, 1974, p. 101.
Spanos, P. K., Simmons, R. L., Lampe, E., et al.: Complications of related kidney donation. Surgery *76*:741, 1974.
Stirrat, G. M.: Prescribing problems in the second half of pregnancy and during lactation. Obstet. Gynecol. Surv. *31*:1, 1976.
Strickler, R. C., Woolever, C. A., Johnson, M., et al.: Serum gonadotropin patterns in patients with chronic renal failure or hemodialysis. Gynecol. Invest. *5*:185, 1974.
Tagatz, G. E., Arnold, N. I., Goetz, F. C., et al.: Pregnancy in a juvenile diabetic after renal transplantation (Class T diabetes mellitus). Diabetes *24*:497, 1975.
Thaysen, J. H., Olgaard, K., and Jensen, H. G.: Ovarian cysts in women on chronic intermittent hemodialysis. Acta Med. Scand. *197*:433, 1975.
Thiery, D. M., Vandkerckhove, D., Ringoir, S., et al.: Zwangerschap na niertransplantatie. Ned. T. Geneesk. *114*:1411, 1970.
Thomson, A. M., Billewicz, W. Z., and Hytten, F. E.: The assessment of fetal growth. J. Obstet. Gynaecol. Br. Commonw. *75*:903, 1968.
Trebbin, W. M.: Hemodialysis and pregnancy. J.A.M.A. *241*:1811, 1979.
Vestergaard, B. F., Hornsleth, A., and Pedersen, S. N.: Occurrence of herpes and adenovirus antibodies in patients with carcinoma of the cervix uteri: Measurement of antibodies to herpes virus hominis (Types 1 and 2), cytomegalovirus, EB virus, and adenovirus. Cancer *30*:68, 1972.
Walsh, A., and O'Dwyer, W. F.: The current use of immuno-depressive drugs in kidney transplantation. *In* Bertelli, A., and Monaco, A. P. (Eds.): Pharmacological Treatment in Organ and Tissue Transplantation. Amsterdam, Excerpta Medica, 1970, p. 47.
Waltzer, W. C., Coulam, C. B., Zincke, H., et al.: Pregnancy in renal transplantation. Transplant. Proc. *12*:221, 1980.
Warne, G. L., Fairley, K. F., Hobbs, J. B., et al.: Cyclophosphamide-induced ovarian failure. N. Engl. J. Med. *289*:1159, 1973.
Weinberg, A.: Side effects of immunosuppressants with special reference to thiopurines. *In* Brent, L., and Holborrow, J. (Eds.): Progress in Immunology II. Clinical Aspects II. Amsterdam, North-Holland, 1974, p. 253.
Williams, P. F., and Jelen, I.: Eclampsia in a patient who had had a renal transplant. Br. Med. J. *2*:972, 1979.

38

URINARY CALCULI IN PREGNANCY

J. D. SCHMIDT, M.D.

Urinary tract stones are a common problem in the general population, occurring most frequently in males 20 to 50 years of age. In fact, in the endemic "stone belt" areas of this country (southeast and mid-Atlantic), renal and ureteral calculi are the most common reason for emergency admissions to hospitals. Urinary stones can be classified according to etiology, e.g., metabolic (uric acid, cystine, calcium phosphate as in hyperparathyroidism), infection (struvite), and idiopathic (calcium oxalate). This chapter deals with those urinary stones diagnosed during pregnancy.

INCIDENCE

Urolithiasis in the pregnant patient is an unusual occurrence. The reported incidence of this combination of events has been variable, ranging between 1 in 286 (0.35 per cent) (Semmens, 1964) to 1 in 3800 (0.03 per cent) (McVann, 1964; Arnell and Getzoff, 1942; Prather and Crabtree, 1934) pregnancies. Incidence rates reported by various authors include 1 per 1000 pregnancies (0.1 per cent) (Ferris, 1975), 1 per 1430 (0.07 per cent) (Strong et al., 1978), 0.14 per cent (King et al., 1967), and 1 per 1027 (0.1 per cent) (Lattanzi and Cook, 1980). The incidence of urolithiasis in the pregnant patient is probably no greater than in the nonpregnant patient (Ferris, 1975).

Although the combination of pregnancy and urolithiasis is unusual, the clinician should be alert to the possibility. Early detection can avoid the complications of impairment of renal function, urinary tract infection, and possible loss of the pregnancy (Marcus and Brandt, 1957).

ETIOLOGIC FACTORS

Pregnancy-Induced Hydroureteronephrosis

For many years, the physiologic hydroureteronephrosis of pregnancy with resultant stasis and infection was thought to be the major etiologic factor in the formation of upper urinary tract stones. If this were so, the majority of such stones should appear on the right side. However, a review of reported series reveals that there is no tendency to right-sided predominance. In fact, neither right nor left side predominates.

Trimester of Pregnancy and Parity

There has been considerable debate whether the incidence of urinary tract stones is related to the specific trimester of pregnancy (Folger, 1955; Harris and Dunnihoo, 1967) or to a woman's parity (Semmens, 1964; McVann, 1964). Current evidence indicates that neither of these variables is directly related to the etiology of urinary tract stones in pregnancy. The finding of urolithiasis more often in multigravid women may only reflect the tendency of stone disease to increase with age (Lattanzi and Cook, 1980).

Recently the incidence of calcium urolithiasis in spontaneous aborters has been shown to be significantly higher than that found in comparable-aged women with either gynecologic or nongynecologic disease (Honoré, 1980). The basis for such an association in young women is yet unclear.

Underlying Disease

Probably the same underlying factors that lead to the development of urolithiasis in the nonpregnant female are operative in the woman who is pregnant. For example, a specific disorder such as primary hyperparathyroidism may be uncovered in the evaluation of such a patient (Conger et al., 1976).

SYMPTOMS AND SIGNS

The pregnant female with a urinary tract stone may present with the same symptoms as those of the nonpregnant woman: typical acute lateralizing pain with microscopic hematuria. However, there are some specific exceptions to this general rule. First, hematuria is generally not as indicative for calculi in pregnancy, since it may be present from other causes; second, at five to eight months, the pain is very atypical for urinary tract stones; and third, the problem of infection may be the most obvious symptom (Ferris, 1975; Klempner et al., 1960).

In their review, Lattanzi and Cook (1980) noted that only 12 per cent of cases were diagnosed in the first trimester, whereas in 88 per cent of women with urinary calculi the diagnosis was made in the second and third trimesters. These authors postulate that the ureteral dilatation seen in late pregnancy allows renal and upper ureteral stones to be passed into the distal ureters, where symptoms result.

DIAGNOSTIC EVALUATION

History, Physical Examination, and Urinalysis

The physician caring for the pregnant patient must first consider the possibility of a urinary tract stone in the woman who has any suggestive symptoms or signs. Her past history may include the documentation and treatment of urinary stones or a background of urinary tract infections. Any pregnant patient with severe pyelonephritis, whether it be recurrent or poorly responsive to usual treatment for urinary tract infection, must be suspected of having some type of obstructive uropathy including a urinary tract stone. Physical examination may reveal unilateral tenderness and muscle guarding; the urinalysis may show variable amounts of hematuria or pyuria, or both, and bacilluria. A urine culture is mandatory.

Radiologic Studies

Abdominal X-Ray Film. An abdominal x-ray film is indicated to look for a radiopaque calculus (Byrd and Given, 1963). The exposure of one such film is equivalent to 0.2 rad to the fetus. By comparison, an intravenous pyelographic study consisting of four to six films represents a hazard of 0.4 to 1.6 rads to the maternal and fetal gonads (Rigby and MacEwan, 1976; Zerner, 1975).

Excretory Urography. Whether or not the abdominal scout film is indicative of a urinary tract stone, a modified excretory urogram (IVP) should be obtained, with a single film exposed at 20 minutes following the intravenous administration of iodinated contrast (Ferris, 1975). If there is still any doubt as to the possibility of a urinary tract stone, a second film should be exposed about one hour following the administration of the contrast material. Typical findings include delayed visualization and ureteral columnation of contrast to the obstructing calculus (Zerner, 1975). Rigby and MacEwan (1976) believed that excretory urography can be delayed for at least 24 hours following admission of the pregnant woman suspected of having urolithiasis.

Radionuclide Renography. The radionuclide renogram has been promulgated by some authors for the diagnosis of urinary tract stones in pregnancy. However, by itself it will not detect the location or the actual etiology of the obstruction seen in the study (McVann, 1964).

Ultrasonography

Abdominal ultrasonography is useful as a non-invasive screening test for a patient with indeterminate symptoms. However, echography cannot distinguish between the physiologic hydronephrosis of pregnancy and that obstruction due to an acquired stone. However, one interesting fringe benefit of the ultrasound technique late in pregnancy is the detection of hydronephrosis and other urinary tract anomalies in the fetus (Chapter 31).

Serum Determinations

For patients with a history of urinary tract stones, or when a stone is identified during pregnancy, serum samples should be obtained for the determination of calcium, phosphorus, uric acid, and alkaline phosphatase concentrations. Parathormone level should be determined in women with recurrent calcium phosphate or oxalate calculi.

MANAGEMENT

The treatment of the pregnant woman with a urinary tract stone in many ways is similar to that of the nonpregnant female. Whereas at least 80 per cent of stones will pass without operative intervention in the nonpregnant patient, at least one half will pass spontaneously in the state of pregnancy (Harris and Dunnihoo, 1967). Treatment usually consists of increased hydration and appropriate analgesics. However, when surgery (either endoscopic or open procedures) has been performed in such cases, maternal and fetal complications have been rare (Lattanzi and Cook, 1980).

Cystoscopic Manipulation

Cystoscopic attempts at manipulation may be indicated if the stone appears impacted and large and if it causes an undue amount of pain and impairment of renal function. Manipulative efforts may consist of simply inserting a ureteral catheter past the calculus to relieve the obstruction, or of attempts at basket extraction.

Operative Intervention

Occasionally, open operative intervention is necessary to relieve the obstruction and remove the calculus during pregnancy. Should the calculus be large and impacted in the upper ureter, a ureterolithotomy may be indicated. In rare cases, a percutaneous or formal surgical nephrostomy may help to relieve the obstruction temporarily. Nephrectomy is rarely needed in the treatment of a patient with underlying severe renal disease with complicating stones. Termination of pregnancy as treatment for an obstructing calculus is no longer tenable (Solomon, 1954).

Timing of Surgery. The timing of any operative intervention, whether endoscopic or open, is critical (Crabtree, 1942). Depending on the specific situation, this intervention may be either during the pregnancy or in the postpartum period. When intervention is necessary during pregnancy, it is generally considered that the middle trimester is the safest.

SPONTANEOUS ABORTION AND PREMATURE LABOR. Spontaneous abortion is more likely with the stress of anesthesia and surgery in the first trimester; premature labor is more likely during the third trimester (Amar, 1966).

Indications. The factors influencing the decision for any type of operative intervention are manifold (Klempner et al., 1960). These include the location of the calculus, the degree of urinary obstruction, the presence or absence of infection, the patient's general condition, the duration of pregnancy, and the availability of obstetrical expertise, as well as the presence of an anesthesiologist equipped to perform fetal monitoring (Szczerbo et al., 1972). In general, the presence of a stone 1 cm. or greater that has not progressed and is complicated by infection or sepsis in an ill patient is indication for immediate operative intervention.

Related Studies

Subsequent to either the spontaneous passing of a urinary tract stone or its removal via endoscopic or open surgical techniques, the patient should be considered for studies related to the etiology of the stone. Depending on a past history of recurrent urinary tract stones or other complicating factors, a metabolic investigation may be undertaken. Repeat serum biochemical determinations, as well as 24-hour urine collections for cystine, uric acid, calcium, and oxalate, can usually be deferred until the postpartum period. Identification of etiologic factors such as hereditary cystinuria (Gibson, 1965) or primary hyperparathyroidism (Rubin et al., 1968) can lead to specific treatment and, it is hoped, prevention of further urolithiasis.

Medical Therapy

Medical therapy includes the use of the xanthine oxidase inhibitor allopurinol for patients with uric acid stones and either hyperuricemia or hyperuricosuria, as well as for patients with these biochemical abnormalities and recurrent calcium oxalate calculi. Thiazide diuretics are helpful to decrease urinary calcium excretion in the patient with recurring calcium oxalate stones. At present there are insufficient data regarding these and other medical treatments for urolithiasis to determine the risks, if any, to the pregnant patient and her fetus.

CASE REPORTS

The recent experience with urinary tract stones in pregnancy at the University of Iowa Hospitals and Clinics was reviewed. In the ten-year period between 1966 and 1975, a total of 287 women of child-bearing age with urinary tract stones were evaluated. Two hundred and sixty-nine charts were available for retrospective review. Nine of this group or 3.4 per cent of the total were pregnant. These nine patients represent 0.045 per cent of all deliveries in the same interval. A brief clinical history of each of the nine patients follows.

Patient 1. A 24-year-old woman presented at 24 weeks' gestation with pain, fever, chills, and gross hematuria. She had a past history of three renal calculi. Her urine culture grew out *Proteus* species, and a 2 × 5 mm. opaque calculus was noted in the area of the distal left ureter. A single 20-minute IVP film revealed partial hydroureteronephrosis to the calculus and a physiologic right hydronephrosis. She was treated with antibiotics and fluids, and the calculus passed spontaneously a few days later. The remainder of her pregnancy was uncomplicated, and delivery was normal.

Patient 2. A 41-year-old woman presented with pain and hematuria at 20 weeks' gestation. An abdominal x-ray film revealed two opacities in the area of the distal right ureter, and a single IVP film demonstrated bilateral hydroureteronephrosis. She underwent two attempts at cystoscopic manipulation without success and was treated with intravenous fluids and analgesics. Shortly thereafter both calculi passed spontaneously; the remainder of the pregnancy and delivery were uneventful.

Patient 3. A 36-year-old multiparous woman presented at 32 weeks with nausea, vomiting, flank pain, hypertension, proteinuria, and pyuria. An abdominal x-ray film and single IVP film demonstrated a marked right hydronephrosis with stones in the lower pole of the right kidney. She was treated with antihypertensive medications; she passed a few calculi spontaneously during the pregnancy. Two months following an uncomplicated delivery, she underwent a right nephrectomy for a congenital hydronephrosis complicated with calculi. Her blood pressure thereafter fell to normal levels.

Patient 4. A 31-year-old woman presented with a history of having passed a urinary tract stone spontaneously at age 24. Retained calculi had been documented. In the seven years intervening, she had had two pregnancies, the first terminating in a stillbirth with fetal deformity and the other resulting in a spontaneous abortion at 12 weeks. Evaluation revealed multiple stones in the upper pole of the left kidney, along with severe chronic inflammatory changes. A left upper pole partial nephrectomy was carried out without incident. Postoperatively, she became pregnant but remained free of infection or recurrent stones. The pregnancy and delivery were uneventful.

Patient 5. A 24-year-old woman presented at 28 weeks' gestation with right flank pain, fever, chills, nausea, vomiting, and pyuria. She recalled passing a kidney stone at age 8. Her urine culture grew out a *Klebsiella* species. An abdominal x-ray film revealed a 5 × 5 mm. opaque density in the area of the right kidney, and a single IVP film showed the calculus to be in the right inferior calyx. Bilateral hydronephrosis, more severe on the right, was present. She was treated conservatively with fluids and antibiotics, and the remainder of her pregnancy and delivery were uncomplicated. She was rehospitalized three weeks following her delivery at which time bilateral renal calculi were present. The diagnosis of medullary sponge disease with complicating nephrolithiasis was made. The patient was advised to consider sterilization but refused.

Patient 6. A 34-year-old multigravida presented at 16 weeks' gestation with right flank pain and hematuria. An abdominal x-ray film revealed radiopaque densities in the area of the right kidney and true pelvis. A single IVP exposure demonstrated delayed visualization of the right kidney. Her right hydronephrosis was drained with a ureteral catheter. Four days later cystoscopic manipulation was attempted but was unsuccessful. At 24 weeks' gestation, she spontaneously passed one stone analyzed as containing calcium oxalate, carbonate, and phosphate. She subsequently developed left renal colic, and a repeat abdominal x-ray film revealed a calculus in the area of the proximal left ureter. A ureteral catheter was passed to relieve the obstruction. She spontaneously passed this stone a few days after removal of the catheter. She underwent an uncomplicated right pyelolithotomy after delivery.

Patient 7. A 23-year-old multigravida presented at 24 weeks' gestation with a history of recurrent stone and infection. Her past history included three ureterolithotomies. She was treated conservatively and, after an otherwise uncomplicated pregnancy and delivery, was treated via a right pyelolithotomy and repair of a ureteropelvic junction obstruction.

Patient 8. A 28-year-old woman presented at 28 weeks' gestation with left flank pain. She recalled the passage of multiple urinary tract stones since age 15. The analysis of these calculi revealed the presence of calcium phosphate as well as calcium magnesium ammonium phosphate. She also recalled stones and infections with other pregnancies. An abdominal x-ray film and a single IVP film showed a large right renal pelvic stone. She was treated conservatively and underwent an otherwise uncomplicated pregnancy and delivery. Six months later, a left pyelolithotomy was performed.

Patient 9. A 20-year-old woman presented at 20 weeks' gestation with left renal and ureteral colic requiring a left ureterolithotomy during the pregnancy. She later had an uncomplicated delivery. She appeared again at age 24, again at 20 weeks' gestation, with right ureteral colic. A ureteral catheter was passed for relief of symptoms. She did not pass the stone and presented once again at 32 weeks' gestation with right ureteral colic. Again she was treated via the passage of a ureteral catheter. She later passed this stone and underwent an uncomplicated delivery. Metabolic evaluation demonstrated both hypercalcemia and increased levels of parathyroid hormone activity. She underwent exploration of her neck at which time a parathyroid adenoma was removed. Serum calcium levels have been normal since, and she has formed no new calculi.

It is important to note that this experience reflects a skewed population group representing a selected set of complicated obstetrical cases in a tertiary care center rather than the large general obstetric population. Many of these women were referred to a university hospital setting because of problems that could not be managed adequately by their primary physicians.

In a recent review from a large general military hospital, 14 women with renal calculi were detected in 22,495 deliveries, representing an incidence of 0.062 per cent (Strong et al., 1978). These women ranged in age between 15 and 34 with an average of 25 years. Gestational stage at the time of presentation ranged between 16 and 36 weeks, with an average of 25.5 weeks. Parity averaged 2.5 pregnancies per patient. Two women had a past history of urolithiasis, and three had a family history of urinary tract stones. One patient presented with two separate stones in the same pregnancy.

In this group of 14 women, 11 passed their stones spontaneously, 10 during the pregnancy and one in the postpartum period. Three patients required surgical intervention, two antepartum and one postpartum. The authors reported no maternal or fetal complications. Surgical intervention included one basket extraction at 16 weeks' gestation and two ureterolithotomies. Metabolic evaluations in all women were normal, although only a few stones were analyzed. All urinary stones were solitary, there being nine on the left and five on the right.

Strong and co-workers (1978) believed that management required individualization based on the location of the stone, its degree of obstruction, and the presence of infection, as well as the general condition of the patient and the state of pregnancy. They found no contraindications to surgical intervention to remove a symptomatic obstructing calculus during pregnancy. Radiographic findings and brief representative histories are included in Figures 38–1 through 38–8.

Coe and associates (1978) have reported their experience with 78 women, aged 45 years or younger, who had a total of 148 pregnancies, 90 prior to and 58 following

Text continued on page 571

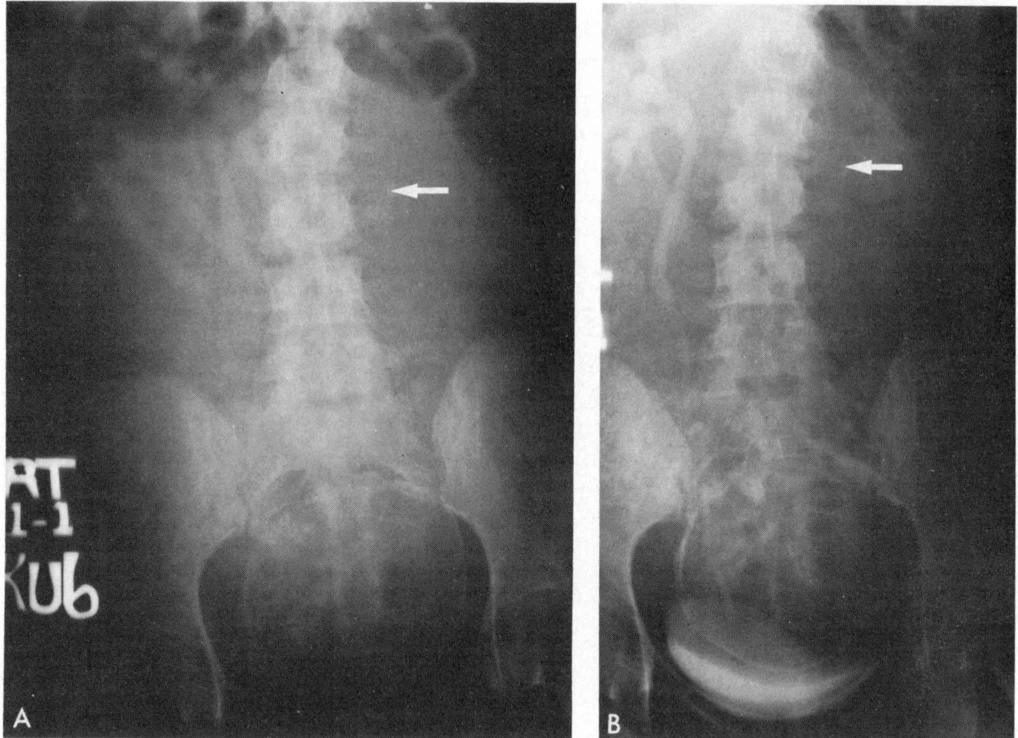

Figure 38–1. *A, Left,* Abdominal x-ray of an 18-year-old patient at 36 weeks' gestation. Opacity suggestive of urinary tract stone is indicated by arrow. Fetal skeleton is apparent.

B, Twenty-minute excretory urogram demonstrates nonfunction of left kidney with probable ureteral calculus. Right hydroureteronephrosis is physiologic.

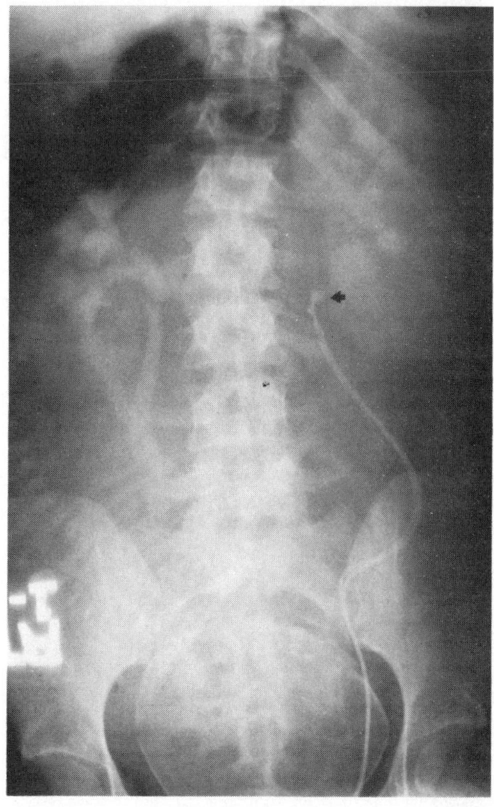

Figure 38–2. Same patient as in Figure 38–1. Left retrograde pyelogram performed with two ureteral catheters; ureteral calculus position indicated by arrow. Patient was treated by ureterolithotomy the next day.

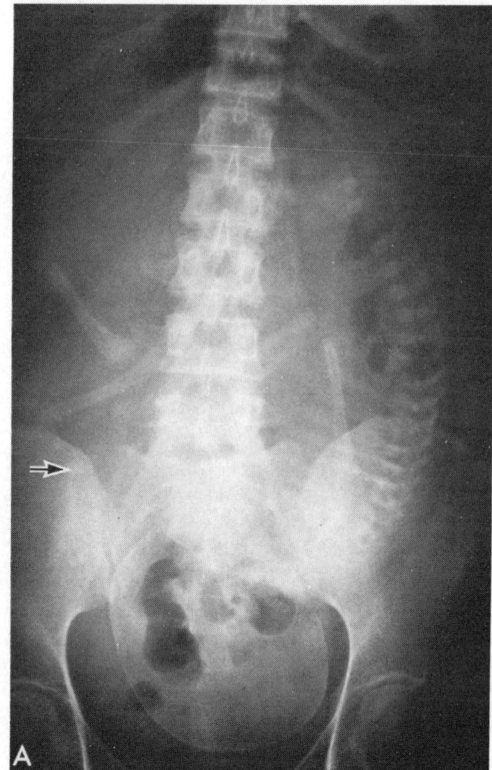

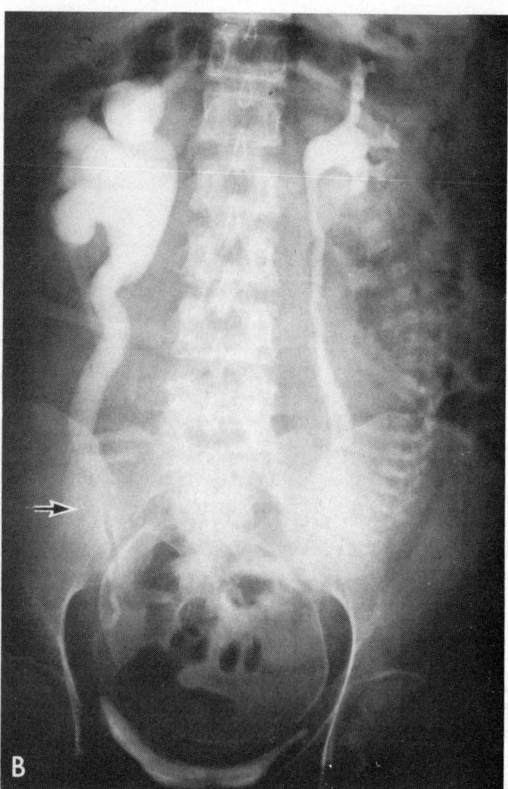

Figure 38–3. *A,* Abdominal x-ray of a 32-year-old patient at 33 weeks' gestation. Opacity suggestive of urinary tract stone is indicated by arrow. Fetal skeleton is apparent.

B, Twenty-minute excretory urogram demonstrates marked right hydroureteronephrosis to level of calculus (arrow); distal right ureter is normal, and left hydroureteronephrosis is physiologic.

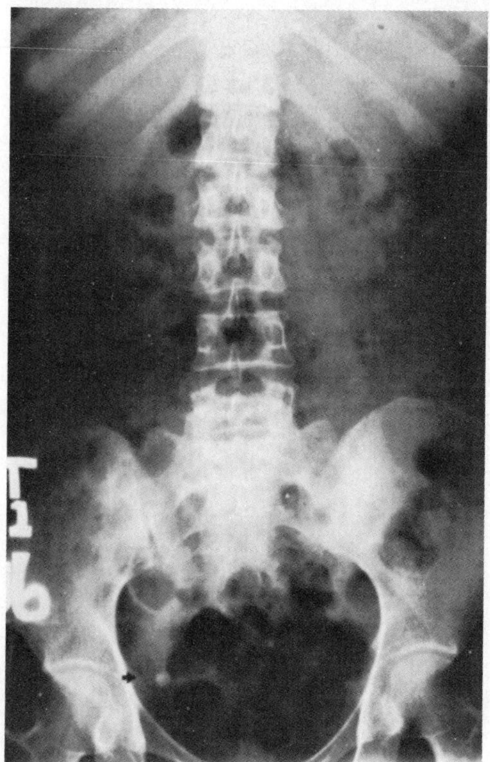

Figure 38–4. Same patient as in Figure 38–3. Abdominal x-ray seven weeks following uncomplicated delivery. Calculus has migrated to distal right ureter (arrow); right ureterolithotomy was performed.

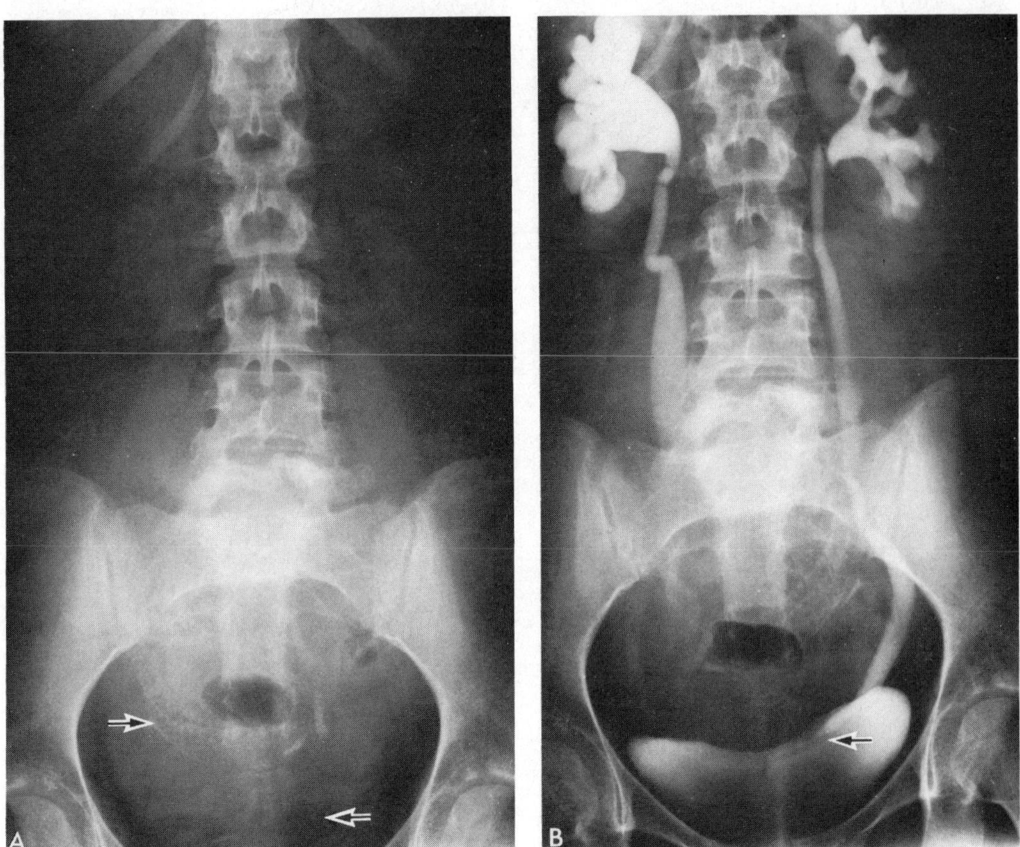

Figure 38–5. *A,* Abdominal x-ray of a 22-year-old patient at 16 weeks' gestation. Opacity suggestive of left ureteral calculus is indicated by bottom arrow; fetal skeleton is indicated by second arrow.

B, Twenty-minute excretory urogram demonstrates moderate left hydroureteronephrosis to level of calculus (arrow); right hydroureteronephrosis is physiologic. This left ureteral calculus passed spontaneously three days later.

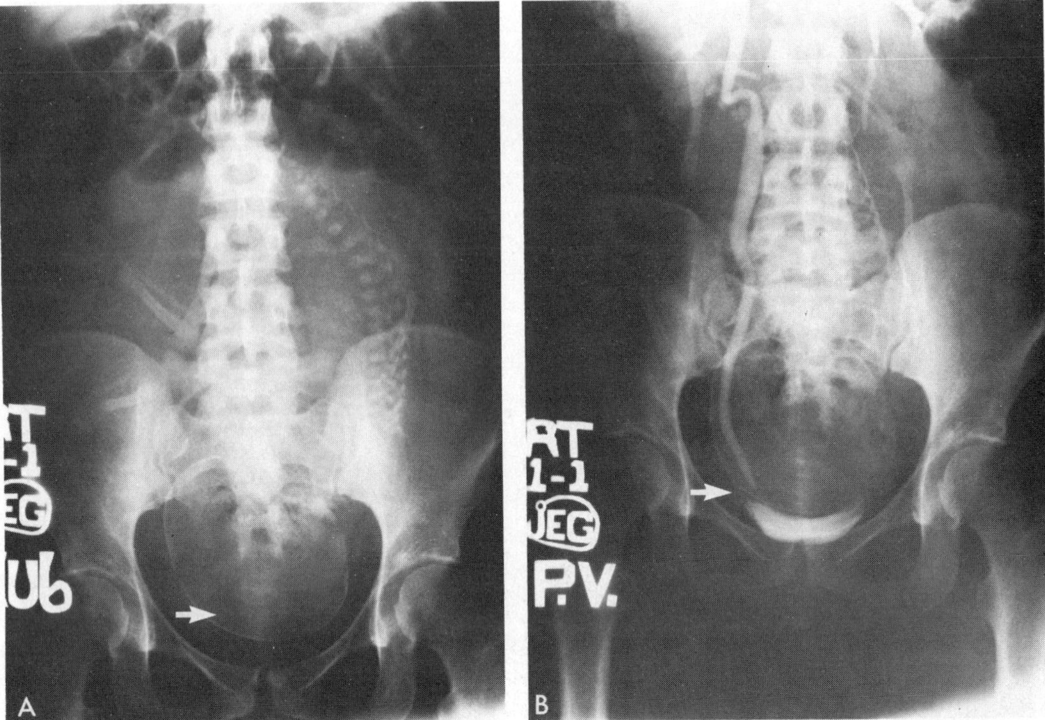

Figure 38–6. *A*, Abdominal x-ray of a 25-year-old patient at 32 weeks' gestation. Opacity suggestive of urinary tract calculus is indicated by arrow. Fetal skeleton is apparent. (This patient required basket extraction of right ureteral calculus at 16 weeks' gestation in the same pregnancy.)

B, Twenty-minute excretory urogram demonstrates right hydroureteronephrosis to level of calculus (arrow); left kidney and ureter are normal. Right ureteral calculus passed spontaneously a few days later.

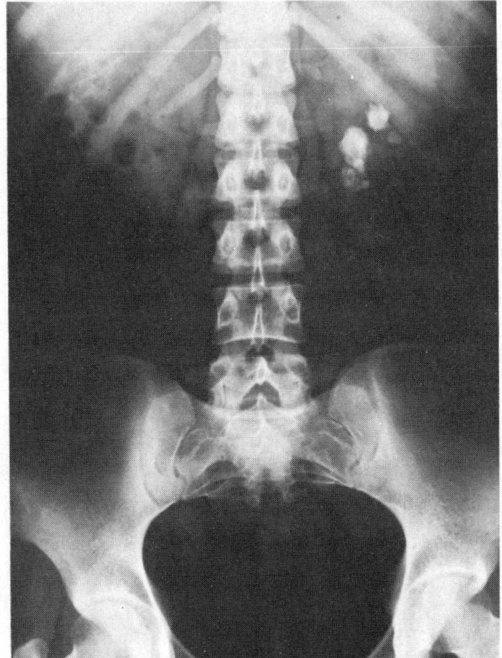

Figure 38–7. Abdominal x-ray of a 19-year-old patient at 12 weeks' gestation. Multiple opacities are seen in area of left kidney. Fetal skeleton is not visualized.

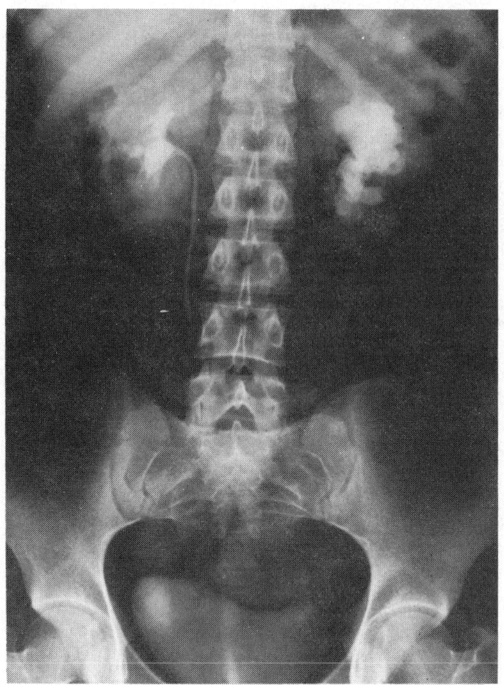

Figure 38–8. Same patient as in Figure 38–7. Twenty-minute excretory urogram demonstrates normal right upper urinary tract and marked left hydronephrosis without visualization of left ureter. Because of uncontrollable infection, the patient was treated by nephrolithotomy at 24 weeks' gestation. The remainder of pregnancy and delivery were uneventful.

the diagnosis of urolithiasis. The principal causes of stone disease were not different from those in their nonpregnant and male patients. Stones were passed during 20 pregnancies of 15 patients. Hospitalization was common but no endoscopic manipulations or open surgery were required. Symptomatic urinary infection, however, was a significant complicating factor, occurring in 11 of the 58 pregnancies that followed the onset of stone disease.

SUMMARY

Although urolithiasis complicating a pregnancy is uncommon, the sequelae of compromised renal function, urinary tract infection, and an endangered conceptus or fetus are real. Once the diagnosis is considered, carefully monitored excretory urography is mandatory. Treatment must then be individualized according to the various factors extant: site and position of calculus, degree of ureteral obstruction and infection, and the proximity to obstetric and anesthesiologic expertise. As in nonpregnant females with urolithiasis, a rational search for the etiology of the calculi can be made safely thereafter.

REFERENCES

Amar, A. D.: Pregnancy and urinary calculi. Calif. Med. *104*:106, 1966.

Arnell, R. E., and Getzoff, P. L.: Renal and ureteral calculi in pregnancy with analysis of 20 cases. Am. J. Obstet. Gynecol. *44*:34, 1942.

Byrd, W. A., and Given, F. T.: Urinary calculi associated with pregnancy. Obstet. Gynecol. *21*:238, 1963.

Coe, F. L., Parks, J. H., and Lindheimer, M. D.: Nephrolithiasis during pregnancy. N. Engl. J. Med. *298*:324, 1978.

Conger, K. B., Crocker, D. W., and De Alvarez, R. R.: Renal diseases and pregnancy. *In* De Alvarez, R. R. (ed.): The Kidney in Pregnancy. New York, John Wiley and Sons, 1976, Chapter 8.

Crabtree, E. G.: Urological Diseases of Pregnancy. Boston, Little, Brown and Co., 1942.

Ferris, T. F.: Renal disease. *In* Burrow, G. N., and Ferris, T. F. (eds.): Medical Complications During Pregnancy. Philadelphia, W. B. Saunders Co., 1975, Chapter 1, pp. 14 and 33.

Folger, G. K.: Pain and pregnancy, treatment of painful states complicating pregnancy with particular emphasis on urinary calculi. Obstet. Gynecol. *5*:513, 1955.

Gibson, J. R. M.: Cystinuria and bilateral calculi in pregnancy. Report of a case. Obstet. Gynecol. *26*:101, 1965.

Harris, R. E., and Dunnihoo, D. R.: The incidence and significance of many calculi in pregnancy. Am. J. Obstet. Gynecol. *99*:237, 1967.

Honoré, L. E.: The increased incidence of renal stones in women with spontaneous abortion: a retrospective study. Am. J. Obstet. Gynecol. *137*:145, 1980.

King, T. M., Griffin, W. T., and Hall, D. G.: Urinary calculi in pregnancy: Case report. Mo. Med. *64*:218, 1967.

Klempner, E., Oppenheimer, G. D., and Glickman, S. I.: Urologic complications. *In* Guttmacher, A. F., and Rovinsky, J. J. (eds.): Medical, Surgical and Gynecological Complications of Pregnancy. Baltimore, Williams & Wilkins, 1960, pp. 262–264.

Lattanzi, D. R., and Cook, W. A.: Urinary calculi in pregnancy. Obstet. Gynecol. *56*:462, 1980.

Marcus, M. B., and Brandt, M. L.: Ureteral calculi complicating pregnancy. N.Y. State J. Med. *57*:3156, 1957.

McVann, R. M.: Urinary calculi associated with pregnancy. Am. J. Obstet. Gynecol. *89*:314, 1964.

Prather, G. C., and Crabtree, E. G.: Impressions relating to urinary tract stones in pregnancy. Urol. Cutan. Rev. *38*:17, 1934.

Rigby, M. R., and MacEwan, D. W.: Urography during pregnancy. J. Can. Assoc. Radiol. *27*:227, 1976.

Rubin, A., Chaykin, L., and Ludwig, G. D.: Maternal hyperparathyroidism and pregnancy. J.A.M.A. *206*:128, 1968.

Semmens, J. P.: Major urologic complications in pregnancy. Obstet. Gynecol. *23*:561, 1964.

Solomon, E. M.: Urinary calculi in pregnancy. Am. J. Obstet. Gynecol. *67*:1351, 1954.

Strong, D. W., Murchison, R. J., and Lynch, D. F.: The management of ureteral calculi during pregnancy. Surg. Gynecol. Obstet. *146*:604, 1978.

Szczerbo, A., Bartoszewski, A., Zwierzynski, T., et al.: Management of urolithiasis during pregnancy, delivery and puerperium. Pol. Med. J. *11*:220, 1972.

Zerner, J.: Ureteral calculus in pregnancy and the puerperium. J. Maine Med. Assoc. *66*:151, 1975.

INDEX

Numbers in *italics* refer to illustrations; numbers followed by a (t) indicate tables.